HEALTH AND WELFARE FOR FAMILIES IN THE 21ST CENTURY

SECOND EDITION

EDITED BY

Helen M. Wallace, MD, MPH
Professor, Maternal and Child Health
Graduate School of Public Health
San Diego University
San Diego, CA

Gordon Green, MD, MPH
Professor and Dean, Allied Health Sciences
The University of Texas Southwestern Medical Center at Dallas
Dallas, TX

Kenneth J. Jaros, MSW, PhD
Director, Public Health Social Work Training Program
in Maternal and Child Health
Department of Behavioral and Community Health Sciences
Graduate School of Public Health
University of Pittsburgh
Pittsburgh, PA

with Contributing Editor
Naomi Morris, MD, MPH
Professor, Maternal and Child Health
Community Health Science Division
School of Public Health
University of Illinois at Chicago
Chicago, IL

JONES AND BARTLETT PUBLISHERS
Sudbury, Massachusetts
BOSTON   TORONTO   LONDON   SINGAPORE

World Headquarters
Jones and Bartlett Publishers
40 Tall Pine Drive
Sudbury, MA 01776
978-443-5000
info@jbpub.com
www.jbpub.com

RA418.5.F3 H428 2003
Health and welfare for
families in the 21st
century.

Jones and Bartlett Publishers Canada
2406 Nikanna Road
Mississauga, ON L5C 2W6
CANADA

Jones and Bartlett Publishers International
Barb House, Barb Mews
London W6 7PA
UK

Production Credits
Chief Executive Officer: Clayton Jones
Chief Operating Officer: Don W. Jones, Jr.
Executive V.P. & Publisher: Robert W. Holland, Jr.
V.P., Sales and Marketing: William J. Kane
V.P., Design and Production: Anne Spencer
V.P., Manufacturing and Inventory Control: Therese Bräuer
Acquisitions Editor: Penny M. Glynn
Senior Production Editor: Linda S. DeBruyn
Associate Editor: Karen Zuck
Manufacturing and Inventory Coordinator: Amy Bacus
Composition: Dartmouth Publishing, Inc.
Cover Design: Philip Regan
Printing and Binding: Malloy, Inc.
Cover Printing: Malloy, Inc.

Library of Congress Cataloging-in-Publication Data

Health and welfare for families in the 21st century / edited by Helen M. Wallace ... [et al.]. – 2nd ed.
   p. ; cm.
   Includes bibliographical references and index.
   ISBN 0-7637-1859-9
   1. Family—Health and hygiene. 2. Family policy. I. Wallace, Helen M.
   [DNLM: 1. Family Health—United States. 2. Child Welfare—United States. 3. Health Policy—United States. 4. Women's Health—United States. WA 308 H4335 2003]
   RA418.5.F3II428 2003
   362.1—de21

                                                                         2002044407

Printed in the United States of America
07 06 05 04   10 9 8 7 6 5 4 3 2

CONTENTS

Unit 2: Social Welfare 115

Unit 3: Health Expenditures and Health Insurance 227

Unit 4: Health Issues

315

Unit 5: Policy Issues   509

DEDICATION

This volume is dedicated to the memory of Vince L. Hutchins, MD, MPH

Vince Hutchins was the Director of the Maternal and Child Health Bureau (MCHB) from 1977 to 1992. Warm, caring, gentle, kind, he was concerned about every child, every family, every community in need of better health care.

From practicing pediatrician to federal administrator with higher and higher levels of responsibility, Vince, as everyone called him, was always available, always willing to make extra time for those who wished to meet with him. He was an exceptionally good administrator. Under his stewardship, the Bureau accomplished many things we now take for granted: standards for prenatal care, for child health supervision, for out-of-home child care, and more. He was always very supportive of the MCH training programs in schools of public health, and other professional education for those who would work to serve families, mothers, and children, including children with special health care needs.

Upon retiring from federal service, Vince worked for the Carnegie Foundation for two years and then joined the National Center for Education in Maternal and Child Health at Georgetown University as Distinguished Research Professor. His final appointment was as Chair, Division of Policy, at the Georgetown Public Policy Institute. He remained active on many MCH-related boards, and received awards recognizing his accomplishments from practically every significant national organization in the field of maternal and child health.

Vince died unexpectedly January 15, 2001. His presence is missed. For those of us who had the opportunity to know him, this book records some of his legacy.

Naomi M. Morris, MD, MPH

FOREWORD

Deanne R. Williams, CNM, MS, FACNM
Executive Director
American College of Nurse-Midwives
Washington, D.C.

Through the eyes of a women's health care professional, the health status of our nation's mothers and babies in the 21st century seems almost incomprehensible. Billions of dollars are destined to be spent on new interventions designed to save lives, yet a dizzying array of public health problems will not be prevented or cured by these medications and machines. The technology brain trust will be generously funded to produce the latest miracle treatment, and marketing agencies will do a record business promoting these treatments directly to consumers. Yet, health care professionals will find it difficult to obtain, in a timely manner, the evidence they need to safely use these new treatments. In addition, a complex series of ethical dilemmas, a higher level of suspicion, and an increasing number of toxic by-products are likely to accompany many of the new interventions. Unfortunately, the HIV/AIDS epidemic, which seems to defy current prevention strategies and is appearing in an alarming number of childbearing age women, will bring a unique set of clinical challenges and an undercurrent of fear to those who commit their professional lives to providing care for pregnant women and their families.

Many will find it hard to reconcile the contrast: billions of dollars spent on production and marketing, sometimes to treat an extremely rare disease, and millions of women and families without health insurance and access to basic health care; basements overflowing with expensive but outdated equipment, yet the maternal and infant mortality and morbidity rates may well remain stagnant at an unacceptably high rate; the cost to educate a specialist physician exceeding hundreds of thousands of dollars while the nation's working poor get less and less preventive health care. In the meantime, dramatic changes in career options will exacerbate the nursing shortage, put patients' lives at risk, make the work of a physician much more difficult, and limit the number of individuals who can become expert providers of direct health care services, such as nurse-midwives, nurse anesthetists, and nurse practitioners.

My colleagues in midwifery are intimately involved in the challenge to find solutions that fit this rapidly changing health care environment. Nurse-midwifery in the

United States grew from a strong foundation of public health and community health nursing. Nurse-midwives are acutely aware that the health status of the family directly mirrors the health status of the mother. Thus, we repeatedly object to actions by policymakers that, in effect, rob the mother bank to make a deposit to the baby bank or vice versa. What is needed, of course, is more dollars for both mothers and babies. Our profession, like so many others in the maternal and child health field, opposes funding for women's health care that is limited to treating the reproductive organs, but we cannot stand quietly by when increased funding does nothing to improve access to quality care for all pregnant women. Nurse-midwives attend over 9% of the vaginal births in the United States and over 96% of these births occur in a hospital. In addition, 20% of the visits to nurse-midwives are from women who are seeking primary health care that is not related to pregnancy. Although nurse-midwives serve all women, a significant number of the women who receive care from nurse-midwives are at risk for poor outcomes because of their age (29% are adolescents), race/ethnicity (50% are non White), immigrant status (27% are immigrants) and lack of insurance coverage (16% are uninsured). These women, along with many others who actively seek the midwifery philosophy of care, know that nurse-midwives prefer to provide care that focuses on the prevention of disease and illness. They are widely recognized for a philosophical approach that emphasizes patient education, informed consent, and respect for individual rights.

In order to face an uncertain and unsettling future, all health care professionals will need to develop a unique set of survival skills. Number one on the list is to learn to work in collaboration with other professionals, including public health colleagues. Pressure to provide more care in less time in systems with shrinking provider-patient staffing ratios will only reward those who can share the burden. The rapid-fire arrival of new information demands that responsibilities and knowledge be redistributed, not hoarded. The consumer who arrives in clinic showing signs of severe information overload or, conversely, lack of essential information needs an expert clinician and a health care professional who enjoys serving in the role of confidante and teacher. The devolution of health care responsibility from the federal to local governments increases the demand for constructive interaction between health care professionals and local policy makers. The rapid privatization of systems of health care delivery that still depend to a large degree on federal sources of funding actually magnifies the need for such constructive interaction, especially between public health officials and those who provide direct patient services. The fact that medical problems and public health problems do not exist in isolation from each other must be reflected in the curriculum and clinical experience required for physicians, nurses, midwives, and public health professionals. Finally, the changing face of the health care consumer is a call to action for each of us to explore our own limitations as we attempt to create a space where all clients can access the care they need.

The 2nd edition of *Health and Welfare for Families in the 21st Century* will help prepare health care professionals who can thrive in the new century. The content, though not always unique, is presented in a context that will help ensure a broad understanding of how health, disease and illness both reflect and define society. Readers will find themselves better prepared to work together to accomplish important and rewarding professional goals.

FOREWORD

Philip R. Lee, MD
Senior Scholar
Institute for Health Policy Studies
School of Medicine
University of California – San Francisco
San Francisco, CA

In the three years since the publication of the first edition of *Health and Welfare for Families in the 21st Century* dramatic changes have occurred that may set a direction for health and welfare policies and services for many years, and possibly decades, to come. The first of these was the election of George W. Bush in November 2000. His highest priority was a tax cut which was enacted in early 2001 by a Republican-controlled Congress. The tax cut of $1.3 trillion was to reduce the future capacity of the federal government to meet domestic needs in health, welfare, and education. The Administration then asked for a second, large tax cut that was called a "stimulus" package. After several efforts to enact it, this package failed in Congress. The tax cut was limited largely to deductions for employers on their investments in new plant and equipment, and it included an extension of unemployment benefits. The impact of the initial tax cut, which largely favored corporations and high-income individuals, will have a growing impact as years pass.

Next, the recession began officially in March 2001, after a decade of economic growth, which had increased tax revenues for the federal, state, and local governments, and beginning in 1997 had produced a federal budget surplus. These revenues and surpluses have disappeared with the recession and the tax cut. Although the recession appears to be ending, the level of recovery is not expected to be robust in the near term. The impact of the recession and the tax cut have been felt particularly by state and local governments, with widespread reductions in expenditures at both levels.

Even more important than these political developments were the terrorist attacks on the World Trade Center and the Pentagon on September 11, 2001, and the subsequent attack of bioterrorism, using anthrax as the agent, in Florida, New York, Washington, D.C., and Connecticut. The results of the terrorist attacks have been a substantial increase in federal funding for rebuilding New York; an increase in spending for the armed forces, particularly since the attack on Afghanistan by the armed forces; an increased funding for intelligence agencies; and potentially increased funding for other domestic antiterrorism programs, including funding for the public health infrastructure. It is likely that major legislation, significantly strengthening the public infrastructure at the federal, state and local levels will be enacted prior to the publication of this new edition. It is too early to predict the long-term impact of these changes on federal funding of other public health, medical care, social welfare and education programs. But it is not too early to recognize the absolute necessity of a revitalized relationship between medicine and public health at the local, state, and national level if the challenge is to be met. Such a revitalized, collaborative relationship that also involves the community could have far-reaching benefits for maternal and child health.

These dramatic changes at the beginning of the 21st century add significantly to the impact of the changes in health and welfare services growing out of the 1980s and 1990s, including the failure of Clinton's health care reform in 1994; the enactment of welfare reform, with a shift from federal to state responsibility in 1996; and the Balanced Budget Act of 1997, which added the Child Health Insurance Program. The changes are affecting government agencies, as well as private and nonprofit organizations and institutions. The changes have been driven by a number of factors—rising costs; the growing role of the ideology in policy, particularly the role of the marketplace in medical care; the impact of technology, including information systems; the need to make these systems more responsive to consumers; fiscal pressures, including the drive to balance the federal budget in the 1990s and the tax cuts in 2001. These forces have affected particularly the government agencies and nonprofit agencies, with the result that downsizing, budget cuts, and privatization of many public health, social welfare, and medical care services have occurred, particularly affecting vulnerable populations.

Medicine, social welfare, and public health are at a critical crossroads as we enter the 21st century. It is not only the move from the industrial age to the information and knowledge age, the globalization of the economy, and the recent terrorist attacks that provide the broad context for these changes, but the consequences of the shift in values and the stress on market values that is affecting policies, programs, services, and people. Services that many of us have long viewed as public goods are now viewed as market goods.

This book provides professionals, both practitioners and academics, as well as policymakers with a rich but practical framework for thinking about the needs of families and children, as well as a wide range of options. In clear, well-documented terms, this new edition of *Health and Welfare for Families in the 21st Century* provides the essential information that is needed to make informed judgements about how best we can meet the needs of families and children in the 21st century. For me, one of the clearest themes to emerge is the need for collaboration in public health, but more importantly, across the sectors of medicine, public health, and social welfare, and within the community.

I hope the book will be widely read and its ideas put to practical use. The issues and action we take are vital to the health and well-being of the nation in the 21st century.

PREFACE

This book was written by recognized maternal and child health leaders. It provides information concerning history, people, policies, legislation, what they mean, how they worked or didn't, what needs fixing, and what matters. This knowledge gives ammunition to existing and potential leaders. It can be used to attract followers who are inspired by the information and its presentation and can share a vision that is worthy and do-able. The data presented importantly support the interpretation of past and current situations and indicate the potential benefits of change. Solid information is basic for accomplishment and its evaluation, especially as we face the health challenges of the 21st century.

The contents of this book are designed to nourish leaders hoping to improve maternal, child, and family health (MCH). MCH leaders may be in academia, teaching, and doing research; in responsible positions at the local, state, or national level of official agencies; in other organizations, task forces, boards, or clinical groups; visible in the development of policy, strategic planning, program evaluation, procuring funding, and influencing legislation; or acting as advocates influencing change at community, state, regional, or national levels. What makes leaders leaders is that they are followed. Their opinions are respected. They are asked to give technical assistance, to help plan change, to advise their peers, to participate in high-level committees in the public or nonprofit sector.

Some leaders are stronger than others. Strong leaders need a vision and the ability to share it; knowledge and the know-how to get things done; self-confidence; experience on which to build; and a personality that attracts followers. The followers are rewarded by the accomplishments they helped to make happen, the support acquired to assure the continuing success of the accomplishment, and the fulfillment of the shared vision.

How do people strengthen their ability to lead? They develop more conviction concerning goals and values, more awareness of the history behind the current situation, more specific knowledge, a more successful way of communicating and persuading others, and maybe more energy and persistence than those they wish to lead.

Not every quality of leadership can be acquired from a book. But in this one there is much food for thought, many suggestions for next steps, and observations that should strengthen the persuasive abilities of current and future leaders motivated to work on behalf of maternal, child, and family health. MCH leaders writing this book have modeled the type of thinking utilized in MCH. Pay attention as you read; you will see yourself filled with new challenges that can be addressed by advocacy and action, and new confidence that you yourself can take the next steps appropriate to your personal goals, values, and position. Should you rise in your level of responsibility, these leaders will have successfully passed on the torch.

Naomi M. Morris, MD, MPH

CONTRIBUTORS

E. Kathleen Adams, PhD
Associate Professor
Center for Public Health Practice
Emory University
Rollins School of Public Health
Atlanta, GA

Greg R. Alexander, MPH, ScD
Professor and Chair
Department of Maternal and Child Health
School of Public Health
University of Alabama at Birmingham
Birmingham, AL

Sarah Arzaga
Institute for Health Policy Studies
University of California - San Francisco
San Francisco, CA

Hani K. Atrash, MD, MPH
Division of Reproductive Health
National Center for Chronic Disease
    Prevention and Health Promotion
Centers for Disease Control and Prevention
Atlanta, GA

Maribeth Badura, MSN, RN
Chief, Healthy Start Branch
Division of Perinatal Systems and
    Women's Health
Maternal and Child Health Bureau
Health Resources and Services
    Administration
US Department of Health and Human
    Services
Washington, DC

Debora Barnes-Josiah, PhD
Assistant Professor
Department of Pediatrics
University of Nebraska Medical Center
Omaha, NE

Donald A. Barr, MD, PhD
Associate Professor (Teaching) of Sociology
Stanford University
Stanford, CA

A. E. Benjamin, PhD
Professor of Social Welfare
School of Public Policy and Social
    Research
University of California – Los Angeles
Los Angeles, CA

Allen Bolton, MPH, MBA
Associate Dean for Administration and
    Finance
School of Medicine
University of Alabama at Birmingham
Birmingham, AL

Paul Boumbulian, DPA, MPH
Associate Professor
Management and Policy Sciences
Dallas Regional MPH Program
University of Texas School of Public Health
Dallas, TX

Mary C. Brucker, CNM, DNSc, FACNM
Director
Parkland School of Nurse-Midwifery
Parkland Health and Hospital System
Dallas, TX

Paul S. Casamassimo, DDS, MS
Professor and Chair
Section of Pediatric Dentistry
College of Dentistry
The Ohio State University
Columbus, OH

Wendy Chavkin, MD, MPH
Professor of Clinical Public Health
Department of Population and Family Health
Mailman School of Public Health
Columbia University
New York, NY

Valire Carr Copeland, PhD, MPH
Associate Professor
School of Social Work
University of Pittsburgh
Pittsburgh, PA

Cathy Cowan
National Health Statistics Group
Office of the Actuary
Centers for Medicare and Medicaid Services
Baltimore, MD

Lucy S. Crain, MD
Department of Pediatrics
University of California – San Francisco
San Francisco, CA

David S. de la Cruz, PhD, MPH
Senior Program Management Officer
Healthy Start Branch
Division of Perinatal Systems and
    Women's Health
Maternal and Child Health Bureau
Health Resources and Services
    Administration
US Department of Health and
    Human Services
Washington, DC

Hazel D. Dean, ScD, MPH
Activity Chief
Applied Surveillance and
    Epidemiology Unit
Division of HIV/AIDS Prevention
Centers for Disease Control and Prevention
Atlanta, GA

Anne Cohn Donnelly, DPH
Resident Fellow and Visiting Scholar in
    Non-Profit Studies
Kellogg School of Management
Northwestern University
Chicago, IL

Laurie D. Elam-Evans, PhD, MPH
Reproductive Epidemiologist
Centers for Disease Control and Prevention
Atlanta, GA

Robert C. Fellmeth, JD
Price Professor of Public Interest Law
Director, Children's Advocacy institute
University of San Diego Law School
San Diego, CA

Kimberley K. Fox, MD, MPH
Epidemiology and Surveillance Branch
Division of STD Prevention
National Center for HIV, STD, and
    TB Prevention
Centers for Disease Control and Prevention
Atlanta, GA

Alison Galbraith, MD
Robert Wood Johnson Clinical Scholars
    Program
University of Washington
Seattle, WA

Shelly Gehshan, MPP
Program Director
National Conference of State Legislatures
Washington, DC

Frederick Green, MD
Kellogg School of Management
Northwestern University
Chicago, IL

Gordon Green, MD, MPH
Professor and Dean
Allied Health Sciences
The University of Texas
Southwestern Medical Center
Dallas, TX

Donald E. Greydanus, MD
Professor
Pediatrics and Human Development
Michigan State University College of
    Human Medicine
Michigan State University/Kalamazoo
    Center for Medical Studies
Kalamazoo, MI

Elizabeth K. Greydanus, BSW
School of Social Work
University of Michigan, Ann Arbor
Ann Arbor, MI

Arden Handler, MPH, DrPH
Associate Professor
Department of Community Health Sciences
MCH Training Program
School of Public Health
University of Illinois - Chicago
Chicago, IL

P. Travis Harker, MD
Research Fellow
Office of the Secretary
US Department of Health and
    Human Services
Washington, DC

Norma S. Harris, PhD, MSPH
Surveillance Branch
Division of HIV/AIDS Prevention
Centers for Disease Control and Prevention
Atlanta, GA

Barbara J. Hatcher, PhD, MPH, RN
Director
Scientific and Professional Affairs
American Public Health Association
Washington, DC

David Heppel, MD
Director
Division of Child, Adolescent, and Family
Health
Maternal and Child Health Bureau
Health Resources & Services Administration
US Department of Health and Human
Services
Rockville, MD

Catherine A. Hess, MSW
Health and Human Services Policy
Consultant
Washington, DC

Sandra L. Hofferth, PhD
Professor
Department of Family Studies
University of Maryland
College Park, MD

Yun-Yi Hung, PhD, MPH
Institute for Health Policy Studies
Univeristy of California – San Francisco
San Francisco, CA

Ellen Hutchins, ScD, MSW
Chief
Perinatal and Women's Health Branch
Health Resources and Services
Administration
Maternal and Child Health Bureau
US Department of Health and Human
Services
Rockville, MD

Dana Hughes, DrPH
Institute for Health Policy Studies
University of California - San Francisco
San Francisco, CA

Solomon Iyasu, MBBS, MPH
Division of Reproductive Health
National Center for Chronic Disease
Prevention and Health Promotion
Centers for Disease Control and Prevention
Atlanta, GA

Kenneth J. Jaros, MSW, PhD
Director, Public Health Social Work Training
Program in Maternal and Child Health
Department of Behavioral and Community
Health Sciences
Graduate School of Public Health
University of Pittsburgh
Pittsburgh, PA

Woodie Kessel, MD, MPH
Assistant Surgeon General
Deputy Assistant Secretary for Disease
Prevention and Health Promotion
Office of Disease Prevention and Health
Promotion
US Department of Health and Human
Services
Washington, DC

Michael D. Kogan, PhD
Director
Office of Data and Information Management
Maternal and Child Health Bureau
Health Resources and Services
Administration
US Department of Health and Human
Services
Rockville, MD

Richard D. Krugman, MD
School of Medicine
University of Colorado Health Sciences
Center
Denver, CO

Helen Lazenby
National Health Statistics Group
Office of the Actuary
Centers for Medicare and Medicaid Services
Baltimore, MD

Philip R. Lee, MD
Senior Scholar
Institute for Health Policy Studies, School
of Medicine
University of California - San Francisco
San Francisco, CA

Laurel K. Leslie, MD
Child and Adolescent Services Research
Center (CASRC)
Children's Hospital – San Diego
San Diego, CA

Katharine Levit
National Health Statistics Group
Office of the Actuary
Centers for Medicare and Medicaid Services
Baltimore, MD

Kimball Lewis
Mathematica Policy Research, Inc.
Princeton, NJ

Marian F. MacDorman, PhD
Division of Vital Statistics
National Center for Health Statistics
Centers for Disease Control and
    Prevention
Hyattsville, MD

Anne Martin
National Health Statistics Group
Office of the Actuary
Centers for Medicare and Medicaid
    Services
Baltimore, MD

T. J. Matthews, MS
Division of Vital Statistics
National Center for Health Statistics
Centers for Disease Control and
    Prevention
Hyattsville, MD

Mary McCoy, MPH
Data Analyst
Injury Prevention Center of Greater Dallas
Dallas, TX

Merle McPherson, MD, MPH
Director
Division of Services for Children with
    Special Health Needs
Maternal and Child Health Bureau
Health Resources and Services
    Administration
US Department of Health and Human
    Services
Rockville, MD

Naomi Morris, MD, MPH
Professor, Maternal and Child Health
Community Health Science Division
School of Public Health
University of Illinois at Chicago
Chicago, IL

Paul W. Newacheck, DrPH
Institute for Health Policy Studies and
    Department of Pediatrics
School of Medicine
University of California – San Francisco
San Francisco, CA

Dilip R. Patel, MD
Associate Professor
Adolescent and Sports Medicine
Pediatrics and Human Development
Michigan State University College of
    Human Medicine
Michigan State University/Kalamazoo
    Center for Medical Studies
Kalamazoo, MI

Magda G. Peck, ScD
CEO/Executive Director
CityMatch
Department of Pediatrics
University of Nebraska Medical Center
Omaha, NE

Donna J. Petersen, MHS, ScD
Associate Dean
School of Public Health
University of Alabama at Birmingham
Birmingham, AL

Brian Quinn
Mathematica Policy Research, Inc.
Princeton, NJ

Irwin Redlener, MD
President
Children's Health Fund
New York, NY

John G. Reiss, PD
Chief
Division of Policy and Program Affairs
Institute for Child Health Policy
Gainesville, FL

Lance E. Rodewald, MD
Director
Immunization Services Division
National Immunization Program
Centers for Disease Control and Prevention
Atlanta, GA

Margo Rosenbach, PhD
Vice President
Mathematica Policy Research, Inc
Princeton, NJ

Patti R. Rosquist, MD
The Children's Hospital
University of Colorado Health Sciences
  Center
Denver, CO

Jeanne M. Santoli, MD, MPH
National Immunization Program
Centers for Disease Control
  and Prevention
Atlanta, GA

Peter Sherman, MD
Medical Director
New York Children's Health Project
New York, NY

Cynthia Smith
National Health Statistics Group
Office of the Actuary
Centers for Medicare and Medicaid
  Services
Baltimore, MD

Jamie Stang, PhD, MPH, RD
Director
MCH Nutrition Training Program
Division of Epidemiology
School of Public Health
University of Minnesota
Minneapolis, MN

Martin T. Stein, MD
Professor of Clinical Pediatrics
University of California
San Diego Medical Center
San Diego, CA

Mary Story, PhD, RD
Professor
Public Health Nutrition and Maternal and
  Child Health
Division of Epidemiology
School of Public Health
University of Minnesota
Minneapolis, MN

Martha Stowe, LMSW
Director
Injury Prevention Center of Greater Dallas
Dallas, TX

Peter C. Van Dyck, MD, MPH
Associate Administrator for Maternal and
  Child Health
Health Resources and Services
  Administration
US Department of Health and Human
  Services
Rockville, MD

Karen VanLandeghem, MPH
Health Policy/Program Consultant
Arlington Heights, IL

Stephanie J. Ventura, MA
Chief
Reproductive Statistics Branch
Division of Vital Statistics
National Center for Health Statistics
Centers for Disease Control and Prevention
Hyattsville, MD

Helen M. Wallace, MD, MPH
Professor, Maternal and Child Health
Graduate School of Public Health
San Diego State University
San Diego, CA

Sandra Wexler, PhD, ACSW
Assistant Professor
School of Social Work
University of Pittsburgh
Pittsburgh, PA

Sabrina T. Wong, PhD, RN
Institute for Health Policy Studies
University of California – San Francisco
San Francisco, CA

Meagan Zimbeck, BA
School of Public Health
University of Illinois – Chicago
Chicago, IL

UNIT 1

FOUNDATIONS

INTRODUCTION

The 20th century was characterized by substantial developments in public health. New technical knowledge, combined with the social welfare movement and growth in governmental programs to promote health and welfare, resulted in remarkable advances in both the length and the quality of life for most Americans. Even the two World Wars added, in a tragic way, to health and social service enhancements.

The United States is a world leader in economic productivity, education, and health. Improved health has been achieved through such factors as vaccine development, new options for family planning, fluoridation of water, and advances in prenatal care. Social conditions also have yielded to new discoveries and new social welfare programs. But many problems remain.

In this unit, health and welfare policy and its relationship to the unique American character are explored in some detail. The unit recounts the rise of federalism and the increasing role of government in health care as these developments took place in halting increments over the 20th century. By the end of the century, however, remarkable changes had taken place, accompanied by upheavals in how health and social services would be funded. Investor-owned programs and managed care began to replace the cottage industries that had constituted the health care system. Behavioral components came to be recognized as increasingly important elements in determining health status. Such documents as Healthy People 2000/2010, and efforts such as the American Public Health Association's Community Health Leadership Institute, both reflected the approaches to health and social services and, in fact, led those approaches.

Remarkable changes in demographics were reflected in population health statistics. Changes in morbidity, mortality, and fertility rates were impressive. Furthermore, variations in these rates by racial, ethnic, socioeconomic, and age groups came to play important roles in policy development. Scientific discoveries (for examples, the polio vaccine, improved contraception) led to changes in the family structure, and consequently in the labor force. The implications for working mothers, for children, and for society as a whole were staggering, and social and health programs struggled to keep up with these changes. Cost-effective efforts in nutrition and education grew to be appreciated as having a direct relationship upon health status, and efforts in various diets, early childhood development programs, and food-assistance programs grew in prominence.

Throughout all these dramatic changes, there came to be a growing appreciation for the importance of surveillance, monitoring, and evaluation of both services and outcomes. The core functions of public health importantly included assessment and assurance efforts, based upon measurable goals. As we entered the new century, the emphasis in health and social welfare programs shifted from simple considerations of costs versus benefits toward outcomes evaluation and "evidence-based" programs.

The Foundations unit offers a broad (and in some cases, deep) view of public health and social welfare at the turn of the century, and it projects those predominant concerns into the first decade of the new century.

ARTICLE 1

HEALTH AND SOCIAL CARE OF WOMEN, CHILDREN, YOUTH, AND FAMILIES

Peter C. van Dyck and Michael D. Kogan

WHERE WE STAND

As the 21st century begins, the United States is the economic giant of the world. Our 2000 gross domestic product (GDP) was more than $9.8 billion[1] and the United States accounted for nearly one-quarter (23%) of the world's production in 2000.[2] The U.S. GDP per capita, a measure of the productivity of our workers, is consistently among the world's highest.[3] We are both the leading destination for exports and the leading source of imports for the world's commodities.[3] We are also the world's leader in the proportion of the population completing higher education, with 27 percent of the adult population (age 25 to 64) completing a university education.[4]

Similarly, at the inception of the 21st century, in many ways the health of America's women and children has never been better. There were stunning achievements in public health and maternal and child health in the 20th century.

TRIUMPHS

The health and life expectancy of people living in the United States have improved significantly since 1900, with the average lifespan lengthening by more than 30 years.

As many as 25 years of this increase are attributable to advances in public health.[5] In 1998, life expectancy at birth reached an all time high of 76.7 years, with a life expectancy for females of 79.5 and for males 73.8 years. And the older a person was in 1998, the greater the overall life expectancy. A 65-year-old, for example, could expect to live on average to 82.8 years old, a 50-year-old to 79.8 years old.[6]

The Centers for Disease Control and Prevention (CDC) suggested the following 10 public health achievements chosen for their opportunity to achieve prevention and an impact on death, illness, and disability. The most important contributors to this expected improvement: vaccination, motor vehicle safety, safer workplaces, control of infectious diseases, decline in deaths from coronary heart disease and stroke, safer and healthier foods, healthier mothers and babies, family planning, fluoridation of drinking water, and recognition of tobacco use as a health hazard.[7] Some of these will be discussed further as triumphs and others as advances, but with lingering concerns that there is still much progress to be made.

Maternal Mortality

Maternal mortality declined precipitously in the 20th century, and this change represents one of public health's greatest achievements, largely due to improved health and social conditions. The maternal mortality rate, defined as maternal deaths occurring to pregnant women and to women up to 42 days postpartum, has fallen from its peak in 1918 of 916 deaths per 100,000 births to 7.1 deaths per 100,000 births in 1998. In the 1940s and 1950s, significant improvement was due in part to an increased percentage of deliveries occurring in hospitals, the introduction of new antibiotics, and improvement in blood typing and transfusion procedures. Much of the decrease in the last 25 years has been attributed to continuing improvements in health care as well as to a decline in infections related to septic abortions, and the legalization of abortion across the country in the early 1970s.[8]

There has been recent discussion about whether the current definition of maternal mortality accurately reflects the complete spectrum of deaths related to pregnancy. The current definition does not include all deaths to pregnant women, but only those deaths reported on the death certificate as complications of pregnancy, childbirth, and the puerperium (ICD codes 630–676). It excludes, therefore, deaths occurring more than 42 days after the end of pregnancy and deaths due to external causes such as accidents, homicides, and suicides.[6] Careful attention should be given to this issue, and agreement should be reached in the near future about a more inclusive definition.

Infant Mortality

The infant mortality rate in the United States continues to improve. In 1999, 27,953 infants died before their first birthday for a rate of 7.1 deaths per 1,000 live births. Preliminary data for 2000 suggests that the rate may fall to 6.9 deaths per 1,000 live births, the lowest ever recorded.[9] Likewise, there were small decreases in the neonatal death rate, from 4.8 deaths per 1,000 live births in 1998 to 4.6 in 2000, and in the postneonatal mortality rate, from 2.4 deaths per 1,000 live births in 1998 to 2.3 in 2000. Although the decline in infant mortality slowed during the 1980s, the decline became more steep in the late 1980s and 90s largely due to the introduction of surfactants to improve the course of respiratory distress syndrome and the national effort partnered by the Maternal and Child Health Bureau (MCHB), the National Institute of Child Health and Development, and the American Academy of Pediatrics to implement the "back to sleep" campaign for prevention of sudden infant death syndrome (SIDS). The SIDS death rate alone declined by 49% between 1988 and 1998.[10] Although the trend in infant mortality for both black and white infants has been a continual decline for the last 85 years, the proportional discrepancy between the rates has remained largely unchanged and will be discussed as an area of concern later.

Child Mortality

The child mortality rate has also continued an exceptional decline in all age groups during the 1990s, except for one group, adolescents aged 15–19, whose rates have leveled off since the late 1950s. In 1900, the death rate for children aged 1–19 was over 3,000 per 100,000 children compared to 35.8 per 100,000 children in 1999,[9] representing a significant achievement in primary and preventive health. In 1999, there were 26,622 deaths of children aged 1–19, 5,249 deaths in children 1–4, 7,595 deaths in children 5–14, and 13,778 deaths for children 15–19.[9,11] The leading cause of death in children aged 1–4 was unintentional injuries, which accounted for 36% of all deaths (2,328), followed by congenital malformations, malignant neoplasms, and homicide. Of the deaths due to injuries in this age group, the most common causes were motor vehicle crashes (4.3 deaths per 100,000 children aged 1–4), drowning (3.2), and fires and burns (2.0). In children 5–14 the leading causes were, in order, unintentional injury, malignant neoplasms, homicide, and congenital malformations. Of the deaths due to injuries (3,826) the most common causes included motor vehicle crashes (4.5 deaths per 100,000 children aged 5–14), firearms (1.1), and drowning (0.9).[11] Although the tremendous decline in childhood mortality is gratifying and represents a triumph, there are still many opportunities for further reductions by continuation and improvement of interventions of proven preventive strategies.

Vaccinations

Since the early 1970s, childhood vaccination has prevented millions of illnesses and tens of thousands of deaths.[12] The National Immunization Survey, sponsored by CDC, provides estimates of vaccination coverage among preschool-aged children for the 50 states.[12] In 2000, the vaccination coverage levels among children aged 19–35 months for 3 doses of any diphtheria and tetanus toxoids and pertussis vaccine (DtaP3) was 94.7%. Coverage for 3 doses of oral poliovirus vaccine (OPV3) changed from 87.9% to 89.5% from 1995 to 2000 with the peak year in 1996 of 91.1%. For 3 doses of *Haemophilus influenzae* type b vaccine (Hib3) the rate increased steadily from 91.7% in 1995 to 93.4% in 2000, and for one dose of measles-mumps-rubella vaccine (1MMR) the rate changed from 87.8% to 90.5% with the peak year in 1998 of 92%. Three doses of hepatitis B vaccine (HepB3) increased steadily from 68% in 1995 to 90.3% in 2000. Varicella vaccine use, which began in 1997 at 25.9%, increased to 67.8% by 2000. National coverage with the combined vaccination series 4:3:1:3:3 (DtaP4, OPV3, one dose of measles-containing vaccine, Hib3, and HepB3) was 72.8% for the year 2000. However, there was significant state variation in this combined series from a high of over 80% to less than 65%. For the continued prevention of illness and death from vaccination coverage to continue, high levels of coverage must be reached for each new birth cohort. Although coverage remains high, efforts must be made to maintain these levels. The slight declines that were seen in coverage for some vaccines between 1995 and 2000 do not pose a major public health risk; however, should these diseases be introduced into low-coverage geographic areas, the accumulation of susceptible persons might serve as a reservoir for disease.[12]

Family Planning

Family planning services, particularly since the 1960s, have allowed couples to better achieve desired birth spacing and family size. Smaller families and longer birth intervals have had a role in contributing to the better health of infants, children, and women, and have improved the social and economic role of women generally.[13] In 1960, both the birth control pill and the intrauterine device (IUD) became available, which resulted in major changes in the way couples practiced contraception. By 1965, the pill had become the most popular birth control method, followed by the condom and contraceptive sterilization.[14] In 1970, the Family Services and Population Research Act, which created Title X of the Public Health Service Act, was established, providing federal funding for family planning services.[15] During the 1980s, contraceptive sterilization became the most practiced form of birth control, and in the last 10 years there has been increasing use of long-acting hormonal contraception.[16]

Fertility rates have changed significantly over the last 80 years from peaks in family size of 3.3 around 1920 to similar peaks in the mid-1950s to the present rate, beginning around 1972 of about 2 children per family.[17] In 1994, 3,119 agencies including health departments, clinics, and hospitals operated 7,122 publicly subsidized family planning clinics for an estimated 6.6 million women.[18] These publicly supported clinics have been effective in supplying contraception and counseling to populations that have high rates of unintended pregnancy and have limited access to private-care providers. In 1988, of the women who obtained reversible contraception, 22.5% received services from public clinics and were most likely adolescents (43%), poor (39%), and never-married women (34%). These services prevented an estimated 1.3 million unintended pregnancies annually.[19] Access to high quality family planning services will continue to be an important adjunct in promoting healthy pregnancies and in improving the overall health of mothers and infants.

Fluoridation of Drinking Water

Fluoridation has had a significant role in reducing tooth decay in children and tooth loss in adults. Fluoridation, first began in 1945, and by 1999 had reached an estimated 144 million people, effectively prevents tooth decay, without regard to socioeconomic status or access to care. A prospective field study conducted in four pairs of cities in Illinois, New York, Michigan, and Ontario, Canada, starting in 1945, first proved the efficacy of adjusting fluoride levels in community water supplies by demonstrating a 50–70% reduction in caries among children in communities with fluoridated water.[20] By 1962, after further epidemiologic studies, a range of 0.7–1.2 ppm was recommended as the optimum range of fluoride concentration, with lower levels for warmer climates (where higher water consumption is expected) and the higher level for colder climates.[21] By the end of 1992, 10,567 public water systems serving 135 million persons in 8,573 communities had instituted water fluoridation.[22] The mean number of decayed, missing, or filled teeth (DMFT) among persons aged 12 years declined 68%, from 4.0 in 1966–1970 to 1.3 in 1988–1994. The percentage of persons aged 45–54 years who had lost all their permanent teeth decreased from 20.0% in 1960–62 to 9.1% in 1988–1994.[23] Fluoride toothpaste also prevents tooth decay, but is dependent on the amount of use by either persons or their caregivers, while water fluoridation reaches all within a community and is particularly advantageous for communities with low overall socioeconomic status who also might have a higher rate of dental disease.

Prenatal Care

The percentage of women beginning prenatal care in the first trimester of pregnancy has risen steadily every year since 1989, from 75.5% to 83.2% in 1999, after having been quite flat in the 1980s. Similar gains were made for all three of the largest racial and ethnic groups with steady and persistent improvements since 1989. For non-Hispanic whites there was an increase from 82.7% to 88.4%, for non-Hispanic blacks from 59.9% to 74.1%, and for Hispanic women from 59.5% to 74.4%.[24] Again, there was significant variation among states, with five states having more than 88% of women begin prenatal care in the first trimester, while two areas were below 75%.[11] Every year since 1983, at least 6% of women initiated care in the last trimester or received no prenatal care at all. However, that figure declined to 4% in 1996 and to 3.8% in 1999, an all time low. Even though the benefits of prenatal care have generated much discussion lately and are difficult to quantify, appropriate care can promote healthier pregnancies by managing pre-existing medical conditions, providing health behavior advice, and assessing the risk of poor pregnancy outcome.[25]

Teenage Birth Rate

The teenage birth rate has been falling steadily since 1991, when a peak of 62.1 per thousand was reached, the highest rate since the early 1970s, and has fallen to an all time low of 49.6 per thousand teens, a decline of 20%. Similar decreases have been recorded for the teenage subgroups as well. For teens aged 15–17 years, the rate has fallen from 38.7 in 1991 to 28.7 per thousand in 1999, a fall of 26% and for teens aged 18–19 years, a decrease from 94.4 per thousand to

80.3 per thousand, a 15% decrease.[24] An even larger drop occurred in non-Hispanic black teenagers for all ages and for each subgroup. For these teens, the rate fell from 118.9 per thousand in 1991 to 83.7 per thousand in 1999, a 30% decrease; for black teens aged 15–17 the rate fell from 86.7 to 53.7, a 38% decrease; and for black teens aged 18–19 the rate fell from 163.1 to 126.8 per thousand, a 22% decrease. Hispanic teenagers also had decreasing rates but of less magnitude, the overall rate falling by 12% between 1991 and 1999, 106.7 to 93.4 per thousand. Much of this decreased rate in the 1990s has been the result of a decrease in first teen birth rates, with first births accounting for almost 4 in 5 teen births.[9] Although the reasons for this marked downturn in teen births is unclear and probably controversial, the proportion of teenagers who are sexually active has stabilized in the 1990s, reversing the increases over the last 15–20 years.[26] Teenagers are also more likely to use contraceptives at first intercourse[27] and many private and now public initiatives and resources have focused attention on the importance of pregnancy prevention through abstinence education, especially for young teens.

AREAS OF CONCERN

Even though there is much that we can point to with pride, there is also much that needs to be accomplished. The United States has continued to rank behind at least 20 other industrialized countries in the rate for infant mortality. In 1997, 27 countries had infant mortality rates better than the United States, with Sweden, Japan, Singapore, Finland, and Hong Kong having the best rates in the world. In fact, Sweden's rate of 3.6 infant deaths per thousand live births is one-half the rate in the United States. Although there are undoubtedly many reasons for these differences, overall the figures reflect differences in the health status of women before and during pregnancy as well as the quality and accessibility of ongoing care for pregnant women and their infants.[11] Further, there are significant differences in the make-up of the populations of each country, particularly relating to racial and ethnic composition and geographic and socioeconomic factors.[28] In addition, there are varying practices in the countries in the reporting of very low birth weight babies dying very soon after birth.[29]

Low Birth Weight

We are also confronted with the problem of a low birth weight (LBW) rate that has continued to rise since 1985 from 6.8% to 7.6% in 1999 when 301,183 infants were born low birth weight or under 2,500 grams.[24] This rise has been gradual, but persistent and steady, and currently is similar to the percentage reported in the 1970s. There has also been a significant increase in the rate for whites, from 5.7% in 1985 to 6.6% in 1999. Interestingly, the rate for blacks has fallen since its peak in 1991 of 13.6% to 13.1 % in 1999, although it is still higher than it was in 1985 at 12.6%. The rate for Hispanics has remained relatively consistent, rising slightly from 6.2% in 1989 to 6.4% in 1999. Although there has been an encouraging decline in the LBW rate for blacks, it is still in the range of twice the rate for whites and Hispanics. There is wide variation among the states, with an LBW rate of over 10% in three states.[24] Much of this increase in the LBW percentage, particularly in the last few years, is impacted by the increasing rates of multiple births, which are often low birth weight. In 1999, 6% of singleton births were low birth weight compared with 57% of multiple births.[24] Multiple births have had the most impact on among whites; in that group the multiple birth rate has risen by 18%. Singleton low birth weight has also increased in this same time period from 4.6% to 4.9%.[24] Low birth weight is the leading contributor to neonatal death, the second leading cause of infant death; it also leads to an increased incidence of long-term disability. In the face of falling infant death rates, the increasing rate of low birth weight is perplexing and challenging. It seems clear that success in dealing with low birth weight would certainly improve the statistics on infant death. Although the causes for the rise in LBW and multiple births are largely unknown, contributing factors include poverty, lack of equal access to primary, preventive, and reproductive care, lack of understanding of the causes of preterm birth (births earlier than 37 weeks gestation), and maternal smoking.

Smoking

Many studies have cited the increased risk of low birth weight among maternal smokers, as well as for other adverse outcomes including infant mortality, SIDS, and intrauterine growth retardation.[9,29,30,31] The rate of low birth weight babies born to maternal smokers in 1999 was 12.1.% compared to 7.2% among nonsmoking women. This significant difference is also true across racial and ethnic groups— whites, 10.8% to 6.1%, blacks, 21.0% to12.4%, and Hispanics, 11.8% to 6.6%.[24] Any use of cigarettes also increases the risk for low birth weight with an 11.1% increase in the lightest smokers (1–4 daily).[24] On a positive note, maternal smoking continues to decline, showing a 35% reduction from 1989 to 1999 (19.5% to 12.6%).[24] In 1999, American Indians had the highest percent (20.2), followed by whites (12.6), Hawaiians (14.7), and blacks (9.3). And the rate declined in all age groups except teenagers. Teens had a decreasing rate until the middle 1990s when a steady increase began that is continuing its upswing. In 1999, teens had the highest maternal smoking rate of any age group, 18.1%, followed by 20–24-year-olds (16.7%), and by 25–29-year-olds (11.0%). Between 1994 and 1996, rates rose for the older teens, those 18–19 years old, as well as for those 15–17. But the rate has leveled off since 1996 for the younger teens while it has increased 7% for the older teenagers.[24] This increasing rate for older teens, as they age, seems to be having an effect on the next age group, those 20–24. Smoking rates have increased for the first time since information was first reported in 1989, rising by 1% to 16.7%, with increases in both non-Hispanic whites and blacks.[24] The increasing smoking rate among teens is troubling and represents both a challenge and an opportunity. It is a challenge because the reasons for this recent upswing are unknown and it always represents a challenge to change teenage behavior. It is also an opportunity because smoking prevention programs are one of the few successful interventions known to reduce a significant cause of neonatal and infant death, not only for teenagers, but for all women who smoke.

Unintended Pregnancy

In the United States, unintended pregnancy, defined as the sum of abortions and of births resulting from pregnancies reported as having been unintended, is a significant problem. Half of all pregnancies (49.2%) were unintended, with 54% of those ending in abortion.[32] There is wide variation among ages as well. Teenagers aged 15–19 years have the highest rate of unintended pregnancy (78%), with a decreasing rate by age cohorts to those women aged 30–34 with the lowest rate (33.1%), and a subsequent increase by age for a rate of 50.7% in women aged 40 or over.[32] Marital status, poverty status, and racial/ethnic background also bear upon the unintended pregnancy rate. Never-married women have the highest rate (77.7%) compared to currently married women (30.7%); women below the poverty level have the highest rate (61.4%) compared to women over 200 percent of the poverty level (41.2%); and blacks have a higher rate (72.3%) than whites (42.9%) or Hispanics (48.6%). When one compares contributory factors among 15 industrialized Western countries, such as Canada and England, the United States has one of the higher rates for both total fertility and abortion, and the highest rate of pregnancy.[33] As noted above, those most likely to have unintended pregnancies—unmarried women, those living in poverty, and those women from a racial or ethnic minority—are also those who have the least ability to navigate the health care system. They are also least likely to get early or adequate prenatal care or ongoing primary and preventive services for themselves or their babies. They also have a higher rate of low birth weight and fewer social and community supports to help with such an infant.

Dental Disease

Oral Health in America: A Report of the Surgeon General declared dental disease the most common health problem affecting children in the United States.[34] Untreated dental decay is found in 25% of all children entering kindergarten and 30% of children in kindergarten have nearly 95% of all tooth decay in that age group. Fifteen percent of fifth graders account for around 80% of all tooth decay in that age group.[35] And in the 1997 National Survey of America's Families undertaken by the Urban Institute, 9.6% of poor children, those under 200 percent of the poverty level, were found to have unmet dental needs, as were 7.2% of all children.[36] Furthermore, 29.5% of poor children and 20.9% of all children made no dental visits in the previous year. Nearly 60% of poor children had not made the two visits per year recommended in the Maternal and Child Health Bureau's Bright Futures Guidelines. Families without dental insurance are over 2.5 times more prevalent than those without health insurance, and more than 30% of children have no dental coverage at all.[37] For the poor, access to publicly financed dental health services seems to be a problem. In 1998, only 19% of children eligible for dental services through the Early and Periodic Screening, Diagnosis, and Treatment program (EPSDT) received a preventive dental service, down from over 25% in 1988.[38] It has been stated that extremely poor oral health harms children physically by hampering growth and development—not just of the mouth and teeth but of the entire body—and that early and extreme disease also predicts long-term disease and dental pain that can actually shape how a child will respond to all painful stimuli. Poor oral health harms kids functionally, behaviorally, and socially. It impacts on family dynamics, peer dynamics, and ability to play and learn.[39]

Racial and Ethnic Disparities

Among the greatest challenges in maternal and child health is reducing the disquieting racial and ethnic disparities that exist for almost every measure of maternal, infant, and child health outcomes. The fact that many of these disparities have been known for decades only makes the following statistics more disturbing to those dedicated to improving the health and social care of women and children. Black and Hispanic women are less likely to begin prenatal care in the first trimester.[24] Black women are almost four times more likely to suffer a pregnancy-associated death compared to white women,[9] and they are almost twice as likely to lose an infant *in utero* or have an infant die in the first year of life.[9,40] Further, black infants are about twice as likely to be born preterm or at low birth weight, both conditions putting them at increased risk for subsequent morbidity or mortality.[24] Disparities are also apparent within broader racial or ethnic categorizations. For example, among Asian Americans, women of Chinese and Japanese ancestry are more likely to have better birth outcomes than Vietnamese or Cambodian women.[24]

Additionally, disparities occur among the most prevalent child and adolescent health conditions. Among other conditions, black and Hispanic youth are more likely to be overweight and obese,[41,42] putting them at higher risk for the future development of diabetes or heart disease. These same groups are more likely to be diagnosed with asthma, the most common chronic disease of childhood. There is further evidence that the disparities may be increasing in this area.[43] Differential mortality for children by race and ethnicity is another ongoing concern: black and Hispanic children are more likely to die from injury.[9] Homicide is the leading cause of death for black male children, with their suicide rates increasing more than for other groups.[9]

Lack of Health Coverage

Concomitantly, the United States is faced with the concern that health coverage is lacking for millions of children. Even though both the percentage and number of children without health insurance has declined in the last few years due largely to increases in private insurance and expansion of the State Children's Health Insurance Program, the most recent figures from the Census Bureau indicate that there were still about 8.5 million children, or 11.6% of those younger than 18 years, who lacked health care coverage in 2000.[44] Moreover, some groups of children are significantly more likely to be without health care coverage. Almost 25% of children of Hispanic origin were without coverage in 2000, compared to 13.6% of black children and 7.3% of white non-Hispanic children.[44]

Continuous health care coverage is important for a number of reasons. Children who are covered are significantly less likely to have unmet health care needs or delayed care.[45] Delaying early treatment of children's health problems has been shown to lead to a higher risk of complications requiring hospitalizations.[46,47] Additionally, children with coverage also have lower rates of hospitalizations,[48] and are less likely to have an emergency room visit.[49] They are also more likely to have a medical home, receive more primary and preventive care visits,[48] have improved access to care, and more dental utilization.[50]

The disparities so prevalent among maternal and child health outcomes likewise pervade measures of health services and exacerbate our inability to eliminate these health status gaps. In addition to health care coverage, black and Hispanic children are less likely to have a regular source of care.[51] These groups are also more likely to be hospitalized for preventable conditions—another indicator of limited access to primary care.[52] There is evidence to suggest that black and white children may receive different kinds of treatment for similar conditions.[53] All these factors may contribute to the perception among racial and ethnic minorities that they receive less adequate health care.[54]

Effects of Poverty

Neither disparities in maternal and child health outcomes nor health services can be mentioned without discussing the plight of children living in poverty. Although the percentage of children in poverty in 1999 was at its lowest since 1979, still, there were 11.5 million children living below the Federal poverty level.[55] Furthermore, childhood poverty exceeded that of adults by about 70%.[55] Very young children and black and Hispanic children were particularly vulnerable. Related children under age 6 had a poverty rate of 18.0%, while one in three black and Hispanic children were poor compared to one in eight white children.[11] The deleterious effects of poverty can be manifested in many ways: through poor nutrition, substandard housing, poor environmental conditions, higher exposure to infectious agents, or inadequate health care. Among health outcomes, poor children are more likely to be born low birth weight[56] and to die in the first year of life. Poverty has also been associated with children's developmental levels and their readiness to learn,[57] which has implications through the rest of the life cycle. Poor children were also much more likely to be without health care coverage (21.5%) compared to all children.[44]

Availability of Quality Child Care

Mothers are increasingly joining or remaining in the labor force, relying on paid child care for their children. In 2000, 61% of mothers with children age 5 and younger were employed. In 1995, approximately one-third of children under 5 years old spent their time in the care of a parent while another parent worked or attended school. The remaining children spent their time attending an organized facility such as a day care center, nursery or preschool, or Head Start program (35%), were cared for in their home by a nonrelative (8%), received care in a family day care (20%), or participated in some other arrangement (11%). Many children were in multiple child care arrangements.[58]

The limited availability of affordable and high-quality child care may affect women's employment choices. The cost of care may demand a high proportion of family earnings, especially among low-income and single parent families and families with very young children.[59] Analysis of a national survey found the cost of child care often cited as a reason for not working among low-income families and these families were less likely to participate in formal child care arrangements compared to those with higher income.[60]

When providers adhere to professional standards for quality child care, children experience better outcomes in school readiness, language comprehension, and behavior problems. However, few providers (10% to 34% depending on child's age) met all recommended standards on child to staff ratios, group sizes, caregiver education, and caregiver training.[61] The particularly low wages of child care employees—the median wage and salary income of child care employees was $11,076 in 1997—may adversely impact the ability of the profession to attract well-trained individuals. Limited evidence suggests that among low-income women, higher-quality child care may increase employment, stability of employment, and hours of work.[62]

Asthma

Since 1980, asthma prevalence has increased dramatically. From 1980 to 1995, asthma prevalence among children 0–17 increased by 5% per year.[63] The CDC's National Center for Health Statistics recently released a fact sheet containing the latest prevalence estimates for asthma.[64] In 1998, children had the highest prevalence of an asthma attack or episode of any age group, 53 per 1,000 children aged 0–17, compared to 35 per 1,000 for those over 18 years old and 39 per 1,000 total in 1998. Asthma creates a great demand on the health care system: children aged 0–17 made 5.8 million outpatient visits, over 867,000 emergency room visits, and had over 89,000 hospitalizations. Following the trend in asthma prevalence is made more difficult by a change instituted in 1997 in the National Health Interview Survey (NHIS). A new national trend line using NHIS data from 1997 onward will need to be established, particularly since the epidemiology of asthma is poorly understood. At present, minimal surveillance of asthma is occurring at the state level across the country, and what is needed is the ability of public health workers to accurately identify cases, have access to good data, and have the resources to analyze the data.[65] Translation of these analyses into improved interventions is of great importance.

Obesity

The prevalence of obesity in the United States is increasing at an alarming rate. Data from the most recent National Health and Nutrition Examination Study (NHANES IV) shows that the number of overweight children has continued to increase among all age and racial groups since NHANES II in the 1970s. Approximately 11% of children were overweight during the survey years 1988 to 1994, and an additional 14% had a BMI between the 85th and 95th percentiles, suggesting that they are at high risk for becoming overtly overweight.[42] Data from the 1988–1991 cohort indicates that approximately 14% of all children are overweight.[41] Between NHANES II and III the prevalence of overweight increased among 6-to-11-year-old males from 6.5% to 11.4% and from 5.5% to 9.9% among females.[42] Between 1986 and 1998, overweight increased persistently and significantly to 21.5% in black children, to 21.8% in Hispanics, and to 12.3% among non-Hispanic whites.[41] In fact, overweight prevalence increased by approximately 50% between 1986 and 1998 for non-Hispanic white children.[41] There are no easy solutions to this increasing epidemic, but attention must be targeted towards lack of physical activity and inappropriate eating patterns. Schools should be encouraged to provide for all students to participate in physical education and to provide instruction not just in team sports, but in individual sports that have a greater chance of being continued into later years. Time limits should be placed on television, movies, and computer games. Proper eating habits should be encouraged at home, at school, and in the workplace. Public health workers should be leading many of these efforts.

Violence among Children

In the United States violence among children, particularly among adolescents, has been a persistent challenge. Firearms remain the second leading cause of death, after motor vehicle crashes, in children aged 5–14 and 15–19, and the fourth leading cause for children aged 1–4 years old.[11] In 1999, 17.3% of high school students had carried a weapon—gun, knife, or club—sometime in the last 30 days and almost 5% of these students had carried a gun in the same period. Students also carry these weapons to school. In 1999, nearly 7% brought a weapon onto school property in the last 30 days.[66] The number of firearm deaths has been declining since a peak in 1994, with a decrease of 35% between 1994 and 1998. Even with this decrease, children 19 years old and less, still accounted for 12.3% of all firearm deaths in the nation.[6] Bullying behavior among school-aged students is also becoming recognized as a component of violence, with a definition generally agreed on as a specific type of aggression in which the behavior is intended to harm or disturb, the behavior occurs repeatedly over time, and there is an imbalance of power, with a more powerful person or group attacking a less powerful one.[67–69] A recent national survey of students in grades 6–10 found that nearly 30% of these students reported some type of involvement in moderate or frequent bullying, as a bully (13.0%), a target of bullying (10.6%), or both (6.3%).[67] All students involved in bullying behavior showed poorer psychological adjustment than those not involved. For example, fighting behavior was increased as was smoking and poorer academic achievement.[67] More work needs to determine if early bullying behavior is associated with more significant violence later in the teenage years, is associated with carrying a firearm, or leads to other antisocial behaviors later in life. The Maternal and Child Health Bureau is developing a major educational and intervention program over the next two years aimed at early prevention of bullying behavior.

Health of Women

The recent publication of results from the Agency for Healthcare Research and Quality's Medical Expenditure Panel Survey (MEPS) has shown that women aged 18–29 had the highest rate of perceived excellent/very good health (67.1%), but by age 45–64 that perception had decreased to less than 56.6%.[70] There were racial/ethnic differences as well, with white women more likely to perceive excellent/very good health (62.7%) than black women (50.7%) or Hispanic women (48.6%).[70] Access to regular care for women, particularly young women, whose health habits are being developed, is a concern. Women aged 18–29 were least likely to have a usual source of care (26.4%) than women of other ages, with the rate declining steadily to 9.7% for 65–74-year-old women.[71] Having a usual source of care and use of the health care system may be partly impacted by insurance status. Compared to women with no insurance, women who had either private or public insurance had more Pap smears (over 70% to 54.8%) and more mammograms (58.8%–71.1% to 40.4%) as well as more frequent complete physical exams.[71] Good health for women, throughout their lifespan, encouraged by ongoing and regular preventive and primary care, is the ideal. With the precursors of many later-in-life disorders having their roots in the preadolescent years, emphasis should be placed on beginning care early. Not only will this improve overall health for women, but it will also provide the opportunity for a healthier pregnancy and birth outcome. Fortunately, the health status of women has become more of a targeted issue in the last several years. Many states and local communities have developed specific programs around the health of women, and most federal agencies have an office of women's health. The Maternal and Child Health Bureau not only has major programmatic activities in this area but has made women's health one of several top priorities.

Health of Children

The health of children will also be affected by two demographic trends: changes in the dependency ratio and immigration patterns. The percentage of the total population who are children rose substantially during the baby boom, from 31% in

1950 to 36% in 1960, and has been declining ever since. By 2010, the Census Bureau projects that only 24% of the population will be under age 18. At the same time, the proportion of the population that is elderly (65 and over) will increase as the baby boom generation ages, from 13% in 1995 to a projected 20% by 2030.[72]

Dependency Ratio

The dependency ratio, or the ratio of children and elderly to working-age people, is projected to decline from 63.7 in 1995 to 60.2 in 2010. Then, as the baby boomers begin to reach age 65, the ratio will begin to increase. However, the youthful dependency ratio, representing the ratio of children to the working-age population, will remain stable. Thus, the elderly will represent an increasing proportion of the population of dependents.[72] In addition, the percentage of families without children is increasing, from 43% in 1960 to 52% in 2000.[73,74] This trend as well threatens the nation's focus on the needs of children. These trends require that we work to assure that children's needs are actively represented in discussions of the distribution of the nation's resources.

Immigration Effects

Nearly 14 million children in the United States are immigrants or have immigrant parents. The population of children in immigrant families has grown by almost 50 percent over the course of the 1990s, nearly 7 times faster than the population of children of U.S.-born parents.[75] Nearly 20% of children aged 5 to 17 do not speak English at home.[3] Immigrant children, particularly Hispanic children, are disproportionately likely to lack health insurance, and are less likely than U.S.-born children to have a usual source of care and an annual doctor's visit.[75]

For adolescents, immigration produces stresses that may be reflected in their behaviors and risk factors. Youth born outside the United States, and those born in the United States to immigrant parents, have been found to be more likely to feel peer pressure to engage in substance use, sexual activity, and violence, and to experience less parental support to resist these pressures.[76]

For immigrant youth, linguistic acculturation—that is, the ability to speak English proficiently—may influence the overall level of cultural acclimation, and thus their level of risk. Findings on the effect of linguistic acculturation on educational and psychological outcomes are mixed: while bilingual students with full English proficiency often exceed native English speakers academically, those with limited English proficiency are at highest risk of school dropout.[77] Another study found that, among Hispanics, linguistic acculturation was associated with greater risk of smoking among adolescent girls.[78] A recent review of the literature by the Institute of Medicine found that first-generation immigrant adolescents were in better health and had lower rates of many risk behaviors than native-born youth and later generations of immigrants.[79] However, the psychological adjustment problems and acculturative stress were most likely to be seen in youth with limited English proficiency or those who were not fully bicultural.[75]

These findings emphasize the need for services that build on the strengths of immigrant families while addressing their particular risks. The American Academy of Pediatrics recommends that pediatricians be sensitive to the needs of immigrant children and that training programs provide information about the stresses associated with immigration;[80] culturally and linguistically appropriate services should be available throughout the health care system.

CHALLENGES (WHAT NEEDS TO BE DONE)

The events of September, 2001, have changed the "business as usual" mindset of many of us in the public health family. The weaknesses in the public health infrastructure, the improvement of which so many of us advocated and fought for without much success, has now become an important issue. But the attention now being paid to infrastructure is overwhelmed by the needs to respond to bioterrorism. Although any strengthening is welcomed, we must remain alert to the infrastructure needs in maternal and child health and not let the existing opportunities pass. No longer can we feel comfortable in just advocating for the range of issues mentioned in this article in the traditional ways, but we must now become even more aware of the strengths and needs of families. The Maternal and Child Health Bureau is heavily involved in planning long-term responses to September 11th, particularly the mental health needs of children and their parents. Even though the documented needs are great closest to the New York site, it is becoming clear that in this age of instant communication through television and the Internet, the needs of children and families farther from Ground Zero—in fact, all across the country—may be nearly as great as those in New York. All of us must be responsive to these needs and to acquiring the data necessary to identify and provide those in the MCH community the increased services they deserve and need.

Challenge: Eliminating Racial and Ethnic Disparities in Health Care

Eliminating racial and ethnic disparities in health is a priority goal for our nation. In order to achieve this goal, we must recognize that these disparities are not expressions of an undefined genetic fallibility, nor do they occur in a vacuum. Rather, they are the manifestations of a complex—and still not completely understood—set of intertwined social, economic, and political factors. The reduction, and subsequent elimination, of disparities will most likely occur when we adopt a multipronged approach that includes, among other conditions: the removal of economic, social, and cultural barriers to receiving comprehensive, timely, and appropriate health care; and reduction of the circumstances that increase health risks, such as poverty. Moreover, because the effects of adverse prenatal events may echo throughout adulthood, it is incumbent upon us to mind the health of women through good preventive and primary care.

We are further hampered by the lack of knowledge on this issue among the U.S. population. A recent national survey found that the majority of Americans are uninformed about health care disparities; most were unaware that blacks fared worse than whites on measures such as infant mortality, and that Hispanics were less likely than whites to have health insurance.[81] Views on whether the health system treats people equally were strikingly different by race. Most minority Americans perceive that they get lower quality care than whites, but most whites think otherwise. These findings indicate that efforts to eliminate disparities will also need to focus on public awareness of the problems.

Challenge: Measuring Maternal and Child Health Outcomes

Billions of dollars are spent each year on maternal and child health services by federal, state, and local governments to address some of the previously mentioned issues. Yet, despite these investments, there has been surprisingly little data on maternal and child health outcomes and programs. For example, while racial and ethnic disparities have been well documented, the reasons for these disparities are not understood because the data used is often administrative data or legal records, such as vital records, which have a limited ability to provide in-depth information. Administrative and clinical records frequently miss children who are not receiving program services or care. In other crucial areas, little data exists; basic information on maternal and child health is relatively rare at state and local levels, both for all children and children with special health care needs. Both the Centers for Disease Control and the Maternal and Child Health Bureau have been moving to address these gaps. The CDC has sponsored the Pregnancy Risk and Monitoring Systems (PRAMS) in an increasing number of states. The PRAMS surveys provide state-level data on pregnancy and the first year after birth. The MCHB has sponsored the National Children with Special Health Care Needs Survey that will provide state-level estimates of children with special needs. In addition, the MCHB is developing a National Child Health Survey that will provide state-level estimates on measures of child health and well-being.

Challenge: Determining the Cost Effectiveness of Health Services

There is also insufficient data on the effectiveness and cost of maternal and child health services. The evidence base for many crucial areas in maternal and child health needs to be strengthened. Oftentimes, the "best practices" of caring for women and children may not be based on rigorously tested scientific methods. The practice of prenatal care is emblematic of this issue. Prenatal care is viewed as the cornerstone of our health system for caring for pregnant women and their fetuses, but the relationship between specific prenatal practices and birth outcomes is largely unknown. Likewise, in the child and adolescent health area there are many examples in which strengthening the evidence base would guide the allocation of funds, including such issues as: what is the optimum content of pediatric care; what are the most effective methods to prevent adolescents from using tobacco and alcohol; and what has been shown to be most effective in reducing racial and ethnic disparities? It is our challenge to rigorously examine the components of prenatal and pediatric care so that we promote the most effective procedures of caring for mothers and their fetuses.

Medical practices and technology have changed the ways that women and children are cared for, but the consequences of these changes need to be addressed. As an example, in the United States, pregnancies associated with assisted reproductive technology (ART) or ovulation-inducing drugs are more likely to result in multiple births than spontaneously conceived pregnancies. The contribution of ART is especially pronounced for triplets and higher-order multiple births. Moreover, because multiple births are at greater risk than singleton births to be preterm, low birth weight, or very low birth weight, the nation's rate for these adverse outcomes has been impacted.[82]

Challenge: Building Partnerships

None of the issues and concerns in this chapter can be improved by one program, one agency, or one department alone. Nearly all the problems have multifactorial etiologies, involve and are influenced by families, schools, and communities, and tend to not be episodic, but problems that may persist over the lifespan. Partnerships among federal, state, and local agencies and programs, and across agencies themselves have become more important and necessary. From data acquisition through data analysis, policy formation, implementation of program interventions, and evaluation, partnerships provide the strengths necessary to succeed. Relationships with corporations, the private sector, and families need to be encouraged. There is much to be done.

ACKNOWLEDGMENTS

We would like to thank Kerry P. Nesseler, RN, MS, and Debbie Maiese, MPA, of the Maternal and Child Health Bureau, and Renee Schwalberg, PhD, of Health Systems Research for their contributions to this chapter.

REFERENCES

1. World Bank. United States at a Glance. *http://www.worldbank.org/data.* Posted 19 September 2001.

2. Central Intelligence Agency. *The World Factbook 2001.* Washington, DC: CIA, 2001.

3. US Census Bureau. *Statistical Abstract of the United States, 2000.* Washington, DC: 2001.

4. Organization for Economic Cooperation and Development. *Education at a Glance.* Paris, France, 1998.

5. Bunker JP, Frazier HS, Mosteller F. Improving health: measuring effects of medical care. *Milbank Quarterly* 1994;72:225–258.

6. Murphy SA. Deaths: Final data for 1998. *National vital statistics reports,* 48(11). Hyattsville, Maryland: National Center for Health Statistics, 2000.

7. CDC. Ten Great Public Health Achievements—United States, 1900–1999. *MMWR* 1999;48(12):241–243.

8. Guyer B, Freedman MA, Strobino DM, Sondik EJ. Annual summary of vital statistics: Trends in the health of Americans during the 20th century. *Pediatrics* 2000;106:1307–1317.

9. Hoyert DL, Freedman MA, Strobino DM, Guyer B. Annual summary of vital statistics 2000. *Pediatrics* 2001;108:1241–1255.

10. MacDorman MF, Atkinson JO. Infant mortality statistics from the 1997 period linked birth/infant death data set. *National vital statistics reports*; vol 47 no 23, supp. Hyattsville, Maryland. National Center for Health Statistics. 1999.

11. *Child Health USA 2001.* Office of Data and Information Management, Maternal and Child Health Bureau, Health Resources and Services Administration, 2001.

12. CDC. National, State, and Urban Area Vaccination Coverage Levels Among Children Aged 19–35 Months—United States, 2000. *MMWR* 2001;50(30); 637–641.

13. Maine D, McNamara R. *Birth spacing and child survival.* New York: Columbia University Center for Population and Family Health, 1985.

14. Forrest JD. Contraceptive use in the United States: past, present and future. *Advances in Population* 1994;2:29–48.

15. Dryfoos JG. Family planning clinics: A story of growth and conflict. *Fam Plann Perspect* 1988;20:282–287.

16. Chandra A. Surgical sterilization in the United States: prevalence and characteristics, 1965–1995. Hyattsville, Maryland: US Department of Health and Human Services, Public Health Service, *National Center for Health Statistics*, 1998;20:1–33. Vital and health statistics—Series 23.

17. CDC. Achievements in Public Health, 1900–1999: Family Planning. *MMWR* 1999;48(47);1073–1080.

18. Frost JJ. Family planning clinic services in the United States, 1994. *Fam Plann Perspect* 1996;29:92–100.

19. Forrest JD, Samara R. Impact of publicly funded contraceptive services on unintended pregnancies and implications for Medicaid expenditures. *Fam Plann Perspect* 1996;28:188–95.

20. Burt BA, Eklund SA. *Dentistry, dental practice, and the community.* 5th ed. Philadelphia, Pennsylvania: WB Saunders, 1999.

21. Public Health Service. *Public Health Service drinking water standards—revised 1962.* Washington, DC: US Department of Health, Education, and Welfare, 1962. PHS publication no. 956.

22. CDC. *Fluoridation census 1992.* Atlanta, Georgia: US Department of Health and Human Services, Public Health Service, CDC, National Center for Prevention Services, Division of Oral Health, 1993.

23. CDC. Achievements in public health, 1900–1999: fluoridation of drinking water to prevent dental caries. *MMWR* 1999;48(41):933–940.

24. Ventura SJ, Martin JA, Curtin SC, Menacker F, Hamilton BE. Births: Final data for 1999. *National vital statistics reports*; vol 49 no. 1. Hyattsville, Maryland: National Center for Health Statistics, 2001.

25. US Public Health Service. *Caring for our future: The content of prenatal care.* Washington, DC: US Department of Health and Human Services, 1989.

26. Abma JC, Sonenstein F. Sexual activity and contraceptive practices among teenagers in the United States, 1988 and 1995. *Vital Health Stat* 23(21). 2001.

27. Abma JC, Chandra A, Mosher WD, Peterson LS, Piccinino LJ. Fertility, family planning, and women's health: New data from the 1995 National Survey of Family Growth. National Center for Health Statistics. *Vital Health Stat* 23(19). 1997.

28. Liu K, Moon M, Sulvetta M, Chawala J. International infant mortality rankings: A look behind the numbers. *Health Care Financing Rev.* 1992;13:4105–18.

29. Pollack HA. Sudden infant death syndrome, maternal smoking during pregnancy, and the cost-effectiveness of smoking cessation interventions. *Am J Public Health.* 2001;91:432–36.

30. Kleinman JC, Madans JH. The effects of maternal smoking, physical stature, and educational attainment on the incidence of low birth weight. *Am J Epidemiol.* 1985;121:843–55.

31. Fox SH, Koepsell TD, Daling JR. Birth weight and smoking during pregnancy—Effect modification by maternal age. *AM J Epidemiol* 139(10):1008–15. 1994.

32. Henshaw SK. Unintended pregnancy in the United States. *Fam Plann Perspect* 1998;30:24–29.

33. Alan Guttmacher Institute. *An international comparison of unintended pregnancy, contraceptive practice and family planning services.* New York: Alan Guttmacher Institute, 1987.

34. *Oral Health in America: A Report of the Surgeon General.* Rockville, Maryland. National Institute of Dental and Craniofacial Research, National Institutes of Health; 2000.

35. Mofidi M, Rosier RG, King RS. Problems with access to dental care for Medicaid-insured children: What caregivers think. *Am J Public Health* 2002;92 no 1;53–58.

36. Kenney GM, Ko G, Ormand BA. Gaps in preventon and treatment: Dental care for low-income children. *National Survey of America's Children.* Series B, no B–15. Washington, DC: the Urban Institute.

37. Mouradian WE. Why children's oral health? An ethical commentary. *J Southwestern Soc Ped Dentistry* 2000;6 no 2:10.

38. Center for Medicaid and State Operations (2001). *Annual EPSDT Participation Report: FY 1998.* Baltimore, Maryland: CMS.

39. Edelstein B. Talking to policy makers about kids' oral health. *J Southwestern Soc Ped Dentistry* 2000;6 no 2:7.

40. Mathews TJ, Curtin SC, MacDorman MF. *Infant mortality statistics from the period linked birth/infant death data se*t; vol 48 no 12. Hyattsville, Maryland: National Center for Health Statistics. 2000.

41. Strauss RS, Pollack HA. Epidemic increase in childhood overweight, 1986–1998. *JAMA* 2001;286(22):2845–2848.

42. Troiano RP, Flegal KM. Overweight children and adolescents: Description, epidemiology, and demographics. *Pediatrics* 1998;101:497–504.

43. CDC. Measuring childhood asthma prevalence before and after the 1997 redesign of the National Health Interview Survey—United States. *MMWR* 2000; 49(40);908–911.

44. Mills RJ; U.S. Census Bureau; "Health Insurance Coverage: 2000;" September 2001; *www.census.gov/prod/2001pubs/p60-215.pdf*

45. Lave JL, Keane CR, Chyongchiou JL, Ricci EM, Amersbach G, LaVallee CP. Impact of a children's health insurance program on newly enrolled children. *JAMA* 1998;279:1820–1825.

46. Maurer HM. Growing neglect of American children. *AJDC* 1993;147:529.

47. Braveman P, Oliva G, Miller MG, Reiter R, Egerter S. Adverse outcomes and lack of insurance among newborns in an eight-county area of California, 1982 to 1986. *N Engl J Med* 1989;321:508–513.

48. Szilagyi PG, Zwanziger J, Rodewald LE, Holl JL, Mukamel DB, Trafton S, Shone LP, Dick AW, Jarrell L, Raubertas RF. Evaluation of a state health insurance program for low-income children: Implications for state child health insurance programs. *Pediatrics* 2000;105(2):363–71.

49. Rosenbach ML, Irvin C, Coulam RF. Access for low-income children: is health insurance enough? *Pediatrics* 1999;103(6 Pt 1):1167–74.

50. Keane CR, Lave JR, Ricci EM, LaVallee CP. The impact of a children's health insurance program by age. *Pediatrics* 1999;104(5 Pt 1):1051–8.

51. Simpson G, Bloom B, Cohen RA, Parsons PE. Access to health care. Part 1: Children. *Vital Health Stat* 10 1997 Jul;(196):1–46.

52. Gaskin DJ, Hoffman C. Racial and ethnic differences in preventable hospitalizations across 10 states. *Med Care Res Rev* 2000;57 Suppl 1:85–107.

53. Park CH, Kogan MD, Overpeck MD, Casselbrant ML. Black-white differences in health care utilization among children with frequent ear infections. *Pediatrics* 2002;109(5):951.

54. Weech-Maldonado R, Morales LS, Spritzer K, Elliott M, Hays RD. Racial and ethnic differences in parents' assessments of pediatric care in Medicaid managed care. *Health Serv Res* 2001;36(3):575–94.

55. Dalaker J, Proctor BD. US Bureau of the Census, *Current Population Reports*, Series P60-210, Poverty in the United States: 1999. Washington, DC: US Government Printing Office.

56. Shiono PH, Rauh VA, Park M, Lederman SA, Zuskar D. Ethnic differences in birthweight: The role of lifestyle and other factors. *Am J Public Health* 1997;87(5): 787–93.

57. Miller JE. Developmental screening scores among preschool-aged children: The roles of poverty and child health. *J Urban Health* 1998;75(1):135–52.

58. Smith K. Who's Minding the Kids? Child Care Arrangements Fall 1995. *Current Population Reports*, P70-70, October 2000.

59. Giannarelli L, Barsimantov J. *Child Care Expenses of America's Families.* Washington, D.C., The Urban Institute, December 2000.

60. Tout K, Zaslow M, Papillo AR, Vandivere S. *Early Care and Education: Work Support for Families and Development Opportunities for Young Children.* Washington, DC: The Urban Institute, 2001.

61. NICHD Early Child Care Research Network. Child Outcomes When Child Care Center Classes Meet Recommended Standards of Quality. *Am J Pub Health* 1999;89(7):1072–1077.

62. Vandell DL, Wolfe B. *Child Care Quality: Does It Matter and Does It Need to Be Improved?* Institute for Research on Poverty, University of Wisconsin-Madison. 2000.

63. CDC. Surveillance for asthma—United States, 1960–1995. In: CDC Surveillance Summaries, April. *MMWR* 1998;47(no SS-1).

64. CDC. *New asthma estimates: tracking prevalence, health care, and mortality.* Fact Sheet (10/5/01). Hyattsville, Maryland: National Center for Health Statistics, Division of Data Services. 2001.

65. Boss LP, Kreutzer RA, Luttinger D, Leighton J, Wilcox K, Redd SC. The public health surveillance of asthma. *J Asthma* 2001;38(1):83–9.

66. CDC. CDC Surveillance Summaries: Youth Risk Behavior Surveillance—United States, 1999. *MMWR* 2000;49(SS05):1–96.

67. Nansel TR, Overpeck M, Pilla RS, Ruan WJ, Simons-Morton B, Scheidt P. Bullying behaviors among US youth: prevalence and association with psychosocial adjustment. *JAMA*. 2001 Apr 25;285(16):2094–100.

68. Boulton MJ, Underwood K. Bully/victim problems among middle school children. *Br J Educ Psychol.* 1992 ;62 :73–87.

69. Olweus D. *Aggression in the Schools: Bullies and Whipping Boys.* Washington, DC Hemisphere Publishing Corp; 1978.

70. Altman BM, Women in the health care system: Agency for Healthcare Research and Quality; 2001. MEPS research findings no 17. AHRQ Pub no 02-0004.

71. Kass-Bartelmes BL, Altman BM, Taylor AK. *Disparities and gender gaps in women's health, 1996.* Rockville, Maryland: Agency for Healthcare Research and Quality; 2001. MEPS Chartbook no 8. AHRQ Pub no 02-0003.

72. Day JC. *Population Projections of the United States by Age, Sex, Race, and Hispanic Origin: 1995 to 2050.* US Bureau of the Census, Current Population Reports, P25-1130, US Government Printing Office, Washington, DC, 1996.

73. Office of the Assistant Secretary for Planning and Evaluation. *Trends in the Well-Being of Children and Youth, 1999.* Washington, DC: GPO, 2001.

74. Fields J, Casper L. *America's Families and Living Arrangements.* Current Population Reports, P20-537, US Census Bureau, Washington, DC, 2001.

75. Hernandez DJ and Charney E, eds. *From Generation to Generation: The Health and Well-Being of Children in Immigrant Families.* Washington, DC: National Academy Press, 1998.

76. Blake SM, Ledsky R, Goodenow C, O'Donnell L. Recency of immigration, substance use, and sexual behavior among Massachusetts adolescents. *Am J Public Health* 2001;91(5):794–798.

77. Zhou M. Growing up American: The Challenge Confronting Immigrant Children and Children of Immigrants. *Annual Review of Sociology.* 1997; 23: 63–95.

78. Epstein JA, Botvin GJ, Diaz T. Linguistic acculturation and gender effects on smoking among Hispanic youth. *Prev Med* 1998;27(4):583–9.

79. Harris KM. The health status and risk behaviors of adolescents in immigrant families. In Hernandez DJ, ed. *Children of Immigrants: Health, Adjustment, and Public Assistance.* Washington, DC: National Academy Press, 2000.

80. American Academy of Pediatrics Committee on Community Health Services. Health care for children of immigrant families. *Pediatrics* 1997;100(1).

81. Lillie-Blanton M, Brodie M, Rowland D, Altman D, McIntosh M. Race, ethnicity, and the health care system: Public perceptions and experiences. *Med Care Res Rev* 2000;57 Suppl (1):218–235.

82. Kogan MD, Alexander GR, Kotelchuck M, MacDorman MF, Buekens P, Papiernik E. Trends in twin birth outcomes and intensive prenatal care utilization in the United States, 1981–1997. *JAMA* 2000;283:335–341.

ARTICLE 2

HEALTH CARE AND HEALTH CARE POLICY IN A CHANGING WORLD

Donald A. Barr, Philip R. Lee, and A. E. Benjamin

The organization of medicine is not a thing apart which can be subjected to study in isolation. It is an aspect of culture, whose arrangements are inseparable from the general organization of society.[1]

Walter H. Hamilton

INTRODUCTION

Understanding the structure of a health care system first requires understanding the society in which that system exists. The health care system that has evolved in the United States reflects not only the impact of science and technology but also the politics, cultural values, and priorities that have deep historical roots. In other texts, we have described characteristics of American society and policy that have had powerful influences on the evolution of the health care system, including the American character (e.g., individualism) federalism, pluralism, and incremental-ism.[2,3] We will briefly describe each of these and will then offer a historical perspective of how they have shaped health care policies over time and how each of them has contributed to the problems our health care system now faces.

THE AMERICAN CHARACTER

The concept of autonomy—along with its related ethical principle of respect for autonomy—has been one of the fundamental building blocks of public policy since the founding of the nation. The policies that established the nation were built on the strongly held view that the right of individuals to their own beliefs and values should be protected by government and protected from the government. To this day the principles of individual choice, confidentiality, and privacy are strongly held. In 1990, the Patient Self Determination Act (P.L. 101-508) translated the concept of autonomy into public health policy concerning the individual's right to make decisions with respect to his or her own medical care, to refuse treatment, and to prepare advanced directives regarding care.

Along with the concept of autonomy has been a deeply held distrust of government. Although the distrust of government waxes and wanes, it is ever present and is reflected in the limited role of government in dealing with such issues as the financing of health care. Distrust of government was one of the factors that resulted in the lack of action by the United States Congress on the health care reforms proposed by President Clinton in 1993. In 1993, the President raised the issue of health care reform to the top of the domestic policy agenda, but the United States Congress ended more than a year of deliberation without taking action. In this case, it was in part the concentrated interests of those who opposed reform (insurance industry, small business) that tapped into the broad distrust of government to sap public support and generate opposition to the proposed reforms. The creation of three branches of government by the founding fathers reflected in part the distrust of government and the need to create the necessary checks and balances to prevent the abuse of power by any branch of government or by the majority of the populace.

Throughout the history of the country there have been shifts toward a strong federal role, originally advocated by Alexander Hamilton, and away from such a role. During the 20th century, periods of public action (1900s, 1930s, and 1960s) were preceded and followed by periods of private action (1890s, 1920s, 1950s, and 1980s).

FEDERALISM AND THE ROLE OF GOVERNMENT IN HEALTH CARE

Government at all levels plays an important role in planning, financing, organization, and delivering health services in the United States. At the federal level, Medicare is the dominant program for financing health care for the elderly. The Departments of Veterans Affairs, Defense, and Health and Human Services all maintain large, complex health care delivery systems to meet the needs of veterans, the military and their dependents, and American Indians and Alaska Natives.

The federal government, particularly through the U.S. Public Health Service, funds a range of categorical public health and medical care programs, largely through grants in aid to state and local governments.

At the state level, Medicaid has become the largest medical care program, financed with federal, state, and, in some cases, local government matching funds. The states have historically had the major role in public health programs in the financing and provision of care for the chronically mentally ill and in substance abuse prevention and treatment.

Local governments, particularly in urban areas, have often been major providers of medical care for the indigent, largely through public hospitals and clinics.

Much of the modern infrastructure for health care has been funded or subsidized with public funds during the past 50 years, including the construction of public and most voluntary hospitals, the training of most of the health professions, and the bulk of basic biomedical research. Currently, approximately 40% of all health care expenditures are provided by the federal, state, and local governments.

Although government's role in financing health care is a major one, this role is not the result of a consistent or comprehensive plan for the organization of health care services, but it is instead an episodic response to market failures (e.g., Medicare). Over time, as the private sector has been unable or unwilling to meet the health care needs of specific segments of the population, government has stepped in to fill the gap. Initially, the needs were met largely by local government and voluntary efforts. Later, states stepped in to meet the needs of the mentally ill. The federal government played a limited role, except for specific beneficiary groups such as veterans and specific public health problems (e.g., venereal disease, tuberculosis), until the enactment of Medicare and Medicaid in 1965. The Balanced Budget Act of 1997 includes some of the most significant changes ever made in the Medicare and Medicaid programs, providing states with greater flexibility in the administration of Medicaid and individuals greater choice of competing plans in Medicare. The result of this piecemeal approach to the development of health policy has been a proliferation of federal categorical programs administered by more than a dozen government departments and agencies (e.g., Departments of Health and Human Services, Transportation, Agriculture, and Energy and the Environmental Protection Agency).

The role of government, particularly the federal government, has been at the heart of this debate about the future of health care in the United States since President Truman proposed a program of federally financed national health insurance in 1947.

This evolving role of government in the financing organization and delivery of health care reflects the role of federalism in the United States. The concept of federalism, and the concomitant role of the federal government in social policy, has evolved in the 200 years since the American Revolution and the drafting of the U.S. Constitution. After the failure of the Articles of Confederation, the drafters of the Constitution saw a need for a central government with clear but delineated authority in areas of common concern such as national defense and foreign policy. Functions such as education, police protection, and health care were left under state and local authority. The lines between federal and state authority were clearly drawn. It was not until after the Civil War, however, that state governments began to play a significant role in health care and public health policy.

This arrangement worked well so long as two conditions were met:

1. There was consistency between the levels of administrative authority and financial accountability.
2. The various levels of government involved had the appropriate resources and other capacities to carry out their responsibilities.

In health care, it is clear that these conditions have not been consistently maintained. The result often has been an increase in federal responsibility for health care, particularly in the financing of care. In some areas, such as Medicare, the shift to federal responsibility has included both administrative authority and financial accountability. In others, such as Medicaid and family planning, the disjunction between authority (i.e., federal) and accountability (i.e., states) has led to dysfunctional outcomes, including funding cutbacks, eligibility restrictions, low levels of payment to providers of care, and programmatic restrictions. The success of the federalist system depends on maintaining this balance between administrative authority and financial responsibility and between federal, state, and local responsibility.

There have been a number of reasons why state and local governments were not able to maintain their historical authority over social policy, not the least of which has been the lack of political will to extend government authority into new or controversial areas (e.g., civil rights). In parallel with the variation among states in the political will to assume responsibility for social needs have been variations in the ability of states to generate sufficient revenue through taxation and in the capacity to plan and administer complex programs. An important pattern has emerged as to how states respond to health programs that are initiated by the federal government for vulnerable populations but left to states to establish local eligibility and funding criteria: States will vary widely around a median level of benefits. Any federal attempt to guarantee a basic level of benefits using this decentralized approach will succeed for only a certain segment of the intended population.

One final consequence of the approach to health policy that decentralizes responsibility over health care programs has been the vulnerability of local governments and agencies to state funding cutbacks. These local entities are important providers of many health services, particularly hospital, outpatient, and emergency services for the poor; mental health and substance abuse services; and a variety of public health services. When local governments are mandated to provide these services (either by regulation or court order) but are not provided the supplemental resources to do so, both the quality of the local programs and the fiscal health of the local agency can be compromised. Although this does not usually occur during periods of sustained economic growth and low unemployment, quality of programs can vary strikingly from one community to another during economic downturns.

PLURALISM AND THE ROLE OF SPECIAL INTERESTS

In addition to establishing a central government with delineated authority, the founders of this country established a legislative and regulatory system based on pluralism in order to protect the individual from the power of government. Decision-making power in a pluralistic society is spread among many groups so that no one group gains excessive power. Over time, pluralism has become not only a mechanism for making decisions but also an ideology that shapes our perceptions of the proper role of government. In order for their voices to be heard, individuals have increasingly organized into groups with interests as broad as the political parties and as narrow as single issues (e.g., abortion). These groups not only are allowed to influence the legislation process, they are encouraged to do so. During the first half of this century, the groups that dominated the health policy process were characterized as an iron triangle, including legislative committees, executive branch agencies, and private interest groups (e.g., the American Medical Association [AMA]). More recently, the process has become more complex and the iron triangles replaced by policy networks. Peterson has observed that the health policy community today "is heterogeneous and loosely structured, creating a network whose broad boundaries are defined by shared attentiveness of participants to the same issues in the policy domain."[4]

The influence of special interests as a manifestation of our pluralistic system is clearly seen throughout the health policy process. In this century, the American Medical Association has exerted a powerful influence on health policy, although its influence has diminished significantly since the enactment of Medicare. Other influential interests have been the hospitals, the insurance industry, and the pharmaceutical companies. Although groups representing patients (e.g., American Association of Retired Persons, organized labor) have exerted influence over specific programs, it has been these four general groups (the medical establishment, hospitals, insurance companies, and pharmaceutical companies) that have tended to shape health policy in the period after World War II. More recently, business interest groups (e.g., Business Group on Health) have begun to be more influential.

Since the late 1960s, as the cost of health care has become a predominant issue, power over health policy has shifted from the providers to the purchasers (e.g., large employers). Regardless of this realignment of power among interest groups, the power of special interests over the process of establishing and implementing health policy has remained intact. The effectiveness of many of these interest groups (e.g., small businesses, insurance) was very evident in President Clinton's ill-fated attempt at health care reform. It is extremely difficult to achieve broad consensus or to implement broad health policy—or even to convince Congress to make minor changes in policy—in the face of the power of special interests. This inhibition inherent in the pluralistic system in the United States has shaped and continues to shape the health policy process.

INCREMENTALISM AS THE PRINCIPAL MEANS OF HEALTH POLICY REFORM

Kingdon[5] and more recently Longest[6] have provided a model for understanding how policy decisions are made. In Longest's model, the process includes policy formulation and policy implementation phases, with both influenced by a policy modification phase. It is very clear that although President Clinton played the key role in placing national health insurance on the policy agenda in 1993, he did not control the process after that. When a policy issue rises to the top of the agenda, two other factors must then be present for successful reform to take place: a policy solution that is broadly seen as successfully addressing the issue, and political circumstances that allow for reform to take place. When all three (agenda, solution, political circumstances) are present simultaneously, a "window of opportunity" exists for significant policy reform. If any one of the three is absent, the potential for significant reform is diminished substantially. A number of analysts have suggested that just such a window for major health care reform existed in the early Clinton years, but his policy solution proved unacceptable to a majority in Congress. Later the success of the "Republican Revolution" in 1994 fundamentally altered the political circumstances, thus removing one of the factors and dooming any efforts at major health care reform.

Once a policy has been enacted, a second process of implementation takes place, usually involving the executive branch agency responsible for establishing the necessary guidelines and regulations. In the case of Medicare, this is the Centers for Medicaid and Medicare Services (CMS), Department of Health and Human Services (HHS). The CMS also has a major role in approving state Medicaid regulations. For many categorical public health programs, although the authority is ultimately vested in the Secretary of HHS, the implementation is provided by the agencies (e.g., National Institutes of Health, Food and Drug Administration, Centers for Disease Control and Prevention). In addition to having the potential to influence all phases of the policy formulating phase, special interest groups can also play an important role in guiding policy implementation. Through ongoing relationships with the implementing agencies, they are able to influence the rules by which policy programs will operate. The AMA, for example, works closely with CMS to influence Medicare regulations.

A third phase of the policy process as it affects health care—policy modification—has also been described by Longest.[6] Part of the responsibility of the legislative process is in oversight of the implementation of programs in achieving their intended goals. Oversight will become increasingly important in the future view of the strict limits set on discretionary spending and in Medicare and Medicaid spending during the next five years.

When policies either do not have clear goals by which to measure them or have not been successful in attaining their stated goals, they often enter back into the legislative process for further modification. From this perspective, the policy process becomes cyclical: Policy formation leads to implementation, which leads to modification, which feeds back into the formation phase. In fact, many key health policies have been modifications to previously existing policies. For example, Medicare and Medicaid were amendments to the Social Security Act and were actually extensions of earlier programs (the Old Age, Survivors' and Disability Insurance program and the Kerr-Mills program to provide medical care for the elderly poor). Medicare, in turn, was shaped by major amendments affecting hospital payments (1983) and physician payments (1989), largely because of the rising costs of health care. The Balanced Budget Act of 1997 represented yet another major shift in Medicare policy, following years of oversight hearings.

The complexity of the policy-setting process, the susceptibility of policy implementation to outside influence, and the cyclical nature of policy modification all have led to a phenomenon that is characteristic of the United States government: the incremental approach to decision-making. Whether for health care or any other social issue, policy is usually made in this country in small steps (increments). An exception was welfare reform, which did call for sweeping changes. One of the reasons for the failure of Clinton's health care reform plan was that it did not propose an incremental approach to change.

Incrementalism has come to be understood by most of the players as the way things are to be done. There is a general hesitance to take anything but a small bite out of a major policy issue, both because of a general comfort with the status quo and because of the risk of unforeseen and unintended consequences of major policy modifications. It appears that only at times of crisis, when there is broad consensus that the need for major action overshadows the risk of unintended outcomes, is our governmental system able to adopt major policy reform. (It should be pointed out that the failed Clinton health care reforms were followed by incremental health insurance reform in the Kennedy-Kassebaum bill and the incremental expansion of health insurance coverage to a portion of uninsured children.)

HISTORICAL DEVELOPMENT OF AMERICAN HEALTH POLICY

Throughout most of the nation's history, the federal government played a minor role in health policy; most of the policy interventions in public health were at the state and local levels, and most of medical care was left to the private sector. At times of crisis, such as the Civil War, the Great Depression, or, more recently, the Civil Rights Movement, quantum shifts in authority from the state level to the federal level or from the private sector to the public sector take place.

In a series of earlier books,[1,2,7] we have reviewed the historical development of health policy in the United States. Others, including Rosemary Stevens[8,9] and Paul Starr,[10] have dealt with the sweeping changes in Medicare and Medical care, and Mullen[11] has provided a history of the U.S. Public Health Service.

We have described four distinct periods in the evolution of health policy:

1. A limited role for the federal government (1798–1862)
2. The emergence of a larger federal role (1862–1932)
3. The expansion of the federal role (1935–1969)
4. New federalism (1969–present)

In the early years of the republic, the Elizabethan poor laws of England were the foundation of most policies for the poor, the aged, and the infirm. In 1798, Congress passed the Act for the Relief of Sick and Disabled Seamen, imposing a twenty-cent-per-month tax on seamen's wages to pay for their medical care. This legislation represented the first step in establishing the U.S. Public Health Service.[11]

After the Civil War, the development of the germ theory of disease by Pasteur was the most powerful force affecting both public health and medical care. In public health, progress was more rapid than in medical care, with policies related to environmental sanitation, clean water, the pasteurization of milk, and expanded programs of quarantine grounded largely in the police power of state and local governments. The first federal law directly related to public health broadly was the Biologies Control Act of 1902 (P.L. 57-244), followed by the

Pure Food and Drug Act (P.L. 59-384) in 1906.

In addition to the gradual increase in federal authority during this period, significant shifts were taking place in the private sector's role in health care. During the latter half of the 19th century, there was a rapid growth in the number and in the role of hospitals. During this period, there was also the establishment of proprietary medical schools (replacing apprenticeship training) and the development of state and local public health agencies. The fragmentation of the hospitals' governance and management began with the growing number of voluntary, nonprofit, often religious hospitals in addition to local public hospitals and the proliferation of proprietary hospitals, usually owned by physicians. As medicine began to be rooted in science, and physicians gained more respect, physicians began to replace the hospital trustees in determining who was and was not admitted to the hospital.

Late in the 19th century and early in the 20th century, hospitals gradually shifted from places for the poor to come to die to centers of medical, but particularly surgical, care for the general public. Two general types of hospitals emerged: public hospitals financed largely at the local level, and private, community-based, nonprofit hospitals, many of them operated by religious institutions. Both the proprietary, hospital-based medical schools and physician-owned proprietary hospitals gradually disappeared in the early decades of the 20th century, largely due to the efforts of the American Medical Association, stimulated by the Flexner Report in 1910.[12]

It was also during this time that state governments, at the urging of state medical societies, became involved in licensing practitioners and supporting medical education. Thus, while government was becoming increasingly involved in guiding health policy during this period, most of this activity was at the state and local rather than the federal level, and the public role in health policy was still quite limited compared with that of the private sector.

Substitution of Public Services and Financing for Private Efforts (1935–1969)

The crisis presented by the Great Depression brought action by the federal government in areas that previously had been left to state and local control. From banking regulation to support for small businesses, from public employment to old age security, there was a broadly held perception that the federal government should do what the state governments had been unable or unwilling to do to respond to the crisis. Over the span of a few years, the role of the federal government vis-a-vis the states changed fundamentally. American federalism evolved from a pattern of limited federal responsibility for domestic policy to a cooperative relationship between federal and state governments with a strong, often leading role for the federal government.

This new relationship is seen nowhere more clearly than in the Social Security Act. Included within the Act was the new principle of federal aid to the states for public health and welfare assistance, including grants for maternal and child health and crippled children's services (Title V) and for general public health programs (Title VI). The Old Age, Survivors' and Disability Insurance (OASDI) program included in the original Act provided the philosophical and fiscal basis for the Medicare program enacted 30 years later. Of particular importance to children and families was the establishment of the Aid to Families with Dependent Children (AFDC) program, which formed the later basis (in 1965) for medical eligibility.

During this period of transformation, the National Cancer Institute was established (1938); the authority of the Food and Drug Administration (FDA) was greatly strengthened (1938), requiring pharmaceutical companies to seek approval of drugs for safety before marketing them; and the Nurse Training Act was passed (1941), providing schools of nursing with direct federal aid to permit them to increase their enrollments and improve their physical facilities.

After World War II, there was a growing federal role in the support of medical research, mental health research, and treatment programs, and the construction of community hospitals (Hill-Burton Act of 1946). In 1946, Congress also created the National School Lunch Program in response to the finding of widespread malnutrition of recruits during World War II. The establishment of the Department of Health, Education, and Welfare in 1953 (now the Department of Health and Human Services), including the U.S. Public Health Service, the then separate FDA, and the Social Security Administration, firmly established the federal government's role in the nation's health care system. This role was not, however, the result of any comprehensive or coordinated plan to develop a national health care policy. Rather, it was the amalgamation of a variety of incremental steps taken for a variety of reasons at a variety of times.

In the 1960s, there was further expansion of this new federal role in health policy. Through the "creative federalism" followed by Kennedy and Johnson Administrations, the federal government became increasingly involved in a number of areas, including environmental health (e.g., air pollution control), community mental health centers, neighborhood health centers, health professions training, family planning, and the other efforts to improve health care delivery to underserved communities. Many of these programs were financed through direct federal support for local governments and local nonprofit agencies. One of the most important laws enacted in the 1960s was the Civil Rights Act of 1964, later used as the means to desegregate the hospitals in the South. A further extension of the federal government's direct regulatory authority came with the 1962 amendments to the Food, Drug, and Cosmetics Act, which specified that manufacturers must demonstrate that a drug is both safe and effective before marketing it. Congress, between 1965 and 1967, enacted more new health legislation than all the previous congresses in the nation's 175 years.

The most dramatic expansion of federal authority in health policy was through the Social Security Amendments of 1965, establishing the Medicare and Medicaid programs to finance health care for all people older than 65 and all people receiving cash welfare assistance. The Medicaid program was particularly important to women and children because recipients of the Aid to Families with Dependent Children (AFDC) program were eligible for Medicaid. These policies marked one of the first times that major health care programs were enacted over the objection of the American Medical Association, fundamentally altering the power relationship between physicians and the federal government. Never again was the medical profession able to exercise veto authority over federal health policy.

In addition to Medicaid, a number of programs were designed to provide greater access to medical care for the poor. Neighborhood health centers and family planning services were funded by the Office of Economic Opportunity, and the Children and Youth and Maternal and Infant Care projects targeted to low-income areas were funded by the Bureau of Maternal and Child health. In addition, the food stamp program was established in 1964, the Head Start Program in 1965, the School Breakfast Program in 1966, and the Child Nutrition Act authorized the Women, Infant and Children's (WIC) program in 1966 and the Early and Periodic Screening, Diagnosis and Treatment (EPSDT) was added to Medicaid in 1967. These initiatives represented a broad-based approach to maternal and child health, well beyond Medicaid's financing of medical care.

These programs of the Kennedy and Johnson years had a profound effect on intergovernmental relationships and on federal expenditures for domestic social programs. The combination of direct federal payments for Medicare and Medicaid and federal grants-in-aid helped lead to a ballooning of the federal budget, which, in the face of the strain on the domestic economy caused by the Vietnam War, created a new crisis and a dramatic shift in the role of the federal government.

The trend away from community involvement in health care was temporarily reversed with an effort in the Great Society era to base health care for vulnerable, underserved populations in community controlled programs (e.g., neighborhood health centers, community mental health centers). Other efforts to strengthen the communities' role in the 1970s include health planning and the beginning of the "health cities" movement. Market forces, which began to play an increasingly important role in health care in the 1970s and 1980s, can have either a positive or negative impact on the role of the community, but their initial impact has been to shift control away from communities.

Entering the Era of Limited Resources: The "New Federalism" (1969–1997)

First coined by President Nixon, the term "New Federalism" described a movement to reverse the swing of government power to the federal government, transferring authority over policy and program to the states. The Nixon and Ford administrations favored block grants to the states for the support of local policy initiatives, with relatively little federal oversight. Congress resisted this move, favoring instead the continued use of categorical grants requiring detailed provisions regulating the type and level of services to be provided.

While Congress and the President argued over the issue of block versus categorical grants in the 1970s, the federal government confronted the problem of skyrocketing health care costs, largely a result of the Medicare and Medicaid programs. Federal and state governments had become third parties that underwrote the costs of a fee-for-service-based health care system that included few if any mechanisms to constrain costs. Coupled with a growing physician work force and increasing specialization, the explosion of new technology catalyzed by the enactment of the Medicare and Medicaid systems and the rapid expansion of biomedical research funded by the National Institutes of Health helped to lead to a rapid upward spiral in health care costs and thus in federal expenditures.

The federal response to rapidly rising health care expenditures assumed a variety of forms, ranging from the elimination of federal subsidies for hospital construction and health professions education to price controls for a limited period and more permanent limits on hospital and physician payments by Medicare.

Although the Nixon Administration advocated a greater role for the private sector, the President proposed a national health insurance plan that would require an employer mandate, greatly expanded family programs (Title X of the Public Health Service Act), created the National Health Services Corps, expanded and consolidated environmental quality and environmental health programs while creating the Environmental Protection Agency (EPA) in the process, and established the Supplemental Security Income (SSI) program for the aged, blind, and disabled. In many respects, the programs established or expanded from 1969–1974 resembled a continuation of the Great Society program of President Johnson, rather than the New Federalism advocated by President Nixon.

Additionally, in a step that was to have profound effects on the direction that later market-based reforms would take, the federal government stimulated the development and expansion of health maintenance organizations (HMOs) through the Health Maintenance Organization Act of 1972. Historically an anathema to most physicians and especially to the American Medical Association, HMOs had grown very slowly.

The movement away from federal responsibility for domestic social policy accelerated when Ronald Reagan was elected President in 1980. The most prominent changes enacted by the Reagan Administration that directly affected health care included (1) a sharp reduction in federal expenditures for social programs, including elimination of the revenue-sharing program initiated by President Nixon; (2) decentralization of regulatory and programmatic authority to the states, particularly through the use of block grants that came with a few strings attached; (3) an increasing reliance on market forces and private institutions to stimulate needed reforms and control rising costs; and (4) through the across-the-board federal tax reductions, a substantial decline in the ability of the federal government to fund new health programs. One of the three major programs that was converted from a formula grant, with strong federal direction, to a block grant was Title V (Maternal Child Health and Crippled Children's Services) of the Social Security Act. Seven categorical programs were consolidated into a block grant with considerable state discretion in how the funds were allocated. In 1989, Congress greatly limited this state flexibility and required a plan that related to needs and required that 30 percent of the funds be allocated to prevention and another 30 percent to children with special health care needs (formerly crippled children). Contrary to the "deregulatory" philosophy of the administration, it established the means to regulate hospital costs, using prospective payment through the diagnosis-related group (DRG) system as an alternative to Medicare's cost-based reimbursement for hospital costs in 1983. In addition, the Reagan Administration initiated major programs in research, prevention (through the Centers for Disease Control and Prevention) and treatment and care through the Ryan White Care Act. Finally with sponsorship by the Reagan Administration, Congress expanded Medicare to include long-term care and a prescription drug benefit through the Medicare Catastrophic Coverage Act of 1988. In the first year of the George H.W. Bush Administration, Congress eliminated the prescription drug benefits and many of the long-term care benefits.

No longer was the federal government to be the unquestioning payer for health services. No longer did the federal government have the capacity, even if the political will were present, to fund new health care programs. The rising budget deficit, not health care, became foremost on the national agenda. The George H.W. Bush Administration followed in 1989 with its support for a congressionally initiated Medicare fee schedule, to be set by the government, to control Medicare payments to physicians specified in the Omnibus Budget Reconciliation Act of 1989 (P.L. 101-239).

At the state level, increasing policy authority brought with it increasing financial burdens. As states became more responsible for establishing and implementing their own programs, they also became increasingly responsible for the costs of those programs. In the area of health care, the spiral of rising costs of Medicaid continued largely unabated, leading to increasing strain on state budgets. Once again a situation was created in which there was a mismatch between authority over a policy program and the capacity to finance that program.

A number of states turned to the private market and to market-based competition as a means of holding down costs, both the costs of publicly financed programs and the costs of health care overall. An initial change that was to have profound effects on our system of health care was an increasing reliance on for-profit corporations to operate within the health care system. Traditionally functioning as nonprofit, community-based institutions, many hospitals were taken over by for-profit chains financed through the sale of stock. A number of organizations involved in the direct provision of care, such as home health agencies and kidney dialysis centers, shifted from community control or nonprofit status to a for-profit basis. The requirement that HMOs operate on a nonprofit basis, included in the original HMO Act, was removed, opening the market to for-profit companies to become directly involved in the financing and provision of care. A number of states chose to rely on private HMOs to provide care to Medicaid beneficiaries, leaving it to the HMO to determine what constitutes "medically necessary" care.

The continued increase in health care costs seen in the late 1980s coupled with the growing role of private markets in providing access to health care services led to a new awareness of what is really an old problem: the rising number of uninsured individuals and families. Currently as many as 44 million Americans have no insurance to pay for needed health care. The number of uninsured is increasing about 1 million per year despite the growing economy with its, low levels of unemployment.

The dilemma that confronted the Clinton Administration when it took office in 1993 was that Americans want to have their health care cake and eat it too. They want health care made more available to the uninsured, and they want the cost of health care to come under control, but only if these actions don't diminish the ability of the average American to get whatever treatment he or she perceives to be necessary or appropriate in a timely manner. This perhaps is the fundamental American health policy dilemma. President Clinton and Congress in 1993 faced conflicting needs and expectations with neither a mechanism to establish a broad-based consensus on how to reconcile them nor a mechanism to enact that consensus if it was achieved. President Clinton had campaigned on the need for the federal government to reassert itself in the area of health policy. With the broad goals of expanding coverage to the uninsured while simultaneously controlling health care costs, the Clinton health reform plan would have given broad new authority to the federal government to regulate the market for health insurance, while maintaining a reliance on market-based competition. It sought a new balance between the market-based delivery of care and a broad umbrella of federal oversight. In her thoughtful analysis of the Clinton Health Plan, Glied noted: "President Clinton's plan combined elements from two well-known policy proposals: single payer and managed competition."[13] She described the supporters of the single-payer plan as "medicalists" and the supporters of managed competition as "marketists." She attributed the failure of the plan to the fact that these two groups differed so strongly in their view that compromise was impossible. Second, she noted that "both groups based their policy prescription on false assumptions about health spending and the health sector," and finally neither group squarely or successfully faced the financing of health care reform (pages 8–9).[13] In addition, the high priority accorded reduction of the federal deficit by President Clinton and his leading economic advisors made it impossible to expand health insurance coverage to 40 million uninsured without politically unacceptable reductions to the Medicare program.

The idea was an attempt to redefine the role of federalism in health policy, but it was seriously out of synch with the continued movement in the evolution of federal authority. As pointed out by Theda Skocpol,[14] the ebbing tide of federal authority over social policy had not yet run its course. With an irony that has not yet been fully appreciated, the country was ready for one part of the Clinton proposal but not the other. Although Congress rejected an increased role for the federal government in regulating the market for health insurance, the deliberations surrounding the Clinton proposal nevertheless opened the door even more widely for market-based competition among health plans to become the principal paradigm for American health care at the end of the 20th century. Although it is happening in some areas of the country more rapidly than others, there has been a clear shift to the evolving concept of managed care for the financing, provision, and oversight of health care to most Americans. The shift comes, however, without any organized system of oversight or regulation and with an increasing role for for-profit companies. As a reaction, many states have proposed a variety of "consumer protective" laws (more than 400 bills introduced in state legislatures in 1997) to begin to place some limits on private sector managed care plans, and several leaders have proposed a "Patient's Bill of Rights." At the same time, states are increasingly mandating the enrollment of Medicaid beneficiaries (e.g., mothers and children) in managed care plans, and Medicare is poised to significantly expand the role of managed care plans.

Reductions in care, financial incentives that pit physicians' needs against those of patients, and a disavowal of responsibility for caring for the uninsured all are characteristics of this new American system of health care. In the words of one of the most vigorous advocates of for-profit health care plans,

> *Investor-owned health plans are a driving force behind this transformation [of the health care delivery system in America], and nonprofit health plans, in my view, are a byproduct of the past .... There is an appropriate role for nonprofit plans, but it is not in the operation of competitive health plans.*[15]

Was this the health care system that the American public intended to have? Did the United States get here as a result of a well-thought-out policy deliberation? As with much of the history of American health policy, the answer to both questions is no. Once again the separation of the authority over health policy and the financial responsibility for it has led to an outcome that was unintended and, as many believe, is not in the best interest of the American people.

While the private sector was moving rapidly, without adequate federal or state ground rules to "level the playing field," there was near paralysis of health policy making at the federal level after the failure of President Clinton's health care reform proposals in 1993–1994. For the first time in almost 40 years, the Republicans in 1994 captured both houses of Congress. There followed a period of confrontation as the Republicans pushed their "Contract with America," and President Clinton resisted major cutbacks in Medicare, federal regulations, and a variety of programs. The end result was a shutdown in the federal government in December 1995 and early January 1996 over a budget impasse. Subsequent to this battle, when President Clinton clearly emerged victorious, there began a period of incremental reform with passage of the Health Insurance Portability and Accountability Act of 1996 and the Personal Responsibility and Work Opportunity Reconciliation Act of 1996. This second Act fundamentally changed the welfare system that had existed for more than 60 years. It ended federal entitlement, particularly the Aid for Families with Dependent Children (AFDC) program, and replaced it with state programs called Temporary Assistance to Needy Families.[16]

The Balanced Budget Act of 1997 (P.L. 105-33) included the most significant reforms in the Medicare Program since its enactment in 1965. It placed greater emphasis on the choice of managed care plans available to beneficiaries and established tighter regulation of hospital and physician payments, including a reduction in payments to providers by $115 billion over five years. In addition, the Balanced Budget Act added Title XXI to the Social Security Act establishing the Child Health Insurance Program (SCHIP), a capped entitlement that added $48 billion to states over the next ten years to expand health insurance for low-income children either through expanded Medicaid or private health insurance options. The Balanced Budget Act also restored Medicaid benefits for disabled children who lost SSI eligibility as a result of the welfare reform of 1996.

The Balanced Budget Act of 1997 reflected a remarkable political consensus that had arisen from the ashes of the rancorous stalemate of 1995–1996 that followed the Republican capture of Congress. The Medicare reform process it established reversed almost every aspect of the failed partisan debates of the previous two years. The impact of the changes was similar to the successful Medicare payment reforms of 1984 and 1989 and the expansion of Medicaid eligibility for children in poverty in the early 1990s.

In 1997, the federal budget began to generate a surplus, particularly in the Medicare and Social Security Trust Funds. So thereafter, there was also a surplus in general revenues. This remarkable turnaround from the huge deficits of the Reagan-Bush years was the result of the severe limitations placed on federal spending by President Clinton beginning in 1993, the remarkable growth of the economy, and the ability of the Federal Reserve to control interest rates. Inflation remained low despite the lowest levels of unemployment in almost 30 years.

The Balanced Budget Act of 1997 attempted to reduce the federal health care budget through substantial reductions in the amount paid to providers, especially physicians and hospitals. There were additional reductions in supplemental payments to hospitals that care for a disproportionately high number of low-income patients and reductions in the amount Medicare pays to teaching hospitals to support graduate medical education. In addition, the Act changed the formula used to calculate payments to HMOs that enrolled Medicare beneficiaries. The previous formula to pay HMOs had been found to be overly generous, based on the tendency of healthy beneficiaries to select HMOs more often than sicker beneficiaries. The new formula led to substantial reductions in payments to HMOs in many areas of the country.

It did not take long after the enactment of the Balanced Budget Act for its effects to be felt. Hospitals were among the hardest hit by the changes. Many reported severe financial problems as a direct result of the payment reductions, especially teaching hospitals and those that served low-income patients. Physicians also experienced substantial reductions in Medicare payments. Hospitals and physicians came together to protest the reductions to Congress. As it turned out, the cost savings resulting from the payment reductions mandated by the Balanced Budget Act were greater than expected. Congress responded to the protests by passing the Balanced Budget Refinement Act in the Fall of 1999. It increased payments to providers by about $16 billion over five years.

An unintended consequence of the Balanced Budget Act was the massive involuntary disenrollment of many Medicare beneficiaries from HMOs and the increased cost of HMO care for those beneficiaries who stayed. As a result of the payment reductions, HMOs in many regions of the country simply pulled out of the Medicare market altogether. Between 1998 and 2001, 1.7 million Medicare beneficiaries (out of a total of about 6 million in HMOs) were notified that their HMO enrollment was being canceled. For those who remained in HMOs, the out-of-pocket HMO premium increased by as much as 300%. What was intended as a correction in a payment formula resulted in massive changes in the attractiveness of HMOs and other market-based options, putting at risk the future success of the entire "Medicare+Choice" program created by the Balanced Budget Amendment in 1997.

As we move into the 21st century, there is a very conservative Republican President, George W. Bush, who successfully advocated for a $1.35 trillion tax cut, largely benefiting the very wealthy; a limited prescription drug benefit for the poor elderly that was "dead on arrival" in Congress; a reduction of environmental regulations and expanded energy production; and a limited expansion of the federal role in education. In mid-2001, the Democrats regained a slim control of the U.S. Senate for the first time in seven years. It is difficult to predict the future for children's health and health care, but it seems clear that the factors that have shaped health policy, particularly in the past 50 years will continue to do so:

1. The American character
2. Federalism
3. Pluralism and the role of special interests
4. Incrementalism as the principal means of health policy reform[17]

REFERENCES

1. Hamilton W.H. *Medical care for the American people: The final report of the Committee on the Cost of Medical Care.* Adopted October 31, 1932. Chicago: University of Chicago Press, 1932.

2. Lee P.R. and Benjamin A.E. Health policy and the politics of health care. In S.J. Williams and P.R. Torrens (eds), *Introduction to health services*, 4th ed. Albany: Delmar Publishers, 1993.

3. Lee P.R., Benjamin A.E., and Weber, M.A. Policies and strategies for health care in the United States. In *Oxford textbook of public health*, 3rd ed. Oxford: Oxford University Press, 1996.

4. Peterson M.A. Political influence in the 1990s: From iron triangle to policy network. *Journal of Health Politics, Policy and Law,* Summer, 1993;18:395–438.

5. Kingdon J.W. *Agendas, alternatives, and public policies.* Boston: Little, Brown, 1993.

6. Longest B. *Health policymaking in the United States.* Ann Arbor, MI: Health Administration Press, 1994.

7. Lee P.R. and Silver G.A. Health planning—A view from the top with specific reference to the U.S.A. In J. Fry and W.A.J. Farndale (eds), *International medical care*. Oxford: MTP Medical and Technical Publishing, 1972.

8. Stevens R. *American medicine and public interest.* New York: Basic Books, 1971.

9. Stevens R. *In sickness and in wealth: American hospitals in the twentieth century.* New York: Basic Books, 1989.

10. Starr P. *Social transformation of American medicine: The rise of the sovereign profession and the making of a vast industry.* New York: Basic Books, 1982.

11. Mullen F. *Plague and politics.* New York: Basic Books, 1989.

12. Flexner A. *Medical education in the United States and Canada.* New York: Carnegie Foundation for the Advancement of Teaching, 1910.

13. Glied S. *Chronic condition: Why health reform fails.* Cambridge, MA: Harvard University Press, 1997.

14. Skocpol T. *Boomerang: Clinton's health security effort and the turn against government in U.S. politics.* New York: W.W. Norton, 1996.

15. Hassan M. Let's end the nonprofit charade. *New England Journal of Medicine,* 1996; 334:1055–1057.

16. Declercq E. The health and welfare policy process: The case of the 1996 welfare reforms. In *Health and welfare for families in the 21st century,* edited by Helen M. Wallace, et al. Sudbury, MA: Jones and Bartlett Publishers, 1998 (pages 68–71).

17. Lee P.R. and Estes C.L. (eds). *The nation's health,* 6th ed. Sudbury, MA: Jones and Bartlett Publishers, 2001.

ARTICLE 3

THE MATERNAL AND CHILD HEALTH COMMUNITY LEADERSHIP INSTITUTE: PUTTING THE HEALTH FOR ALL FRAMEWORK INTO ACTION

Barbara J. Hatcher

INTRODUCTION

The Health for All policy and framework was originally proposed at the International Conference on Primary Health Care held in Alma-Ata (Kazakhstan) in 1978. The Declaration of Alma-Ata provided the rationale and support of health care as an integrated systems approach to attaining the goal of health for all. Subsequently, at the first international Conference on Health Promotion, participating member nations endorsed the Ottawa Charter for Health Promotion. The Ottawa Charter specified five priorities: advancing public health policy, creating supportive environments, strengthening community action, developing personal skills, and reorienting health services. More recently and here in the United States, Healthy People 2010 seeks to address two central goals: increase quality and years of healthy life and eliminate health disparities.

The attainment of health for all is predicated on the following key elements: (1) elimination of both relative and absolute poverty and social and economic disparities, (2) sustainable economic development within stable ecosystems, (3) development and implementation of healthy public policies, (4) assurance of human and reproductive rights, (5) empowerment of women, youth, and communities, and (6) provision of health care that is accessible, affordable, culturally acceptable, and part of an integrated system.[1] Underlying all these various efforts is the need for strong public health leadership for policy and practice and a global response to health inequalities.

THE NEED

Global and local disparities exist with respect to the burden of disease and the allocation of resources. This is particularly true for women and children. All agree that the health status of mothers and children is a barometer for our present and our future. The health and well-being of mothers and children is inseparable as is their health of paramount importance to our global future. Despite tremendous improvements in maternal and child health, worldwide, significant disparities persist by race and ethnicity as well as by social class. The growing disparities are evident among and between communities and countries. Poor maternal and child health status knows no boundaries and many communities, globally, cannot assure a healthy and fair start for their children. In disenfranchised communities across the globe, poor maternal and child health is still too familiar, and there are still too many preventable deaths and disabilities.

Nationally, despite the tremendous decline in infant and maternal mortality over the past century, racial/ethnic disparities persist and are increasing particularly between Black and White women and infants. The higher infant mortality among Blacks is attributed to the higher incidence of low birth weight (LBW), preterm births, which also contributes to the higher risk of death even among infants of normal weight. Further, Black women are twice as likely to die of pregnancy-related causes than white women. There is also evidence of disparity among infants from other major ethnic groups. For example, American Indian/Alaska Native infants have a higher death rate than white infants because of higher SIDS rates and Hispanics of Puerto Rican origin have higher deaths rates because of higher LBW rates.[2] It is important to note that on measures such as low birth weight, Hispanics fare better than other groups.[3]

A retrospective cross-sectional comparison of death certificates of women of reproductive age, live birth and fetal death records, and medical examiner records in Maryland found that pregnant or recently pregnant women in the state are more likely to die by homicide than by any other cause, according to a study in a special issue of the Journal of the American Medical Association devoted to women's health. Pregnancy-associated death was defined as "death from any cause during pregnancy or within one year of delivery or pregnancy termination." A total of 247 pregnancy-associated deaths were ascertained in Maryland between 1993 and 1998. Of those deaths, 50 (20%) were homicides.[4] By contrast, homicide accounted for less than 12% of deaths among nonpregnant women in the state during the same time period.[5] Cardiovascular disorders were the second-leading cause of death at 19%.[6] The term "pregnancy-associated" was developed to "capture more completely all deaths occurring during or after pregnancy," including those that may be "socially related" and not solely "biologically" associated, according to an accompanying editorial by Victoria Frye of the Center for Health and Gender Equity.[7]

In 1998, nearly 80% of all births in Hartford, Connecticut, the capital of this nation's wealthiest state, were to single mothers, double the national average and 10 times the state's average. Single parenthood all too often is a precursor to a cycle of poverty and poor health status. Even Montgomery County, Maryland, a thriving and wealthy Washington, D.C., suburb, has released data showing that African American infants in that county are four times more likely to die before their first birthday than Whites.[8] In cities like Washington D.C. the infant mortality rate is comparable to that of developing countries.

In contrast, the global scene shows the ravaging impact of infectious and emerging diseases as well as barriers to good health such as inadequate primary health care systems and unsupportive political contexts. HIV and AIDS continue to present dramatic health challenges, particularly to mothers and children who are increasingly vulnerable. More than one million children are currently infected with the virus and at risk of dying from AIDS, despite recent medical advances that have all but eliminated the transmission of HIV to the unborn child in the United States and other western countries. New infections continue to strain available resources worldwide. The major cause of HIV/AIDS in children under 15 years of age is the transmission of HIV from mother to child during pregnancy, delivery, and breastfeeding; 90% of such transmissions occur in Africa. This problem is most acute in urban centers in southern Africa. However, recent medical advances and information have not been widely accessible to providers and HIV infected populations outside the United States, Canada, and Western Europe. It is estimated that only 20% of the estimated 250,000 women affected in South Africa, for example, will be reached through the recent availability of the drug nevirapine. More important, there are thousands of young women who are HIV negative, who are in need of counseling and support to prevent such infection.

Access to health care, including public health measures, is not the only determinant of health. Health is strongly and consistently related to income and other measures of socioeconomic status at the individual and societal level. The distribution of many goods—income, education, political participation, control over life and work—also affects the health of populations. The unequal distribution of these goods results in the excess mortality and morbidity previously described above. These descriptions also point out, somewhat graphically in the case of Montgomery County, that the degree of inequality among people and communities is more important than average income. These reported outcomes suggest that income inequality is linked to the distribution of social goods, including but not limited to access to health care and outcomes such as low reading scores and high infant mortality.[9] Income inequality affects health by undermining social cohesion and accounts for 25% of the variance in mortality among U.S. states.[10] Clearly local, state, or national wealth does not ensure well-being.

Hartford and other chronically impoverished communities and Montgomery County and other thriving communities with marginalized neighborhoods across the world struggle to correct the social and economic problems that are decades long. Many of these communities are trying to bridge social capital and build community capacity.

THE STATE OF MATERNAL AND CHILD HEALTH

As previously indicated, despite significant medical advances and improved health status in the United States over the past century, much remains to be done. One key maternal and child health indicator—infant mortality—is still higher than that of many "Western" countries and disproportionately impacts ethnic/racial minority populations. Maternal and child health status in the United States remains well behind that of other industrialized nations and even some Third World countries with the United States' infant mortality rate, ranked 21st. Wide gaps in infant and child mortality, low birth weight and preterm birth, illness and disability, and teen pregnancies occur across racial and ethnic groups, social classes, and geographical/jurisdictional boundaries. For example, in 1997 and 1998, the infant mortality and low birth rates among African American infants was at least twice that of Hispanic, Asian, and/or White infants.[11,12] The rates in American Indian/Alaska Native infants are also significantly higher.[13] Thus, in selected communities across this country, many do not enjoy the same level of health as other Americans. The reported health status indicators for most disenfranchised and minority communities clearly demonstrate that our country has not fully realized the promise of an optimal quality of life for all. Some of this is due in part to our failure to capitalize on the growing body of social and behavioral research that could help in designing appropriate strategies that would improve the public's health and to address public health needs. Clearly, biomedical interventions alone cannot improve the health status of populations. Health is influenced by not only biologic and genetic factors, but by the broader social, political, and economic context.

In light of this growing evidence, there is a need to improve evidence-based practice and promote the health and well-being of individuals, families, and communities by putting in place interventions that not only address "downstream" individual-level phenomena (e.g., physiologic pathways to disease, individual and life-style factors) but also "mainstream factors" (e.g., population-based interventions) and "upstream" societal-level phenomena (e.g., public policies).[14] Although many interventions are in place to address downstream issues, less attention has been given to addressing mainstream and upstream factors. Finally, the nation cannot meet its goal of eliminating health disparities without addressing a broad range of underlying causes.[15]

Thus, the need for effective and boundary-spanning leadership is important to improved health status in communities across the country and world. The Maternal and Child Health (MCH) Community Leadership Institute is designed to assist state MCH directors and the American Public Health Association (APHA) state affiliates to work in partnership with community and civic leaders to achieve the Healthy People 2010 objectives in selected communities across the United States. Through their collaborative work, these professional and community leaders will create sustainable efforts to improve the quality of life for mothers and children in their communities and ultimately nationwide.

THE MATERNAL AND CHILD HEALTH COMMUNITY LEADERSHIP INSTITUTE

Funded by the Colgate Palmolive Company, the Maternal and Child Health Community Leadership Institute offers health officials and advocates the opportunity to look at recent research on the effects of social systems, community context, social capital, and economic inequality and to examine how findings may be applied to change social systems and to enhance the well-being of women and children. The Institute also attempts to expose participants to concepts, models, and tools such as geographic information systems, qualitative mathematic logic, neighborhood indicator systems, community-based public health, measurement of social capital, communication with health policy makers, enhancing diversity, and consideration of the social determinants of health. Using an approach that addresses a community's "social and human capital" and is intersectoral, the Institute trains citizens and communities to become active participants in solving our nation's health problems by diffusing and applying social scientific knowledge.

The Institute is in part a reaction to the ongoing practice in health to approach individuals and communities as beneficiaries, clients, or patients and not as agents of change. It is also a reaction to the current emphasis that programs and training efforts place on data and quantitative measures, a traditional epidemiological approach, to the exclusion of qualitative, sociological, and economic data. Further, in part the Institute is a refocusing on earlier approaches. As a reaction against recent practices, the Institute seeks to help leaders go beyond "lip service" to action as it relates to eliminating racial and ethnic disparities. The Institute is APHA's effort to help leaders and policymakers design and support policies and actions that place a priority on reducing poverty and promoting economic and racial justice and opportunity. It also is a refocus on earlier and ongoing initiatives such as Healthy Start and the underpinnings of public health—equity and fairness. Initiatives like Healthy Start have taught us that community involvement creates positive changes in individual behaviors, enhanced community infrastructure, and new mechanisms of civic participation and accountability.[16]

THE INSTITUTE'S CORE PRINCIPLES

The Institute's core principles are based on the belief that public health must promote the design and implementation of mainstream and upstream interventions. To accomplish this, the focus of health interventions must shift to the health-promoting attributes of the social context. One such attribute is social capital. Communities gain social capital through collaborative social relationships and through increased community empowerment and control. Communities may best achieve social capital though a process called community building.

Social Capital

Social capital builds community strength and well-being. These qualities are often described as social connectedness, social trust, and community identity.

Social capital, then, is trusting cooperative relationships and social interactions. These interactions allow persons and communities to mobilize greater resources and achieve the common good. In poorer and disenfranchised communities, income inequality, social exclusion, and poor networks result in inadequate resources and most importantly lack of access to evidenced-based information and care. (See appendix A.)

In recent publications, Robert Putnam, Professor, Harvard University's Kennedy School of Government summarizes the importance of social capital:[17]

> *Research shows how powerfully social capital, or its absence, affects the well-being of individuals, organizations, and nations. Economic studies show that social capital makes workers more productive, firms more competitive, and nations more prosperous. Psychological research suggests that abundant social capital makes individuals less prone to depression and more inclined to help others. Epidemiological reports show that social capital decreases the rate of suicide, colds, heart attacks, and even infant mortality and improves individuals' ability to fight or recover from illness once they have struck. Sociological studies demonstrate that social capital reduces crime, juvenile delinquency, teenage pregnancy, child abuse, welfare dependency, and drug abuse. From political science we learn that social capital makes government agencies more responsive, efficient, and innovative. From our own personal experience we know that social capital makes navigating life a whole lot easier: friends & family cheer us up when we are down, bring us chicken soup when we're sick ... give us loans when we are broke ....*

Community Building

Efforts such as the Aspen Roundtable make a case for both social capital and community-building. As defined by the Roundtable,[18] *community building* is the process of improving the quality of life in a neighborhood by building capacity in neighborhood institutions, strengthening ties among residents, and developing individual capacities in order to work individually and collectively toward neighborhood change. It may simply mean reprioritizing programmatic strategies not starting a new program. Essential to community building is leadership development and a learning community.

Social Justice

Public health has profound moral and political implications. The pursuit of good health is both an obligation and a right. The ethicist, Norman Daniels,[19] states that fairness and equity are important to heath because maintaining normal functioning contributes to opportunities for all and the fair distribution of goods would eliminate health disparities.

CONCLUSION

The American Public Health Association's effort to train leaders who can build or bridge social capital by helping marginalized communities gain the necessary links to mainstream resources and information is powerful. Given its current depletion, improved social capital can help people to access health and information, design better health care delivery systems, build and improve infrastructure, advance prevention efforts, and address cultural norms that are detrimental to health.[20] An investment in health, like education, is an investment in human capital. Targeted health investments can help to break cycles of poverty and political instability around the world and contribute to national and global economic development.[21] This effort is also consistent with the focus of Healthy People 2010 that encourages:

> ... *local and state leaders to develop community-wide and statewide efforts that promote healthy behaviors, create healthy environments, and increase access to high-quality health care* .... *[G]iven the fact that individual and community health are virtually inseparable, it is critical that both the individual and the community do their parts to increase life expectancy and improve quality of life.*[22]

APPENDIX A: SOCIAL CAPITAL

Social capital refers to the institutions, relationships, and norms that shape the quality and quantity of a society's social interactions. Increasing evidence shows that social cohesion is critical for societies to prosper economically and for development to be sustainable. Social capital is not just the sum of the institutions that underpin a society—it is the glue that holds them together.

Horizontal Associations

A narrow view of social capital regards it as a set of horizontal associations between people, consisting of social networks and associated norms that have an effect on community productivity and well-being. Social networks can increase productivity by reducing the costs of doing business. Social capital facilitates coordination and cooperation.

Vertical and Horizontal Associations

A broader understanding of social capital accounts for both the positive and negative aspects by including vertical as well as horizontal associations between people; social capital also includes behavior within and among organizations, such as firms. This view recognizes that horizontal ties are needed to give communities a sense of identity and common purpose, but also stresses that without "bridging" ties that transcend various social divides (e.g., religion, ethnicity, socioeconomic status), horizontal ties can become a basis for the pursuit of narrow interests. Horizontal ties without bridging ties can actively preclude access to information and material resources that would otherwise be of great assistance to the community (e.g., tips about job vacancies, access to credit).

Enabling Social and Political Environment

The broadest and most encompassing view of social capital includes the social and political environment that shapes social structure and enables norms to develop. This analysis extends the importance of social capital to the most formalized institutional relationships and structures, such as government, the political regime, the rule of law, the court system, and civil and political liberties. This view not only accounts for the virtues and vices of social capital, and the importance of forging ties within and across communities, but also recognizes that the capacity of various social groups to act in their interest depends crucially on the support (or lack thereof) that they receive from the state as well as the private sector. Similarly, the state depends on social stability and widespread popular support. In short, economic and social development thrives when representatives of the state, the corporate sector, and civil society create forums in and through which they can identify and pursue common goals.

Source: http://www.worldbank.org/poverty/scapital/whatsc.htm (3/21/01).

REFERENCES

1. Messias D.K.H. (2001). Globalization, nursing, and Health for All. *Journal of Nursing Scholarship*, 33(1):p. 9.
2. ____. (October 01, 1999). Achievements in Public Health, 1900–1999: Healthier Mothers and Babies. *MMWR Weekly*. 48(38):849–858. [*http://www.cdc.gov/epo/mmwr/preview/mmwrhtml/mm4838a2.htm* 11/18/99]
3. ____. Trends Among Hispanic Children, Youth, and Families. *http://childtrends.org/HomePg.asp*
4. Horon I.L. and Cheng D. (2001). Enhanced surveillance for pregnancy-associated mortality—Maryland, 1993–1998. *JAMA*. 285:1455–1459.
5. Huggins A. (20 March 2001). Homicide: Common cause of death in pregnant women. *Reuters Health Professional Medical News*.
6. Horon I.L. and Cheng D. (2001). Enhanced surveillance for pregnancy-associated mortality—Maryland, 1993–1998. *JAMA*. 285:1455–1459.

7. Frye V. (2001). Examining homicide's contribution to pregnancy-associated deaths. *JAMA*. 285. Commentary.

8. Becker J. (14 March 2001). Montgomery Finds Racial Gap in Child Health Care. *The Washington Post*, pp. B1, B8.

9. Kawachi I., Kennedy B., Lochner K., and Prothrow-Stith D. (1997). Social capital, income inequality, and mortality. *American Journal of Public Health*, 87, pp. 1491–1498.

10. Daniels N., Kennedy B., and Kawachi I. (2000). Justice is good for our health. In symposium with replies to comments. *Boston Review* 25(1):4–19.

11. America's Children 2000. (*http://www.childstats.gov*)

12. *Healthy People 2010*, Volume I and II, U.S. Department of Health and Human Services, January 2000.

13. America's Children 2000. (*http://www.childstats.gov*)

14. Smedley, B.D. and Syme, S.L. (Eds.). (2000). *Promoting Health: Intervention Strategies from Social and Behavioral Research*. Institute of Medicine. Washington, D.C.

15. Levins R. and Awerbuch T.E. Human Ecology and its value for population health papers and populations. *Investigators Awards in Health Policy Research Author Series* (Volume 1 Issue 14.1 April 2000). *http://www.ihhcpar.Rutgers.edu/rwjf/author_series_detail.asp*

16. Thompson M., et al. (June 2000). *Community Involvement in the Federal Healthy Start Program*. (Summary Document). PolicyLink.

17. Putnam R.D. (2000). *Bowling alone: The collapse and revival of American community*. New York: Simon & Schuster.

18. ___. Getting Started: Findings from Comprehensive Community Initiatives Practices. *Voices from the Field. http://www.aspenroundtable.org/voies/32.htm*.

19. Daniels N. Why justice is good for our health. *Investigators Awards in Health Policy Research Author Series* (Volume 1 Issue 15 December 2000) *http://www.ihhcpar.Rutgers.edu/rwjf/author_series_detail.asp*

20. ___. *Social Capital and Health, Nutrition, and Population* (3/14/01). *http://www.worldbank.org/poverty/scapital/health1.htm*

21. ___. Informing the future: *Critical issues in health*. Institute of Medicine, p. 86.

22. U.S. Department of Health and Human Services. *Healthy People 2010* (Conference Edition, in Two Volumes). Washington, DC: January 2000.

A R T I C L E   4

DEMOGRAPHIC FACTORS AFFECTING FERTILITY PATTERNS IN THE UNITED STATES

Stephanie J. Ventura

INTRODUCTION

The size and composition of the American population have been affected by trends in fertility, mortality, and immigration, but the most critical changes in the last half-century have been the result of dramatic swings in fertility patterns. In turn, fertility patterns are shaped by trends in marriage and family formation and the factors that affect them. In this chapter we will review the long-term and recent changes in these key areas and consider how they may affect future population change in the United States. Much of the data presented here is drawn from information collected through the National Vital Statistics System (NVSS), operated by the Centers for Disease Control and Prevention's (CDC) National Center for Health Statistics (NCHS). The NVSS collects data on births (and deaths) through the Vital Statistics Cooperative Program (VSCP). All the states and the District of Columbia as well as the territories furnish data to NCHS based on 100% of the birth certificates filed in their jurisdictions. Detailed technical information on birth certificate data is presented in NCHS reports.[1-3]

FERTILITY RATES

The fertility rate is the key summary measure that describes trends and variations in childbearing. It is defined as the number of births per 1,000 women of reproductive age (women aged 15–44 years). Following wide swings in the U.S. fertility rate from the early part of the twentieth century until the mid-1970s, the rate has changed very little in the last quarter-century (Figure 1 and Table 1). The trends in the fertility rate and the number of births were essentially parallel until the mid-1970s. Then the fertility rate flattened out, while the annual number of births rose fairly steeply, jumping about 1 million (a nearly one-third increase) from the mid-1970s (3.14 million per year) to 1990 (4.16 million).[4] The number of births increased so substantially in large part because of the concomitant increase in the number of women of reproductive age; the "baby-boom" generation (representing women born during 1946–64) accounted for a 23% jump in this population.[5,6]

TABLE 1 SELECTED MEASURES OF CHILDBEARING, UNITED STATES, SELECTED YEARS, 1940–2000

Year	Total Births	Fertility Rate[1]	Marital Birth Rate[2]	Nonmarital Birth Rate[3]	Births by Age % under 20	% 30+
1940	2,559,000	79.9	—	7.1	12.9	28.3
1945	2,858,000	85.9	—	10.1	10.4	32.7
1950	3,632,000	106.2	141.0	14.1	12.0	27.4
1955	4,097,000	118.3	153.7	19.3	12.1	28.7
1960	4,257,850	118.0	156.6	21.6	13.9	26.9
1965	3,760,358	96.3	130.2	23.4	15.9	23.9
1970	3,731,386	87.9	121.1	26.4	17.6	17.7
1975	3,144,198	66.0	92.1	24.5	18.9	16.5
1980	3,612,258	68.4	97.0	29.4	15.6	19.8
1985	3,760,561	66.3	93.3	32.8	12.7	25.0
1990	4,158,212	70.9	93.2	43.8	12.8	30.2
1995	3,899,589	65.6	83.7	45.1	13.2	35.0
2000	4,058,814	67.5	89.3	45.2	11.8	36.4

[1]Live births per 1,000 women aged 15–44 years.
[2]Live births to married women per 1,000 married women aged 15–44 years.
[3]Live births to unmarried women per 1,000 unmarried women aged 15–44 years.

FIGURE 1

Live births and fertility rates: United States 1910–2000

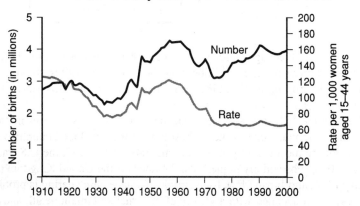

Note: Beginning with 1959, trend lines for rates are based on registered live births; trend lines for 1910–59 are based on live births adjusted for underregistration.

FERTILITY BY AGE

Let's examine the components of the recent changes in fertility, beginning with a summary review of age-specific birth rates (Table 2). Trends in two age groups in particular have captured the attention of researchers, the public, and policymakers over the last quarter-century. These are the rates for teenagers and the rates for women in their thirties and older. Birth rates at the younger ages have generally fallen since the late 1950s, except for a brief upward spike in the late 1980s (Figure 2). The teenage birth rate in 2000, 48.5 births per 1,000 women aged 15–19 years, was about half the peak rate reported for 1957 (96.3).[1,4] Partly as a result of the falling teenage birth rate, the proportion of all births that are to teenagers has fallen in the United States, from a high of 19 percent in 1975 to 12 percent in 2000 (Table 1).

FIGURE 2

Birth rates for teenagers by age of mother: United States 1960–2000

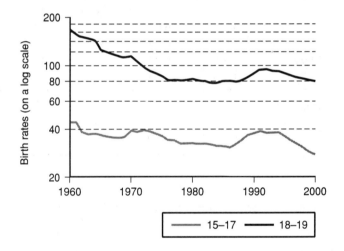

The declines in teenage childbearing since 1991 reflect declines in both first-birth rates and rates of repeat childbearing. Since the mid 1990s, the reductions have been primarily in the first-birth rate. First births account for nearly 80% of births to teenagers.[7]

Although the U.S. teenage birth rate has dropped considerably in the last decade, it still remains one of the highest among the developed countries of the world.[7-9] For the most recent year with comparable data, 1997, the U.S. rate was 52.3 per 1,000, substantially higher than the rates for the United Kingdom (30.2), Norway (12.8), and Japan (4.3), for example. Teenage childbearing is problematic because it is associated with a variety of maternal and infant health and social risks.[7,10] Teenage mothers are less educated, are more likely to be unmarried, have

TABLE 2 Live Births, General Fertility Rates, Birth Rates by Age of Mother, and Total Fertility Rates, by Race and Hispanic Origin of Mother: United States, 2000

Race/Hispanic Origin	Live Births	General Fertility Rate[1]	Age-Specific Birth Rates									Total Fertility Rate[2]
			10–14 Years	15–17 Years	18–19 Years	20–24 Years	25–29 Years	30–34 Years	35–39 Years	40–44 Years	45–49 Years	
Total[3]	4,058,814	67.5	0.9	27.4	79.2	112.3	121.4	94.1	40.4	7.9	0.5	2,130.0
White	3,194,005	66.5	0.6	23.6	72.7	107.9	124.3	97.4	40.7	7.8	0.4	2,113.5
Black	622,598	71.7	2.4	50.4	121.3	144.2	105.3	67.5	32.2	7.2	0.4	2,193.0
American Indian/Alaska Native	41,668	71.4	1.3	39.6	113.1	135.6	106.9	68.3	32.5	7.3	0.4	2,100.5
Asian/Pacific Islander	200,543	70.7	0.3	11.5	37.0	72.0	125.8	120.8	60.4	12.7	0.9	2,072.5
Total Hispanic	815,868	105.9	1.9	60.0	143.6	184.6	170.8	109.0	48.7	11.6	0.6	3,108.0
Mexican	581,915	115.1	2.1	65.0	154.5	197.9	175.4	112.4	50.7	12.2	0.7	3,265.5
Puerto Rican	58,124	84.3	1.9	63.2	143.1	181.3	121.3	74.2	34.1	6.7	0.3	2,584.0
Cuban	13,429	57.3	—*	16.5	42.2	74.2	138.9	84.1	42.0	8.5	—*	1,871.0
Other Hispanic[4]	113,344	94.3	1.3	47.0	118.0	154.5	180.2	117.7	50.2	12.4	0.7	2,969.5
Non-Hispanic White	2,362,968	58.5	0.3	15.8	56.8	89.6	112.8	94.0	39.0	7.2	0.4	1,879.0
Non-Hispanic Black	604,346	73.7	2.5	52.0	125.1	148.6	108.2	69.3	33.0	7.3	0.4	2,256.0

*Figure does not meet standards of reliability of precision; based on fewer than 20 births.

[1]Births per 1,000 women aged 15–44 years in specified group.

[2]Sum of birth rates in 5-year age groups times 5.

[3]Includes other Hispanic origin and non-Hispanics of other races.

[4]Includes births to Central and South American and Other and Unknown Hispanic women

fewer financial resources and more limited social support. Babies born to teenagers are more likely to be low birth weight and preterm, and they are at greater risk of infant morbidity and mortality.[1,11]

Birth rates for women in their twenties are especially important because these women account for such a large share of births. In 2000, for example, 52% of U.S. births were to women aged 20–29 years.[1] During the peak baby-boom year of 1957, birth rates were as high as 261 per 1,000 for women aged 20–24 and 201 per 1,000 for women aged 25–29 years (Figure 3). The rates are now running about half of the peak levels: In 2000, the rates were 112 and 121 per 1,000, respectively, for ages 20–24 and 25–29 years. Birth rates for these age groups have been remarkably stable since the mid to late 1970s.

FIGURE 3

**Birth rates by women aged 20 and older by age of mother:
United States 1960–2000**

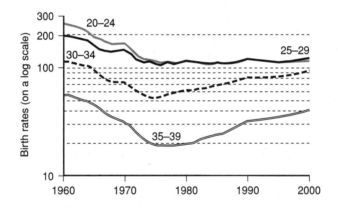

Birth rates for women in their thirties (and older) have been the only rates that have shown sustained and steady increases in the last quarter century and the increases have been quite substantial (Figure 3).[1,12] The current rates, however, are not as high as they were in the 1950s and early 1960s. For example, the birth rate for women aged 30–34 years in 1957 was 119 per 1,000. It dropped steeply over the next two decades, and by 1975, it had fallen by more than half, to 52 per 1,000. Since then the birth rate has risen 80%, reaching 94 per 1,000 in 2000. The trends for women aged 35–39 and 40–44 have been similar. The combination of rising birth rates by age along with tremendous growth in the number of women in these age groups has largely accounted for the steep increase in the proportion of all births that are to women aged 30 and older, which more than doubled from 17% in 1975 to 36% in 2000 (Table 1).

The increases in birth rates for women aged 30 and older over the last quarter-century have reflected principally the sizeable increases in *first- and second-*

order birth rates, a result of the postponement of births from younger reproductive ages. Birth rates for high-order births (for example, fourth- and higher-order births) have generally declined. For example, the birth rate for fourth births to women aged 30–34 years was about three times higher in 1957, the peak baby-boom year, than in 2000. The postponement of first births is considered later in this chapter.

VARIATIONS IN FERTILITY AMONG RACIAL AND ETHNIC POPULATION GROUPS

One of the striking trends in fertility in the last decades of the 20th century has been the narrowing of disparities among racial and ethnic population groups (Figure 4). The gap between the fertility rates of white and black women had widened considerably during the late 1950s before beginning to narrow. With the exception of rates for Hispanic women, fertility rates now vary little by race, rang-

FIGURE 4

Birth rates by race and Hispanic origin: United States 1920–2000

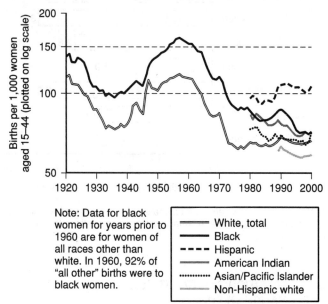

Note: Data for black women for years prior to 1960 are for women of all races other than white. In 1960, 92% of "all other" births were to black women.

White, total
Black
Hispanic
American Indian
Asian/Pacific Islander
Non-Hispanic white

ing in 2000 from 59 to 74 births per 1,000; the rate for Hispanic women was 106.[1] Another way to compare fertility patterns is to examine variations in the total fertility rate (TFR), a measure of lifetime fertility. Estimates of lifetime fertility are based on the total fertility rate, which shows the potential impact of current fertility patterns on completed family size (Figure 5). The current fertility patterns are measured from age-specific birth rates (Table 2). The total fertility rate is computed by summing rates for five-year age groups multipled by 5. The result is divided by 1,000 to yield an estimate of lifetime births per woman. The "replacement" level for the total fertility rate is the level at which a given generation can exactly replace itself; that rate is 2.1 births per woman. Figure 5 shows a wide range in the total fertility rates, from 1.9 births per woman for Cubans to 3.3 births for Mexican women in 2000. Rates are below "replacement" for non-Hispanic white and Cuban women; at replacement for American Indians and Asian or Pacific Islanders; and above replacement for non-Hispanic black, Puerto-Rican, Mexican, and other Hispanic women.

FIGURE 5

Total fertility rates by race and Hispanic origin, 2000

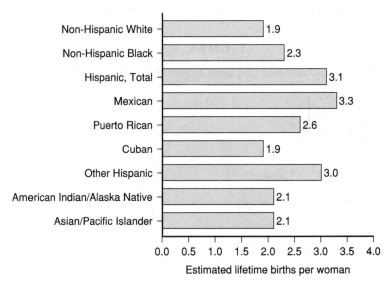

Estimated lifetime births per woman

Note: Total fertility rates are estimates of the number of live births a woman will have if she experiences the age-specific birth rates observed in a given year.

POPULATION COMPOSITION, MARITAL STATUS, AND FAMILY FORMATION SHIFTS

How did the swings in age-specific birth rates affect overall U.S. fertility levels? To answer this question, we must consider changes in the composition of the female population of reproductive age and in marriage and family formation patterns. The overall number of women of childbearing age (defined for this purpose as ages 15–44 years) has increased much more rapidly (by 66%) than the total population (53%) since 1960.[13,14] The number of women in their late teens and twenties rose steeply during the 1960s and 1970s as the "baby-boom" generation (women born in the late 1940s through the early 1960s) came of age. Because fertility rates plummeted in the late 1960s and 1970s, the numbers of women in these key childbearing ages fell by the 1980s and the fertility rates are only recently increasing again, due to the upward spurt in birth rates for all ages in the late 1980s (Figure 6).

FIGURE 6

Number of women by age:
United States 1950–2000, and projections to 2010

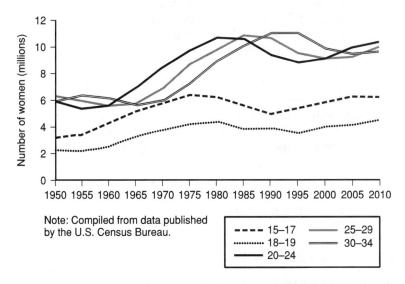

Note: Compiled from data published by the U.S. Census Bureau.

- - - - 15–17
.... 18–19
——— 20–24
——— 25–29
═══ 30–34

Marriage patterns underwent remarkable changes as well. Beginning in the mid-to-late 1960s, women (and men) began postponing marriage. For example, among those women who are aged 20–24, the percentage unmarried more than doubled from 1960 to 2000, rising from 31% to 75%. Increases were even more dramatic for women aged 25–29 years (up from 13% to 45%), and for women aged 30–34 years (rising from 11% to 32%).[15,16] Among men and women in the early childbearing ages, especially, the decline in the married population reflects delays in the timing of first marriage; the proportions of unmarried women who are never-married have soared.[16] Moreover, the marriages that did occur have been less stable, although the steep increases in divorce rates have leveled off in the 1990s.[16–18]

Cohabitation is an increasingly common living arrangement in the United States, growing especially as marriage has been delayed and divorce increased.[16,19] A substantial proportion of nonmarital births in recent years have occurred to cohabiting couples, about 4 in 10 during 1990–94.[20]

A recent analysis of the March 2000 Current Population Survey data showed striking changes in household and family formation and composition over the last three decades.[16] Nonfamily households have become increasingly common, while family households have declined. In particular, the proportion of all households comprised of married couples with children has dropped from 40% in 1970 to 24% in 2000. Married couples without children remained a stable fraction of all households, about 3 in 10. Single-parent households with children accounted for about 16% of households in 2000 compared with 11% in 1970. The growth of single-parent households during the last third of the 20th century is due to the increase in nonmarital childbearing and the rise in divorce.

Family composition has changed as well. Married couples with children accounted for 69% of all families in 2000, down from 87% in 1970. Single-mother families represented 26% of families in 2000, more than double the 1970 level, 12%, while single-father families grew from 1% to 5%.[16]

Recent analyses of data from the Current Population Survey found that the proportion of children living in single-parent households has stabilized or possibly declined since the mid 1990s.[21,22] The percentage of children living in these households remained at 29% during 1996–1999 before declining slightly to 28% in 2000.[21] The stability in this measure may reflect the much slower rate of increase in out-of-wedlock births since the mid-1990s, modest declines in the divorce rate, as well as increases in marriage.[16,23]

During the last three decades, family size has declined, especially reflected in reductions in larger families: In 1990 and 2000, only about 6% of families had four or more children, about one-third the level in 1970, 17%.[16] Trends in marriage rates, delayed childbearing, and out-of-wedlock childbearing have all played a role in these changes in family size. We will review how these trends have affected fertility in the next sections.

DELAYED CHILDBEARING

As would be expected, the tendency to delay marriage has been associated with a tendency to delay childbearing; married women still account for the majority of births (about two-thirds in 2000).[1] In fact, the proportions of women who were childless at ages 25, 30, and 35 years about doubled between 1960 and the mid-1990s, reaching record levels, and have since stabilized (Figure 7).[4,24–26] For example, since 1988, one in five women reaching age 35 was childless, compared with one in ten in the early to mid-1970s.

Because the tendency to delay first births occurred among women who themselves were born during the baby-boom years of 1946 to 1964, the impact of the trend was accentuated, affecting large numbers of women and causing substantial shifts in the age patterns of childbearing in the United States. Women aged 30 and older accounted for 24% of first births in the U.S. in 2000, compared with only 4% in 1970.[1,12]

Since the 1990s, childlessness levels have leveled off. The numbers of women in their thirties have begun to decline and in the next few years, the only sizeable population increases among women in the "older" years of childbearing will be among women in their forties.[27] At the same time the numbers of women in the younger ages of childbearing, which had fallen as a result of the declining birth

FIGURE 7

Percent of childless women aged 25, 30, and 35 years: United States, 1960–2000

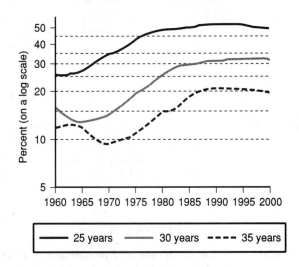

rates, have now begun to increase, because of the upward spurt in fertility at all ages during the late 1980s. Thus, over the next few years, the age distribution of women in the childbearing ages will again shift to younger ages (Figure 6). Although there is no evidence that the ongoing tendency for women to delay marriage and childbearing will reverse, there will be fewer women and thus fewer babies born to women in the older ages.

We can examine the trends in delayed childbearing by using a special series of birth rates, referred to as *cohort fertility rates*.[4,12,25] With these rates, we can look at a refinement of the first-birth rate, which is computed on the basis of women "at risk," that is, women who have not had any children.[12] This measure helps to sort out the two main factors behind the increase in first-birth rates, the change in the proportion of women childless at a given age and the change in the likelihood that a childless woman will give birth. As noted above, the upward trend in the proportion childless has leveled off in the 1990s. In contrast, the first-birth rate for childless women in their early thirties has risen considerably, by a third from 1990 to 2000. Thus essentially all of the increase in first-birth rates among older women in the 1990s is due to the increase in the likelihood that a childless woman will give birth.

One of the fascinating aspects of delayed childbearing is the rapid growth in the number of multiple deliveries to older women during the last two decades of the 20th century. While the numbers are still relatively small overall, the ratio of multiple births for women in the older ages of childbearing have increased tremendously. In 2000, for example, among births to women aged 45 to 54 years, 18.2% were part of a multiple delivery, compared with 2% to 3% for women in their twenties.[1]

BIRTHS TO MARRIED AND UNMARRIED WOMEN

As mentioned earlier, more than two-thirds of U.S. births are to married women. The overall birth rate for married women dropped substantially in the last half of the 20th century, with sustained declines until the mid 1990s (Table 1). Birth rates for married women in their twenties have changed relatively little in the last two decades. In contrast, rates have increased considerably for women 30 and older, although the rates for older women are much lower than for women in their twenties. Moreover, birth rates for married women by age have not increased as rapidly as rates for unmarried women.[23]

One of the striking trends of the late 20th century was the tremendous increase in childbearing among unmarried women (Figure 8).[23] The birth rate for unmarried women in 2000 (45 per 1,000 aged 15–44) was 5 times the rate in 1940 (7 per 1,000) (Table 1). The rate tripled from 1940 to 1960 (22 per 1,000), moderated its increase for the next two decades, reaching 29 in 1980, and then resumed steep increases from 1980 to 1994, when the rate increased 60%, or more than 3% per year.

FIGURE 8

Number of births, birth rate, and percentage of births to unmarried women: United States, 1940–2000

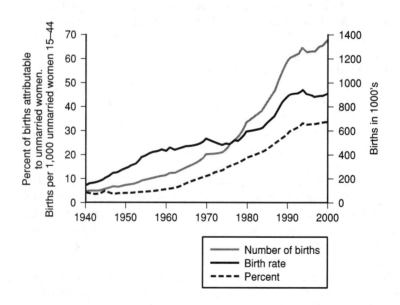

Another critical trend was the explosion in the size of the unmarried female (and male) population of reproductive age. The impact on the baby-boom generation of declining marriage rates was dramatic. A growing proportion of a growing population was delaying marriage, with the result that the number of unmarried women of reproductive age skyrocketed. The total number of unmarried women aged 15–44 years increased 2.5 times from the mid-1960s to 2000.[15,16] The details by age are even more extraordinary. For example, the number of unmarried women aged 25–29 years rose more than fivefold, from 750,000 in 1965 to more than 4 million in 2000. And the number of unmarried women aged 30–34 rose six times, from about 500,000 in 1965 to 3.2 million in 2000.[15,16,23]

These changes in marriage and fertility among married and unmarried women have led to a steep rise in the proportion of all births that are to unmarried women, from 4% in 1940 to 33% in 2000.[6,23] This upward trend was across the board in terms of large increases among women in all age, race, and ethnicity groups. Until the mid-1990s, the proportion of births to unmarried women rose because births and birth rates for unmarried women were increasing while childbearing among married women was declining. More recently, births to married women have begun to increase modestly, but increases in nonmarital births are continuing, so the overall proportion of out-of-wedlock births continues to inch up.

Although differentials in overall fertility by race and ethnicity have narrowed over the last quarter-century, racial disparities persist in rates by marital status. Among married women, rates are highest for Hispanic women (113 per 1,000 in 2000) followed by non-Hispanic white women (85 per 1,000), and black women (70 per 1,000). Among unmarried women, the birth rates were highest for Hispanic women (97 per 1,000), followed by black women (73 per 1,000) and non-Hispanic white women (28 per 1,000).[1,24]

FACTORS CONTRIBUTING TO FERTILITY PATTERNS

Educational Attainment

Many factors contribute to the trends in fertility and family formation. One of the key factors in the last 25 to 30 years has been the increasing educational level of the U.S. population. Education has long been shown to be one of the best measures of socio-economic status to consider in accounting for trends in fertility and fertility-related behavior.[28] The educational attainment of all women in the U.S. population has increased substantially over the last 25 years.[29,30] But the educational level of first-time mothers has continued to exceed that of the general population. For example, among all women aged 30–34 years, the proportion with college degrees increased from 16% in 1975 to 30% in 2000.[29,30] Among women of the same age who gave birth to their first child during those years, the proportion with four years or more of college increased from 40% to 59%.[12,24] Similarly, among all women aged 35–39 years, the proportion with college degrees increased from 12% to 27% in this period, while the comparable proportion among first-time mothers rose from 32% to 56%.

Some of the rise in educational attainment among first-time mothers is clearly related to the general increase in the educational attainment of the population during the last 25 years. But the far higher level of college completion among first-time mothers probably reflects the particular characteristics of those postponing the start of their families as well as a greater increase in first-birth rates among these women than among their lesser educated counterparts. First-birth rates for college educated women aged 30–34 years more than doubled between 1975 and 1994 (the most recent year for which these rates are available), rising from 20 first births per 1,000 women aged 30–34 years with four years or more of college in 1975 to 46 in 1994.[12,31] For women aged 35–39 years, the rate tripled from 5 per 1,000 in 1975 to 16 in 1994. First-birth rates for less educated women in their thirties increased during this period, but their rates are substantially lower than for college-educated women. More evidence of the postponement of childbearing by well-educated women is seen in the first-birth rates for college educated women aged 25–29 years, which changed relatively little during this period.[31,32]

There is some evidence that the upward trend of couples making up for previously postponed childbearing has recently abated. The evidence for this is in several areas. The proportion of women in the older range of the childbearing years who are childless has stabilized in the 1990s (Figure 7). The proportions childless at younger ages have also stopped increasing. The proportions of women reporting impaired fecundity increased across all age groups according to the National Survey of Family Growth, but the percentages seeking treatment did not change.[33] The numbers of women seeking treatment increased because of the growth in the size of the older cohort.

Over the next several years, we should know the extent to which women who have postponed the start of their families will actually make up the births that they have delayed. It is worth noting that about 28% of college-educated women aged 35–44 years in 2000 were childless, compared with about 20% of all women in that age group.[34] This suggests that permanent childlessness may increase. About one in five women who were childless in 1995 indicated that they expect to remain childless. In the next few years, as women born in the first decade of the baby boom reach the end of their reproductive years, we will be able to assess the extent to which women's birth expectations and their actual childbearing were in agreement.

Immigration

Another important factor affecting U.S. fertility patterns throughout the 20th century was immigration. More than 26 million immigrants entered the United States during the period 1901–70.[35] In the last three decades, about 19 million persons have immigrated to the United States. Recent immigrants have hailed mainly from Mexico, Asia, and Latin America. Just released statistics from the U.S. Census Bureau show even more rapid increases in immigration during the 1990s.[36]

Although fertility rates overall have been fairly stable in the United States in recent years, rates have increased among Hispanic and Asian or Pacific Islander populations. Moreover, the rates for some subgroups within these population groups are relatively high. For example, in 2000, the birth rate for Mexican women was 115 per 1,000, and for Puerto Rican women, it was 84, compared with 68 for all groups combined.[1] The combination of higher birth rates and considerable immigration among these groups has resulted in a growing number and proportion of births that are to women who were born outside the 50 states and the District of Columbia. The number increased one-third from 1990 to 2000, and the percentage of all births occurring to immigrants rose from 15.5% to 21.4% during the decade.[1,37] Most of the increase in births since the mid-1990s is due to increasing numbers of births to Hispanic and Asian or Pacific Islander women. Births to non-Hispanic white and black women have declined.

Contraception

The National Survey of Family Growth (NSFG), conducted by CDC/NCHS, collects information on contraceptive use from a representative sample of women of childbearing age. Data for the surveys conducted in 1982, 1988, and 1995 show that use of contraception increased from 56% in 1982 to 64% in 1995.[38] Methods used changed little during these years—the three most prevalent were female sterilization, the contraceptive pill, and the male condom. Pill use has declined in recent years while condom use rose, probably because of concerns about HIV/AIDS and other sexually transmitted diseases. These changes were especially notable among sexually experienced teenagers.[39]

A recent study also based on the NSFG found that unintended pregnancy has declined in the United States since the early 1980s.[40] This decline is probably linked to greater use of contraception and the use of more effective methods. Relatively large proportions of teenagers at especially high risk of unintended pregnancy—that is, teenagers who have already had one child—are using the highly effective new hormonal methods (implants and injectables).[39,41]

Pregnancy and Abortion

Not all pregnancies end in live births. According to the most recent estimates, 63% of pregnancies in 1997 ended in live births, 21% in induced abortions, and 16% in fetal losses (miscarriages or stillbirths).[42] There are considerable differences in pregnancy, birth, and abortion rates by age and by marital status as well as by race and ethnicity. As shown in Figure 9, pregnancy and abortion rates are highest for women aged 20–24 years. The rates in 1997 were 182 and 49 per 1,000, respectively. Abortion rates are also high for women aged 18–19.

Pregnancy rates differ considerably by race and Hispanic origin. In 1997, the rates were 85 per 1,000 for non-Hispanic white women, 151 for non-Hispanic black women, and 156 for Hispanic women (Figure 9). Although overall pregnancy rates for black and Hispanic women are similar, rates by outcome are quite different; birth rates are lower and abortion rates are higher for black than for Hispanic women. Differences in pregnancy rates and outcomes by marital status are also very large: In 1997, the birth rate for married women was about double that for unmarried women, whereas the abortion rate for unmarried women was more than four times the rate for married women.

We have a consistent series of national abortion estimates since 1976. The proportion of pregnancies ending in abortions rose from 24% in 1976 to 26% in

FIGURE 9

Pregnancy and birth rates by age (in years), by race/Hispanic origin, and by marital status: United States, 1997

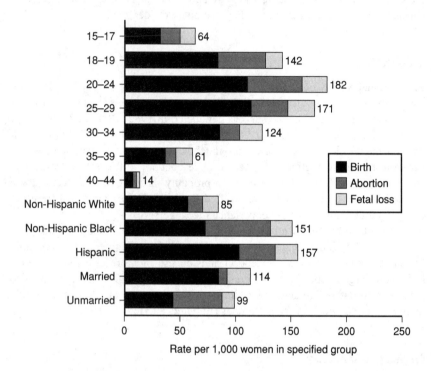

Rate per 1,000 women in specified group

1980 and then stabilized before beginning to decline in the late 1980s.[41,42] The overall abortion rate fell 19% from 1990 to 1997. Rates by age fell steeply for teenagers, by nearly a third, followed by rates for women in their early twenties, down 13%. Abortion rates for women in their late twenties and older have declined much less. The decline in abortion rates is more evidence that unintended pregnancy rates have fallen.[40]

Multiple Deliveries

An emerging trend that has played an important role in recent fertility trends, especially among women in the older reproductive ages, is the upward trend in multiple births, reflecting the role of fertility therapies (drugs and fertility techniques). Although multiple births account for only about 3% of all births, they do comprise larger proportions for older women, as much as one in five births to women aged 45–54 years.[1] A recently created data file now makes it possible to examine the characteristics of women having multiple deliveries. To put it another way, the data file makes it possible to analyze sets of multiple births, in addition to analyzing the routinely available data on individual babies who are part of a multiple delivery.[43]

LOOKING AHEAD

As we consider some of the possible fertility trends in the next few years, several factors should be considered. Based on the increase in births that occurred in the late 1980s, we know that the largest growth in the female population in the childbearing ages will be among women aged 18–29 years.[27] These women accounted for 37% of women aged 15–44 years in 2000, but 60% of the births in that year.[6,14] By 2010, it is projected that they will account for 41% of women in the reproductive ages. Even though the total number of women aged 15–44 is projected to increase less than 1%, the number aged 18–29 will rise by about 13%.[27] If we assume that birth rates by age remain at their 2000 levels throughout the current decade, the number of births could be expected to rise by about 5%, from 4.06 million in 2000 to 4.28 million in 2010. Thus substantial shifts in the number of women in the peak years of childbearing alone will account for a sizeable increase in the number of births, even if birth rates by age remain unchanged. The projected drop in the number of women aged 30 and older is expected to keep the total number of births from increasing more, but these projections could also be conservative, in part because they do not take account of the impact of the growing Hispanic population with accompanying higher fertility levels.[1,36,44]

Births to unmarried women may be expected to rise as well because of the growth of the population in the peak ages of out-of-wedlock childbearing, absent increases in marriage rates.[23] But, nonmarital births may increase more slowly if teenage childbearing continues to decline. Pregnancies and births that occur in the teenage years are much more likely to take place out of wedlock than those to older women. As births are deferred from the teenage years to early or late twenties or even thirties, they will be more likely to occur to married women.

Fundamental changes in behavior and attitudes as well as societal trends may play important roles. For example, birth rates for teenagers have likely been affected by changing attitudes about premarital sex. The large array of public and private initiatives at the federal, state, and local levels have focused teenagers' attention on the importance of pregnancy prevention through abstinence and responsible behavior.[45] Even though large proportions of teenagers are sexually experienced, teenage sexual activity has leveled off according to several national surveys.[39,46] Also important has been the introduction of effective new birth control methods (implant and injectable contraceptives), especially for sexually active teenagers and adult unmarried women. To the extent that young peoples' educational and career aspirations continue to grow, they may be deterred from early and out-of-wedlock childbearing, and encouraged to begin their families when they are ready for the emotional, physical, and economic responsibilities of parenthood.

REFERENCES

1. Martin JA, Hamilton BE, Ventura SJ, Menacker F, Park MM. Births: Final Data for 2000. *National Vital Statistics Reports.* National Center for Health Statistics (NCHS). 2002;50(5).

2. National Center for Health Statistics. Technical Appendix. *Vital Statistics of the United States, 2000. Volume 1, Natality.* Hyattsville, Maryland: National Center for Health Statistics, 2002. Available at: http://www.cdc.gov/nchs/births.htm.

3. National Center for Health Statistics. Technical Appendix. *Vital Statistics of the United States, 1999. Volume 1, Natality.* Hyattsville, Maryland: National Center for Health Statistics, 2001. Available at: http://www.cdc.gov/nchs/births.htm.

4. National Center for Health Statistics. *Vital Statistics of the United States, 1998, Volume I, Natality.* Hyattsville, Maryland: National Center for Health Statistics, 2001. Available in CD-ROM and on the Internet at: http://www.cdc.gov/nchs/datawh/statab/unpubd/natality/natab98.htm.

5. U.S. Bureau of the Census. Preliminary estimates of the population of the United States, by age, sex, and race: 1970 to 1981. *Current Population Reports.* P-25(917). Washington, DC: U.S. Department of Commerce, 1982.

6. Hollmann FW. U.S. population estimates, by age, sex, race, and Hispanic origin: 1980 to 1991. *Current Population Reports.* P-25(1095). Washington, DC: U.S. Bureau of the Census, 1993.

7. Ventura SJ, Mathews TJ, Hamilton BE. Births to Teenagers in the United States, 1940–2000. *National Vital Statistics Reports.* National Center for Health Statistics (NCHS). 2001;49 (10).

8. Singh S, Darroch JE. Adolescent pregnancy and childbearing: Levels and trends in developed countries. *Family Planning Perspectives* 32(1):14-23, 2000.

9. Department of Economic and Social Affairs, Statistical Office, United Nations. Demographic Yearbook, 1998. New York, NY: United Nations, 1998.

10. Maynard R, ed. *Kids Having Kids: Economic costs and social consequences of teen pregnancy.* Washington, DC: The Urban Institute, 1997.

11. Mathews TJ, MacDorman MF, Menacker F. Infant Mortality Statistics from the 1999 Period Linked Birth/Infant Death Data Set. *National Vital Statistics Reports.* National Center for Health Statistics (NCHS). 2002;50(4).

12. Ventura SJ. Trends and Variations in First Births to Older Women, 1970–86. *Vital and Health Statistics* 21(47). Hyattsville, Maryland: National Center for Health Statistics, 1989.

13. U.S. Bureau of the Census. Estimates of the population of the United States, by age, sex, and race: April 1, 1960 to July 1, 1973. *Current Population Reports.* P-25(519). Washington, DC: U.S. Department of Commerce, 1974.

14. U.S. Census Bureau. Unpublished estimates of the July 1, 2000 United States population by age, sex, race, and Hispanic origin. 1990-based estimates. Washington, DC: U.S. Census Bureau.

15. U.S. Bureau of the Census. Marital Status and Family Status: March 1965. *Current Population Reports.* P-20(144). Washington, DC: U.S. Department of

Commerce, 1965.
16. Fields J, Casper L. America's Families and Living Arrangements. *Current Population Reports.* P-20(537). Washington, DC: U.S. Department of Commerce, 2001.
17. Bramlett MD, Mosher WD. First Marriage Dissolution, Divorce, and Remarriage: United States. *Advance Data* 323. Hyattsville, Maryland: National Center for Health Statistics, 2001.
18. Clarke SC. Advance Report of Final Divorce Statistics, 1989 and 1990. *Monthly Vital Statistics Report.* Hyattsville, Maryland: National Center for Health Statistics (NCHS). 43(9, supplement), 1995.
19. Raley RK. Recent Trends and Differentials in Marriage and Cohabitation in the United States. In: Waite L, Bachrach C, Hindin M, Thomson E, and Thornton, eds. *Ties That Bind: Perspectives on Marriage and Cohabitation.* New York, Aldine de Gruyter, 2000.
20. Bumpass L, Lu HH. Trends in Cohabitation and Implications for Children's Family Contexts in the U.S. *Population Studies*; 54, 2000.
21. O'Hare W. The Rise—and Fall?—of Single-Parent Families. *Population Today* 29(5):1,4, July 2001. Additional data available at: http:www.prb.org/pt.
22. Dupree A, Primus W. Declining Share of Children Lived With Single Mothers in the Late 1990s. Washington, DC: Center on Budget and Policy Priorities; 2001.
23. Ventura SJ, Bachrach CA. Nonmarital Childbearing in the United States. 1940–99. *National Vital Statistics Reports*; National Center for Health Statistics (NCHS). 2000; 48(16).
24. National Center for Health Statistics. Unpublished tabulations. 2001.
25. Heuser RL, *Fertility Tables for Birth Cohorts by Color: United States, 1917–73.* DHEW Pub. No. (HRA) 76-1152. Health Resources Administration. Washington, DC: U.S. Government Printing Office, 1976. Available at: http://www.cdc.gov/nchs/data/misc/fertiltbacc.pdf
26. National Center for Health Statistics. *2000 Natality Data Set.* CD-ROM Series 21(14) (SETS 2.0 version). Hyattsville, Maryland: National Center for Health Statistics, 2002.
27. Population Projections Program, Population Division, U.S. Census Bureau. Projections of the Resident Population by 5-Year Age Groups, and Sex with Special Age Categories: Middle Series, 2006 to 2010. Washington, DC: U.S. Department of Commerce. Internet release NP-T3-C. December 1999. Available at: http://www.census.gov/population/www/projections/natdet-D1A.html.
28. Kiser CV, Grabill WH, Campbell AA. *Trends and Variations in Fertility in the United States.* Vital and Health Statistics Monographs, American Public Health Association. Cambridge, MA: Harvard University Press, 1968.
29. Newberger EC, Curry A. Educational Attainment in the United States (Update), March 2000. *Current Population Reports.* P-20(536). Washington, DC: U.S. Department of Commerce, 2000.
30. Waite LJ. Educational Attainment in the United States, March 1975. *Current Population Reports.* P-20(295). Washington, DC: U.S. Government Printing Office, 1976.

31. Mathews TJ, Ventura SJ. Birth and Fertility Rates by Educational Attainment: United States, 1994. *Monthly Vital Statistics Report.* Hyattsville, Maryland: National Center for Health Statistics (NCHS). 45(10, supplement), 1997.

32. Lewis CT, Ventura SJ. Birth and Fertility Rates by Education, 1980 and 1985. *Vital and Health Statistics* 21(49). Hyattsville, Maryland: National Center for Health Statistics, 1990.

33. Chandra A, Stephen EH. Impaired Fertility in the United States: 1982–1995. *Family Planning Perspectives*; 30(1):34–42. 1998.

34. Bachu A, O'Connell M. Fertility of American Women, June 2000. *Current Population Reports.* P-20(543RV). Washington, DC: U.S. Department of Commerce, 2001.

35. U.S. Census Bureau. *Statistical Abstract of the United States, 2000* (120th Edition). Washington, DC: U.S. Department of Commerce, 2000.

36. U.S. Census Bureau. *Census 2000 Supplementary Survey Summary Tables.* Available at: http://factfinder.census.gov.

37. National Center for Health Statistics Advance Report of Final Natality Statistics, 1990. *Monthly Vital Statistics Report.* Hyattsville, Maryland: National Center for Health Statistics. 40(9, supplement), 1993.

38. Piccinino LJ, Mosher WD. Trends in Contraceptive Use in the United States: 1982 to 1995. *Family Planning Perspectives*; 30(1):4–10,46. 1998.

39. Abma JC, Sonenstein F. Sexual Activity and Contraceptive Practices Among Teenagers in the United States, 1988 and 1995. *Vital and Health Statistics* 23(21). Hyattsville, Maryland: National Center for Health Statistics, 2001.

40. Henshaw S. Unintended Pregnancy in the United States. *Family Planning Perspectives*; 30(1):24–29;46. 1998.

41. Ventura SJ, Mosher WD, Curtin SC, Abma JC, Henshaw S. Trends in Pregnancies and Pregnancy Rates by Outcome: Estimates for the United States, 1976-96. *Vital and Health Statistics* 21(56). Hyattsville, Maryland: National Center for Health Statistics, 2000.

42. Ventura SJ, Mosher WD, Curtin SC, Abma JC, Henshaw S. Trends in Pregnancy Rates for the United States, 1976-97: An Update. *National Vital Statistics Reports*; National Center for Health Statistics (NCHS). 2001;49(4).

43. National Center for Health Statistics. 1995–97 *Matched Multiple Birth Data Set.* CD-ROM Series 21 (12) (ASCII version). Hyattsville, Maryland: National Center for Health Statistics, 2000.

44. Mathews TJ, Ventura SJ, Curtin SC, Martin JA. Births of Hispanic Origin, 1989–95. *Monthly Vital Statistics Report.* Hyattsville, Maryland: National Center for Health Statistics. 46(6, supplement), 1998.

45. U.S. Department of Health and Human Services. *National Campaign to Prevent Teen Pregnancy. Mission and Goal.* Available at: http://www.teenpregnancy.org/about/atc.asp (Accessed December 19, 2002).

46. Centers for Disease Control and Prevention. Trends in Sexual Risk Behaviors Among High School Students—United States, 1991–1997. *MMWR* 47(36):749–52, 1998.

ARTICLE 5

THE AMERICAN FAMILY: CHANGES AND CHALLENGES FOR THE 21ST CENTURY

Sandra L. Hofferth

DEMOGRAPHIC CHANGES

During the last third of the 20th century, enormous demographic and economic changes occurred in American families. These include

1. A decline in marriage and an increase in cohabitation
2. Increased marital dissolution due to divorce
3. An increase in nonmarital births
4. Increased incidence of single-parent family structures
5. Increased maternal employment outside the home

Although children's living arrangements have changed, increased parental education, increased earnings, and smaller families have improved the lives of children over the past five years. In addition, changes in attitudes and values towards parenting have meant that children in two-parent families spend increased time with their parents in the late 1990s compared with the time they spent in the early 1980s.

WHAT IS A FAMILY?

A family is a group of two or more persons who are related by birth, marriage, or adoption. A household, on the other hand, consists of all the persons who occupy a housing unit, often defined by sharing cooking facilities or direct access to outside. The housing unit can be a house, an apartment, group of rooms, or a single room, but intended as separate living quarters and can include related and unrelated persons. A single household can contain several families. A family, in contrast, can be scattered over several households. For the most part, data that describe families refer to what are often called "family households," related persons sharing living quarters. In 1999 there were about 104 million households, 71 million family households, and 71 million families.

Families Now and Then

What is the particular past to which we compare today's families? The family of the past is often described as being large, multigenerational, and self-sufficient, with marriage that is universal and young and does not end in divorce. Contrary to this picture of a big, happy family, historians have generally found most families to be small and not extended or self-sufficient. Marriages did not last forever. There were some differences certain, including higher fertility; however, the classical family of Western nostalgia is largely a myth (Goode, 1982).

In this chapter we compare today's families with families created in the 1950s, right after the end of World War II. That was the peak of what we know as the "baby boom," when men and women were marrying and raising children in large numbers and times were good. However, the baby boom ended a unique long-term trend toward increased age at marriage and lower fertility (Cherlin, 1992). Thus many of the trends we describe below continue trends established over the previous 100 years rather than initiate a new direction. It is convenient to compare these numbers to the numbers from the 1950s because that was the most recent peak in family building. In cases in which we have data, we go back further in time.

Marriage

Compared with the 1950s, more men and women now are delaying marriage. In 1955, 11% of females 25–29 had never married. By 1999 the number was 39%. Sixty percent of black females 25–29 had never married by 1992, compared with 29% of white females. Among males 25–29, in 1955 28% had never married. By 1999 that number was 52%. Sixty-five percent of black males had never married, compared with 46% of white males (U.S. Census Bureau, 2000).

Another way to look at marriage is to examine the age at which half of young people have been married. The median age at first marriage was 22 for women and 26.1 for men in 1890. It dropped to 20.1 and 22.5, respectively, in the 1950s and rose again to 24 and 26 in 1990. In the late 1990s, the median age at first marriage continued to rise, to 25 for women and 27 for men (Bianchi & Casper, 2001).

Cohabitation and Union Formation

Cohabitation is becoming a common precursor to marriage. Half of all males and females 25–29 have ever cohabited (U.S. Census Bureau, 2000). Even though they are delaying legal marriage, young men and women are not delaying the formation of coresidential sexual unions. When we sum the proportion who have ever cohabited and who have ever married, rates of first-union formation have declined only slightly. Three-quarters (76%) of women born in 1960–64 had formed a union by age 25, compared with 83% of those born in 1940–44 (Moore, 1995).

Births

Between 1920 and 1935 the total fertility rate dropped dramatically, from about 3.2 children per woman to about 2.2 children per woman. It rose dramatically in the 1950s to 3.6 children per woman, but dropped again to about 1.8 in 1974. Since then it rose to about 2 and then has been stable at that level for the past decade. The number of births has risen because of the increasing number of women of childbearing age born during the baby boom. School enrollments have risen as the large cohort of baby-boom babies have their own children (U.S. Census Bureau, 2001c). The median age at first birth for women was 23.7 years in 1989. Childlessness has risen only slightly; in 1980 10% were expected to be childless; today 19% may be. Most women will eventually bear children.

Out-of-Wedlock Births

The proportion of children born to unmarried mothers has increased, partly as a result of declines in marital fertility. In 1960–64, 8.5% of births to unmarried white women, 42.4% to black women, and 19.2% to Hispanic women were out-of-wedlock. In 1985–89, 22% of first births to white women 15–34 occurred before first marriage. This was 70% for black women and 38% for Hispanic women. In 1998, 33% of all births were to unmarried women (26% of births to unmarried white women, 69% of births to unmarried black women, 42% of births to unmarried Hispanic women) (U.S. Census Bureau, 2000). Marital fertility is lower than nonmarital fertility for blacks. The birth rate per 1,000 unmarried women was 44 for all women, 38 for white, 73 for black, and 95 for Hispanic women. The rate for all women was 64 for white, 71 for black, and 104 for Hispanic women. Out of wedlock fertility rose during the 1980s but has been declining in the late 1990s for all race/ethnic groups.

Childbearing in Cohabiting Unions

About one-quarter of out-of-wedlock births occurs to cohabiting couples. This includes 29% of births to non-Hispanic whites, 18% to blacks, and 40% to Mexican Americans (Moore, 1995). Although children in these relationships may be better off than if they were living with only their mother, the relationships are less stable (Hofferth & Anderson, 2001). Fewer than 40% marry within three years, and rates of divorce are higher for the marriages that result.

Divorce and Remarriage

Divorce is a 20th century phenomenon. Until the 1940s, the most common reason for ending a marriage was the death of one partner. However, following World War II, divorce has increased dramatically as death rates have fallen. The rates rose in the 1960s–1970s and leveled off in the 1980s, declining slightly in the 1990s. Divorce rates are at about 20 per 1,000 married women who are in the age range 15–44. Remarriage rates are higher than first marriage rates, but also have been declining. Even though the numbers have stabilized, today it is estimated that two-thirds of first marriages will end in divorce, more than twice as many as two decades ago (Martin & Bumpass, 1989).

Maternal Employment

A major family change has been a sharp increase in levels of maternal employment (Hofferth & Phillips, 1987). Women are much more likely to be working in the 1980s and 1990s than in previous periods. In the 20th century in the United States, married mothers were traditionally least likely to work. Their labor force participation rose in the 1970s and 1980s, leveling off in the 1990s. Although 40% of married mothers with children under age 18 were in the workforce in 1970, 70% were in the workforce in 1999 (U.S. Census Bureau, 2000). Rates have traditionally been lower for married mothers of children under 6, but they rose as well, from 30% in 1970, to 45% in 1980, to 59% in 1990, and to 62% in 1999. Unmarried mothers were the least likely to work. The availability of public assistance as a source of economic support for unmarried mothers has been cited as the reason for the low levels of employment. In the 1990s, public policies that were implemented to increase work effort and a good economy resulted in large increases in the employment of unmarried mothers. Labor force participation rates rose from 44% in 1980, to 48% in 1990, to 68% in 1999, an increase of 50%. The labor force participation of these mothers is now above the level of married mothers with young children. These trends have led to a record proportion of the mothers of infants in the workforce, 59% in 1998 (U.S. Census Bureau, 2001b).

Attempts to identify the consequences that loss of maternal time may have for children have shown few effects (Hayes, Palmer, & Zaslow, 1990). It may be that the extra income brought into the family offsets the loss of maternal time (Garfinkel & McLanahan, 1986; Furstenberg, Nord, Peterson, & Zill, 1983). However, there is some concern that too early employment of mothers out of the home for many hours when children are infants may be associated with greater emotional problems for children later on, though it may also be associated with greater cognitive development (Han, Waldfogel, & Brooks-Gunn, 2001; NICHD Early Child Care Research Network, 2001). Research has begun to sort out the mechanisms, such as the quality of the home environment (Desai, Chase-Lansdale, & Michael, 1989), child care (NICHD Early Child Care Research Network, 1997), or characteristics of the job (Parcel & Menaghan, 1994), through which maternal employment affects children or subgroups of children.

Earnings of Workers

The real earnings of men who worked full-time, year-round increased during the latter part of the 1990s after declining for the previous decade (Levy, 1998). As a result, households experienced real income increases of from 2% to 3% (U.S. Census Bureau, 2001a). The earnings of females were flat, after having risen through the late 1980s and early 1990s (Spain & Bianchi, 1996). Finally, low unemployment (5.4% in 1996) and low inflation rates characterized the U.S. labor market in the late 1990s (Goodman & Ilg, 1997).

IMPLICATIONS FOR CHILDREN'S FAMILY EXPERIENCE

In 1997, 28% of all children, 22% of white children under 18, 57% of black children, and 31% of Hispanic children in 1996 were living with one parent (Fields, 2001). Although the proportion of children living only with the father has increased over the past decade from 4% to 5%, the great majority were living with the mother. Five percent of white, 31% of black, and 12% of Hispanic children were living with a never-married mother.

As described above, 33% of white, 70% of black, and 41% of Hispanic children are currently born to unmarried mothers (U.S. Census Bureau, 1996). This, plus the experience of divorce, leads to a very high proportion of children—60% according to some estimates—who are expected to spend at least part of their childhood with only one parent (Hernandez, 1993). Although many divorced parents remarry, three in five children in such families spend more than five years with only one parent (Bumpass, 1984). Parental divorce has been identified as a risk factor for school failure, school drop-out, early parenthood, and becoming a female family head (McLanahan, 1985, 1988; McLanahan & Bumpass, 1988). One explanation for this is insufficient economic and social support from absent fathers (Weiss & Willis, 1993; Garfinkel & McLanahan, 1986; Furstenberg et al., 1983). Since having a stepparent does not necessarily increase resources to children up to the level experienced with the natural parent, parental remarriage may also have risks for children (Mclanahan, 1989). On the bright side, new research suggests that many problems experienced by the children of divorce actually existed before the family breakup occurred. Divorce per se may not be the cause of children's problems, but merely a marker for it (Cherlin et al., 1991; NICHD, 1993).

As a result of increased earnings and income, poverty rates declined over the past several years. In 1999, the poverty rate of children was the lowest since 1979, 16.9% (U.S. Census Bureau, 2001a). In 1969 only about 14% of U.S. children lived in families with incomes below the official poverty line. Throughout the 1980s and 1990s the incidence of childhood poverty exceeded 20% and, for blacks, childhood poverty had become more persistent as well (Duncan & Rodgers, 1988). Even though overall poverty rates declined, poverty rates of single mother households were still over 50% in 1999. Other research shows that in spite of the increased employment of women and single mothers, their incomes have not risen (Hofferth, Pleck, Stueve, Bianchi, & Sayer, 2001). Increased poverty reflected the growing number of mother-only families, lower real wages of young adult workers, and falling real benefits in transfer programs such as Aid to Families With Dependent Children (AFDC) and its successor program, Temporary Assistance for Needy Families (TANF). The implementation of public policies reducing access to public assistance and encouraging work, supported by the excellent economy of the 1990s, may have actually contributed to the employment of more single mothers; however, many still experience financial difficulties (Hofferth et al., 2001).

Two other positive trends include higher schooling levels of parents and smaller family size. About one-fifth of mothers had some college in the 1950s, compared with 40% in the 1980s. Under 10% of black mothers and fathers had some college in the 1950s. In the 1980s that percentage had climbed to one out of three black fathers and one out of four black mothers (Hernandez, 1993). These changes suggest that a larger proportion of children are better off today than several decades ago. Fewer than 8% of families whose head had at least some college were poor in 1994. This may be offset by the large number of immigrant children entering U.S. schools. In contrast to the U.S.-born, immigrants often have lower educational levels. They also bring diverse cultural habits and languages. Besides monetary advantages, education also affects the values, knowledge, experience, time allocation, and aspirations that parents bring to childrearing. Consequently, children's educational attainments have consistently been found to be related to those of their parents.

Reduced fertility might influence children and families in a positive way. The number of children born to the average woman has declined substantially. Each woman born after 1945 is expected to bear about two children by the time she completes childbearing (U.S. Census Bureau, 1988). In contrast, the average woman born between 1930 and 1939 had about three children. Children in small families do consistently better academically than those in larger families and it has been argued that this is due to the greater time and resources that can be devoted to the former (Blake, 1989; Polit, 1982; Zajonc & Markus, 1975). Family size is not independent of the other demographic changes. One-parent and working-couple families tend to have fewer children than two-parent one-earner families.

Recent research has found that between 1981 and 1997 children's time spent with their parents increased, in spite of the change in maternal employment and other factors. Although increased education and reduced family size explain some of this, most of the change appears to result from actual changes in parental behavior that could result from shifts in attitudes and values. There was an increase of 6 hours per week of time spent with mothers and 4 hours per week of time spent with fathers between 1981 and 1997 (Sandberg & Hofferth, 2001). It turns out that most of the increase occurred in family time, time both parents and child are together. The only discouraging aspect is that there was no increase in the time of children with their single mothers over the period, and, of course, such children do not have as much access to father time. Consequently, children of single mothers are still disadvantaged.

CONCLUSIONS

In the late 20th century, family change resulted in a large proportion of female-headed families and increased female labor force participation. This change was also accompanied by increased levels of education and reduced family sizes. Because of changes in public assistance policy there was considerable concern that families would be much worse off and, as a result, they would be unable to care for their children. This has not happened. As a result of increased labor force participation of single mothers and the good economy in the late 1990s, families are actually a bit better off than they were. However, single mothers' earnings have not risen and poverty rates are still very high. There is also a positive note in the increased time children are spending with their fathers and mothers. Again, children of single mothers are not benefiting from these changes in parental behavior, both because single mothers' time is constrained and because fathers are less available to nonresidential children.

Finally, there is a record proportion of mothers of young children who are employed outside the home. The well-being of infants of mothers working extensively continues to be of concern to those interested in social policy. The United States is one of the few Western countries that has no national system of paid maternity leave. And public policies have not exempted mothers of infants from work requirements. This issue is likely to be raised in the policy arena in the coming years.

REFERENCES

Bianchi S. M., and Casper L. M. (2001). *American Families*. Washington, DC: Population Reference Bureau.

Blake J. (1989). *Family Size and Achievement*. Berkeley, CA: University of California Press.

Bumpass L. (1984). Children and marital disruption: A replication and update. *Demography, 21*, 71-82.

Cherlin A. (1992). *Marriage, Divorce, Remarriage*. Cambridge, MA: Harvard University Press.

Cherlin A. et al. (1991). Longitudinal Studies of the Effects of Divorce on Children in Great Britain and the United States. *Science, 252*, 1386–1389.

Desai S., Chase-Lansdale P., and Michael R. T. (1989). Mother or Market? Effects of Maternal Employment on the Intellectual Ability of 4-year-old Children. *Demography, 26*(November), 545–562.

Duncan G. J., and Rodgers W. L. (1988). Longitudinal aspects of childhood poverty. *Journal of Marriage and the Family, 50*, 1007–1021.

Fields J. (2001, April). Living Arrangements of Children 1996. *Current Population Reports, P70*(74), 1–16.

Furstenberg F. F., Jr., Nord C., Peterson J., and Zill N. (1983). The life course of children of divorce: Marital disruption and parental contact. *American Sociological Review, 48*, 656–668.

Garfinkel I., and McLanahan S. (1986). *Single Mothers and their Children: A New American Dilemma*. Washington, DC: The Urban Institute.

Goode W. J. (1982). *The Family*. New York: Free Press.

Goodman W. C., and Ilg R. E. (1997). Employment in 1996; Jobs Up, Unemployment Down. *Monthly Labor Review, 120*(February), 3–15.

Han W. J., Waldfogel J., and Brooks-Gunn J. (2001). The Effects of Early Maternal Employment on Later Cognitive and Behavioral Outcomes. *Journal of Marriage and Family, 63*(2), 336–354.

Hayes C., Palmer J., and Zaslow M. (1990). *Who Cares for America's Children? Child Care Policy for the 1990s*. Washington, DC: National Academy Press.

Hernandez D. J. (1993). *America's Children: Resources from Family, Government and the Economy*. New York: Russell Sage.

Hofferth S. L., and Anderson K. (2001, February 9–10). *Biological and Stepfather Investment in Children*. Conference on Measuring Father Involvement. Bethesda, MD.

Hofferth S. L., Pleck J., Stueve J., Bianchi S., and Sayer L. (2001). *The Demography of Fathers: What Fathers Do*. In K. Tamis-Lemonda and N. Cabrera (Eds.), *Handbook of Father Involvement*.

Hofferth S., and Phillips D. (1987). Child care in the United States, 1970–1995. *Journal of Marriage and the Family, 49*, 559–571.

Levy F. (1998). *The New Dollars and Dreams*. New York: Russell Sage Foundation.

Martin T. C., and Bumpass L. L. (1989). Recent trends in marital disruption. *Demography*, 26, 37–51.

McLanahan S. (1985). Family structure and the reproduction of poverty. *American Journal of Sociology, 90*, 873–901.

McLanahan S. (1988). Family structure and dependency: Early transitions to female household headship. *Demography, 25*, 1–16.

McLanahan S. (1989, August). *The Two Faces of Divorce: Women's and Children's Interests*. Paper presented at the American Sociological Association Annual Meeting, San Francisco, CA.

McLanahan S. and Bumpass, L. (1988). Intergenerational Consequences of Family Disruption. *American Journal of Sociology* 94(1): 130–152.

Moore K. A. (1995). Nonmarital Childbearing in the United States. In K. Moore (Ed.), *Report to Congress on Out-of-Wedlock Childbearing* (pp. v–xxii). Washington, DC: U.S. Department of Health and Human Services.

NICHD Early Child Care Research Network. (1997, April). *Mother-child interaction and cognitive outcomes associated with early child care* Symposium presented at Biennial Meeting of the Society for Research in Child Development. Washington, DC.

NICHD Early Child Care Research Network. (2001). *Early Child Care and Children's Development Prior to School Entry*. Paper presented at. Biennial Meeting of the Society for Research in Child Development, Minneapolis, MN.

NICHD. (1993). *Children of Divorce*. Bethesda, MD: Center for Population Research.

Parcel T., and Menaghan E. (1994). *Parents' Jobs and Children's Lives*. New York: Aldine de Gruyter.

Polit D. (1982). *Effects of Family Size: A Critical Review of Literature since 1973.* Washington, DC: American Institutes for Research.

Sandberg J. F., and Hofferth S. L. (2001). Changes in Parental Time with Children. *Demography.*

Spain D., and Bianchi S. (1996). *Balancing Act: Motherhood, Marriage, and Employment among American Women.* New York: Russell Sage Foundation.

U.S. Census Bureau. (1988). Fertility of American Women: June 1987. *Current Population Reports, P-20(427).*

U.S. Census Bureau. (1996). How we're changing. *Current Population Reports, P23(191),* 1-4.

U.S. Census Bureau. (2000). *Service Industries, New Economy's Biggest Generator of Jobs: Mississippi Leads States,* Census Bureau Reports. Available: www.census.gov/epcd/ec97sic (Accessed 7/7/2000).

U.S. Census Bureau. (2001a). *Poverty Rate Lowest in 20 years, Household Income at Record High,* Census Bureau Reports. Available: www.census.gov/press-release/www/2000/cb00-158htn.

U.S. Census Bureau. (2001b). *Record Share of New Mothers in Labor Force,* Census Bureau Reports.Available: www.census.gov/press-release/www/2000/cb00-175htn

U.S. Census Bureau. (2001c). *Children of 'Baby Boomers' and Immigrants Boost School Enrollment to Equal All-Time High,* Census Bureau reports. Available: www.census.gov/press-release/www/2000/cb01-52htn.

Weiss Y., and Willis R. (1993). Transfers among Divorced Couples: Evidence and Interpretation. *Journal of Labor Economics, October,* 629–679.

Zajonc R. B., and Markus G. B. (1975). Birth order and intellectual development. *Psychological Review, 82,* 74–88.

ARTICLE 6

NUTRITION ISSUES FOR MOTHERS, CHILDREN, YOUTH, AND FAMILIES

Jamie Stang and Mary Story

INTRODUCTION

Nutrition is essential for growth, development, health, and well-being throughout the life cycle. Nutrition directly impacts many health conditions such as overweight, hyperlipidemia, hypertension, and bone density, which in turn increase the risk of certain chronic diseases such as cardiovascular disease, stroke, type 2 diabetes, and osteoporosis.[1,2] The nutritional status of mothers, infants, youth, and their families is of exceptional importance, as it serves as a predictive indicator of the health status of the next generation. The sufficiency of energy and nutrient intakes among infants, children, and adolescents is known to affect rates of growth and development, risk for obesity, resistance to infection, and future chronic diseases.[3] Nutritional status of women prior to and during pregnancy directly impacts maternal and infant outcomes, and may impact future risk of chronic diseases among offspring.[4]

The Healthy People 2010: Objectives for Improving Health[1] outlines priority areas of need for public health efforts aimed at improving the health and well-being of women, youth, and families. The first section of this chapter discusses key nutrition-related 2010 health objectives that pertain to pregnant women, children, and adolescents (Table 1). The second section of the chapter summarizes key federal food assistance programs.

PRIORITY NUTRITION CONCERNS

Overweight

Obesity has been named as the single most pervasive public health nutrition problem in the United States.[5] National data suggest that over half of the U.S. adult population and more than 10% of children and adolescents are overweight.[6]

80

TABLE 1 HEALTHY PEOPLE 2010: SELECTED KEY NUTRITION-RELATED OBJECTIVES FOR MOTHERS AND CHILDREN

Objective	Target
Reduce the proportion of adults who are obese.	Reduce to 15% prevalence
Increase the proportion of adults who are at a healthy weight.	Increase to 60% prevalence
Reduce the proportion of children and adolescents who are overweight or obese.	Reduce to 5% prevalence in children aged 6–19 years
Reduce growth retardation among low-income children under age 5.	Reduce to 5% prevalence
Increase the proportion of persons aged 2 and older who consume less than 30% of calories from fat and less than 10% of calories from saturated fat.	Increase to 75% prevalence
Increase the proportion of persons aged 2 and older who consume at least two daily servings of fruit.	Increase to 75% prevalence
Increase the proportion of persons aged 2 and older who consume at least three daily servings of vegetables, with at least one-third of servings being dark green or deep yellow vegetables.	Increase to 50% prevalence
Increase the proportion of persons aged 2 and older who consume at least six daily servings of grain products with at least three servings being whole grains.	Increase to 50% prevalence
Increase the proportion of persons aged 2 and older who met dietary recommendations for calcium.	Increase to 75% prevalence
Reduce iron deficiency among young children and women of childbearing age.	Reduce to 5% prevalence in children aged 1–2 years; to 1% prevalence in children aged 3–4 years; to 7% prevalence in nonpregnant females aged 12–49 years
Reduce anemia among low-income pregnant females in their third trimester.	Reduce to 20% prevalence
Increase the proportion of mothers who breastfeed their babies.	Increase to 75% prevalence in women who breastfeed in the early postpartum period; to 50% prevalence in women who will breastfeed at 6 months; to 16% prevalence in women who will breastfeed at 1 year
Increase the proportion of mothers who achieve recommended weight gain during their pregnancies.	Developmental
Increase the proportion of pregnancies begun with an optimum folic acid level.	Increase to 80% prevalence in women aged 15–44 years who will consume at least 400 μg of folic acid each day; the median red blood cell folate level among women aged 15–44 years will be 220 ng/ml
Increase the proportion of children and adolescents aged 6–19 whose intake of meals and snacks at schools contributes proportionally to good overall dietary quality.	Developmental
Increase food security among U.S. households and in so doing reduce hunger.	Increase to 94% prevalence

Source: U.S. Department of Health and Human Services. Healthy People 2010: Objectives for Improving Health, Volume 2. Washington D.C.: Public Health Service, 2000.

Overweight adults experience increased rates of many acute and chronic health conditions, including hypertension, hyperlipidemia, cardiovascular disease, type 2 diabetes mellitus, gallbladder disease, respiratory disorders, some forms of cancer, gout, and arthritis.[6]

The prevalence of overweight among youth and adults varies considerably by age, gender, and race (Table 2). The most recent data on the prevalence of overweight in the United States are derived from the Third National Health and Examination Survey (NHANES III) 1988–1994 and from NHANES 1999, conducted by the National Center for Health Statistics.[6,7] Among adults, 61% were overweight (Body Mass Index [BMI] > 25, and 20% of men and 25% of women were obese [BMI ≥ 30]).[7] Obesity is particularly prevalent among women of color. Twenty-three percent of non-Hispanic white adult women were obese, whereas 38% of non-Hispanic blacks and 35% of Mexican Americans were overweight.[7] Poverty is also related to overweight in women. In NHANES III, 35% of women with incomes below the poverty level were obese compared with 23% of those with incomes above the poverty level.[1] Obesity is also prevalent among American Indians and is associated with the epidemic of type 2 diabetes.[8]

TABLE 2 PREVALENCE OF OVERWEIGHT AMONG CHILDREN, ADOLESCENTS, AND ADULTS, NHANES III, 1988-1994

	Children (%)			Adolescents (%)	Adults (%)
	2–3 y	4–5 y	6–11 y	12–17 y	> 20 y
Both sexes	3	8	14	12	35
Males	2	5	15	12	33
White, Non-Hispanic	1	3	13	12	34
Black, Non-Hispanic	3	9	15	13	33
Mexican-American	6	1	19	15	36
Females	5	11	13	11	36
White, Non-Hispanic	3	9	12	10	34
Black, Non-Hispanic	6	11	18	16	52
Mexican-American	11	13	16	14	50

*Overweight definition:
- For 2- to-5-year-olds: Weight-for-stature above the 95th percentile of the NCHS reference growth curves.
- For 6- to-17-year-olds: BMI at or above the sex- and age-specific 95th percentile from National Health Examination Survey cycles 2 and 3.
- For adults (> 20 years): BMI > 27.8 for men and > 27.3 for women (85th percentiles from NHANES II for ages 20–29 years).

Adapted from: National Center for Health Statistics. Prevalence of Overweight Among Children, Adolescents and Adults: United States, 1988–1994. MMWR, 1997, 46(9): 199–201.

National Center for Health Statistics. Prevalence of Overweight Among Children and Adolescents: United States, 1999.

http//:www.cdc.gov/nchs.products/pubs/pubd/hestats/overwght99.htm.

In NHANES III, 8% of 4- to 5-year-olds, 11% of children aged 6–11 years, and 11% of adolescents aged 12–17 years were overweight (Table 2).[6] In NHANES 1999, 13% of children between 6 and 11 years old were overweight, while 14% of adolescents were overweight, representing a 2–3% increase over the 5-year period.[7] The prevalence of overweight is particularly high among Mexican-American and American Indian youth and African-American adolescent girls. Overweight during childhood and adolescence has been associated with an increased risk of obesity during adulthood. Data suggest that the risk of adult obesity increases with age among overweight youth.[9–11]

Overweight is a complex condition in which genetic, metabolic, environmental, cultural, and socio-economic factors are involved. Genetic influences largely determine whether a person has the potential to become obese, whereas environmental influences determine the manifestation and extent of the obesity. Overweight occurs as a result of a positive shift in energy balance, when energy intake exceeds energy expenditure. It is not clear why the prevalence of obesity has increased substantially over the past several decades, but low levels of physical activity combined with the consumption of high fat and high sugar foods are likely to be predisposing factors. Results from NHANES III also documented a high prevalence of physical inactivity among adults. Rates of inactivity appear to be greater for women than men and for non-Hispanic blacks and Mexican Americans than non-Hispanic whites.[7] These trends in physical activity correlate highly with rates of obesity within the U.S. adult population. Many children are less physically active than recommended, and physical activity declines during adolescence.[1]

To reverse the trend of increasing rates of overweight in the U.S. population, dual actions are needed in the areas of nutrition and physical activity. Interventions that target specific behaviors such as reducing consumption of foods high in fat and sugar; increasing consumption of fruit, vegetables, and whole grains; reducing portion sizes; and increasing physical activity are crucial to reducing the trend toward increasing rates of obesity. Since overweight disproportionately affects low-income families and people of color, such as African American females, Hispanics, and American Indians, the development of culturally sensitive prevention and intervention programs is essential. The increasing prevalence of overweight among children indicates that prevention activities aimed at encouraging healthy food choices and increased physical activity need to begin during early childhood.

Guidelines on the evaluation and treatment of obesity among children and adolescents recommend that children be screened annually for weight and height status.[12,13] Youth at risk for overweight (BMI between 85th–95th percentile for age and sex) or who are overweight (BMI $\geq$ 95th percentile for age and sex) should be referred for a complete medical examination to determine the presence of obesity-related complications, such as hypertension, hyperlipidemia, or orthopedic disorders. The course of treatment for overweight youth should be determined by age, growth, and development on an individual basis. Family involvement in weight management programs for youth is crucial to the success of the program, since many of the behaviors that predispose youth to becoming overweight are shared by family members and are often modeled by parents.

Inadequate or Excessive Dietary Intakes

Dietary Fat. Current dietary recommendations indicate that all healthy people over the age of 2 should strive to consume no more than 30% of calories from fat, with less than 10% of calories comprised of saturated fat.[1] Diets that are high in fat have been associated with increased risk of obesity, cardiovascular disease, some types of cancer, and gallbladder disease. A strong relationship exists between saturated fat intake, high blood cholesterol, and increased risk for coronary heart disease.[1,2] The current dietary fat recommendations for children over the age of 2 have been criticized because of the possibility of deleterious effects on growth and development. However, large-scale studies of children consuming diets in which from 28% to 30% of calories were derived from fat found that growth, sexual maturation, iron stores, and nutritional adequacy were not affected by the lower level of fat intake.[14,15]

Intakes of total and saturated fats appear to have decreased in recent years. National data indicate that the proportion of calories in the U.S. diet provided by total fat is about 33%, saturated fat is about 11%. The primary sources of saturated fat are meats and dairy products that contain fat.[1] Although improvements have been made for all age groups, intakes of total fat and saturated fatty acids remain above recommended levels for a substantial proportion of the population. For example, one-quarter of children 6–17 years of age meet guidelines for percentage of calories from fat and only 16% meet recommendations for saturated fat intake.[16]

Racial and ethnic differences exist with regard to meeting dietary guidelines for calories from fat. A comparison of changes in dietary intake among children from the CSFII 1998–91 to CSFII 1994–96 found that a significantly higher percentage of white children met guidelines for intakes of total and saturated fats over time, while the proportion of black and Hispanic children meeting the guideline for total fat intake decreased slightly.[16] The proportion of black and Hispanic children who met guidelines for saturated fat intake remained unchanged.

Fruits and Vegetables. Public health recommendations are that people aged 2 and older consume a minimum of two servings of fruits and three servings of vegetables a day. Higher intakes of fruits and vegetables are associated with reduced risk of a variety of cancers.[1,2] Increasing the consumption of fruits and vegetables is also likely to reduce overall fat intake. The most recent national estimates reveal that only 32% of adults and from 10% to 20% of children and adolescents consume five or more servings of fruits and vegetables per day.[16–19]

Fruits tend to be consumed less frequently than vegetables. Current estimates suggest that children consume an average of 2.6 servings of vegetables each day and 1.4 servings of fruit each day, for a total of 4.1 servings of fruit and vegetables each day.[16] Over a three-day period, about 30% of adolescent and adult males and 24% of adult and adolescent females did not eat any fruits, and about 6% of individuals did not eat any vegetables.[2] Moreover, nearly 25% of all vegetables consumed by young people were french fries.

Lower intakes of fruits and vegetables are even more pronounced in low socio-economic groups, where cancer incidence among adults is higher.[2] Although average intake of vegetables has increased overall among youth, the greatest increases have occurred among white and Hispanic youth.[16] Fruit intake has remained largely unchanged among youth during the past decade. Only white youth have shown small increases in fruit intakes.

Future public health campaigns need to promote awareness of the importance of consuming adequate amounts of fruit and vegetables and need to incorporate age-appropriate behavior change strategies. Special efforts and resources should be directed to low-income and minority populations, addressing personal and environmental barriers to healthy eating, such as accessibility, cost, and quality issues.

Calcium. Calcium is essential for the formation and maintenance of bones and teeth. The level of bone mass achieved at skeletal maturity (peak bone mass) is a factor modifying the risk for developing osteoporosis.[1] Achieving peak bone mass appears to be related to adequate calcium intake in adolescence and early adulthood.

Calcium intake varies by gender, age, racial and ethnic background, and household income. Population-based survey data indicate that while 79% of girls and 89% of boys aged 2–8 years met recommended levels of calcium intake, only 19% of girls and 52% of boys aged 9–19 years met calcium recommendations.[1] Less than half (40%) of adult females 25–50 years met recommended intakes of calcium.[1] Comparison data from the CSFII 1988–91 and 1994–94 surveys show that consumption of milk and milk products by children decreased from 2.4 to 2.0 servings per person per day.[16] At the same time, intakes of soft drinks rose from 1.0 to 1.4 servings per day and intakes of fruit drinks rose from 0.5 to 0.8 servings per day, suggesting that these beverages are replacing milk in the diets of American youth.[16]

Low calcium intakes by many adolescents and adults, particularly females, suggest that many Americans are not getting the calcium they need to achieve and maintain optimal bone health and prevent age-related bone loss. In general, white and Hispanic persons are more likely to meet recommended daily intakes of calcium than black persons, and individuals with family incomes at or below 130% of the poverty threshold have lower calcium intake than do individuals from higher income households.[1] Among children, only Hispanic youth did not show significant decreases in numbers of servings of milk/milk products consumed each day.[16] Increases in soft drink consumption were noted most commonly among white children and adolescents, while increases in consumption of fruit drinks were most noticeable among black children and adolescents.

About 75% of calcium in the U.S. food supply comes from milk products. Milk products contain about 300 mg of calcium per serving (for example 8 oz of milk or yogurt or 1.5 oz of cheddar cheese). Other calcium-rich foods include calcium-set tofu, Chinese cabbage, kale, broccoli, lime-processed tortillas, and calcium-fortified foods such as fruit juices, breads, pancakes, and crackers. Calcium supplements may be appropriate for children, adolescents, young adults, and pregnant and lactating women who are unable or unwilling to increase calcium intake through food sources.

The Institute of Medicine[20] dietary reference intakes (DRIs) for calcium have been set at levels associated with maximum retention of body calcium. For several sex-age groups, the recommended calcium intakes are higher than the previous Recommended Dietary Allowances. The DRIs for calcium for youth aged 9–18 years are 1,300 mg/day and for adults 19–50 years are 1,000 mg/day. The DRI for pregnant and lactating women is 1,300 mg/day for women under age 19 and 1,000 mg/day for women older than 19 years.

Given the importance of calcium to bone development, public health efforts are needed to increase awareness about the importance of calcium to lifelong health, recommended intakes (in terms of servings), and food sources of calcium. Culturally appropriate food sources of calcium should be recommended for ethnic and racial minority groups. Educational efforts that also address the increase in soft drinks and fruit beverages that replace milk in the diets of American youth are also needed. High-risk groups, such as adolescent girls, should be the focus of targeted education efforts.

Folic Acid. Birth defects known as neural tube defects (NTDs) affect approximately 2,500 to 3,000 infants born each year in the United States. Clinical trials and case control studies have documented that folic acid can reduce the risk of NTDs.[21] In general, NTDs occur 15 to 28 days after conception, at a time most women are unaware of their pregnancy.[21] Setting an optimal intake of folic acid that promotes health and reduces the risk of NTDs has been a controversial issue in the past decade. Some health professionals worry that setting recommended levels of folate intake at too high a level would mask the rare, but potential, diagnosis of pernicious anemia.[22] But because almost half of pregnancies in the United States are unplanned, it is necessary to recommend that all women who are capable of becoming pregnant consume adequate amounts of folic acid daily in an effort to reduce NTDs. The Daily Reference Intake for folate among females of childbearing age has been set at 400 µg/day, a level thought to offer protection against the occurrence of NTDs in most pregnancies.[23] Intakes of 600 µg/day have been recommended during pregnancy, with 500 µg/day recommended during lactation.

Three complementary strategies to increase intakes of folic acid have been recommended: a) eating more folate-rich foods; b) multivitamin/folic acid supplementation; and c) food fortification. A diet rich in folate can be achieved by increased consumption of green leafy vegetables, citrus fruits, legumes, and fortified grain products, such as pasta, bread, and breakfast cereals. Consumption of fortified foods appears to offer the best dietary strategy, since folic acid, the form of folate used during fortification, is much more bioavailable than naturally occurring forms of folate found in foods.[24] A diet that is rich in folic acid also provides a variety of nutrients and would exert multiple health benefits beyond the prevention of NTDs. Indeed, adequate intakes of folic acid and other B vitamins have been suggested to lower homocysteine levels, thus reducing the risk of car-diovascular disease.[25] However, increasing folate intake by improving dietary intake would require a major change on a population level.

Increased intakes of folic acid can also be achieved with multivitamin supple-mentation (most multivitamin preparations contain 400 µg or more of folic acid). Although women planning a pregnancy may take a folic acid supplement prior to conception, most women of childbearing age do not consume folic acid supple-ments on a regular basis throughout their childbearing years.

The most effective public health strategy to date appears to be fortification of grain products with folic acid. In 1996, the U.S. government authorized food for-tification of all "enriched" grain products with folic acid; compliance with this rule was mandated to occur by 1998. Recent data suggest that the number of chil-dren born with NTDs dropped by 19% as a result of folic acid fortification.[26] According to this study, levels of NTDs occurred at a rate of 37.8/100,000 live births prior to folic acid fortification. This rate dropped to 30.5/100,000 live births after folic acid fortification was mandated. This finding is consistent with nutri-tion surveillance data that have shown increases in serum and red blood cell folate levels since folic acid fortification was mandated. Data from NHANES III (1988–94) and NHANES 1999 show that serum folate levels have increased among women of childbearing age from 6.3 ng/ml to 16.2 ng/ml, while red blood cell folate levels increased from 181 to 315 ng/ml.[27] These findings suggest that the Healthy People 2010 objective for improving folate status among women of childbearing age has been met, a result that has largely been attributed to food fortification.

Iron Deficiency. Iron deficiency is the most prevalent nutritional deficiency dis-order in the United States and worldwide. Iron deficiency refers to a lack of iron that is severe enough to impair the production of red blood cells but not neces-sarily to the extent that health is impaired or that hemoglobin concentration falls below the normal reference range.[1] Iron deficiency can progress to iron deficien-cy anemia, which is associated with health consequences such as impaired ener-gy metabolism, temperature regulation, and immune function. However, the con-sequence of greatest concern for infants and young children is impairment of mental and psychomotor development, which is associated with even mild iron deficiency anemia.[1] Infants and toddlers who are diagnosed with iron deficiency anemia consistently perform less well on tests of mental and motor development than their peers whose body iron stores are replete.[28] Compared to controls, preschoolers and school-age children with iron deficiency scored lower on cog-nitive tests and performed less well on school tests. Iron supplementation led to significantly improved performance on measures of overall intelligence and on tests of specific cognitive processes among iron-deficient children. Another area of great concern is the increased risk of lead poisoning among iron deficient chil-dren, due to increased absorption of lead.[29] Prevention of iron deficiency anemia is a cost-effective method for decreasing the risk of lead poisoning.

Adults with iron deficiency experience increased lactic acid levels and tachy-cardia with exercise, and impaired work performance. Among pregnant women, studies have shown that anemia is associated with prematurity and low birth weight, which are the most common causes of infant morbidity and mortality.[1] Iron deficiency anemia may also be associated with poor maternal weight gain during pregnancy.[28,29]

The most vulnerable populations for iron deficiency include infants and young children, women of childbearing years, and pregnant women.[1,28,29] Among infants and young children, iron needs are primarily based upon growth. Women of childbearing age are at increased risk for iron deficiency because of iron loss in menstruation and dietary intakes of iron that fall below recommended daily requirements. Pregnancy imposes increased iron needs for the growth of the fetus and for expansion of maternal blood volume.

U.S. population-based data on iron deficiency anemia from NHANES III (1988–94) suggest that 9% of children 12–24 months old, 4% of children 36 to 48 months old, and 11% of nonpregnant women of childbearing age were iron-deficient.[28,29] National population survey data on iron deficiency anemia are not available for pregnant women. However, data on low-income women, which are available through the Pregnancy Nutrition Surveillance System (PNSS, 1996), suggest a prevalence of iron deficiency anemia of 29% during the third trimester of pregnancy.[30]

The prevalence of iron deficiency is substantially higher among minority and low-income children. For women between 20–44 years of age, a higher prevalence of iron deficiency anemia is associated with poverty, low educational attainment, black or American Indian/Alaskan Native racial ethnicity, and high parity.[3] The prevalence of iron deficiency among infants and young children has declined over the past two decades. The improvements are attributed to changes in infant feeding practices, specifically, the later introduction of cow's milk, and greater use of iron-fortified formula and cereal.[1,3,29] The incorporation of iron-fortified formula in the WIC food package for infants is believed to have played a major role in the decline of anemia among infants from low-income families. Although substantial progress has been made in preventing iron deficiency anemia among infants and children during the past two decades, the prevalence of iron deficiency anemia among women of childbearing age increased while the prevalence remained unchanged among pregnant women.[1]

The prevention of iron deficiency merits a high priority because of its high prevalence and serious consequences. Prevention programs should be targeted to those populations at greatest risk, such as women and children living in poverty, women and children of color, and recent immigrants. Two approaches can be used to reduce the prevalence of iron deficiency anemia: a population-based approach and an individual-based approach.[29] The population-based approach seeks to lower the population's risk by enriching and fortifying the food supply and by modifying individual food choices through education and dietary change programs. The individual-based approach seeks to identify those at highest risk and provide preventive interventions and treatment. Both approaches are complementary means of achieving lower rates of iron deficiency anemia. A reduction in the prevalence of iron deficiency among infants and young children can be achieved by increasing the proportion of women who breastfeed postpartum, increasing the use of iron-fortified formulas when formulas are used, and delaying the introduction of whole cow milk feedings until 9–12 months.[1] For children and women, dietary iron intakes can be improved by increasing the consumption of iron-rich foods (meat, fish, poultry, iron-fortified cereals). Consuming foods that contain vitamin C (e.g., citrus fruits/juice, strawberries, green pepper, broccoli) during meals increases the absorption of nonmeat sources of iron by maintaining iron in its reduced, more soluble form. Items that inhibit absorption of iron (tea, coffee, whole grains [particularly bran], and dried beans) should be consumed separately from iron-rich foods. For prevention of iron deficiency anemia and protection of maternal iron stores in pregnant women, supplementation with 30 mg of elemental iron per day is recommended for all women during the second and third trimesters of pregnancy.[31]

Adequate Weight Gain and Nutrition during Pregnancy

Nutrition plays a critical role in maternal health, and attention to diet and nutritional status both before and during pregnancy may reduce the risk of adverse pregnancy outcomes. An infant's birth weight is a major determinant of survival potential. Nutrition-related risk factors for low infant birth weight include prepregnancy weight status, gestational weight gain, and iron deficiency anemia.[3] Women who begin pregnancy underweight are at greater risk for the delivery of a low birth weight infant than those who are normal weight or overweight. Inadequate weight gain during pregnancy also increases the risk of low birth weight. A low prepregnancy weight in combination with inadequate gestational weight gain is associated with the highest incidence of low birth weight.[32] About 14% of low-birth-weight births in the United States can be attributed to inadequate gestational weight gain.[3] The National Academy of Sciences[32] has established prenatal weight gain recommendations based on prepregnancy body weight (Table 3). Weight gains at the higher end of the range are recommended for young adolescents and African American women, as both groups are at increased risk for having a low-birth-weight infant. Pregnant adolescents who have not completed physical growth and development may require additional weight gain to accommodate their own growth and development as well as that of the fetus.

During pregnancy, increased energy and nutrients are needed for the growth and maintenance of the fetus, maternal tissues, and the placenta. Therefore, healthy eating practices during pregnancy are important to ensure a healthy outcome for the pregnant women and her developing fetus. Data on the dietary intakes of pregnant women in the United States indicate that mean intakes from food were lower than recommended levels for several key nutrients (folate, calcium, vitamin B_6, iron, zinc, and magnesium).[2] The Dietary Guidelines for Americans are appropriate guidelines to meet the nutrient needs of pregnant women. A recommended daily food guide for pregnancy may include 6–11 servings of grain products, 2–4 servings of fruit, 3–5 servings of vegetables, 2–3 servings of meat or meat alternatives, and 3 or more servings of dairy products. With the exception of iron, the increased nutrient needs of a singleton pregnancy can be met by most women with a nutritionally balanced diet.[32]

TABLE 3 GESTATIONAL WEIGHT GAIN RECOMMENDATIONS BASED ON PREPREGNANCY BMI*

BMI	Weight Gain (lbs)
Low (< 19.8) (underweight)	28–40
Normal (19.8–26.0)	25–35
High (26.1–29.0) (overweight)	15–25
Very High (> 29) (obese)	> 15

*BMI = Body Mass Index (wt/ht²)

Source: Institute of Medicine: Nutrition During Pregnancy: Part I. Weight Gain, Part II. Nutrient Supplements Committee on Nutrition Status During Pregnancy and Lactation, Food, and Nutrition Board, Washington D.C., National Academy Press, 1990.

Breastfeeding Promotion

The policy statement on Breastfeeding and Use of Human Milk from the American Academy of Pediatrics (AAP)[31] summarizes the considerable advances that have occurred in breastfeeding research and set forth principles to guide health care providers in the initiation and maintenance and support of breastfeeding. The AAP statement concludes that "human milk is the preferred feeding for all infants including premature and sick newborns, with rare exceptions." Exceptions to breastfeeding include women with active tuberculosis, those who are HIV positive, women who use illicit drugs, and women who take prescription medications that are contraindicated during lactation. The AAP report further stated, "exclusive breastfeeding is ideal nutrition and sufficient to support optimal growth and development for approximately the first 6 months after birth. It is recommended that breastfeeding continue for at least 12 months and thereafter for as long as mutually desired."[31]

The advantages of breastfeeding range from biochemical, immunologic, enzymatic, and endocrinologic, to psychosocial, developmental, hygienic, and economic.[1] Human milk is uniquely superior for infant feeding and contains the ideal balance of nutrients, enzymes, immunoglobulin, anti-infective and anti-inflammatory substances, hormones, and growth factors to provide physiologic benefits for the newborn infant. Research shows that human milk and breastfeeding of infants provide advantages with regard to general health, growth, and development, while decreasing the risk for a large number of acute and chronic diseases.[31] For example, a longitudinal analysis of infant morbidity and the extent of breast-feeding in the United States found that breastfeeding protects infants against the development of diarrhea and ear infections in a dose-response manner.[31] The more breast milk an infant received in the first six months of life, the less likely that diarrhea or an ear infection developed. Breastfeeding also provides a time of intense maternal-infant interaction. There is emerging evidence that breastfeeding may reduce the risk of overweight among children later in life.[33,34]

Breastfeeding rates declined dramatically from the 1940s to the 1960s, following the introduction of infant formulas. Beginning in the early 1970s, breast-feeding rates steadily increased, reaching a peak in 1982 (62%) and then declining to 52% in 1989.[30] During the 1990s there was resurgence of breastfeeding in the United States. In 1998, 64% of mothers initiated breastfeeding in the early postpartum period, while 29% continued breastfeeding at least to 6 months of age.[1] Rates of breastfeeding at one year were 16% in 1998.

Breastfeeding rates are highest among women who are 35 years of age or older, college educated, live in households with income well above the poverty line, and live in the western states. Among those least likely to breastfeed are women who are low-income, black or Hispanic, with a low level of education, and less than 21 years old. The greatest increases in the initiation and duration of breastfeeding have occurred among groups of women who traditionally have been the least likely to breastfeed. For example, there was a 65% increase in breastfeeding initiation and an 81% increase in breastfeeding rates at 6 months postpartum among African American women between 1988 and 1997.[1]

The increase in breastfeeding seen among less educated and younger women is due in large part to the WIC program[35] which has developed community-based breastfeeding promotion programs for program participants. Continued efforts must be made to encourage more mothers to initiate breastfeeding and to breast-feed longer. A major barrier to meeting the Healthy People 2010 objective for breastfeeding is likely to be the lack of workplaces promoting breastfeeding. Given the large percentage of mothers of young children who work outside the home, efforts to support breastfeeding must focus on work and school policies to provide assistance such as extended maternity leave, part-time employment, provision of facilities for pumping and storing breast milk or breastfeeding, and on-site child care. Finally, there is a need to provide resources (home visits by lactation consultants, breast pumps) and social support (such as peer counseling) for low-income women.

Growth Retardation

Retardation in linear growth in preschool children serves as an indicator of overall health and development, but may especially reflect the adequacy of a child's diet.[1] While inadequate nutrition is generally the first cause considered in growth retardation, other factors include infectious diseases, chronic diseases, or extreme psychosocial stress. Inadequate weight gain during pregnancy and low birth weight may also affect the prevalence of growth retardation among infants. Growth retardation or stunting is defined as height-for-age below the fifth percentile of children in the National Center for Health Statistics' reference population.[3] Given this definition, 5% of healthy children are expected to be below the fifth percentile of height for age due to normal biological variation. A prevalence of more than 5% indicates that on a population level, full growth potential is not being reached.[1]

The CDC Pediatric Nutrition Surveillance System (PedNSS) is designed to monitor the nutritional status of low-income children served by various publicly funded health and nutrition programs, with WIC being the largest program represented. Recent PedNSS data showed that about 10% of children less than 2 years old and almost 6% of 2–5 year olds fell below the fifth percentile in height for age.[36] Rates of growth retardation remain largely unchanged for children less than two years of age over the past decade, while it has decreased significantly for children 2 to 5 years old.[1]

Among black infants less than 12 months old, the prevalence of short stature for age is almost 15%. Black infants have the lowest height for age status at birth; however, by age 2 years, they are, on average, as tall or taller than children of other racial and ethnic groups.[1,37] These findings suggest that the prevalence of short stature among black infants is a result of the increased rates of low birth weight. The prevalence of stunting is highest among Asian and Pacific Islander children between the ages of 2 and 5 years old.[36] Among Asian children, primarily Southeast Asian refugees, there has been a drastic decrease in the prevalence of low height-for-age since the 1980s. This improvement in height suggests a positive change in the nutritional, health, and socio-economic status of Southeast Asian refugee families since their arrival in the United States in the late 1970s and early 1980s.

Even though growth retardation is not a problem for the vast majority of young children in the United States, the consequences of growth stunting and malnutrition are serious. Chronic undernutrition during infancy and early childhood has significant adverse effects on subsequent cognitive development and school performance.[29] Studies have shown that supplementary feeding during pregnancy and during the first two years of postnatal life enhances the development of nutritionally at-risk children and improves cognitive competence as measured 10 years later.[37]

Interventions to reduce growth retardation in children include prevention of low birth weight; better nutrition; improvements in the prevention, diagnosis, and treatment of infectious and chronic diseases; and universal access to fully adequate health services.[1] Special attention should be given to poor and homeless children, and children with disabilities and other special needs. Good nutrition is a first step in ensuring that children reach their full growth potential, both in terms of physical health and cognitive development. Given the importance of adequate nutrition and the higher prevalence of growth retardation among low-income children, health professionals need to advocate for continued funding of the federal child nutrition programs.

Hunger and Food Insecurity

Food security is defined as "access by all people at all times to enough food for an active, healthy life."[38] Households that are considered food insecure are uncertain of having or being able to attain sufficient food to meet the fundamental needs of individuals or families at least some time during a year, due to a lack of resources to obtain food. Households that report food insecurity with *hunger* are homes in which the level of food shortage is so serious that at least one household resident experiences hunger due to the lack of adequate resources to purchase enough food.[38,39] National prevalence estimates of food insecurity and hunger appear to have declined slightly during the past decade. In 1995, it was estimated that 12% of all U.S. households were food insecure (with or without hunger), while in 1999, 10% of households were classified as food insecure.[38,39] Poverty and family income are major determinants of households that experience food insecurity. While 5% of U.S. households with incomes greater than 130% of the poverty line were considered food insecure in 1999, 32% of households with incomes below 130% of the poverty line were food insecure.[39] Interestingly, rates of food insecurity are higher among families living in poverty that receive food stamps (48% of U.S. citizens and 53% of noncitizens) than among low-income families that do not participate in the food stamp program (27% of citizens and 34% of noncitizens). Rates of food insecurity are highest among female-headed households with children, two-parent households with children, black and Hispanic households, and in central city areas.

Hunger is experienced by 3% of all households in the United States.[39] As with food insecurity, poverty is a major determinant of which families experience hunger. In 1999, 11% of households with incomes below 130% of the poverty line reported hunger compared to 1% of households with incomes above 130% of the poverty line. Households headed by noncitizens are slightly more likely to experience hunger than households headed by U.S. citizens.[39] Higher rates of food insecurity and hunger among families headed by noncitizens have been attributed in part to changes in welfare reform.

A recent study[40] investigated associations between family income, food insufficiency, and health among U.S. preschool and school-aged children. Results showed that low-income children had a higher prevalence of poor/fair health status and iron deficiency than high-income children. Food-insufficient children were more likely to have poorer health status and to experience more frequent stomachaches and headaches than food-sufficient children. This research underscores the importance of food security as a critical component of child health policy.[40]

Healthy School Nutrition Environments

School nutrition environments exert a great deal of influence over student's food choices. Students are increasingly faced with a variety of competitive food options as alternatives to meals served though the National School Breakfast and Lunch programs, such as a la carte foods, vending machines, and snack bars. Although meals served through federal child nutrition programs are mandated to comply with the Dietary Guidelines for Americans, these standards are not required of competitive food products. Youth obtain a significant proportion of energy and nutrients through foods purchased and consumed at school. Public health efforts aimed at improving the quality of diets consumed by children and adolescents must therefore include policy changes that improve school nutrition environments.

One of the key areas of concern among public health professionals and school health officials is that of increasing commercial activities within schools. An increasing number of school districts see a la carte or commercial food sales as a means of generating profit that can be used in areas of the school other than the food service operation. A report by the General Accounting Office[41] on commercial activities in schools reported the pervasive presence of such activities as product sales under exclusive contracts. These include soft drink sales; direct advertising on vending machines, scoreboards, textbooks, school buses, and banners and signs placed in prominent places within the school; direct advertising through media companies, such as Channel One that offer free televisions and videocassette recorders to schools that air its news show and advertisements, and ZapMe!, a corporation that offers free computer equipment along with Internet delivery of advertisements; and indirect advertising through corporate sponsored curricula or gifts to schools. These commercial activities largely promote food products that are high in energy, fat, and sugar and of low nutrient density. Such foods do not promote a healthy school nutrition environment.

FOOD ASSISTANCE PROGRAMS

The United States Department of Agriculture (USDA) administers the nations major domestic food-assistance programs. These programs provide a nutritional safety net to people in need and play an important role in reducing food insecurity in U.S. households. Federal outlays for USDA's food-assistance programs totaled $32.9 billion in 1999.[42] The food-assistance programs can be categorized into four general areas: (a) the Food Stamp program; (b) child nutrition programs; (c) WIC program; and (d) food donation programs.

Food Stamp Program

The Food Stamp program was created in 1964 to help low-income households obtain a more nutritious diet by using government issued stamps to purchase foods in the marketplace. Approximately 1 in every 15 Americans (18 million) participated in the Food Stamp program in 2000, at a cost of $15 billion, or $73 per participant.[42] Slightly more than half (55%) of households receiving food stamps in 1999 contained children. Participation in the food stamp program by families with children declined significantly during the 1990s, with larger decreases in program participation seen in urban areas than in rural areas.[42] Despite reductions in participation rates, the Food Stamp program remains the single largest federal food-assistance program.

Child Nutrition Programs

The child nutrition programs were designed to subsidize meals served to children in schools and a variety of other institutions and consist of five programs: the National School Lunch, School Breakfast, Child and Adult Care, Summer Food Service, and Special Milk programs. In the year 2000, $9.5 billion was allocated to federal child nutrition programs.[43] The largest of these programs is the National School Lunch Program (NSLP).

The NSLP was created in 1946 as "a matter of national security" when it was discovered that many young recruits to the armed forces during World War II exhibited signs of nutritional deficiency or poor nutrition. The NSLP operates through federal reimbursements as cash and commodity foods to schools for lunches that meet federally defined meal pattern requirements. In 2001, The NSLP received $5.6 billion of federal funding.[43] Each school day, about 27 million children in 97,000 schools participate in the program. About half of these children receive a free school lunch, while approximately one in 12 receive a reduced-price lunch. A 1993 study of meals served through the NSLP found that youth who participated in the NSLP were twice as likely to consume milk or milk products, almost twice as likely to consume vegetables, and one-and-a-half times as likely to consume fruit or fruit juice at lunch.[44] Participants in the NSLP were also found to consume more total and saturated fat, however. Youth who did not participate in the NSLP were almost three times as likely to consume sweetened beverages, candy and other sweets, sugar, crackers, and high-sodium snack foods.

The findings on increased fat consumption from school meals prompted the USDA to enact legislation that mandated schools participating in the NSLP meet the goals in the Dietary Guidelines for Americans of no more than 30% of calories from fat and no more than 10% of calories from saturated fat. Initial results from several states that have evaluated changes in school lunches as a result of the mandate to meet the Dietary Guidelines for Americans suggest that school lunches now average from 30% to 32% of calories from fat and from 10.5% to 10.8% of calories from saturated fat.[45]

Congress established the School Breakfast program in 1966, to provide funding for breakfast in "poor areas and areas where children had to travel a great distance to school." In 2001, government spending for the program was almost $1.5 billion.[44] Over 7 million children in 72,000 schools participated in the School Breakfast program in 2001.[44] Studies have shown improvements in academic functioning among low-income elementary School Breakfast program participants.

Other child nutrition programs serve children and their families during the early childhood years through childcare centers, during after-school care programs, or during summer months when school meals are not available. In 1998, the USDA authorized the provision of free or reduced price snacks to low-income children who participate in after school care programs;[44] however, data on participation rates in this program are not yet available. The Child and Adult Care Food program received more than $2.5 billion in funding during 2001,[44] serving meals to more than 2.6 million children who were enrolled in childcare programs.

During the summer of 2000, more than 2.1 million low-income children who might otherwise have gone hungry were served meals during summer school vacation under the Summer Food Service program.[44]

WIC Program

The Special Supplemental Food Program for Women, Infants and Children (WIC) is targeted to low-income pregnant or lactating women and infants and children up to age 5 who are certified as having health or nutritional risks. The program was initially created in 1972 and made permanent in 1974. Its main purpose is to supplement diets in specific nutrients by providing milk or cheese, iron-fortified cereal, vitamin C juice, eggs, and peanut butter or dry beans. Iron-fortified formula is provided to infants who are not breastfed. In addition to the specified packet of supplemental foods, the program provides nutrition education.

WIC program costs totaled $3.9 billion in 1999.[46] Since WIC is not an entitlement program, federal funding levels limit participation. In 1999, WIC served 7.3 million participants per month, half of who were children. Almost half of U.S. infants and one-quarter of children between 1 and 4 years old currently participate in the WIC program.[46]

Numerous studies have documented the effects of prenatal WIC participation on increasing newborn birth weight and preventing low birth weight, preventing preterm delivery, and reducing Medicaid costs. A 1990 five-state study found that a savings of $3.13 in Medicaid costs for infants within two months of birth for each $1 spent on the WIC program.[46] A more recent study by the USDA Economic Research Service found that children who participated in WIC increased their intakes of iron by 21% of the RDA, increased intake of vitamin B_6 by 23% of the RDA, and increased their intakes of folic acid by 91% of the RDA.[46] Increases in intakes of vitamins C and A and protein were also found; however, these increases were not statistically significant.

Food Donation Programs

Food donation programs consist of six separate government programs: Food Distribution on Indian Reservations, Emergency Food Assistance, Food Distribution for Charitable Institutions and Summer Camps, Food Donations to Soup Kitchens and Food Banks, Disaster Feeding, and Nutrition for the Elderly. Over the past decade, these programs have been reduced substantially. Modifications in the price stabilization and surplus removal programs have resulted in less surplus food being available for distribution through these programs.

Nutrition and Food Assistance Programs under Welfare Reform

Federal food assistance programs are an important means of assuring that all Americans have access to an adequate, safe, and nutritious food supply at adequate cost. These programs were cut back, however, under the welfare reform law, P.L. 104-193, the Personal Responsibility and Work Opportunity Reconciliation Act (PRWORA) of 1996. Although states assumed authority over many programs, the federal government remained custodian of the food assistance programs. PRWORA changed the basic set of safety-net programs for families with children in fundamental ways that jeopardize the entire safety-net concept.[47]

Changes in the food assistance programs as a result of PRWORA have been noted in federal food assistance programs, most notably among the Food Stamp program. From 1996 to 2000, Food Stamp program expenditures declined by 33%, with average monthly participation rates also falling from 25.5 million to 17.2 million recipients per month.[42] It should be noted that some of the reductions in participation in the Food Stamp program may have resulted from a booming economy in the late 1990s. It is estimated that approximately 35% of the decline in Food Stamp program participation was the result of increased economic opportunity between 1994 and 1998.[42]

IMPROVING NUTRITION FOR THE 21ST CENTURY

While Americans are slowly changing their eating patterns toward more healthful diets, considerable gaps remain between public health recommendations (Healthy People 2010 objectives, the Food Guide Pyramid, and the Dietary Guidelines for Americans) and actual practices. Progress has been made in decreasing intakes of total and saturated fatty acids; however, intakes still remain above recommended levels. Fruit and vegetable consumption has not increased substantially in recent years and remains below recommended levels. Mean calcium intakes from food also have not changed appreciably over the past decade and are below recommended values, particularly for adolescents, and adult females.[2]

In addition to dietary intakes, nutritional status continues to be of public health concern. The prevalence of overweight has increased dramatically over the past few decades among all age groups, but is especially high among low-income women and black and Mexican-American adolescent and adult females. Most of the increase in the prevalence of overweight has occurred among those individuals classified as obese, that is, those who are the most severely overweight. While improvements have been made in decreasing the rates of iron deficiency among infants and young children, prevalence rates have not changed among pregnant women and have increased among nonpregnant women of childbearing age. Progress has also been made in the proportion of women who breastfeed. There has also been a positive change in the prevalence of low-income children who are low height-for-age, especially among Asian children. Progress towards healthier eating practices and nutritional status will depend on improvements for people of color and low-income populations; two subgroups that are at greatest risk for nutrition-related problems and conditions.

The challenge for health professionals is to implement public health programs and policies that protect and promote healthy eating and nutritional health of

Americans. Kumanyika[47] stresses that health professionals need to advocate more aggressively for adherence to dietary recommendations within federal agencies, for example, by ensuring the healthfulness of all foods served within schools and foods distributed to low-income women and children as well as the inclusion of nutrition education in core services provided in publicly funded health clinics. Advocacy efforts are also needed to strengthen in-kind safety-net programs to better meet children's and families needs for adequate food. Health and social service professionals need to advocate that all Americans be guaranteed food security. All American children and families should be ensured an adequate food supply. Programs such as WIC, which has been found to be effective in improving the health and nutritional status of pregnant women and infants, should be guaranteed full funding.

Health professionals also need to help individuals become aware of and implement the dietary guidelines. Providers such as obstetricians, pediatricians, and nurse practitioners can educate women of childbearing age on choosing healthy diets, new mothers about breastfeeding their infants, and children and their parents on healthful food choices to support growth and development. Since many people in low-income and minority communities have limited reading skills or may consider English their second language, targeted educational programs that address cognitive and language barriers are needed in health care and community settings. More evaluative research and demonstrative projects are needed to guide future development of behavior change intervention and prevention programs. A better understanding of barriers to behavior change among high-risk populations is also needed.

Continued work is needed toward the development and implementation of nutrition surveillance and monitoring systems at the local, state, and national levels. Data are currently lacking on the nutritional status of youth with chronic and disabling conditions, youth and women in correctional facilities, families in homeless shelters, children in childcare facilities, and Native American families on reservations. To improve surveillance and research efforts more sensitive dietary assessment methods are needed. An increase in the number of public health nutrition professionals with training in nutrition surveillance techniques and epidemiology is also needed.

If Americans are to meet dietary recommendations, sufficient food choices must be available. Considerable progress has already been achieved by the food industry in increasing the availability of food products with lowered sodium and fat, and these efforts need to be continued. These products, along with quality fruits and vegetables need to be made available to schools and other institutions and low-income families. With food safety issues receiving national attention, ensuring a safe and wholesome food supply will be of high priority.

REFERENCES

1. US Department of Health and Human Services. *Healthy People 2010: Conference Edition, Vol. II.* Washington, DC: US Department of Health and Human Services, 2000.

2. Federation of Associated Societies for Experimental Biology. *Third Report on Nutrition Monitoring in the United States.* Washington, DC: US Government Printing Office, 1995.

3. Wilcox L, Marks JS. *From data to action. CDC's public health surveillance for women, infants and children.* Washington, DC: US Department of Health and Human Services/Public Health Service, Centers for Disease Control and Prevention, 1995.

4. Brown JE, Kahn ES. Maternal nutrition and the outcome of pregnancy. A renaissance in research. *Clin Perinatol* 1997;24:433–49.

5. Centers for Disease Control and Prevention. Achievements in public health, 1900–1999: Safer and healthier foods. *Morb Mortal Wkly Rep* 1999;48:905–912.

6. National Center for Health Statistics. Prevalence of overweight among children, adolescents, and adults: United States, 1988–1994. *Morb Mortal Wkly Rep* 1997:199–201.

7. National Center for Health Statistics. *Prevalence of overweight among children and adolescents: United States, 1999.* http://www.cdc.gov/nchs/products/pubs/pubd/hestats/ovrwght99.htm 1999;Viewed May 6, 2001.

8. Broussard BA, Johnson A, Himes JH, et al. Prevalence of obesity in American Indians and Alaska Natives. *Am J Clin Nutr* 1991;53:1535S–1542S.

9. Garn S, La Velle M. Two-decade follow-up of fatness in early childhood. *Am J Dis Child* 1985; 139:181–185.

10. Rimm I, Rimm A. Association between juvenile onset obesity and severe adult obesity in 73, 532 women. *Am J Public Health* 1996;66:479–481.

11. Guo SS, Roche AF, Chumlea WC, Gardner JD, Siervogel RM. The predictive value of childhood body mass index values for overweight at age 35 y. *Am J Clin Nutr* 1994;59:810–819.

12. Himes J, Dietz W. Guidelines for overweight in adolescent preventive services: Recommendations from an expert committee. *Am J Clin Nutr* 1994;59:307–316.

13. Barlow SE, Dietz WH. Obesity evaluation and treatment: Expert Committee recommendations. The Maternal and Child Health Bureau, Health Resources and Services Administration and the Department of Health and Human Services. *Pediatrics* 1998;102:E29.

14. DISC Collaborative Writing Group. Efficacy and safety of lowering dietary intake of fat and cholesterol in children with elevated low-density lipoprotein cholesterol. The Dietary Intervention Study in Children (DISC). The Writing Group for the DISC Collaborative Research Group. *J Am Med Assoc* 1995;273:1429–35.

15. US Department of Agriculture, US Department of Health and Human Services. *Nutrition and your health: Dietary guidelines for Americans.* 5th ed.

Washington, DC: US Dept. of Agriculture: US Dept. of Health and Human Services, 2000.

16. Gleason P, Suitor C. *Changes in children's diets: 1989–1991 to 1994–1996*, CM-01-CD2. Alexandria, VA: US Department of Agriculture, Food and Nutrition Service, Office of Analysis, Nutrition and Evaluation, 2001.

17. Breslow RA, Subar AF, Patterson BH, Block G. Trends in food intake: The 1987 and 1992 National Health Interview Surveys. *Nutr Cancer* 1997;28:86–92.

18. Krebs-Smith SM, Cook A, Subar AF, Cleveland L, Friday J, Kahle LL. Fruit and vegetable intakes of children and adolescents in the United States. *Arch Pediatr Adolesc Med* 1996;150:81–6.

19. Krebs-Smith SM, Cook A, Subar AF, Cleveland L, Friday J, Kahle LL. Fruit and vegetable intakes, 1989 to 1991: A revised baseline for the Healthy People 2000 objective. *Am J Public Health* 1995;85:1623–9.

20. Institute of Medicine, Food and Nutrition Board, Standing Committee on the Scientific Evaluation of Dietary Reference Intakes. *Dietary reference intakes for calcium, phosphorus, magnesium, vitamin D, and fluoride.* Washington, DC: National Academy Press, 1997.

21. Czeizel AE. Folic acid containing multivitamins and primary prevention of birth defects. In: Bendich A, Deckelbaum RJ, eds. *Preventive nutrition: The comprehensive guide for health professionals.* Totowa, NJ: Humana Press, 1997.

22. Mills JL. Fortification of foods with folic acid: How much is enough? *N Engl J Med* 2000;342:1442–1445.

23. Institute of Medicine, Standing Committee on the Scientific Evaluation of Dietary Reference Intakes, Panel on Folate Other B Vitamins and Choline, Subcommittee on Upper Reference Levels of Nutrients. *Dietary reference intakes for thiamin, riboflavin, niacin, vitamin B6, folate, vitamin B12, pantothenic acid, biotin, and choline: A report.* Washington, D.C.: National Academy Press, 2000.

24. Brown J, Jacobs D, Hartman T, et al. Predictors of red cell folate levels in women attempting pregnancy: Results from the Diana Project. *J Am Med Assoc* 1997;277:548–552.

25. Christen WG, Ajani UA, Glynn RJ, Hennekens CH. Blood levels of homocysteine and increased risks of cardiovascular disease: causal or casual: *Arch Intern Med* 2000;160:422–34.

26. Hyonein MA, Paulozzi LJ, Mathews TJ, Erickson JD, Wong LY. Impact of folic acid fortification of the US food supply on the occurrence of neural tube defects. *J Am Med Assoc* 2001;285:2981–2986.

27. Centers for Disease Control and Prevention. Folate status in women of childbearing age: United States, 1999. *Morb Mortal Wkly Rep* 2000; 49:962–965.

28. Food and Nutrition Board, Institute of Medicine. *Iron deficiency anemia, recommended guidelines for the prevention, detection, and management among US children and women of childbearing age.* Washington, DC: National Academy Press, 1993.

29. US Department of Health and Human Services. *Surgeon General's report on nutrition and health.* US Department of Health and Human Services, Public Health Service, 1988.

30. Centers for Disease Control and Prevention. *Pregnancy nutrition surveillance, 1996 full report.* Atlanta: US Department of Health and Human Services, Centers for Disease Control and Prevention, 1998.

31. American Academy of Pediatrics Work Group on Breastfeeding. Breastfeeding and the use of human milk. *Pediatrics* 1997;100:1035–9.

32. Institute of Medicine, Committee on Nutrition Status During Pregnancy and Lactation. *Nutrition during Pregnancy.* Washington, DC: National Academy Press, 1990.

33. Dietz WH. Breastfeeding may help prevent childhood overweight. *J Am Med Assoc* 2001; 285:2506–2507.

34. Hediger ML, Overpeck MD, Kuczmarski RJ, Ruan WJ. Association between infant breastfeeding and overweight in young children. *J Am Med Assoc* 2001;285:2453–2460.

35. Ryan AS. The resurgence of breastfeeding in the United States. *Pediatrics* 1997;99:E12.

36. Centers for Disease Control and Prevention. *Pediatric nutrition surveillance survey, full report, 1997.* Atlanta, GA: US Department of Health and Human Services, Centers for Disease Control and Prevention, 1999.

37. Task Force on Reconceptualization and Behavioral Development of the International Dietary Energy Consultative Group. A reconceptualization of the effects of undernutrition on children's biological, psychosocial and behavioral development. Social policy report. In: Politt E, ed.: *Society of Research in Child Development*, 1996.

38. US Department of Agriculture, Food and Consumer Services, Office of Analysis and Evaluation. *Household food security in the United States in 1995.* Executive summary. Washington DC: US Department of Agriculture, 1997.

39. Nord M. Food stamp participation and food security. *Food Review* (electronic journal) 2001;24:13–19.

40. Alaimo K, Olson CM, Frongillo EA, Briefel RR. Food insufficiency, family income, and health in US preschool and school-aged children. *AM J Public Health* 2001;91:781–786.

41. US General Accounting Office. *Public education: Commercial activities in schools.* Report to congressional requesters. GAO/HEHS-00-156: US General Accounting Office, 2000.

42. US Department of Agriculture Food and Consumer Services. *Nutrition assistance in the United States: 30 years after the White House conference on food, nutrition, and health.* FNS-318: US Department of Agriculture, 2000.

43. US Department of Agriculture. United States Department of Agriculture Web page.

44. Burghardt J, Gordon A, Chapman N, Gleason P, Fraker T. *The School Nutrition Dietary Assessment Study: School Food Service, Meals Offered, and Dietary Intakes.* October, 1993 ed. Princeton, NJ: Mathematic Policy Research, Inc., 1993.

45. Griffith P, Sackin B, Bierbauer D. *School meals: Benefits and challenges.* National Nutrition Summit. Alexandria, VA: American School Food Service Association, 2000.

46. Oliveira V, Gundersen C. WIC increases the nutrient intake of children. *Food Review* 2001;24:27–30.

47. Kumanyika S. Improving our diet–still a long way to go. *N Engl J Med* 1997;335:738–740.

Article 7

Integrating the Roles of Health Surveillance, Performance Monitoring, and Systems Evaluation

Donna J. Petersen and Greg R. Alexander

INTRODUCTION

Public health, health care, and welfare reform efforts of the 1990s challenged public health agencies to monitor and evaluate the effects of various system-level reforms on populations, families, and in particular children, including children with special health care needs. Although evaluation has long been seen as a critical element to program development and management, state maternal and child health programs have been hindered by the lack of a framework for identifying and using data to assess the effects of these programs, much less for assessing the impact of greater system-level change that is occurring around them. In recognition of similar problems at a more global public health level, recent efforts, such as the Turning Point initiative funded by the Robert Wood Johnson Foundation,[1] and the reconvening of a public health committee by the Institute of Medicine,[2] have tried to galvanize the public health profession and its diverse infrasructure to adapt in an ever-changing world. It is essential that maternal and child health professionals enhance their understanding of evaluation principles—and their application to assessing program performance and monitoring system-level change—if they are to continue to pursue success in their endeavors.

EVALUATION

Evaluation is indispensable to the core assessment and assurance functions of public health. Evaluation should be a component of any public health activity, serving as the objective assessment of whether or not a particular service, intervention, program, or system has succeeded in achieving its aims. By comparing actual accomplishments of an intervention or program to the original expecta-

103

tions, objectives, or a targeted desired state, evaluation also provides feedback for continuously improving operations and performance.[3]

The basic steps in evaluation are inextricably linked to program planning. These steps include: (1) articulating measurable objectives, (2) planning and implementing specific activities to achieve those objectives, and (3) collecting information to determine whether the planned activities were carried out and whether the pre-selected objectives were reached.[3] In public health, needs assessment is typically the initial step in establishing objectives and is a fundamental part of evaluation; current health status and health care utilization indicators are compared against stated objectives or goals.[4] The national Year 2001 health objectives provided for such comparisons and allow public health programs to assess discrepancies between current levels of health status and stated national goals and to plan activities to reduce discrepancies.[5]

Evaluations can be relatively simple or can involve sophisticated and complex designs. The issues involved in the design and conduct of evaluation research have been elegantly described in several outstanding texts and will not be addressed here.[3,6–8] However, it is important to note that in addition to clearly stated and measurable objectives, any good evaluation design also considers both the nature and scope of activities conducted as part of the intervention or program (i.e., process evaluation) and the results of those activities (i.e., outcome evaluation).[3] A good design will also assess the accuracy of the implementation of the program plan (i.e., For an implementation evaluation, did we do what we said we were going to do?). Finally, evaluation should be viewed as an ongoing process that provides feedback on the headway we are making toward attaining our long-term program objectives and goals (i.e., For progress evaluation, are we on course and do we need mid-course corrections?).

PERFORMANCE MONITORING

The importance of evaluating specific interventions has been well understood in public health and other related fields. The federal inclusion of recognized "performance measures" to improve accountability across states for state use of federal grant funds is a recognition that evaluation of broad-based programs is also important. Performance monitoring is rooted in the basic concepts of evaluation, (i.e., assessing progress against stated objectives). Indeed, interest on the part of Congress to understand the results of their legislative and allocation decisions resulted in the passage of the Government Performance and Reporting Act of 1995, which requires each federal agency to establish performance measures that can be reported as part of the budgetary process, thus linking funding decisions with performance. State health agencies together with various federal partners have developed National Public Health Performance Standards in response to this call for accountability.[9] In the guidance material for state Maternal and Child Health (MCH) Block Grant applications, states are directed to list program priorities derived from required needs assessments and to describe their planned efforts to address their identified needs.[10] These plans must specify capacity, process, risk factor, and outcome indicators. States are further required both to develop a set of negotiated performance measures specific to their needs, data capacity, and priorities and to report on a set of outcome measures reflecting overall MCH goals. Finally, states must report annual budgets according to expenditures by specific categories of activity. Reporting progress toward performance measures, reporting budgets according to service categories, and monitoring progress toward national health goals are three mandated levels of accountability for state MCH programs.

As in any evaluation effort, the selection of measurable objectives and the indicators of whether or not they have been achieved is dependent upon the availability of relevant and accurate data. This is also true for performance monitoring. Here we propose some basic criteria for selecting health status indicators as performance measures. Such measures should reflect health conditions for which: (1) the etiology of the disease is fairly well understood, (2) there is a well-established prevention or intervention approach that is cost-effective, affordable, and socially acceptable, and (3) improvement in the indicator can be reasonably anticipated within three to five years. Health status indicators that do not meet these basic criteria for performance monitoring may still be important items for surveillance efforts.

EVALUATION OF SYSTEMS

Although much attention has been placed on service, intervention (process), and program evaluation and performance monitoring, the evaluation of entire systems of care is an important and ongoing area for public health in general and MCH in particular. There are limited examples of attempts to evaluate the impact of systems. Recent efforts to evaluate State Child Health Insurance programs have of necessity considered broader system components in assessing the impact of these programs, not only on insurance coverage of children but on increasing access to comprehensive services and on improving the quality of those services.[11–12] An examination of the impact of the New Jersey Healthy Mothers, Healthy Babies Coalitions, entailed assessing the effectiveness of everything from clinical services, health education, and outreach to community-based coalitions and health professional collaborations.[13] Each of these system-level initiatives contributes to the infrastructure that supports population-based improvements in health outcome indicators. Among the component parts that support achievement of targeted outcome objectives that are essential to systems evaluation are (1) the documentation of those elements of the system components that facilitate successful interventions and (2) the articulation of those interrelationships. Not unexpectedly, the availability of timely, high quality data is also critical for the success of system-level evaluation. A strong monitoring system not only helps assess the level to which desired outcomes were achieved and sustained, it also provides a systems-based data system, providing information on emerging needs, trends, declining needs, and targeted evaluations of specific interventions.

A major barrier to the evaluation of systems is the characterization and measurement of the purpose, attributes, structure, provision, and interactions of the system. In addition to descriptives of the personnel, facilities, range, and availability of services, the following dimensions have been proposed as attributes of primary care systems for children: continuous, coordinated, comprehensive, community-oriented, family-centered, accessible, culturally competent, developmentally appropriate, and accountable.[14–17] As primary care systems for children exist within a larger system of health care that in turn operates within the public health system, attributes of the overall system, the level of development, the interrelationships and the level of coordinated functioning are important added characteristics. Hence, systems evaluation also entails the development of a taxonomy for the characterization of the functioning of the entire health system and the other social systems that exist within a community and state. Platt has proposed the following dimensions for use as a framework for analyzing the functioning of systems: communication, decision-making, boundary-setting, conflict resolution, mutual support, resource distribution, and external relations.[18]

In all, the evaluation of the emergence, reformulation, and impact of systems represents a complex undertaking. The evaluation of the impact of a system can take the form of comparison against stated target objectives, a historical comparison of outputs of a system at two points in time, or comparison of the outputs of two different systems. It is the overall system that is being assessed along various dimensions, but it is important to determine whether or not the system collectively and its component parts individually are to be judged against the stated goals, against past performance, or against another system or system components. Several possibilities exist for designing a system evaluation.

Historical comparisons of health status and health care utilization indicators depend upon the availability and quality of trend data. Pre–post contrasts require knowledge of the factors that may have led to changes in the selected process and outcome measurements, independent of changes in the particular system or system components under study. Because historical comparison studies are among the weakest evaluation designs and are subject to numerous biases that threaten the validity of results,[3] they may be among the least attractive approaches for evaluating systems.

Contemporary comparisons between operating systems represent another possible approach for systems evaluation, although this design may be difficult due to the growing statewide and multistate operations of many health care organizations. Because large and integrated systems possess singularly unique characteristics, the opportunities to compare systems with similar characteristics and service populations may be increasingly limited. A design that monitors progress toward stated goals and objectives may be the most fruitful starting place for system evaluation. As such, *system monitoring* is best undertaken prospectively, given the weaknesses of historical designs.

Rossi and Freeman (1989) define monitoring as "a set of quality assurance activities directed at maximizing a program's conformity with its design."[6] Unlike program evaluation, which seeks to determine whether or not a particular intervention in fact achieved its intended goals, monitoring is broader—it complements and supports program implementation. The function of monitoring is also entirely consistent with public health responsibilities, as it provides the means to continually assess needs and changes in those needs; the availability and accessibility of resources; the short- and long-term products of those resources; and the effects, positive or negative, on health outcomes of interest.

Monitoring is a data-driven effort, dependent upon the timely availability of high-quality data, that directly relate to and reflect the original hypotheses that led to system-level or programmatic interventions. Rossi and Freeman also note that "a few items of data gathered consistently and reliably are generally much better for monitoring purposes than a more comprehensive set of information of doubtful reliability and inconsistent collection ...."[6]

As in any evaluation, monitoring requires the development of clearly articulated objectives, reasonable data collection strategies, and consistent and accurate data reporting. Monitoring within a systems context encompasses the basic notion of a system: a set of component parts that regularly communicate and interrelate toward a common purpose or shared goal. Articulating these goals and the objectives that flow from them, identifying and defining the component parts, explicating the communication pathways among the parts, and placing the overall system in its appropriate context are all necessary to ensure successful and useful monitoring.

As illustrated in the classic model described by Donabedian (1980), the overall system, and to some degree each of the entities within it, consists of components that can be categorized into four domains: inputs, processes, outputs, and outcomes.[19] For purposes of developing and establishing a system for monitoring the system, the elements of each of these domains must be clearly explicated so that indicators and data measurement strategies can be devised for each activity. The general model has been described as follows.

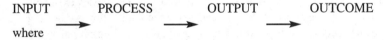

INPUT   PROCESS   OUTPUT   OUTCOME

where

- INPUT = legislative authority, budget authority, staff, equipment, supplies, information and data systems, community support

- PROCESS = data collection, research, analysis, problem or needs assessment, planning and policy development, methods development, standard setting, program development and coordination, grant-making, or contract awards

- OUTPUT = service delivery, training, technical assistance, demonstrations, guidelines, knowledge and skill building, coalitions

- OUTCOME = access to services, improved utilization, improved quality of life, lower mortality/morbidity, improved health status

Health Status Surveillance

Monitoring and surveillance are fundamental functions of public health and have become well-established tools to support health promotion, disease prevention, and epidemiological research efforts, in addition to being important to program planning, implementation, evaluation, and advocacy. These activities provide the means to assure that health status is maintained or improved within populations and communities; that emerging health problems are identified early; that necessary health and related services are available, accessible, and of high quality; and that expenditures are justified by documented results in the form of process, output, and outcome objectives achieved.[20] The basic elements of monitoring and surveillance include the *ongoing* and *systematic* steps: (1) collection of data; (2) evaluation, consolidation, analysis, and interpretation of data; and (3) prompt dissemination of the synthesized results to the public, relevant stakeholders, and decision/policymakers.[20,21]

Although public health surveillance has traditionally been used in efforts to control infectious disease, there has been growing appreciation of its use for the broad domains of public health: describing and measuring shifts in population demographic structures and dynamics, health systems, and in a broad array of health outcomes.[21] This larger view of public health surveillance encompasses an expanded conceptualization of public health as extending beyond just disease occurrence and risk exposure to include population characteristics and the "services, resources and policies that constitute the organized social response to health conditions."[21] A broad-based model for public health monitoring and surveillance should describe not only health status and individual and family predictors of health outcomes but also characteristics of the broader health system and patterns of health care utilization. In some instances, data bases exist to provide insights into these areas; in others, traditional data collection methods such as surveys are needed; while in still others, qualitative and empirical methods should also be explored for studying the overall status of health and the health system.

Ironically, public health has an immensely rich supply of vital record and other population-based data on births, deaths, immunizations, newborn screening, and communicable diseases, amidst a persistent dearth of information on many other important aspects of family life and child development. Despite decades of efforts to develop stronger, more comprehensive data systems, we continue to mainly rely on existing data bases, patching together weak assemblages of program management data created for the administration of public health service programs. Obviously, the time and expense involved in developing and implementing reliable and valid survey instruments is the limiting factor for states embarking on systematic and ongoing surveillance efforts. Few, if any, states are fortunate in having available population-wide surveillance systems that provide the breadth of data needed to fully assess health status within the state. This continues in spite of numerous efforts to focus attention on this blind spot in our nation's focus on health. In regard to child health surveillance, Dr. Mary Grace Kovar made the following and still relevant observation nearly a quarter of a century ago: "A great deal of data has been gathered, but there has not been a research plan or a coordinated plan to direct what was being collected and why. As a result, there are gaps and missing pieces; data have not been tabulated to investigate a set of hypotheses; information is not presented in a unified body of knowledge so that the public, the legislature, and the administrative bodies can use it."[22]

CASE EXAMPLES

In Arizona and Minnesota, efforts to develop statewide surveillance systems to monitor the health status of children were undertaken during the era of reform in the 1990s. In 1995, the Arizona MCH developed a model of child health surveillance (see Figure 1) that articulated four domains: "child health status," "health care utilization," "the health care system," and "population/contextual factors."[23] Using this model a variety of potential indicators were identified that could be drawn from available databases.

Figure 1

Public health surveillance system model

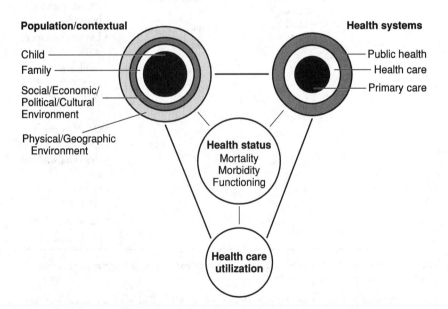

In 1996, following several years of state- and market-driven health care reforms, the Minnesota Department of Health envisioned a dynamic monitoring system to strengthen its capacity in the surveillance.[24] Using the "Arizona Model," a group of experts developed a set of indicators within the four domains and these are listed in Table 1. The potential uses and interpretations of these data for needs

TABLE 1 PROPOSED CHILD HEALTH INDICATORS FOR EVALUATION, PERFORMANCE MONITORING, AND SURVEILLANCE IN THE STATE OF MINNESOTA

Health Status	Health Utilization	Health Systems	Population Context
• Mortality rates	• Immunizations	• Health insurance coverage	• Children in poverty
• Incidence of communicable diseases	• Barriers to utilization	• Type and number of pediatric providers available	• Children in special ed
• Mental health	• ER visits		• School drop-out rate
• Youth risk behavior	• School screening	• Type and number of specialty providers available	• Adolescent arrest rate
• Adolescent pregnancy	• Well-child visits		• Community violence
• Low birth weight	• EPSDT	• Type and number of support services available	• Pre-1970 housing units
• Confirmed cases of child abuse and neglect	• School clinic use	• Perceived availability of care	• Housing % of income
• Incidence of injuries	• Mental health service use	• Denials of service	• Urgent care facilities
• Nutritional deficiency	• Specialty services used by children with special health care needs	• Uncompensated care	• Public libraries, books
	• Community resources used by children with special health care needs	• Out-of-pocket expenditures	• Law enforcement level
			• Adult CE programs
			• Youth vocational ed
			• Open/green spaces
			• Bike and walking paths
			• Voting in elections
			• Alcohol outlets
			• Food shelf use

Note: EPSDT = Early and Periodic Screening, Diagnosis, and Treatment Program (a part of the federal Medicaid program)

Source: Petersen, Donna J. Monitoring the Health of Minnesota's Children and Families in an Era of Reform: The Minnesota MCH Indicators Project, under contract from the Minnesota Department of Health, June 1997.

assessment and systems development include, but are not limited to: (1) documenting various factors related to the child, the family, the community and the environment that individually or collectively impact health status, regardless of health care utilization or system factors; (2) documenting various health care system factors that affect utilization; (3) documenting various utilization measures that affect health status and that also impact the health system itself; (4) monitoring trends in indicators of interest over time and across geographic areas; (5) providing preliminary evidence regarding the potential impact of various program interventions operating currently or in the future; (6) advocating for needed policy initiatives as indicated and supported by these data; (7) advocating for program initiatives across various sectors, both public and private; and, (8) supporting the public health role in fostering accountability across the health system for health outcomes and health service availability and quality.[24]

Welfare reform efforts have spawned another wave of systems evaluation efforts in that the goals of reducing welfare rolls and increasing employment among former welfare recipients must not be achieved at the expense of declines in the well-being of children. Like health care, welfare systems are complex and interact with other complex systems, including mental health, education, childcare, and justice. Again, accountability is being shifted from individuals to systems requiring the development of parallel data structures that allow for the analysis of these complex interactions.[25]

CONCLUSIONS

Given the growing emphasis on needs assessment and health status monitoring as essential components of public health practice and on performance measurement as a way to ensure system- and unit-level accountability, it is critical that public health professionals become well versed in the design and implementation of health status and performance monitoring and surveillance systems. Evaluation has long been considered an essential component of good program planning and should be built into any program development and implementation effort, but the ongoing systemic changes in welfare, public health, and health care systems suggest an equally critical need for broad-based performance and health status monitoring and surveillance strategies. These efforts are needed to support the continuation within the evolving greater U.S. health system of a population-based public health approach and to enhance the ability of public health programs to be accountable for their overall performance. Indeed, a strengthened capacity in the area of public health performance and health status monitoring and surveillance, as well as further emphasis on program and system evaluation, is fundamental to assure the vitality of the health care system and the optimal health status of populations.

ACKNOWLEDGEMENT

This work was supported in part by DHHS, HRSA, MCHB grant 5T78MC00004-06.

REFERENCES

1. Robert Wood Johnson Foundation. *Turning Point: Advancing Community Public Health Systems*, www.turningpointprogram.org, January 2001.

2. Institute of Medicine. *Assuring the Health of the Public in the 21st Century.* Washington, D.C. www.iom.edu, June 2001.

3. Isaac S, Michael WB. *Handbook in Research and Evaluation.* EdITS, San Diego, 1990.

4. Petersen, DJ and GR Alexander. *Needs Assessment in Public Health: A Practical Guide for Students and Professionals.* Kluwer Academic/Plenum Publishers, New York, 2001.

5. US Department of Health and Human Services. *Healthy People 2001: Understanding and improving health*, 2nd ed. Washington, D.C. US Government Printing Office, November 2000.

6. Rossi PH, Freeman HE. *Evaluation: A systematic approach.* Sage Publications, Newbury Park, 1993.

7. Shadish WR, Cook TD, Leviton LC. *Foundations of program evaluation.* Sage Publications, Newbury Park, 1991.

8. Weiss CH. *Evaluation research.* Prentice Hall, Englewood Cliffs, NJ, 1972.

9. Centers for Disease Control and Prevention. *National Public Health Performance Standards Program*, www.phppo.cdc.gov/nphpsp/, July 2001.

10. *Maternal and Child Health Services Block Grant Application Guidance*, issued August 2001, Maternal and Child Health Bureau, Health Resources and Services Administration, US DHHS, Rockville, Maryland.

11. Starfield, B. Evaluating the State Children's Health Insurance Program: Critical considerations. *Annu Rev Public Health* 2000 21:569–85.

12. Shi, L, Oliver, TR and Huang, V. The Children's Health Insurance Program: Expanding the framework to evaluate state goals and performance. *Milbank Q* 2000 78(3):403–46, 340–1.

13. Petersen, Donna J. with L. Klerman and N. Eisen. *Developing a Strategy for Monitoring New Jersey's Perinatal System*, Health Systems Research, Inc. under contract with the Maternal and Child Health Bureau, HRSA, USDHHS, for the New Jersey Department of Health, November 1997.

14. Grason H, Wigton A. *Review of the Literature and Measurement Strategies Related to Key Principles in the Development of Systems of Care for Children and Youth.* Child and Adolescent Health Policy Center, The Johns Hopkins University, Baltimore, MD, 1995.

15. *Primary Health Care for Children and Adolescents: Definitions and Attributes. Maternal and Child Health Bureau*, HRSA, US PHS, DHHS, Rockville, MD, 1994.

16. Starfield B. *Primary Care: Concept, Evaluation and Policy.* Oxford University Press, New York, 1992.

17. Johansen AS, Starfield B, Harlow J. *Analysis of the Concept of Primary Care for Children and Adolescents: A Policy Research Brief.* Child and Adolescent Health Policy Center, The Johns Hopkins University, Baltimore, MD, 1994.

18. Platt LJ, Hill I. *Measuring Systems Development in Wyoming: Instruments to Assess Communities' Progress.* Health Systems Research, Inc., Washington, D.C., June, 1995.

19. Donabedian, A. Explorations in quality assessment and monitoring. *The Definition of Quality and Approaches to its Assessment, 1980*, Chapter 3, Vol. 1, Health Administration Press, Ann Arbor, Michigan.

20. Thacker SB, Berkelman RL. Public Health Surveillance in the United States. *Epidem Reviews* 1988; 10: 164–190.

21. Sepúlveda J, López-Cervantes M, Frenk J, de León JG, Lezana-Fernández MA, Santo-Burgoa C. Keynote Address: Key Issues in Public Health Surveillance for the 1990s. Proceedings of the 1992 Symposium on Public Health Surveillance. *MMWR* 1992; 41 (Suppl): 61–76.

22. Walker DK, Richmond JB, Eds. *Monitoring Child Health in the United States: Selected Issues and Policies.* Harvard University Press, Cambridge, Massachusetts, 1984.

23. Alexander GR. *A Population-based Maternal and Child Health Status Surveillance System for the State of Arizona.* Technical report prepared for Health Systems Research, Inc. and the Community and Family Health Section of the Arizona Department of Health Services, January, 1996. (Available on HRS WWW site)

24. Petersen, Donna J. *Monitoring the Health of Minnesota's Children and Families in an Era of Reform: The Minnesota MCH Indicators Project*, under contract from the Minnesota Department of Health, June 1997.

25. Usher, CL, Wildfire, JB, Gibbs, DA. Measuring performance in child welfare: secondary effects of success. *Child Welfare* 1999 Jan–Feb: 78(1):31–51.

U NIT 2

SOCIAL WELFARE

INTRODUCTION

Income, housing, employment, education, and the availability of child care are all among the many factors affecting the overall health and welfare of families. Any examination of the well-being of families in the United States must take into consideration the range of social welfare and economic security programs that are supported at the federal, state and local levels. Although the health care and social welfare systems are typically funded and administered as separate entities, they are closely intertwined. For both systems the legislative and policy making process is heavily influenced not only by the availability of resources, but by various political and social factors as well. One recent major piece of federal legislation, the 1996 Personal Responsibility and Work Opportunity Reconciliation Act (PRWORA), fundamentally altered the existing welfare system and subsequently changed the lives of many low-income families. This legislation not only affects employment and welfare payments, but also affects health insurance coverage, access to child care, and the eligibility for many other health and social welfare services. The long-term impact of the PRWORA is as yet not clear. Although there are many apparent positive aspects of the program, other less favorable outcomes are beginning to emerge as well. The down-turn in the economy since 2000 and the associated increases in unemployment are also beginning to complicate the situation.

This unit gives the reader an overview of the history of social welfare programs and policies in the United States and provides the background and philosophy underlying federally supported maternal and child health services. Special attention is given to the details of the 1996 Temporary Assistance to Needy Families (TANF) legislation, with an examination of the impact of this legislation on income and employment. The unit provides an in-depth analysis of the relationship of TANF to the reproductive health of women and considers two selected topics—child care services and health care of children in foster care—within the framework of the existing TANF and Medicaid systems. Finally, the unit highlights two major initiatives, Head Start and Healthy Start, and discusses the role of this type of successful initiative in the overall social welfare system. In each article the authors attempt to focus on the future, giving the reader a prospective view of the health and social welfare systems as they continue to evolve and impact on families.

117

ARTICLE 1

COMBATING FAMILY POVERTY: A REVIEW OF THE AMERICAN WELFARE SYSTEM

Sandra Wexler and Valire Carr Copeland

INTRODUCTION

For much of this century, public health and social work practitioners have been major players in efforts to combat poverty and its effects on mothers and children. Research demonstrates a strong, consistent relationship between poverty and negative maternal and child health outcomes (Geronimus, 2000; Longest, 2001). This complex relationship requires an understanding of the fundamental link between health and welfare at both macro and micro levels. A review of the development of the American welfare state provides insight into how our country has vacillated from a priority of relieving poverty to one of eliminating dependency.

The history of American efforts to alleviate poverty is one of shifting attitudes, beliefs, interventions, and loci of responsibility. The programs and policies formulated, both now and in the past, have reflected explicit or implicit theories of causation and have incorporated answers to such questions as: Who are the poor? Why are they poor? What type of assistance is needed? Responses also have both mirrored and influenced societal views of gender, race, and social class (Davidson, 1994; Gordon, 1994). Central to any discussion of poverty and public policy is whether assistance is an act of charity or an entitlement of citizenship.

This chapter examines American policy responses to poor mothers and their children. It begins with a brief historical review of the forms of aid available before 1935. The chapter then describes the Social Security Act of 1935 that created the modern American welfare state. Next, it traces the debates about and the modifications in the income maintenance system to the present time. Finally, it offers some thoughts about public health and social work practice in the new, "post-welfare" context.

ASSISTANCE FOR POOR FAMILIES BEFORE 1935

American responses to poverty are rooted historically in the Elizabethan Poor Law of 1601, from which the distinction between worthy and unworthy poor derives (DiNitto, 2000; Karger & Stoesz, 1997; Leiby, 1978; Reid, 1995). From the colonial period through the end of the 1700s, "outdoor" relief—that is, assistance provided in the home—was the common way of assisting worthy, poor families (Trattner, 1999). Although other methods (i.e., poorhouses, auction, contract) also were used (Katz, 1996), outdoor relief was especially favored in the United States (Davidson, 1994). Outdoor relief, administered locally by an appointed overseer of the poor and funded through local taxes, included the provision of clothing, food, coal, other supplies, and sometimes an allowance (Leiby, 1978; Trattner, 1999).

Poor families were much like their neighbors, sharing common heritage, religion, and hardships. "Distinctions between the family and the community were often vague; in many ways, the home and the community were one" (Baker, 1990, p. 56). Being poor, in itself, was not a cause for shame; rather, neediness was seen as beyond the control of the individual, as a result of unavoidable circumstances—unfavorable weather, death of the provider, old age, or injury—and as an inevitable feature of society (Trattner, 1999).

Not all needy residents, however, were deemed worthy of aid. Drunkards, loafers, and "sturdy beggars" (Trattner, 1999, p. 22) were defined as unworthy and were thought to deserve their fate. "Strangers" (i.e., nonresidents), Native Americans, and African Americans were denied relief, too (Karger & Stoesz, 1997; Reid, 1995). And whereas widows merited assistance, unmarried mothers were viewed as unfit and unworthy. Children were placed with local families— boarded out if they were under the age of 6 and indentured or apprenticed if they were older (Davidson, 1994).

The 19th century was a time of ideological and political debate, rapid population growth, and geographic expansion (Axinn & Levin, 1997). The Civil War revealed deep national divisions and produced massive social dislocation. Urbanization and industrialization were transforming American society. Ideas about how to provide assistance also began to change, paralleling and reflecting these other societal changes (Trattner, 1999).

Outdoor relief was criticized for fostering laziness, for contributing to immorality, and for increasing public costs (Katz, 1996). "Social provision," it was argued, "would validate debased manhood by servicing it" (Mink, 1990, p. 100). Outdoor relief as a public function was said to create dependency; aid by private charities was thought to avert this problem (Abramovitz, 1996).

"Indoor" relief—almshouses, poorhouses, workhouses, and orphanages— became the preferred response. Institutions were proposed as a less costly alternative, providing care more cheaply and making assistance less attractive to those who might apply (Katz, 1996). The number of institutions rose sharply in the pre-Civil War years (Trattner, 1999), with some designated for specific racial, ethnic, and religious groups. A variety of specialized institutions—reformatories, homes for unwed mothers, orphanages, schools for the disabled, and asylums for the mentally ill—were created, as well (Liebmann, 1993).

The poor of the 1800s no longer necessarily shared the characteristics of their better-off neighbors. The six million European immigrants, who arrived between 1800 and 1860 and congregated in the growing northern industrial cities (Trattner, 1999), differed from the majority in their religion, customs, and language. Institutions, it was believed, could reform their immoderate ways and instill in them the virtues of work (Katz, 1996), as well as impose a degree of social control (Jansson, 2001) on these potentially "dangerous classes" (Brace, 1872/1973).

Whereas being poor had been thought to be a matter of God's will, it was now considered to be evidence of deficits in one's character and family-of-origin (Abramovitz, 1996). Reformers attempted to distinguish poverty from pauperism: those in poverty—widows, the orphaned, the aged, and the incapacitated—suffered from misfortune and were worthy of aid, while paupers were unworthy, having brought about their own downfall (Katz, 1996; Leiby, 1978). Relief efforts embraced the 1834 English Poor Law Reform concept of less eligibility—benefits should be less than that earned by the poorest laborer (Patterson, 1994; Reid, 1995). Thus even the worthy poor faced lives of enormous hardship and deprivation.

Criticisms of indoor relief mounted during the second half of the 19th century. Some "child-saving" activists challenged the use of large institutions, arguing that children's development required a family environment (Katz, 1996; Liebmann, 1993). Women's associations pressed for social reforms and for legislation to protect mothers and children for the vagaries of the industrial system (Skocpol, 1992).

Reform in the late 1800s involved two contrasting approaches: (1) Charity Organization Societies, whose friendly visitors adjudged the eligibility of the poor for aid and offered them moral guidance to change their ways and (2) settlement houses, which stressed direct involvement with communities as a way to improve individual situations and environmental conditions (Brieland, 1995). The emergent Progressive movement, which has been called a "uniquely American movement" (Reid, 1995, p. 2212), set out a diverse reform agenda that influenced turn-of-the-century social and political thought (Jansson, 2001; Karger & Stoesz, 1997).

Further momentous changes were sweeping the country at the beginning of the 20th century. Industrial capitalism and large corporations dominated the economic landscape. Wealth and income became more concentrated, and labor unrest grew (Abramovitz, 1996). Rural to urban migration and the immigration of 22 million people between 1890 and 1920 dramatically changed America's cities (Karger & Stoesz, 1997). Following the 1896 Supreme Court decision in *Plessy v. Ferguson,* which upheld the doctrine of "separate but equal" (Brieland & Lemmon, 1985), the segregation and repression of African Americans went unchecked (Axinn & Levin, 1997).

Progressive reformers promoted the idea that children should not be removed from their family because of poverty alone. To preserve families, the 1909 White House Conference on the Care of Dependent Children recommended providing financial assistance by means of mothers' pensions (Katz, 1996; Liebmann, 1993;

Nelson, 1990). The conference recognized the societal service performed by married women who remained at home to raise children (Trattner, 1999), and mothers' pensions were designed to limit the intrusions on motherhood caused by employment and poverty (Mink, 1990).

The appropriateness of mothers' pensions was vigorously debated, with proponents arguing for public sponsorship and opponents countering that assistance was better provided by private charities (Axinn & Levin, 1997). Public sponsorship ultimately prevailed, although private charities often delivered the programs locally. Illinois and Missouri passed the first mothers' pension laws in 1911, and enactment of such statutes spread rapidly among the states. By 1935 all but two states—South Carolina and Georgia—had authorized mothers' pensions (Katz, 1996; Nelson, 1990; Skocpol, 1992; Trattner, 1999).

Each state's legislation set its own level of benefits and conditions for assistance (Nelson, 1990). Within the state, the decision to provide aid, along with administrative and financial responsibilities for the program, was vested in the counties (Trattner, 1999). Wide variation resulted, with some counties in a state providing financial assistance and some not. In fact, before the 1935 Social Security Act less than half of the nation's counties provided mothers' pensions (Abramovitz, 1996).

Potential beneficiaries had to meet behavioral as well as economic criteria (Gordon, 1994; Nelson, 1990; Skocpol, 1992). Applicants typically had to show proof of residency and citizenship. "Suitable home" provisions were common, and mothers had to demonstrate that they were "fit"—that they did not drink or smoke, kept a tidy home, went to church, did not have boarders, and maintained proper hygiene (Trattner, 1999). Charity workers exercised discretion in determining "fitness" and "suitability," and many impoverished families were excluded on these grounds.

Mothers' pensions were principally intended for widows, who were regarded as the deserving poor (Davidson, 1994; Nelson, 1990). Unmarried mothers, African Americans, and Mexican Americans often were excluded (Mink, 1990), or were granted lower amounts (Gordon, 1994). Although amendments broadened many of these statutes (Trattner, 1999), marital status remained a criterion in all but ten states (Skocpol, 1992). Yet despite their limitations, mothers' pension programs served to legitimate the government's role in providing financial assistance to poor families (Gordon, 1994).

THE 1935 SOCIAL SECURITY ACT— THE CREATION OF THE "WELFARE SYSTEM"

The Great Depression, which began in 1929, plunged the United States into social and economic crisis. Mothers' pension programs were never adequate to provide aid to all who could qualify or to allow those who received assistance to give up employment completely (Axinn & Levin, 1997; Skocpol, 1992). The Depression caused some of these programs to shrink significantly and led others to suspend the distribution of aid periodically (Gordon, 1994). Temporary financial support for these programs came in 1933 from the Federal Emergency Relief Act (Gordon, 1994), one of President Franklin D. Roosevelt's first New Deal enactments (Axinn & Levin, 1997).

Swept into the office by a landslide in 1932, President Roosevelt instituted a variety of emergency relief programs to help individuals and state governments, many of which were themselves almost bankrupt. Although these emergency efforts helped to relieve the immediate crisis, the Roosevelt administration moved to formulate more permanent measures. In June 1934, the President appointed a Committee on Economic Security to draft legislation (Jansson, 2001).

The result was the Social Security Act of 1935, characterized as "the foundation of the American welfare state" (Jansson, 2001, p. 199). It included two major programmatic areas: social insurance (e.g., Old Age Insurance and Unemployment Compensation) and public assistance (e.g., Old Age Assistance, Aid to Dependent Children, and Aid to the Blind). The Act also contained provisions for maternal and child health, crippled children, and child welfare programs, and state and local public health services (Axinn & Levin, 1997).

The public assistance programs of the Social Security Act were state-administered and financed through a combination of federal and state funds. To be eligible for assistance, an individual had to belong to one of the defined categories and had to demonstrate need. In contrast, the two social insurance programs were federally administered and funded through a payroll tax to which both employers and employees contributed (Axinn & Levin, 1997). Farm laborers, domestic workers, and government employees, however, were not covered by these social insurance programs, resulting in the exclusion of many women and persons of color (Abramovitz, 1996). Moreover, the distinctions drawn between the social insurance and public assistance programs in many ways reified the historical division of worthy and unworthy poor: Social insurance program beneficiaries merited coverage by virtue of their work histories, whereas public assistance program recipients had not necessarily "earned" their benefits (Reid, 1995).

Title IV of the Social Security Act created the Aid to Dependent Children (ADC) program, commonly termed "welfare." ADC replaced the state-sponsored, locally administered mothers' pensions with an expanded federal–state program (Gordon, 1994). To reduce the intra-state variability common to the mothers' pension programs, the ADC program had to be offered statewide (Abramovitz, 1996).

ADC grants were based on the number of children in a family, with federal funds matching up to a maximum of $18 for the first child and up to $12 for each additional child (Axinn & Levin, 1997; Gordon, 1994). These allowances were based on the amounts given to "families of servicemen who had lost their lives in the World War" (Leiby, 1978, p. 232). The $30 monthly stipend received by veterans' widows, however, was not considered by the congressional committee responsible for the legislation (Leiby, 1978).

ADC incorporated many of the elements and assumptions of the mothers' pension programs, including the belief that worthy mothers should be occupied fully raising their young children (Abramovitz, 1996; Gordon, 1994). Many of its original architects viewed ADC as a short-term program that would become obsolete as families qualified for social insurance benefits (DiNitto, 2000; Plotnick,

2000). Starting in 1939, many widows and their children did leave ADC to become beneficiaries of Survivors' Insurance (Abramovitz, 1996).

Compared to the 50% share it paid under Old Age Assistance, the federal government originally contributed one-third of the funding for ADC, with the states responsible for the rest (Jansson, 2001). In 1939 the federal contribution was raised to "$1 for $1 of state money" (Patterson, 1994, p. 67). Each state had to designate a single agency to administer ADC and had to define a standard of need that reflected a subsistence budget (Gordon, 1994). Each state was also required to establish eligibility criteria and benefit levels within broad federal guidelines, although benefits did not have to be large enough to equal the state's standard of need. Not surprisingly, significant variation occurred among the states, and no state had payments high enough to lift a family out of poverty (Levitan, 1990).

By 1940 only one-third of eligible children received ADC (Patterson, 1994). Public discourse in the 1940s focused on economic recovery, the situation in Europe, war production and World War II, and post-war prosperity, rather than on poverty (Reid, 1995). Yet despite the more positive economic situation, "low pay and joblessness among women," especially African American women, "led them to ADC" (Abramovitz, 1996, p. 320).

The 1950s were characterized by economic growth, rising wages, and a pervasive sense of complacency: Poverty was no longer a major problem in the new "classless" American society (Axinn & Levin, 1997; Trattner, 1999). The Civil Rights movement was in its formative stages (Katz, 1996). The 1950s were also an era of heightened social conservatism. The perceived threat of Communism was attacked domestically by the McCarthy hearings and internationally by increased military might. Over $40 billion a year—about 75% of the national budget—went to military spending (Jansson, 2001).

The number of ADC recipients rose steadily in the 1950s, increasing 13% during the decade. Program costs expanded more rapidly, exhibiting a 60% rise over the decade (Axinn & Levin, 1997). Moreover, the composition of ADC clientele began to change. By the mid-1950s, a program designed for white widows was serving increasing numbers of African American and unmarried mothers (Abramovitz, 1996; Trattner, 1999).

The contradictions and tensions of the 1950s were reflected in the policies of the decade. In 1950, ADC was expanded to permit grants to the adult caretakers (most often the mothers) of dependent children. That year, as well, Aid to the Permanently and Totally Disabled was created; in 1956, Disability Insurance was introduced. Social services were added to the ADC program in 1956, but funding was not appropriated (Abramovitz, 1996; Trattner, 1999).

Parallel to these expansions, "an attack on public welfare began to take shape" (Axinn & Levin, 1997, p. 234). Many states, particularly those in the South, implemented punitive administrative policies to reduce ADC rolls and to deter new applications. These policies commonly involved residency requirements, "suitable-home" criteria, and "man-in-the-house" or "substitute-father" rules (i.e., any man living in an ADC home was assumed to contribute financially to the family) (Abramovitz, 1996; Trattner, 1999).

THE WAR ON POVERTY AND THE BEGINNING OF THE "WELFARE PROBLEM"

"The relative quiet of the 1950s gave way to the quasi-revolutionary spirit of the 1960s" (Karger & Stoesz, 1997, p. 66). Rural and urban poverty was rediscovered (Trattner, 1999). Various social movements demanded "rights" for African Americans, Mexican Americans, Native Americans, women, juveniles, and gay men and lesbians (Axinn & Levin, 1997). Welfare recipients and their supporters formed the National Welfare Rights Organization in 1966 to advocate for the rights of welfare recipients (Patterson, 1994; Piven & Cloward, 1977/1979).

Two new explanations were offered for poverty. One argument, which drew on Oscar Lewis's anthropological work, cited a "culture of poverty," or a set of attitudes, beliefs, and behaviors among the poor themselves that distinguished them from mainstream society and that was transmitted intergenerationally. The other perspective, derived from Richard Cloward and Lloyd Ohlin's writings on juvenile delinquency, highlighted structural factors, particularly limitations to opportunities (Patterson, 1994).

President Kennedy's New Frontier and President Johnson's Great Society programs changed the social policy landscape dramatically. Major health, welfare, and economic development initiatives expanded the welfare state to an unprecedented degree. Legislation from this period include: the Manpower Development and Training Act of 1962; the Community Mental Health Centers Act of 1963; the Civil Rights Acts of 1964 and 1965; the Food Stamp Act of 1964; and the 1965 Title XVIII (Medicare) and Title XIX (Medicaid) amendments (Dickinson, 1995; Trattner, 1999).

The ADC program was not immune from this groundswell of legislative activity. Significant changes were made by the Public Welfare Amendments of 1962, commonly referred to as the Social Service Amendments (Abramovitz, 1995). One thrust of the amendments was to respond to charges that the program contributed to family breakup by encouraging fathers to leave. States, therefore, were given the option of providing benefits to two-parent families in which the main earner was unemployed. Although no more than half of the states at any given time offered AFDC-UP ("UP" for Unemployed Parent) benefits, those that did could require unemployed adult recipients (typically fathers) to 'work off' their public assistance grant" (Abramovitz, 1996, p. 333). Moreover, ADC was renamed Aid to Families with Dependent Children (AFDC) to affirm the program's emphasis on the family unit (DiNitto, 2000; Mason, Wodarski, & Parham, 1985).

The second thrust of 1962 amendments, drawing on the culture of poverty thesis, expanded the scope and funding of social services to ameliorate the deficits of poor, "multiproblem" beneficiary families (Mason, Wodarski, & Parham, 1985; Patterson, 1994). Smaller caseloads were recommended to complement this rehabilitative approach (DiNitto, 2000). States could provide these social services not only to current AFDC recipients but also to former clients and to those deemed at-risk of becoming recipients. The federal share of funding was high—fully $3 for every $1 of state money, making provision of these services attractive to the states (Axinn & Levin, 1997; Katz, 1996; Trattner, 1999).

Demonstration funding also was provided to the Community Work and Training program to assist AFDC recipients to become self-supporting (Goodwin, 1989).

The optimism of the early 1960s gave way to growing conflict and skepticism. Between 1965 and 1968 cities across the nation were shaken by riots (Schram & Turbett, 1983). Criticism of the Vietnam War mounted and thousands took to the streets in anti-war protests. Some liberal reformers argued that the war was being carried on at the expense of domestic anti-poverty programs (Jansson, 2001).

Meanwhile, the welfare rolls continued to rise, climbing from 3.5 million in 1961 to 5.0 million in 1967. Never-married mothers accounted for 40% of the increase. About half of the recipients were members of racial or ethnic minorities. By 1967, AFDC costs had reached $2.2 billion (Abramovitz, 1996).

The 1967 Social Security Amendments marked yet another shift in societal attitudes about welfare (Gueron, 1987). The developers of ADC had recognized the societal function performed by mothers staying at home to raise their young children (Aaronson & Hartmann, 1996). By the late 1960s, however, "as more mothers with infants entered the job market, the argument that welfare mothers should earn their living gained broad support" (Levitan, 1990, p. 53).

The 1967 amendments separated cash assistance from social services, which had been added only five years earlier. Welfare advocates applauded this change, reasoning that the separation would counter the pejorative assumption that all recipient families needed services (DiNitto, 2000; Miller, 1983). "Soft" services, such as counseling, lost favor to "hard" services, such as day care or vocational rehabilitation, that could promote self-sufficiency. The amendments allowed the states to purchase services from non-governmental sources (Trattner, 1999).

Two provisions of the 1967 amendments were designed to encourage employment. Prior to 1967, an adult recipient who obtained employment would have her or his grant reduced by a dollar for every dollar earned. To make work more attractive, the "30 plus one-third" rule required states to exclude a portion of recipients' monthly income (i.e., the first $30 and a third of the remainder earned) and certain work-related expenses from the income/assets base used to compute the AFDC grant (Axinn & Levin, 1997; DiNitto, 2000; Levitan, 1990; Patterson, 1994).

Workfare, in contrast, required that employable adult recipients, except single parents with children below the age of 6 or those exempted for other reasons, engage in work or employment training (Axinn & Levin, 1997; Dickinson, 1995). The Work Incentive program (WIN) was designed to assist recipients to learn job search skills, to obtain training, and to gain work experience (Goodwin, 1989; Levitan, 1990). Child care and other supportive services were to be made available to WIN participants (Abramovitz, 1995). Those who did not comply with WIN requirements could have their grants reduced or suspended for three months (Abramovitz, 1996).

A series of judicial rulings also significantly influenced AFDC policies and procedures. Between 1968 and 1970, the U.S. Supreme Court handed down three landmark decisions in AFDC-related cases (Levy, 1992). Of greatest consequence was the opinion rendered in *Goldberg v. Kelly* in 1970, in which the Court held that the Fourteenth Amendment's due process clause entitled AFDC recipients to an administrative hearing prior to being terminated from the program. Welfare, the Court wrote, "was a 'right' or . . . a 'statutory entitlement' "; that is, welfare recipients had "a valid reason to expect that, if they meet certain requirements, they should get AFDC" (Levy, 1992, p. 225).

By the close of the decade, public and political interest intensified to reform welfare, which was viewed as a failure and a mounting burden to taxpayers (Day, 1989; Karger & Stoesz, 1993). Critics charged that welfare discouraged work, fostered family dissolution, and encouraged childbearing outside of marriage, especially among teens (DiNitto, 2000). Varying benefit levels allegedly contributed to migration from low- to high-benefit states (Dear, 1989). Meanwhile, the welfare rolls continued to increase, spurred by liberalized eligibility requirements, more generous benefits, increased numbers of households headed by never-married and divorced mothers, and a new sense among the poor of their entitlement to benefits that was stimulated by the Welfare Rights Movement.

In 1969, the Nixon administration proposed the Family Assistance Plan (FAP) as a substitute for AFDC and AFDC-UP (Jansson, 2001). The FAP proposal guaranteed a minimum income to all poor American families with children (Dickinson, 1995). It required participation in employment or job training by all able-bodied individuals whose children were over the age of three (Axinn & Levin, 1997; Karger & Stoesz, 1997). To encourage employment, families would have been allowed to keep the first $60 plus half of their monthly income without losing their governmental subsidy, until an income maximum, or break-even point, was reached when aid would end (Patterson, 1994).

The FAP proposal was controversial among liberals and conservatives alike. With little support in Congress, FAP was abandoned in 1972. However, a portion of President Nixon's general welfare reform plan was enacted that year: Old Age Assistance, Aid to the Blind, and Aid to the Permanently and Totally Disabled were combined into a new federally administered program, Supplemental Security Income (DiNitto, 2000; Jansson, 2001). Thus, of the Social Security Act's public assistance programs, only AFDC remained under state administrative control.

Legislative modifications to the WIN program in 1971 and 1975 heightened the emphasis on job placement over training and imposed additional penalties for nonparticipation (Abramovitz, 1995; Goodwin, 1989). Recognition of absent parents' financial obligations to their children led to the creation in 1975 of the Office of Child Support Enforcement, whose mission was to encourage states to pursue vigorously paternity establishment and child support collection (DiNitto, 2000). That same year, the Earned Income Tax Credit was passed, representing the first use of "the tax system as a vehicle for giving resources to the poor" (Jansson, 2001, p. 286).

President Carter, who took office in 1977, proposed to supplant the AFDC, SSI, and food stamp programs with the Better Jobs and Income program. The proposal entailed a negative income tax and public jobs creation plan that applied to all poor individuals and families. Its controversial provisions and high annual costs—projected at $30.7 billion a year, or $2.8 billion above what was then spent (Trattner, 1999)—contributed to its failure (Day, 1989; Dickinson, 1995; Gueron, 1987).

THE REAGAN YEARS AND THE FAMILY SUPPORT ACT OF 1988

The economic growth of the 1950s and 1960s ended in the 1970s. Ronald Reagan's 1980 campaign themes of lower taxes, higher military spending, a balanced budget, and a return to "traditional" values struck a responsive chord among many voters (Jansson, 2001). Reagan's victory over Carter legitimated neoconservative politics and policies.

The Reagan administration profoundly transformed discourse on social policy issues (Rose, 1989; Stoesz & Karger, 1990, 1993). The problem was no longer poverty, but dependency; the cause was neither structural features of the economic system nor characteristics of the poor, per se, but the very government programs that had been implemented to help the poor (Funiciello & Schram, 1991). As President Reagan asserted: "In 1964, the famous War on Poverty was declared. . . . 'Poverty won the War.' Poverty won, in part, because instead of helping the poor, government programs ruptured the bonds holding poor families together" (Danziger, 1990, p. 18).

Capitalizing on a growing popular disillusionment with the federal government's ability to resolve social problems (Axinn & Levin, 1997), President Reagan called for less "big government" in domestic matters. In the economic arena, this meant reduced federal regulation of business and decreased taxes, especially for the wealthy—supply-side prescriptions to stimulate economic growth (Jansson, 2001). In the social policy arena, the emphasis was on transferring social welfare authority to state and local governments and on reducing means-tested social programs (Stoesz & Karger, 1993). The federal government's role in welfare-related matters was to be a "safety net," a last resort when charities, volunteerism, the private sector, and individual initiatives failed (Katz, 1996).

President Reagan launched his effort to dismantle the liberal welfare state soon after assuming office (Patterson, 1994). The Omnibus Budget Reconciliation Act (OBRA) of 1981 eliminated some programs and replaced 57 other categorical programs with seven block grants, which were given reduced funding (Dickinson, 1995). OBRA also restricted eligibility for food stamps (Jansson, 2001).

OBRA imposed stricter eligibility requirements for AFDC; broadened the definition of assets for eligibility and benefit-setting purposes; limited to four months the earned income disregard for employed recipients; capped child care and work-related deductions; added further work requirements; and reduced WIN training funds (Abramovitz, 1995; Moffitt & Wolf, 1987; Stoesz & Karger, 1990). These changes reflected the Reagan administration's views of individual and public responsibility: "those who have children should support them" and "should be required to work" (Mason, Wodarski, & Parham, 1985, p. 199), with government aid available only to the truly needy (Gueron, 1987).

"The impact of the 1981 amendments was immediate and dramatic. In the following year, during the worst recession since the Great Depression, the number of families receiving AFDC declined by 8%" (Levitan, 1990, p. 54). By 1983, OBRA had resulted in about $1.1 billion in federal and state savings and a 2%

increase in poverty (Patterson, 1994). The percentage of families disqualified for AFDC benefits ranged from 8% to 60%, depending on the state, with an additional 8% to 48% having their benefits reduced (Moffitt & Wolf, 1987).

President Reagan, re-elected in 1984 by a decisive majority, continued to push for reductions in domestic spending, particularly in means-tested programs, as a way to alleviate the rising federal deficit (Jansson, 2001). Attacks on the AFDC system and its recipients were bolstered by "poverty-by-choice" theories, which posited that the poor choose values, attitudes, and behaviors that keep them impoverished (Rose, 1989, p. 87). Rhetoric focused on the question of "reciprocity"—what welfare recipients owed to society in return for public financial support (Stoesz & Karger, 1990).

Welfare reform again was placed on the political agenda in 1987 and both the Senate and the House considered bills to restructure AFDC. The Family Support Act (FSA) of 1988 was hailed as the most important revision in welfare policy since the Social Security Act (Segal, 1989; Stoesz, 1989). The FSA was favored by both liberals and conservatives, who, for different reasons, saw it as a way to resolve the welfare dilemma (Chilman, 1992; Nichols-Casebolt & McClure, 1989).

The legislation changed AFDC "from an income support to a mandatory work and training program" (Stoesz, 1989, p. 133), now emphasizing short-term cost savings over long-term human capital investment (Goodwin, 1989). Its major thrusts were paternity establishment, child support collection, and mandatory work. These provisions reflected the Administration's arguments that the obligation to support children resides first with the parents (Dickinson, 1995; Stoesz & Karger, 1990) and that encouragement of economic self-sufficiency must replace dependency on public stipends (Nichols-Casebolt & McClure, 1989).

Mandatory work (i.e., workfare) provisions were the centerpiece of the legislation. WIN was replaced by the Job Opportunities and Basic Skills Training (JOBS) program, which states were to implement by October 1990 (Chilman, 1992). JOBS required AFDC recipients whose children were at least three years of age (or, at the state's option, at least one year of age) to participate in a training or employment preparation program or to locate work (Abramovitz, 1996). The legislation identified three groups for special consideration: young parents (i.e., under age 24) who lacked a high school diploma and work experience; long-term recipients (i.e., with more than three years in any five-year period); and those nearing the end of their eligibility based on the age of the youngest child (Harris, 1989). States could exercise considerable latitude in the design of their JOBS programs (Dickinson, 1995).

To encourage the transition from welfare to employment, the FSA included provisions for supportive services for JOBS participants and for time-limited, post-AFDC child care services and Medicaid coverage (Harris, 1989). The AFDC-UP program, which then existed in 27 states (Chilman, 1992), was made mandatory nationwide. Participation of one parent, or at the state's option both, in workfare was required. Recipients who did not comply with JOBS program requirements would lose the parent's portion of the AFDC grant for a specified period, although aid to the children would continue (Harris, 1989).

George Bush succeeded Ronald Reagan to the presidency in January 1989. President Bush called for a "kinder, gentler nation" and for volunteers to be "a thousand points of light" in eradicating domestic social problems. Like his predecessor, President Bush emphasized military spending, "no new taxes," and a transfer of responsibility for social programs to the states (Axinn & Levin, 1997; DiNitto, 2000; Jansson, 2001). Bush also inherited "a staggering $2.6 trillion debt . . . a crisis in the scandal-ridden savings and loan industry . . . and an economy with various structural weaknesses that, by 1990, would lapse into an increasingly serious recession" (Trattner, 1999, p. 379).

President Bush did not initiate any major federal-level modifications to the AFDC program. He did, however, encourage state experimentation and characterized the "states as laboratories" (DiNitto, 2000, p. 52). States, seeking to reduce their welfare expenditures, applied for and received waivers to institute policies and procedures that did not comply with the existing federal rules (DiNitto, 2000). The "devolution revolution" (Kamerman, 1996, pp. 453–454) was set in motion, wherein ever greater authority for welfare programming shifted from the federal government to state and local governments.

THE 1990s AND THE END OF THE WELFARE ENTITLEMENT

The United States entered the final decade of the 20th century facing a decline in economic productivity, continued unemployment and underemployment, and an increase in the concentration of income and wealth among the richest five percent (Axinn & Levin, 1997). The number of Americans living in poverty in 1992 was the highest it had been since 1962 (Patterson, 1994). Members of racial and ethnic minorities; children; and single-parent, mother-headed families were especially vulnerable to impoverishment (Axinn & Levin, 1997).

Although the JOBS program was in the early stages of implementation and its impacts were far from certain, the dismantling of the welfare system became a prominent theme in the 1992 presidential campaign (Trattner, 1999). Bill Clinton, the Democratic challenger, promised to "scrap the current welfare system and make welfare a second chance, not a way of life" (Patterson, 1994, p. 225). Clinton's victory in the 1992 election placed a Democrat in the White House; the 1994 elections gave Republicans control of Congress, with many of those in the House claiming their victory as a mandate for the policies outlined in their Contract with America (Axinn & Levin, 1997).

Democrats and Republicans alike vilified AFDC and its beneficiaries (Sidel, 1996). Myths about welfare mothers became popular reality; scant attention was given to the realities of life on welfare or to the declining value of welfare grants (Axinn & Levin, 1997; Funiciello & Schram, 1991). Responsibility for everything from gang violence to drug addiction to teenage pregnancy to the changing composition of American families began to be attributed to the welfare system and to "dependent" welfare mothers (Withorn, 1996).

By the mid-1990s welfare "reform" meant "reducing expenditures of public money, increasing labor-force participation of single parents (largely women), and changing the social and sexual behavior of women" (Axinn & Levin, 1997, p. 313). The Personal Responsibility Act, based on the Republican's Contract with America, was introduced in the House in 1995. After a year of political wrangling, a final welfare bill emerged that incorporated elements of the Personal Responsibility Act and suggestions made by the National Governors' Association (Axinn & Levin, 1997). President Clinton's promise to "end welfare as we know it" came to fruition on August 22, 1996, when he signed into law the Personal Responsibility and Work Opportunity Reconciliation Act (PRWORA).

The PRWORA modified a number of long-standing U.S. social policies and fundamentally changed the system of welfare that existed in America for 60 years. It replaced the AFDC, AFDC-UP, and JOBS with the Temporary Assistance to Needy Families (TANF) program (Office of the Assistant Secretary, 1997; Super, Parrott, Steinmetz, & Mann, 1996). TANF ended poor families' entitlement to welfare. It created a five-year lifetime limit on benefits, although it allowed states to exempt up to 20% of their cases from this limit (Plotnick, 2000). It established strict, escalating work-participation targets. Block grants replaced matching grants as the mechanism for allocating federal funds to the states (Super et al., 1996).

Although general oversight responsibility is retained by the federal government, TANF permits states' significant latitude in program design and administration. States can adopt any one of a number of optional features included in the federal legislation (e.g., special requirements for teen parents, lifetime participation ban for those convicted of drug-related felonies) (Office of the Assistant Secretary, 1997). They can decide "whether to aid all qualifying families" and how long beneficiaries will receive aid (Plotnick, 2000, p. 111). States can use surplus block grant funds, which should result as welfare rolls decline, for related purposes.

One provision of TANF gave states the option to pay differential benefit amounts based on length of residence. States that chose to adopt this provision could base the TANF payments of recipients who lived in the state less than 12 months on the amount paid by the state in which they formerly resided. This, in effect, allowed states to implement a "two-tiered" benefit structure, wherein residents new to a state could receive smaller TANF grants than otherwise similar, long-term residents. A California case challenging the state's residency-related benefit levels reached the U.S. Supreme Court in 1999. The Court held that California's two-tiered benefit scheme violated the Fourteenth Amendment's Citizenship Clause (*Saenz v. Roe*, 1999). Other states that had adopted residency provisions withdrew them in the wake of this decision.

TANF's implementation coincided with a time of rising prosperity and low unemployment. The recession of the early 1990s gave way to steady economic growth. Record high 1992 AFDC participation figures began to decline even before the introduction of TANF, such that between March 1994 and October 1996 welfare caseloads decreased by at least 5% in every state but Hawaii (DeParle, 1997). Thus states started their TANF programs with a short-term financial cushion (since TANF block grants were based on federal payments made during the early 1990s when welfare rolls were higher) and a reduced proportion of their caseloads that had to meet the first federal work target (Super et al., 1996).

The number of families receiving TANF fell by 50% between August 1996 and June 2000, from 4.4 million to 2.2 million. More adult TANF recipients were engaged in work in fiscal year 1999 than in fiscal year 1997 (Welfare reform: Progress, 2001). If success is judged simply by caseload reduction, then TANF, at least initially, appears to be successful. But do these data mean that states' "work-first" approaches, wherein recipients are encouraged to take any job and training and education are downplayed, have worked?

As Edin and Lein (1997) have shown, low-wage, dead-end jobs that offer few, if any, benefits do little to promote the economic self-sufficiency of poor families. Their conclusions seem borne out by recent data on former TANF recipients. The 1999 National Survey of America's Families (NASF), which employed a nationally representative sample, found that almost two-thirds (64%) of those who left TANF between 1997 and 1999 were working at the time of the interview. However, the median income of employed former recipients was close to the poverty threshold, and fully 41% fell below the poverty line even after factoring in the Earned Income Tax Credit and food stamps. Fully a quarter worked nights or irregular schedules, increasing the difficulty of securing child care (Loprest, 2001).

Families leaving TANF may still qualify for food stamps and Medicaid, two important anti-poverty measures. A recent U.S. General Accounting Office study of seven states found that "between 44 and 83 percent of the families who left welfare received Medicaid benefits, and between 31 and 63 percent received food stamps" (Welfare reform: Progress, 2001, p. 4). However, many who are eligible for these benefits do not receive them. In the 1999 NSAF, among those who left welfare, only "about 4 in 10 income-eligible families participated" in the Food Stamp program (Zedlewski, 2001, p. 3).

Equally disturbing trends are found for health insurance. Analysis of data from the 1997 NSAF found that 41% of the adults who left welfare between 1995 and 1997 were uninsured at the time of the interview, 23% had private/employer coverage, and 36% received Medicaid. Of those with income below the poverty line, merely 44% received Medicaid, while 14% had private/employer coverage, and 43% were uninsured. Children in families that had left welfare fared somewhat better—overall, half had Medicaid or state-provided health coverage. Yet a fourth were uninsured (Garrett & Holahan, 2000).

Some have suggested that those who left TANF early in its implementation represented "easier" clients—those with more education, better job skills, and fewer obstacles to employment (Welfare reform: Progress, 2001). These "more advantaged" former recipients entered the job market during a period of strong economic performance. Yet even with all of these favorable indicators, the 1999 NSAF found that 22% of those who had left welfare were again receiving TANF (Welfare reform: Progress, 2001).

The economic boom of the late 1990s has given way to fears of a recession. The August 2001 unemployment rate of 4.9% reflected the largest one-month increase in six years (Leonhardt, 2001). Against this backdrop of changing economic circumstance and, perhaps, changing recipient characteristics and needs, two important tests of TANF remain: What will happen when large numbers of recipient families reach the end of their five years' eligibility? and How will the TANF program and its beneficiaries fare in the face of an economic downturn? More fundamentally, however, is the question of how to combat poverty and its sequelae among this nation's children and families.

Congress will soon begin to consider reauthorization of TANF. Future legislative provisions may well depend on how questions such as those above are answered. Historical evidence suggests that states and localities may be ill-equipped to respond to the needs of poor families without the infusion of federal dollars.

CONCLUSIONS

Although the nomenclature has changed since this country was founded, similar themes continue to dominate debate about how to respond to the needs of those in poverty. This review of welfare history suggests three conclusions: First, and most obviously, there is no easy or "quick fix" solution to family impoverishment—responses based on simple, unicausal definitions inevitably prove to be inadequate. Second, most efforts to assist poor families have sustained them, but have not allowed families to escape poverty. An emphasis on maintenance is understandable for the Colonial period, when resources generally were scarce; to make sense of the choices being made today brings us to our third conclusion. Thus, third, American norms, ideologies, and social traditions have given rise to a political culture that has narrowly constructed government's responsibility to its citizens' economic welfare. The right to financial assistance from the modern welfare state has been based on statute and has never been construed as a right of citizenship. As statutes have changed, as they dramatically did in 1996, so have the obligations of government.

In 21st century America, as in the past, much remains to be done to ensure the well-being of families and children, especially those experiencing economic hardship. Those in social work and public health are uniquely situated to give definition to post-TANF realities and to move the discussion beyond simple political expediency, economic vagaries, and moralistic pronouncements. At both the federal and state levels, research, advocacy, and coalition-building will be needed to assure that provisions promoting poverty eradication are included in any new welfare reforms. The expertise of social work and public health practitioners can contribute to future policy decisions and to the lives of those affected by them.

ACKNOWLEDGMENTS

The authors thank Donald Brieland and Kenneth Jaros for their helpful comments on this manuscript.

REFERENCES

Aaronson, S., and Hartmann, H. (1996). Reform, not rhetoric: A critique of welfare policy and charting new directions. *American Journal of Orthopsychiatry, 64*, 583–598.

Abramovitz, M. (1996). *Regulating the lives of women: Social welfare policy from colonial times to the present* (Rev. ed.). Boston: South End.

Abramovitz, M. (1995). Aid to families with dependent children. In the *Encyclopedia of Social Work* (19th ed., Vol. 1, pp. 183–194). Washington, DC: NASW Press.

Axinn, J., and Levin, H. (1997). *Social welfare: A history of the American response to need* (4th ed.). White Plains, NY: Longman.

Baker, P. (1990). The domestication of politics: Women and American political society, 1780–1920. In L. Gordon (Ed.), *Women, the state, and welfare* (pp. 55–91). Madison, WI: University of Wisconsin Press.

Brace, C.L. (1872/1973). *The dangerous classes of New York, & twenty years' work among them.* Washington, DC: National Association of Social Workers.

Brieland, D. (1995). Social work practice: History and evolution. In the *Encyclopedia of Social Work* (19th ed., Vol. 3, pp. 2247–2257). Washington, DC: NASW Press.

Brieland, D., and Lemmon, J.A. (1985). *Social work and the law* (2nd ed.). St Paul, MN: West Publishing.

Chilman, C.S. (1992). Welfare reform or revision? The Family Support Act of 1988. *Social Service Review, 66*, 349–377.

Danziger, S. (1990). Antipoverty policies and child poverty. *Social Work Research and Abstracts, 26*(4), 17–24.

Davidson, C.E. (1994). Dependent children and their families: A historical survey. In F.H. Jacobs & M.W. Davies (Eds.), *More than kissing babies? Current child and family policy in the United States* (pp. 65–89). Westport, CN: Auburn House.

Day, P.J. (1989). *A new history of social welfare.* Englewood Cliffs, NJ: Prentice Hall.

Dear, R.D. (1989). What's right with welfare? *The other face of AFDC. Journal of Sociology and Social Welfare, 16*(2), 5–43.

DeParle, J. (1997, February 2). A sharp decrease in welfare cases is gathering speed. *The New York Times*, Section 1, pp. 1, 12.

Dickinson, N.S. (1995). Federal social legislation from 1961 to 1994. In the *Encyclopedia of Social Work* (19th ed., Vol. 2, pp. 1005–1013). Washington, DC: NASW Press.

DiNitto, D.M. (2000). *Social welfare: Politics and public policy* (5th ed.). Boston: Allyn and Bacon.

Edin, K., and Lein, L. (1997). *Making ends meet: How single mothers survive welfare and low-wage work.* New York: Russell Sage Foundation.

Funiciello, T., and Schram, S.F. (1991). Post-mortem on the deterioration of the welfare state. In E.A. Anderson & R.C. Hula (Eds.), *The reconstruction of family policy* (pp. 149–163). New York: Greenwood.

Garrett, B., and Holahan, J. (2000, March). *Welfare leavers, Medicaid coverage, and private health insurance.* (Assessing the New Federalism Brief B-13.) Washington, DC: The Urban Institute.

Geronimus, A.T. (2000). To mitigate, resist, or undo: Addressing structural influence on the health of urban populations. *American Journal of Public Health,* 90, 867–872.

Goodwin, L. (1989). The work incentive years in current perspective: What have we learned? Where do we go from here? *Journal of Sociology and Social Welfare,* 16(2), 45–65,

Gordon, L. (1994). *Pitied but not entitled: Single mothers and the history of welfare.* New York: The Free Press.

Gueron, J.M. (1987). Reforming welfare with work. *Public Welfare, 45*(4), 13–25.

Harris, S. (1989). *A social worker's guide to the Family Support Act of 1988: Summary, analysis, and opportunities for implementation.* Silver Spring, MD: NASW Press.

Jansson, B.S. (2001). *The reluctant welfare state: A history of American social welfare policies* (4th ed.). Pacific Grove, CA: Brooks/Cole.

Kamerman, S.B. (1996). The new politics of child and family policies. *Social Work, 41,* 453–465.

Karger, H.J., and Stoesz, D. (1997). *American social welfare policy: A pluralist approach* (3rd ed.). New York: Longman.

Karger, H.J., and Stoesz, D. (1993). Retreat and retrenchment: Progressives and the welfare state. *Social Work, 38,* 212–220.

Katz, M.B. (1996). *In the shadow of the poor house: A social history of welfare in America* (Rev. ed.). New York: Basic Books.

Leiby, J. (1978). *A history of social welfare and social work in the United States.* New York: Columbia University Press.

Leonhardt, D. (2001, September 8). Jobless rate rises sharply, to 4.9%; Bush vows to act. *The New York Times,* pp. A1, A9.

Levitan, S.A. (1990). *Programs in aid of the poor* (6th ed.). Baltimore, MD: The Johns Hopkins Press.

Levy, P.A. (1992). The durability of Supreme Court welfare reforms of the 1960s. *Social Service Review, 66,* 213–236.

Liebmann, G.W. (1993). The AFDC conundrum: A new look at an old institution. *Social Work, 38,* 36–43.

Longest, B.B. (2001). Contemporary health policy. Chicago: Health Administration Press.

Loprest, P. (2001, April). *How are families that left welfare doing? A comparison of early and recent welfare leavers.* (Assessing the New Federalism Brief B-36). Washington, DC: The Urban Institute.

Mason, J., Wodarski, J.S., and Parham, T.M.J. (1985). Work and welfare: A reevaluation of AFDC. *Social Work, 30,* 197–203.

Miller, D.C. (1983). AFDC: Mapping a strategy for tomorrow. *Social Service Review, 57,* 599–613.

Mink, G. (1990). The lady and the tramp: Gender, race, and the origins of the American welfare state. In L. Gordon (Ed.), *Women, the state, and welfare* (pp. 92–122). Madison, WI: University of Wisconsin Press.

Moffitt, R., and Wolf, D.A. (1987). The effect of the 1981 Omnibus Budget Reconciliation Act on welfare recipients and work incentives. *Social Service Review, 61*, 247–260.

Nelson, B.J. (1990). The origins of the two-channel welfare state: Workmen's compensation and mothers' aid. In L. Gordon (Ed.), *Women, the state, and welfare* (pp. 123–151). Madison, WI: University of Wisconsin Press.

Nichols-Casebolt, A.M., and McClure, J. (1989). Social work support for welfare reform: The latest surrender in the war on poverty. *Social Work, 34*, 77–80.

Office of the Assistant Secretary for Planning and Evaluation, U.S. Department of Health and Human Services (1997, January). *Summary of provisions: Personal Responsibility and Work Opportunity Reconciliation Act of 1996 (H.R. 3734)*. Washington, DC: Author.

Patterson, J.T. (1994). *America's struggle against poverty, 1900–1994*. Cambridge, MA: Harvard University Press.

Piven, F.F., and Cloward, R.A. (1977/1979). *Poor people's movements: Why they succeed, how they fail*. New York: Vintage Books.

Plotnick, R.D. (2000). Economic support for families with children. In P.J. Pecora, J.K. Whittaker, A.N. Maluccio, & R.P. Barth, with R.D. Plotnick, *The child welfare challenge: Policy, practice, and research* (2nd ed., pp. 95–127). New York: Aldine De Gruyter.

Reid, P.N. (1995). Social welfare history. In the *Encyclopedia of Social Work* (19th ed., Vol. 3, pp. 2206–2225). Washington, DC: NASW Press.

Rose, N.E. (1989). The political economy of welfare. *Journal of Sociology and Social Welfare, 16*(2), 87–108.

Saenz v. Roe, 526 U.S. 489 (1999).

Schram, S.F., & Turbett, J.P. (1983). The welfare explosion: Mass society versus social control. *Social Service Review, 57*, 614–625.

Segal, E.A. (1989). Welfare reform: Help for poor women and children? *Affilia, 4*(3), 42–50.

Sidel, R. (1996). The enemy within: A commentary on the demonization of difference. *American Journal of Orthopsychiatry, 66*, 490–495.

Skocpol, T. (1992). *Protecting soldiers and mothers: The political origins of social policy in the United States*. Cambridge, MA: The Belknap Press of Harvard University.

Stoesz, D. (1989). A new paradigm for social welfare. *Journal of Sociology and Social Welfare, 16*(2), 127–150.

Stoesz, D., and Karger, H.J. (1990). Welfare reform: From illusion to reality. *Social Work, 35*, 141–147.

Stoesz, D., and Karger, H.J. (1993). Deconstructing welfare: The Reagan legacy and the welfare state. *Social Work, 38*, 619–628.

Super, D.A., Parrott, S., Steinmetz, S., and Mann, C. (1996, August). *The new welfare law*. (Available from the Center on Budget and Policy Priorities, 820 First Street, N.E., Suite 510, Washington, DC 20002.)

Trattner, W.I. (1999). *From poor law to welfare state: A history of social welfare in America* (6th ed.). New York: The Free Press.

Welfare reform: Progress in meeting work-focused TANF goals: Hearing before the Subcommittee on Human Resources, of the House Committee on Ways and Means (2001) (testimony of Cynthia M. Fagnoni) (General Accounting Office Report No. GAO-01-522T). Retrieved August 20, 2001 from http://www.gao.gov

Withorn, A. (1996). "Why do they hate us so much?" A history of welfare and its abandonment in the United States. *American Journal of Orthopsychiatry, 66,* 496–509.

Zedlewski, S. R. (2001, April). *Former welfare families and the Food Stamp Program: The exodus continues.* (Assessing the New Federalism Brief B-33). Washington, DC: The Urban Institute.

ARTICLE 2

DID WELFARE REFORM WORK?
IMPLICATIONS FOR 2002 AND BEYOND

Sandra Hofferth

INTRODUCTION

Welfare reform has been widely accepted as a success. New research shows that welfare reform policies led recipients to leave public assistance for work, as hoped. However, many return within two years and a considerable group remain poor. Mothers of very young children have the hardest time becoming self-sufficient. Although public policies worked, the prosperous economy was a critical facilitating factor.

Former President Bill Clinton entered office vowing to "end welfare as we know it." Yet, in 1996, the Clinton Administration was deeply divided into liberal and conservative camps over the welfare reform bill Congress had passed. Would the law's stringent limits encourage welfare recipients to be more self-sufficient, as conservative proponents of welfare reform argued, or would it simply punish them and harm their children, as liberal opponents protested? Clinton bet on the first outcome and signed the act. Several of the architects of the liberal alternative plan resigned in protest. The jury is still out on the great federal welfare reform experiment of 1996, even as a decision to extend it looms in 2002. But states' experiments with welfare policies during the 1990s can tell us much about what works and what does not.

At first glance, the conservative approach seems to have been vindicated; welfare rolls dropped sharply by the end of Clinton's term—49% between 1994 and 1999. But skeptics reply that this felicitous turn of events would not have happened without economic prosperity. The policy may have given people a push, but the economy pulled them into jobs. Some say that it does not matter which was more important; others argue that we need to know whether policies did what they were designed to do and that compassionate citizens will want to know what happened to former recipients.

While some benefitted from economic independence and work, other former recipients, especially the most marginally employable, returned to welfare or remained impoverished off of it. In past years, as many as half of former recipients returned to public assistance within two years of leaving it. And, although employment is high at exit from welfare, family finances may not be greatly improved. Although many left welfare to take jobs, their incomes often rose little. This is because families must substitute earnings and other sources of income for welfare payments. Also, now off of state aid, they may need to pay for the full amount of housing, child care, medical care expenses, and transportation, reducing their net earnings. Ex-recipients would need to earn a lot more to pay for these critical expenses, since their new jobs often do not provide such benefits.

Fortunately, information collected in the early to mid-1990s across the states permits us to follow public assistance recipients before and after leaving the welfare rolls and links their fates to variations in state policies and to economic conditions. Even though it is impossible to determine precisely the parts separately played by policy and economy, what we now know from a national study of women who were on welfare is that public policies were instrumental in encouraging women to leave AFDC in the early 1990s. The economy played only a supporting role. We also know that a substantial proportion of families returned to welfare within two years, that the availability of jobs helped determine how soon they returned, and that a substantial proportion remained poor. High-risk families, such as those with young children, appear to be returning to public assistance faster than other former recipients. What we have learned about the effects of public policy on public assistance recipients and what it implies for the upcoming debate over reauthorization is the subject of this article.

WELFARE REFORMS BEFORE THE WELFARE REFORM

The Personal Responsibility and Work Opportunity Reconciliation Act of 1996 fundamentally altered the federal government's promise to maintain a safety net for low-income families. It did so by repealing the entitlement to cash assistance in the 60-year-old program of Aid to Families with Dependent Children (AFDC). Beginning no later than July 1, 1997, each state was required to assist needy families under the Temporary Assistance for Needy Families (TANF) Block Grant. Cash assistance cannot be given to families in which an adult has received assistance for 60 months in his or her lifetime. Also, recipients must work after two years on assistance or even sooner, if the state prefers.

But welfare reform had started earlier. Most states had obtained waivers to federal requirements in the early 1990s. These state waivers established "natural experiments" in program administration beginning considerably before the TANF program was passed. In essence, TANF formalized what was already in effect in many states prior to 1996. Largely because of the waiver programs implemented in many states, between the peak level in 1994 and mid-1997 there was a substantial decline of 25% in the welfare rolls. Variation from state to state in this waiver period permits researchers to examine which aspects of welfare reform have led to which consequences.

Of particular interest are the waivers that established:

1. Time limits; whether restricting total months on public assistance to 60 or fewer, depending on the state
2. Work requirements; whether the state mandates that recipients work or look for work after a certain amount of time on public assistance
3. Work exemption for children under age 3; whether states require mothers of children under age 3 to work
4. Earnings disregard; whether states allow recipients to disregard some of their earnings in calculating benefits
5. Family cap; whether recipients who have additional children are prohibited from receiving additional benefits
6. Sanctions; whether the state reduces recipients' benefits for failure to meet the work or other requirements

Besides changes in welfare policy in the early 1990s, other policy changes may have given recipients additional incentives to work. For example, the Earned Income Tax Credit (EITC) expanded beginning in 1993. This credit in the income tax code provides money to families in which there is at least one earner and in which earnings are below about $30,000, whether or not that individual owes income tax. In 1998, a working single mother with one child and an income of about $11,000 received a maximum benefit of $2,272, compared with a maximum of $950 in 1990. Since these mothers' earnings would be increased by the amount of the EITC to which they were entitled, it is possible that this credit also encouraged recipients to work. Other social insurance changes probably had little effect on the welfare rolls.

Although it is still too soon to know what happened after 1996, by examining how recipients behaved in states with different policies in the early 1990s under waivers, we can make an educated guess. I base my conclusions not just upon across-state variation, which was considerable, but also upon changes within states over time. States may differ in recipient behavior for many reasons having nothing to do with their public assistance policies, and we have adjusted for these differences.

Four questions arise: Did the new policies get recipients off of welfare? Did they reduce how often ex-recipients returned to welfare? Did economic conditions affect leaving and returning? How well-off were recipients in the two years after leaving welfare? Colleagues and I used a long-established survey of families, the Panel Study of Income Dynamics, which has followed thousands of families over many years, to answer these questions. The story I find, while not surprising, is consistent with stories that have been reported in other places, but I am able to provide numbers and statistical evidence for this story. This gives me some confidence in my conclusions.

Did Public Policies Get Recipients Working?

The new welfare policies did what they were designed to do—they moved people off of AFDC and into work. My reasoning is as follows: First, more families left public assistance in the mid-1990s after waivers were implemented than in the early 1990s. Second, waiver policies designed to get recipients working were associated with increased work. More recipients left welfare in those states that instituted key changes than in those that did not. And they left because of work. For example, in the states that implemented a work requirement between 1993 and 1996, 3% left welfare per month and began working, compared with only 1% in states that did not do so. In work requirement states, 92% of those who left welfare left because they took a job. Fewer than ¹/₂ of 1% left welfare for other reasons, such as marriage or the loss of eligibility because the youngest child reached age 18. Similar results were obtained for recipients in states that implemented more restrictive exemptions for young children; leaving through work tripled. Instead of simply requiring work, some states tried to encourage work by allowing recipients to keep more of their earnings and still get financial aid. As expected, implementing this policy led to lower rates of exit. In such states, leaving through work was cut in half.

Did Public Policies Keep Former Recipients Off Welfare?

Many recipients were unable to remain self-sufficient. One out of three former recipients returned to welfare within two years after leaving. Consistent with the greater proportion of recipients who left, fewer former recipients returned to the welfare rolls in the mid-1990s compared with the early 1990s. Surprisingly, the welfare policies did little to keep recipients off the rolls.

The one rule that affected returning was requiring mothers of very young children to work. In states that required work from such mothers, recipients were 2.5 times as likely to return to AFDC as mothers in other states, though the overall probability of returning was quite low. As described earlier, that rule also encouraged such mothers to leave welfare in the first place. It is likely that the costs of working were simply too high for these mothers and, unable to maintain self-sufficiency without considerable supports, they soon reappeared at the welfare office. Former recipients who left welfare to take a job returned to welfare sooner than those who left for other reasons. Taking an initial job is still very difficult for public assistance recipients, particularly for those with young children, and is no guarantee of continuous employment. Another route off of welfare is finding a partner. However, forming a partnership with a male is also not, by itself, a ticket to self-sufficiency. The most successful at becoming self-sufficient were women who took both a job and a partner for a year or more.

How Much Did Good Times Help?

The overall level of prosperity and availability of jobs in the 1990s were undeniably important contexts for the declines in welfare rolls. In more prosperous states, defined as those with higher family incomes, recipients were somewhat slower to leave AFDC. Such states had higher benefit levels, which encouraged recipients to stay. The research shows, however, that in states requiring work, recipients left AFDC more quickly if the state was prosperous than if it was not. Prosperity helped welfare reform work.

Although it should make it more difficult to get a job, higher unemployment in a state did not appear to hurt recipients' ability to get off AFDC. In fact it did not affect whether welfare recipients left the rolls or not. I suspect that this was because overall levels of unemployment were low and many states assisted recipients in finding jobs, making that first job possible. However, the level of state unemployment substantially affected the chances of staying off of welfare; former recipients in high unemployment states were more likely to return to public assistance than those in low unemployment states.

How Well-Off Are Families after Leaving AFDC?

As the women described here moved off AFDC they entered the workforce and their financial well-being typically improved. At exit, about half were employed; after two years, two-thirds of those still off welfare were employed (Figure 1). For all leavers (including some who returned before 24 months), earnings rose 17%, and family income rose an average of 41% between the first and 24th month off AFDC (Figure 2). For continuous leavers (those who remained off at 24 months),

FIGURE 1

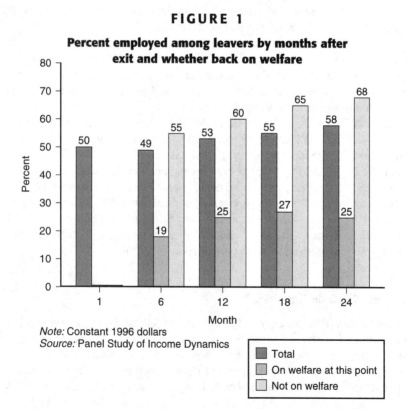

Percent employed among leavers by months after exit and whether back on welfare

Note: Constant 1996 dollars
Source: Panel Study of Income Dynamics

■ Total
▨ On welfare at this point
□ Not on welfare

earnings increased 28% and family income increased 30% over the same two years. But many were still unable to escape poverty (Figure 2). Over half were poor at exit. (Because not all income is counted for determining welfare benefits and because increases in income may result from combining households, not all families are poor at exit.) Two out of five families remained poor two years later. Of course, those who go back on welfare have less income and are highly likely to be poor (Figures 2 and 3).

FIGURE 2

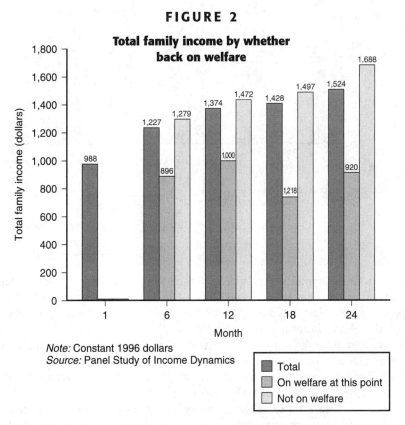

Total family income by whether back on welfare

Note: Constant 1996 dollars
Source: Panel Study of Income Dynamics

Total
On welfare at this point
Not on welfare

How people leave AFDC is important to whether or not they return. Increases in family income and self-sufficiency can occur through either finding a partner or through work. Each one alone is not enough. Mothers who exited AFDC through a combination of work and a partnership had the highest incomes and the lowest rates of poverty.

The kinds of income families receive also affect their chances of returning to AFDC. Receiving child support and supplemental security income (SSI) is associated with staying off AFDC longer, whereas receiving food stamps and private transfers is associated with going back on sooner. Child support and SSI tend to be stable, long-term sources of income. Other research has found child support to be more important than many other sources of support to the well-being of

FIGURE 3

Percent poor by whether back on welfare

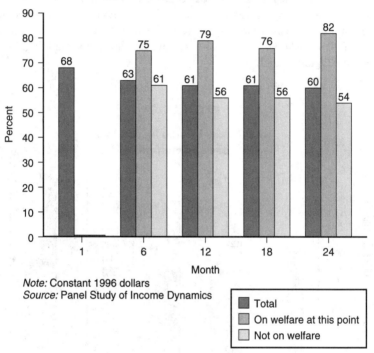

Note: Constant 1996 dollars
Source: Panel Study of Income Dynamics

- Total
- On welfare at this point
- Not on welfare

children. Child support also provides a considerably larger share of income than do other sources. Personal gifts and loans tend to be small and probably not very consistent over time; thus they are not likely to assist a young mother in remaining off welfare. Instead, they may set up a set of obligations that the young woman may have difficulty paying off. Receipt of private transfers and Food Stamps may also be an indicator of financial distress for some. For others off of AFDC, the hassle of continuing to be certified to receive food stamps may outweigh the benefit to be gained. Or they may simply not realize that they remain eligible. The data we used lack information on child care and health insurance coverage, critical support services, so I can draw no conclusions about their likely contribution to self-sufficiency.

WHAT ARE THE EFFECTS OF WORK PROGRAMS ON FAMILIES AND CHILDREN?

In the late 1980s and early 1990s, Canada and states as diverse as Minnesota, Wisconsin, Michigan, California, and Georgia tested a variety of interventions to increase the earnings of welfare families. The results of these earlier projects shed light on what the long-term consequences of the work provisions in TANF may be for families and their children. Women enrolled in programs that included a substantial subsidy for work (which required work of 30 hours or more and which provided substantial support services such as child care) worked more, had higher earnings, and were less likely to be poor. The larger the subsidy, the larger the gains.

None of the programs found significant changes in parents' emotional or physical health, the quality of parent-child interactions, or the home environment.

However, some studies found that children's achievements in school and their behavior improved when they were in the test programs. Minnesota children whose families were in the program did better in school and had fewer behavior problems, probably resulting from the increased financial and emotional security of the family and access to benefits such as health insurance. The achievement of Canadian elementary school-age children in program families also improved more than that of children in nonprogram families. This could possibly be due to the fact that these children were more likely to be in child care and to participate in lessons and sports after school. Adolescent children in program families, however, showed more problem behaviors such as staying out late, smoking, drinking, and using drugs. Lack of supervision may be responsible, as there was no increase in participation in supervised after-school activities among older program youth. Wisconsin boys in the experimental group did significantly better than those in the control group on teacher-reported academic achievement and classroom behavior. These program group boys were more likely to participate in organized out-of-school activities than boys in control families. Children may have more problems if there are no supervised after-school programs.

The conclusion from these early studies is that programs that provide substantial subsidies and services increase family self-sufficiency. Programs that are more modest and that are similar to those the states are now operating post-TANF find very small or no economic effects on families. Numerous state studies of welfare leavers have demonstrated that families subject to these programs do leave welfare, but they improve their economic well-being little. In spite of the lack of economic effects of modest programs, young children do not suffer any harm, though there is some evidence of potential behavioral and emotional adjustment problems, particularly for older children. I conclude that the evidence to date is that, absent large subsidies and support services, the goal of improving family self-sufficiency eludes us still. The fact that such programs do not harm children and at their best may improve their achievement in school is hopeful. The weakest part of the evidence concerns the children; more research is needed.

IMPLICATIONS FOR THE NEXT DECADE

The research reported here describes how welfare policies under state waivers in the 1990s led more recipients to leave AFDC due to work. Since TANF policies passed in 1996 are very similar to waiver policies and since low unemployment played only a supporting role in leaving AFDC in the waiver experience, I would expect this movement to work to have continued through the late 1990s, under TANF. This would be the end of the story except that a substantial fraction of former recipients returned within two years, having failed to become independent. Given what was reported here, it seems quite possible that, absent substantial help for former recipients, returns to TANF may accelerate in the next few years without additional supports for former recipients. Few waiver policies affected returning, but rising unemployment strongly increased the numbers coming back to welfare. In the research described here, raising unemployment by 3 percentage points (from a mean of about 6) doubled reentry. One group of mothers is at especially high risk of failure to become self-sufficient: women with children under age 3. Public policies affect both their risk of leaving and of returning. Attention needs to be paid to their needs. The fraction of eligible children receiving child care assistance is low. Other research has suggested that children's health problems are a major hindrance to their mothers' ability to remain employed since many lack health insurance for their children, in spite of their eligibility. With little job flexibility and accumulated leave time, mothers who have to choose between taking their child to see a doctor and their job are likely to choose the former. It is not surprising that turnover is high and many cycle on and off welfare.

The state waiver experiences suggest changing policies that require mothers of very young children to work. Although the well-being of many former recipient families continues to improve after leaving AFDC, the mothers of very young children are at greater risk of failure because of their greater barriers to self-sufficiency. Their children may also be at risk from poor-quality child care. We could return to a uniform standard exemption from work requirements for TANF mothers of children under age 1. This reduces the cost to mothers of caring for infants and the cost to the government of child care and other support services, as well as dealing with what may become a revolving door. The problem is that, without also instituting paid maternity leave for all mothers, such a policy would not be consistent with other U.S. public policies for nonpoor mothers of infants. Working and nonpoor mothers in America do not receive such a paid maternity leave. The debate over this issue was not fully aired prior to the passage of welfare reform in 1996 and would be worth revisiting with the additional information we have today.

Recipients who leave and stay off AFDC, on average, clearly lead better lives. More get married, find jobs, and increase their household incomes. The bad news is that their own earnings increase only about one-third and 40% of ex-recipients are still poor several years after leaving AFDC. These women may be in precarious situations if their partnerships dissolve. And the good outcomes do not come cheaply; former recipients' incomes do not increase without public subsidies. But supportive public policies can assist low-income families who have exited AFDC. We saw that receipt of child support or SSI was associated with reduced return to public assistance. The next challenge will be to focus upon the highest-risk and most vulnerable group of former AFDC recipients and low-income mothers.

Work was important to the increased well-being of women and their families, and so was partnering, but neither work nor partnering alone substantially increases women's fortunes. Both work and partnering together make women better off. The sticky issue here is what types of partnerships and household sharing are good for women and their children. Conservatives are interested in promoting marriage; however, research suggests that long-term cohabiting relationships may also be good both for the economic stability of the family and for the children. This is clearly an issue to be debated over the next few years.

Based upon recipients' behavior under the waiver experiments of the early to mid-1990s, we conclude that welfare reform encouraged independence within the context of an overall level of a prosperity in which jobs were available for those willing and able to work. We do not know the effects of welfare reform when jobs are scarce, but the results of the waiver experiments predict more returns to public assistance. Policies that would help both former recipients and their working-poor counterparts include stronger work supports and support services. Finally, in the reauthorization debates more thought needs to be given to whether this country really believes that it is cost-effective and desirable to require mothers of infants to work outside the home.

ACKNOWLEDGMENTS

Funding for the research summarized here was provided under a grant from the Economic Research Service, U.S. Department of Agriculture. The interpretations presented are those of the author and do not represent the views of the U.S. Department of Agriculture or its employees.

REFERENCES

Acs, G., and Loprest, P. (2001). *Initial Synthesis report of the Findings from ASPE's "Leavers" Grants.* Washington, DC: The Urban Institute, January 4. http://aspe.hhs.gov/hsp/leavers/synthesis01/

Brauner, S., and Loprest, P. (1999). *Where are they Now? What States' Studies of People who Left Welfare Tell Us* [Issues and Options]. A, No. A-32. Washington, DC: The Urban Institute. http://www.urban.org/

Haskins, R., Isabel Sawhill I., and Weaver K. 2001. *Welfare Reform: An Overview of Effects to Date.* Welfare Reform and Beyond Brief #1. Washington, DC: The Brookings Institution. http://www.brook.edu/wrb/publications/pb/pb01/pb01.htm

Hofferth, S. L., Smith, J., McLoyd, V., and Finkelstein, J. (2000). Achievement and Behavior among Children of Welfare Recipients, Welfare Leavers, and Low Income Single Mothers. *Journal of Social Issues,* 56(4), 749–776.

Hofferth, S. L., Stanhope, S. and Harris, K. M. (2000a, October). *Exiting Welfare in the 1990s: Did Public Policy Influence Recipients' Behavior?* Ann Arbor, MI: Institute for Social Research. http://www.psc.isr.umich.edu/pubs/papers/rr01-469.pdf

Hofferth, S. L., Stanhope, S., and Harris, K. M. (2000b, December). *Remaining Off Welfare in the 1990s: The Influence of Public Policy and Economic Conditions.* Ann Arbor, MI: University of Michigan Institute for Social Research. http://ww.psc.isr.umich.edu/pubs/papers/rr01-468.pdf

Loprest, P. (1999). *Families Who Left Welfare: Who Are They and How Are They Doing?* [Assessing the new Federalism]. Discussion Paper, vol. 99–02. Washington, DC: The Urban Institute. http://www.urban.org/

Moffitt, R., and Roff, J. (2000). *The Diversity of Welfare Leavers* [Policy Brief 00-2]. Baltimore, MD: Johns Hopkins University. http://www.jhu.edu/~welfare/

Morris, P. A., Huston, A.; Duncan, G. J., Crosby, D. A., and Bos, J. M. 2001. *How Welfare and Work Policies Affect Children: A Synthesis of Research.* New York: Manpower Demonstration Research Corporation, March. http://www.mdrc.org/NextGeneration/

ARTICLE 3

THE EFFECTS OF WELFARE REFORM ON THE REPRODUCTIVE HEALTH OF WOMEN

Arden Handler, Meagan Zimbeck,
Wendy Chavkin, and Kathleen Adams

INTRODUCTION

Welfare benefits for women and children in the United States have always come with strings attached.[1] Since the creation of Aid to Families with Dependent Children (AFDC) in 1935, legislators have linked cash benefits to women's reproductive behavior. How to oblige poor women to bear and raise children in marriages (or not at all) has been a central concern of social welfare policy in this country for nearly seventy years.[2] This concern also serves as the foundation for the provisions of the 1996 Personal Responsibility and Work Opportunity Reconciliation Act (PRWORA). The Act ended "welfare as we know it," but left in place moral levers on poor women's reproductive behavior.[3] Poor women's entitlement to income supports has vanished, but strong strings remain attached to the limited benefits they may receive through AFDC's successor, Temporary Assistance to Needy Families (TANF).[4]

This chapter will examine the main mechanisms through which the PRWORA can affect the reproductive health of women: changes in *access to health care* and changes resulting from *reproductive-related provisions* of the PRWORA.

BACKGROUND

AFDC was launched as part of the Social Security Act in 1935 as an alternative to earnings for women whose husbands had either died or abandoned their families. AFDC relieved poor single mothers of the necessity of wage earning so that they could care for their children.[5] The cash benefits provided by AFDC have historically been lower and more restricted than the pensions provided in the Social

Security system.[6] AFDC's low payments have provided a safety net for women and children, but were never enough to lift them out of poverty.[7-9]

This lifetime guarantee of support, however meager, to all eligible families ended on July 22, 1996, with the passage of the PRWORA. The Act replaced the AFDC entitlement program with the block grant program known as TANF. The PRWORA responded to what was viewed as a social problem—the pathological "dependency"—not the poverty—of poor women.[10] This so-called problem was addressed through time limits and work requirements. Women who accept cash benefits through TANF may do so only for five lifetime years. They are also obliged to fulfill work requirements, accepting employment even at very low wages.[11] The PRWORA also prohibited many legal immigrants from gaining access to public benefits and reaffirmed a federal bar that prevents illegal immigrants from utilizing most federal programs.[12]

In a sense, the framers of PRWORA proposed a nostalgic solution to female poverty. Three of the four statutory purposes of the PRWORA sought specifically to make men, rather than the government, responsible for supporting poor women and children.[4] Indirectly, marriage and the two-parent family were heralded as the solution. For example, the PRWORA allows states to sanction benefits for women who bear additional children outside of marriage or who do not disclose the identity of their children's father(s).

The PRWORA has succeeded in reducing poor women's reliance on government benefits. Since 1996, national welfare rolls have dropped more than 44%.[13] There is no evidence, however, that the displaced economic needs of poor women are being taken up by men.[4] Although there has been a decline in the percentage of children living with a single mother since welfare reform, there is concern about the stability of these households.[14] Nor are the economic needs of poor women being met in the low-wage labor market.[15] Many women are moving into low-wage jobs while paying childcare costs and many are not using benefits (e.g., food stamps) for which they still qualify.[11,16] A woman with three children who works full time at the minimum wage earns only 64% of the federal poverty level (FPL) for a family of four.[15] Further, finding employment is not easy. Employment rates among welfare leavers are barely above 50% in some states[17] and nationally equal to 54%.[18]

Research suggests that a major effect of welfare reform has been a deepening of poverty among low-income families.[19,20] Since it is known that low-income individuals are at higher risk of poor health outcomes,[21,22] there is concern that the PRWORA has had additional detrimental effects on health status. Because low-income families are no longer guaranteed the cash to cover basic needs,[7] their risk of stress and other poverty-related health related outcomes may have increased.

Despite this concern, little attention has been paid to the effect of the PRWORA on health or reproductive outcomes. However, there are at least two specific mechanisms through which welfare reform may affect reproductive health. First, poor women may have decreased access to health care due to welfare reform-related changes in the Medicaid program. Second, the reproductive provisions of the PRWORA, including the family cap, "illegitimacy bonus," the funding of abstinence only education, and the requirements by some states for TANF recipients to attend family planning counseling[23] may contribute to changes in sexual activity, contraceptive use, and childbearing among low-income women. These two mechanisms are discussed in detail below.

ACCESS TO HEALTH CARE

Medicaid Enrollment

The PRWORA may have a direct effect on reproductive health through changes in women's access to health care. In an effort to retain access to health insurance for low-income families, the PRWORA decoupled Medicaid eligibility from eligibility for TANF. Although TANF is no longer an entitlement program, low-income individuals are entitled to Medicaid if they meet their state's AFDC income and resource tests as of July 16, 1996 (new category called Section 1931). States can also expand coverage beyond these minimum levels, and an increasing number of states have done so. In addition, the Transitional Medical Assistance (TMA) program provides 12 months of transitional Medicaid coverage to individuals leaving welfare for work.

Yet, this approach was not taken for immigrants who were singled out for particularly harsh treatment under PRWORA. Welfare reform did not alter the situation of undocumented immigrants, who were already ineligible for public benefits including Medicaid.[24] However, legal immigrants can now obtain Medicaid only if they fall into one of the new, more restrictive categories of "qualified immigrants," and this depends on when they immigrated.[25] Qualified immigrants entering post PRWORA are subject to a five-year ban on public benefits, including Medicaid.[26]

The decoupling of Medicaid eligibility from eligibility for TANF had the potential to ensure coverage for most low-income families, but most of the evidence suggests this has not occurred.[27–29] Post PRWORA there have been dramatic reductions in Medicaid enrollment for families and children,[30–32] and it appears that much of this has been inappropriate.[32]

As advocates had warned,[33] many families who were dropped from or failed to enroll in cash assistance have not enrolled in the Medicaid program despite their continued eligibility.[27–30,32] Chavkin and colleagues demonstrated that declines in Medicaid were associated with state's choices to implement diversion policies when individuals apply for TANF.[34] Since in most states there is still a joint application process for Medicaid and TANF, women applying for Medicaid are vulnerable to TANF-related practices such as diversions and sanctions.[34]

In addition, many individuals who lose Medicaid eligibility due to increased wages do not enroll in the TMA program because they are not aware of eligibility or are not encouraged to apply.[29] Furthermore, since the TMA program requires enrollment in Medicaid for at least three of the past six months, women applying for TANF who are immediately placed in work programs may lose Medicaid eligibility before qualifying for TMA.[35]

The declines in Medicaid enrollment for women in particular have been dramatic. In 1998, Medicaid covered 6 million women ages 15 to 44—1.5 million women fewer than in 1994.[31] Low-income single mothers experienced the largest drop; between 1994 and 1998 their enrollment rate dropped from 50% to 39%, and uninsuredness among this group rose from 23% to 30%.[36] A recent Families USA study[37] examined parents' enrollment in Medicaid post PRWORA. In the 15 states with the largest number of uninsured low-income adults, the number of parents on Medicaid, the majority of whom were women, dropped by 27% between 1996 and 1999. However, the most recent data show a turnaround. The number of adults (nonelderly) on Medicaid grew by 100,000 in 2000.[38] This turnaround appears to reflect some very recent state Medicaid expansion efforts and outreach activities associated with the State Children's Health Insurance Program (SCHIP).

Importantly, the general decline in Medicaid coverage since welfare reform has not been compensated for by an increase in private insurance coverage; the percentage of uninsured Americans in 1998 increased to 16.3% from 15.2% in 1994; this was equivalent to 44.3 million in 1998.[31] In 1999, there was a slight decline in the number of uninsured Americans to 42.1 million; yet this was still higher than the 1994 figure of 39.8 million.[39]

Medicaid Enrollment, Well-Woman Care, and Family Planning

Nearly half—46%—of all publicly funded family planning services in 1994 were paid for by the Medicaid program.[40] The aforementioned declines in Medicaid coverage are beginning to negatively affect family planning (FP) providers who serve low-income populations. Many are reporting a decrease in revenues from their Medicaid patients with a simultaneous rise in the number of uninsured patients whose care must be subsidized.[31] If this trend continues, it will jeopardize the ability of FP providers to provide care to all those in need.

More generally, women without health insurance coverage fail to make family-planning or well-woman care visits.[41] As such, they are less likely to access routine prevention services such as pap smears, screenings for genitourinary tract infections and sexually transmitted diseases, as well as screenings for hypertension and diabetes.

States may prevent the decline in the use of Medicaid family planning services through the adoption of Medicaid waivers for family planning. As of August 1, 2001, sixteen states had passed waivers to extend Medicaid coverage for family planning services for women who would not otherwise have been eligible. They either extend Medicaid coverage for family planning services to women who are only covered during pregnancy or postpartum, expand Medicaid eligibility for family planning services solely on the basis of income to individuals (women or men) who were not previously covered, or extend Medicaid coverage for women losing Medicaid for any reason (Delaware).[42] Although early in 2001 the Bush Administration was ready to halt the use of Medicaid family planning waivers, strong criticism led to a reversal of this position.

Medicaid Enrollment, Prenatal Care, and Pregnancy Outcomes

Detecting the impact of changes in Medicaid coverage as the result of welfare reform on access to prenatal care is made more complex by the fact that in the late 1980s and early 1990s there were several expansions in Medicaid coverage for pregnant women. By April 1990 states were required to provide coverage to pregnant women up to 133% of the Federal Poverty Level (FPL). As of October 2000, 39 states had gone beyond this level, including 12 states and the District of Columbia who cover pregnant women at or above 200% of the federal poverty level.[43]

Given these expansions, there should be virtually no effect of welfare reform on prenatal care coverage and use of prenatal care services. However, although the Medicaid expansions have increased the proportion of births paid for by Medicaid to 35% in 1998 from 17% in 1985,[43,44] many women still fail to enroll in Medicaid during pregnancy and consequently may delay or even forgo entry into prenatal care. In fact, (see Table 1) while increasing in the early 1990s, the percentage of pregnant women covered by Medicaid declined from almost 24% in 1993 to only 15% by 1997. The increase in private insurance over this time period was not enough to offset this trend, leaving almost 14% of pregnant women without coverage sometime during pregnancy.[45]

TABLE 1 DISTRIBUTION OF HEALTH INSURANCE COVERAGE AMONG PREGNANT WOMEN, 1990–1997

	Source of Coverage				
Year	Private Insurance	Medicaid	Other	Uninsured	Total (Millions of women)
1997	69.0%	15.2%	2.1%	13.7%	3.4
1996	66.1	18.3	1.9	13.7	3.4
1995	63.2	20.8	2.4	13.6	3.4
1994	63.1	20.0	4.2	12.7	3.4
1993	62.3	23.6	2.9	11.2	3.6
1992	61.4	23.0	3.7	11.9	3.6
1991	61.6	22.2	4.2	12.0	3.5
1990	63.7	21.6	3.7	11.0	3.6

Available: http://www.modimes.org/HealthLibrary2/PubPolicyStudies/Default.htm
Source: Thorpe, Kenneth. *The Distribution of Health Insurance Coverage Among Pregnant Women, 1990–1997.* Washington, DC: March of Dimes, 1999. [45]

Lack of insurance coverage for pregnancy is concentrated among the lowest income women. Over 28% of pregnant women in poverty in 1997 were uninsured versus only 3% of those earning at least three times the poverty level.[45] Yet, over 77% of uninsured pregnant women were eligible for Medicaid in 1997.[45] So, whereas Medicaid paid for an expanding proportion of births during the 1990s (i.e., Medicaid reimbursement was obtained by the hospital to pay for the births of uninsured women), many women remained uninsured for all or part of their pregnancy despite expanded Medicaid eligibility. This may have reduced the potential positive impact of the Medicaid expansions on perinatal outcomes.

Although several studies are under way, there are insufficient data to determine the effect of the PRWORA on prenatal care use and pregnancy outcomes. The few analyses available do not yet suggest a major negative effect. Currie and Grogger, using data from the national Natality files from 1990–1996 (prior to PRWORA), found that decreases in welfare caseloads reduced the use of prenatal care, especially among African Americans, but this had minimal impact on birth weights.[46] Similarly, Korenbrot et al. examined the effect of changes in welfare and immigration policy in California on births to foreign-born women from 1990–1997 and found that the volume of births to foreign-born women using Medicaid declined.[47] However, there was no decrease in the use of prenatal care by foreign-born women, and birth outcomes were no worse. Likewise, an analysis by Joyce et al. compared prenatal care and birth outcomes between U.S. born and foreign-born Latinos between 1995 and 1998 and found no significant changes in the percentage of uninsured, pregnant, foreign-born Latinos and no significant change in their prenatal care initiation and birth outcomes.[48]

All of the analyses published to date utilize data from years prior to when a significant impact of PRWORA might be expected. As such, it will be essential to examine changes in prenatal care utilization and pregnancy outcomes based on data from years substantially after the passage of PRWORA. It will also be important to examine PRWORA's effects on the pregnancy experiences of distinct groups of women: those receiving TANF as well as their low-income counterparts who are no longer receiving TANF, or those who are eligible but have not even applied. Additional studies that examine the pregnancy experience of immigrants and low-income women of color are also needed.

Food Stamps and the WIC Program

Although not thought of as preconceptional or prenatal care per se, access to the Special Supplemental Nutrition Program for Women, Infants, and Children (WIC) and food stamps prior to and during pregnancy can have a significant impact on reproductive health. Women with low pre-pregnancy weights and/or who do not gain a sufficient amount of weight are at higher risk of low birth weight and pre-term delivery.[49] Welfare reform drastically altered the food safety-net, eliminating more funds from the Food Stamp Program (FSP) than from any other program; the Congressional Budget Office (CBO) estimated that cuts in the FSP would generate about $23 billion in "savings" by 2002.[50] Reductions in benefits per person and restrictions on eligibility, along with economic growth, have contributed to a dramatic decline in FSP participation. The FSP caseloads had fallen from 27.5 million people in 1994 to 18.2 million people in 1999.[51] A recent USDA study found that at least 12 million people were not receiving food stamps even though they were eligible.[52] Poor women who, under TANF work requirements, have been forced into low-wage jobs, experience reductions in food stamp benefits as they begin to draw a meager income.[11] Such reductions cause them not only to decrease spending on food, but can also affect their spending on housing, clothing, and medical care.[50]

As the FSP caseloads fall, we might expect participation in the less restrictive WIC program to increase. The WIC program, which provides not only food assistance, but also nutritional counseling and referral services, has been effective in reducing the incidence of low birthweight[53] and other health problems among children.[51] Although not representative of the nation as a whole, an Illinois study found that Food Stamp Program participation fell by 22% while WIC participation increased by 10% between 1993–1996 (years prior to welfare reform).[51] Unlike the FSP, however, WIC is not an entitlement program, and hence, not sufficiently funded to meet the food security needs of all low-income pregnant women.[54] Given the declines in food stamp enrollment and the inherent limitations of the WIC program, the effect of welfare reform on women's nutritional health remains a concern.

SPECIAL PROVISIONS OF PRWORA AIMED AT REPRODUCTIVE HEALTH

Illegitimacy Bonus

Although the rise in nonmarital childbearing leveled off in the 1990s,[55] and the majority of nonmarital births are not to recipients of public assistance,[56] the framers of PRWORA targeted "illegitimacy" as a major social problem. To encourage states to decrease nonmarital births while not increasing abortion rates, Congress included an "illegitimacy bonus." For the four years beginning in 1999, the five states that achieve the greatest decreases in nonmarital births for all women while not increasing abortion rates are to receive a $20 million bonus. In 1999, Alabama, California, the District of Columbia, Massachusetts, and Michigan received the bonuses based on modest changes in their rates.[23] Alabama, Michigan, the District of Columbia, Arizona, and Illinois were recipients in 2000.[57]

Because these first awards were based on data from 1994–1998, it is unlikely that that they are a reflection of initiatives implemented to obtain the bonus. Indeed these changes actually reflect long-standing secular trends. Rates of teen sexual activity have been declining slightly—data from NSFG show that the proportion of teenagers who had ever experienced sex decreased from 52.6% to 51.3% between 1988 and 1995.[58] In addition, contraceptive use has been increasing,[59] rates of abortion have been decreasing,[60] and rates of adolescent childbearing have also been declining for all age and race/ethnic groups.[61]

States have varied in the vigorousness of their efforts to win the illegitimacy bonus and some recipients of the bonus did not even have specific policies or programs in place to achieve this goal.[23] Some states have, however, developed policies to increase contraceptive use among women on welfare, including requiring TANF recipients to attend family planning counseling or to be provided information about family planning. Others have focused on increasing use of prepregnancy family planning services, while others are attempting to use TANF funds to reduce adolescent pregnancy rates.[23,56] Although these efforts may actually increase the availability or use of family planning, they may also serve as ways to penalize women. For example, women on TANF may be required to attend family planning counseling, which usually requires Medicaid coverage; however, failure to comply with this requirement may lead to sanctions including loss of Medicaid.[23] Another negative effect might occur if states further restrict access to abortion as a way to ensure lower abortion rates in order to win the illegitimacy bonus.[62]

Family Cap

The framers of the PRWORA viewed the welfare "problem" as an issue of dependency, furthering the notion that welfare recipients have additional children to receive increased benefits. Even though there is little evidence that payment levels affect childbearing decisions,[63] even prior to welfare reform, 19 states had obtained Section 1115 waivers to enact a family cap,[64,65] a policy which disallows additional benefits when a new child is born in the family. Federal law does not require a family cap, but states have this option; 23 states have some sort of family cap.[64] Data from 16 states show that family cap policies have resulted in more than 83,000 children being capped.[65]

Although the effect of the family cap on women's childbearing decisions is equivocal,[57,63,64] its effect on the economic well-being of families with capped children is not. The family cap is a redundant, noneffective, and directly punitive welfare reform strategy, and advocates in states with a family cap policy should continue to monitor its effects and simultaneously work for its elimination.

Abstinence Education

In light of their belief that nonmarital childbearing is a fundamental cause of welfare dependency, the framers of PRWORA also included an abstinence education provision which affects all families, not just families receiving welfare. Although not the first federal effort to support abstinence education (i.e., the 1981 Adolescent Family Life Act supported such programs),[66] the PRWORA amended Title V of the Social Security Act (Section 510) to include a $50 million program over five years for abstinence education. The amendment outlines eight specific principles of abstinence education, including teaching that "a mutually faithful monogamous relationship in the context of marriage is the expected standard of human sexual activity." As part of Title V, states are required to match every four dollars of federal funds with three dollars in state funds, making the total annual abstinence education expenditure closer to $90 million.[67] States are required to adhere to all eight principles, but they are allowed flexibility in implementation. States have awarded abstinence education funding to a variety of agencies including schools, local health agencies, faith-based organizations, as well as other community-based organizations.

A major concern is the impact these federal dollars may have on a long-standing movement to increase the availability of comprehensive sexuality education in the schools. Importantly, the majority of U.S. adults support such education and believe it should include information about contraception for the prevention of pregnancy, STDs, and HIV.[68] A recent examination of sexuality education policies in a representative sample of schools (825 school districts) found that only 14% have a comprehensive sexuality education policy. Fifty-one percent of the districts have what is called an abstinence-based or abstinence-plus policy. Thirty-five percent of the districts report that abstinence is taught as the only option for adolescents and discussions of contraception are either forbidden or its alleged ineffectiveness in preventing pregnancy or STDs is emphasized.[68] Although not necessarily providing funds for the programs included in this study, the PRWORA has provided strong federal endorsement for such abstinence-only programs.

Even though little emphasis has been placed on evaluation, proponents of abstinence education are quick to claim credit for recent declines in pregnancy and birth rates among teens. However, data show that teen pregnancy and teen birth rates began declining dramatically in the early 1990s after a steep increase in the late 1980s, returning to a long-term trend of steadily declining teen birth rates since the 1960s.[61] In addition, the Alan Guttmacher Institute (AGI) finds that only 25% of the drop in the teenage pregnancy rate between 1988 and 1995 resulted from increased abstinence. About three-quarters of the decline was attributable to decreased pregnancy rates among sexually experienced teens. Importantly, only one-quarter of the decrease among sexually experienced teens was due to a decline in the frequency of sexual intercourse. The other three-quarters was due to a lower pregnancy rate among those having sex, which in turn, is attributed to increased use of long-term contraceptives including injectables.[58]

Those who have been involved in evaluations of teen pregnancy prevention programs for decades question the efficacy of abstinence-only programs. The National Campaign to Prevent Teen Pregnancy in its recently released report *Emerging Answers* reviews studies that evaluate different models of teenage pregnancy prevention programs.[69] According to the report, eight teenage pregnancy programs demonstrated strong evidence of success—five are sex education programs that are not short-term, two are service learning programs, and one is an intensive program that combines sex education, comprehensive health care, and activities such as tutoring.

The *Emerging Answers* report notes that there has been very little rigorous evaluation of abstinence-only programs. Only three studies focusing on abstinence education met the criteria for review and "none of the three evaluated programs showed an overall positive effect on sexual behavior, nor did they affect contraceptive use among sexually active participants." More insights should be forthcoming by 2003, when the results of a well-designed federal study of abstinence education authorized by the Balanced Budget Act of 1997 become available.[69]

The current reality of teen sexual behavior and evidence from rigorous evaluations make it clear that comprehensive sexuality education is the most effective approach to ensure that teens are empowered to make decisions to decrease their risk of unintended pregnancy as well as STDs and HIV. However, until abstinence education falls out of favor with policymakers such as the framers of PRWORA as well as local school boards, abstinence-based rather than abstinence-only education may be the only feasible alternative to enable teens to obtain critical information necessary to protect themselves.

In sum, the reproductive related components of the PRWORA are direct attempts by policymakers to control the reproductive lives of low-income women and, in the case of abstinence education, to promote an agenda for all families that restricts sexual activity to monogamous heterosexual relationships within marriage. Such efforts at social control are at best blatantly hypocritical, given the current devolution of federal responsibility for social programs, and at worst, an aggregious attempt to interfere in women's reproductive decisions with serious potential to negatively affect the health of low-income women and their families.

CONCLUSION

There is a great likelihood that the PRWORA of 1996 will have a substantial effect on the reproductive health status of low-income women. Through its potential to increase economic hardship for women forced into low-wage jobs without adequate child care support, to decrease access to health insurance and health services through changes related to the Medicaid program, and through its specific provisions aimed at women's decisions about sexuality and childbearing, a multitude of effects are possible. For advocates, researchers, and policymakers, the challenge is to disentangle the potential web of effects and to be able to link these outcomes to changes in welfare policy. Although the task ahead is formidable, it is hoped that the scheduled reauthorization of PRWORA in 2002 is based on evidence about the health and well-being of the women and families affected by welfare reform, rather than based on rhetoric that blames and continues to punish low-income women for the fact of their poverty.

REFERENCES

1. Soss, J., Schram, S. F., Vartanian, T. P., and O'Brien, E. (2001). Setting the terms of relief: Explaining state policy choices in the devolution revolution. *American Journal of Political Science 45*(2): 378–395.
2. Lewis, J. (1998). 'Work,' 'Welfare' and Lone Mothers. *Political Quarterly.* 69:4–13.
3. Chavkin, W. and Wise, P. (1998). Welfare reform and women's health. *American Journal of Public Health, 88*(7): 1017–1018.
4. Mink, G. (1998). *Welfare's End*. Ithaca, New York: Cornell University Press.
5. Tilly, L. (1997). Women, work, and citizenship. *International Labor and Working-Class History* (52): 1–26.
6. Kornbluh, F. (1996). The new literature on gender and the Welfare State: The U.S. case. *Feminist Studies 22*(1):171–187.
7. O'Campo, P. and Rojas-Smith, L. (1998). Welfare reform and women's health: Review of the literature and implications for state policy. *Journal of Public Health Policy.* 19: 420–446.
8. Children's Defense Fund (1998). *The State of America's Children, Yearbook, 1998.* Washington, DC: Children's Defense Fund.
9. Fox Piven, F. and Cloward, R. A. (1993). *Regulating the poor: The functions of public welfare.* New York: Vintage Books.
10. Fraser, N. and Gordon, L. (1994). "Dependency" demystified: Inscriptions of power in a keyword of the Welfare State. *Social Politics 1*(1): 4–31.
11. Edin, K. and Lein, L. (1997). *Making ends meet: How single mothers survive welfare and low-wage work.* New York: Russell Sage Foundation.
12. Kaiser Family Foundation (2001). *Medicaid eligibility and citizenship status: Policy implications for immigrant population* [On-line]. Available: http://www.kff.org/content/2001/2241/
13. Golonka, S. (2000). *State Outreach and Enrollment Strategies to Improve Low-Income Families' Access to Medicaid.* Washington, DC: National Governors Association [On-line]. Available: http://www.nga.org/center/divisions/1,1188,C_ISSUE_BRIEF^D_370,00.html
14. Harden, B. (2001). 2-Parent Families Rise After Change in Welfare Laws. *New York Times*, August 12, 2001. Page 1.
15. Lawton, E., Leiter, K., Todd, J., and Smith, L. (1999). Welfare reform: Advocacy and intervention in the health care setting. *Public Health Reports*, 114 (November/December): 540–549.
16. Primus, W., Rawlings, L., Larin, K., and Porter, K. (1999). *The initial impact of welfare reform on the incomes of single mother families.* Washington, DC: Center on Budget and Policy Priorities.
17. Brauner, S. and Loprest, P. (2000). *Where Are They Now? What States' Studies of People Who Left Welfare Tell Us.* Washington, DC: The Urban Institute [On-line]. Available: http://newfederalism.urban.org/html/anf_32.html
18. Loprest, P. (1999). Washington, DC: *Families who left welfare: Who are they and how are they doing?* Washington, DC: Urban Institute, Assessing the New Federalism [On-line]. Available: http://newfederalism.urban.org/html/discussion99-02.html

19. Loprest, P. (2001). *How Are Families that Left Welfare Doing? A Comparison of Early and Recent Welfare Leavers.* Washington, DC: Urban Institute, 2001.

20. Children's Defense Fund (2001). *Families Struggling to Make It in the Workforce: A Post Welfare Report* [On-line]. Available: http://www.childrens defense.org/fair-start-pubs.htm

21. Wise, P. and Meyers, A. (1988) Poverty and child health. *Pediatric Clinics of North America 35*(6): 1171–1186.

22. Starfield, B. and Budetti, P. (1985, Part II). Child health status and risk factors. *Health Services Research.* 19(6): 817–886.

23. Chavkin, W., Draut, T., Romero, D. and Wise, P. (2000). Sex, reproduction and welfare reform. *Georgetown Journal on Poverty Law and Policy 7*(2): 379–393.

24. Fix, M. and Passell, J. (1999). Trends in Non-Citizens' and Citizens' Use of Public Benefits Following Welfare Reform 1994–1997. Washington, DC: The Urban Institute.

25. Kaiser Family Foundation (2001). *Medicaid eligibility and citizenship status: policy implications for immigrant population* [On-line]. Available: http://www.kff.org/content/2001/2241/

26. Ellwood, M. and Ku, L. (1998). Welfare and immigration reforms: Unintended side effects for Medicaid. *Health Affairs*, May/June:137–151.

27. Garrett, B. and Holahan, J. (2000). Health insurance coverage after welfare. *Health Affairs* 19(1): 175–184.

28. Garrett, B. and Holahan, J. (2000). *Welfare Leavers, Medicaid Coverage, and Private Health Insurance.* Washington, DC: Urban Institute [On-line]. Available: http://newfederalism.urban.org/html/series_b/b13/b13.html

29. Guyer, J. (2000). Health care after welfare: *An update of findings from state-level Leaver Studies.* Washington DC: Center on Budget and Policy Priorities; August 16, 2000.

30. Ellwood, M. (1999) The Medicaid eligibility maze: Coverage expands, but enrollment problems persist. Findings from a five-state study. Washington, DC: Kaiser Commission on Medicaid and the Uninsured and the Urban Institute's Assessing the New Federalism Project.

31. Gold, R. B. (1999). Implications for family planning of post-welfare reform insurance trends. *The Guttmacher Report on Public Policy.* December, 1999: 6–9.

32. Families USA (1999). *Losing health insurance: The unintended consequences of welfare reform* [On-line]. Available: http://www.familiesusa.org/unintpdf.htm

33. Rosenbaum, S. and Darnell, J. (1996). An analysis of the Medicaid and health-related provisions of the Personal Responsibility and Work Opportunity Reconciliation Act of 1996. Washington, DC: Center for Health Policy Research at the George Washington University Medical Center.

34. Chavkin, W., Romero, D., and Wise, P. (2000). State welfare reform policies and declines in health insurance. *American Journal of Public Health, 90*(6): 900–908.

35. Dion, M. R. and Pavetti, L. (2000). *Access to and participation in Medicaid and the Food Stamp Program: A review of the recent literature.* Washington, DC: Mathematica Policy Research, Inc. [On-line]. Available: http://www.acf.dhhs.gov/programs/opre/med-fs.htm

36. Wyn, R., Solis, B., Ojeda, V., and Pourat, N. (2001). *Falling through the cracks: Health insurance coverage of low-income women.* Menlo Park, CA: Kaiser Family Foundation.

37. Families USA (2000). *Go directly to work, do not collect health insurance: Low-income parents lose Medicaid* [On-line]. Available: http://www.familiesusa.org/pubs/gowrk.htm

38. Ku, L. and Guyer, J. (2001). *Medicaid spending: Rising again, but not to crisis levels.* Washington, D.C.: Center on Budget and Policy Priorities.

39. Kaiser Commission on Medicaid and the Uninsured (2000). *Health Insurance Coverage in America: 1999 Data Update* [On-line]. Available: http://www.kff.org/content/2001/2222/

40. The Alan Guttmacher Institute (1997). *Issues in Brief: Title X and the U.S. Family Planning Effort.* New York: Alan Guttmacher Institute.

41. Weisman, C. and Poole, V. (1999). Health care services and systems for women of reproductive age. In H. Grason, J. Hutchins, and G. Silver (Eds.) *Charting a Course for the Future of Women's and Perinatal Health: Volume II- Reviews of Key Issues*, pp. 25–40. Baltimore, MD: Women's and Children's Health Policy Center at the Johns Hopkins School of Public Health.

42. The Alan Guttmacher Institute (2001). *State Policies in Brief: Medicaid Family Planning Waivers.* [On-Line], Available: http://www.agi-usa.org/pubs

43. National Governors Association (2001). *Maternal and Child Health (MCH) Update: States have expanded eligibility and increased access to health care for pregnant women and children.* Washington, DC: National Governor's Association.

44. The Alan Guttmacher Institute. (1987). *Blessed Events and the Bottom Line: Financing Maternity Care in the United States.* New York: Alan Guttmacher Institute.

45. Thorpe, K. E. (1999). *The distribution of health insurance coverage among pregnant women, 1990–1997.* [On-line]. Available: http://www.modimes.org/PublicAffairs2/distribution.htm

46. Currie, J. and Grogger, J. (2000). *Medicaid expansions and welfare contractions: Offsetting the effects on prenatal care and infant health?* (working paper) Cambridge, MA: National Bureau of Economic Research.

47. Korenbrot, C. C., Dudley, R. A., and Greene, J. D. (2000). Changes in births to foreign-born women after welfare and immigration policy reforms in California. *Maternal and Child Health Journal 4*(4): 241–250.

48. Joyce, T. (2000, April 4). *Preliminary Findings: Welfare reform and the perinatal health of immigrants.* Paper presented at the 28th seminar on MCHB-funded research projects, Rockford, MD.

49. Worthington-Roberts, B.S. and Klerman, L.V. (1990). Maternal nutrition. In I. Merkatz and J.E. Thompson (Eds.) *New Perspectives on Prenatal Care*, pp. 235–271. Thompson, NY: Elsevier Science Publication Co.

50. Gunderson, C., LeBlanc, M., and Kuhn, B. (1999). The Changing Food Assistance Landscape. *Agricultural Economics Report No. 773.* Washington, DC: US Department of Agriculture.

51. Lee, B.J. Bilaver, L., and Goerge, R. (2001). Health and welfare of Illinois children: Shifting WIC and food stamp use. *Poverty Research News 5*(2): 8–9.

52. Becker, E. (2001, February 26). Millions Eligible for Food Stamps Aren't Applying. *The New York Times*, pp. A1, A11.

53. Avruch, S. (1995). Savings achieved by giving WIC benefits to women prenatally. *Public Health Reports 110*(Jan/Feb): 27–35.

54. Laraia, B. and Dodd, J. (1997) Issues in Maternal and Child Health Nutrition. In *Maternal and Child Health, Programs, Problems and Policy in Public Health,* J. Kotch (ed.), Gaithersburg, Md: Aspen Publishers.

55. National Center for Health Statistics/Centers for Disease Control. Nonmarital Childbearing in the United States, 1940–99, *National Vital Statistics Reports* 48(16), Oct. 18, 2000.

56. Donovan, P. (1999). The "Illegitimacy Bonus" and state efforts to reduce out-of-wedlock births. *Family Planning Perspectives 31*(2): 95–97.

57. Boonstra, H. (2000). Welfare and the drive to reduce "illegitimacy." *Guttmacher Report on Public Policy 3*(6).

58. The Alan Guttmacher Institute. Occasional Report. Why is Teenage Pregnancy Declining? *The roles of abstinence, sexual activity and contraceptive use* [On-line]. Available: http://www.agiusa.org/pubs/or_teen_preg_decline.html

59. Piccinino, L. and Mosher, W. Trends in contraceptive use in the United States: 1982–1995. (1998). *Family Planning Perspectives 30*:4–10, 46.

60. U.S. Department of Health and Human Services (2000, December 8). CDC Surveillance Summaries no. ss-11. *Morbidity and Mortality Weekly Report* vol. 49.

61. National Center for Health Statistics/Centers for Disease Control. Variations in teenage birth rates, 1991–98: National and state trends. *National Vital Statistics reports,* 48(6), April 24, 2000.

62. The Alan Guttmacher Institute (2000). *Facts in Brief: Welfare reform, marriage, and sexual behavior* [On-line]. Available: http://www.agi-usa.org/pubs/

63. Wise, P., Chavkin, W., & Romero, D. (1999). Assessing the effects of welfare reform policies on reproductive and infant health. *American Journal of Public Health, 89*(10): 1514–1521.

64. Center for Law and Social Policy (1999). *Caps on Kids: Family Cap in the New Welfare Era* [On-line]. Available: http://www.clasp.org/pubs/caps_on_kids.htm#top

65. Stark, S. and Levin-Epstein, J. (1999). *Excluded Children: Family Cap in a New Era.* Washington, DC: Center for Law and Social Policy [On-Line]. Available: http://www.clasp.org/pubs/teens/excludedchildren.htm

66. National Abortion Rights Action League (1999). *NARAL Factsheets: The need for comprehensive sexuality education* [On-line]. Available: http//www.naral.org/publications/facts/compresed.html

67. Association of Maternal and Child Health Programs. (1999). Abstinence education in the states. *Implementation of the 1996 Abstinence Education Law: Results of a Survey of State Title V Programs.* Washington, DC: Association of Maternal and Child Health Programs.

68. Landry, D., Kaeser, L., and Richards, C. (1999). Abstinence promotion and the provision of information about contraception in public school district sexuality education policies. *Family Planning Perspectives 31*(6): 280–286.

69. Kirby, D. (2001). *Emerging answers: research findings on programs to reduce teen pregnancy* (summary). Washington, DC: National Campaign to Prevent Teen Pregnancy.

ARTICLE 4

THE SOCIAL SECURITY ACT AND MATERNAL AND CHILD HEALTH SERVICES: SECURING A BRIGHT FUTURE

Woodie Kessel, Kenneth Jaros, and P. Travis Harker

INTRODUCTION

Kasserian ingera? (how are the children?) is the traditional greeting between Masai tribal members. The expected reply, *all the children are well,* conveys the high value the Masai have for protecting their young. It is also a hopeful message about the importance that the Masai have for the future and about the essential role that community plays in maintaining and supporting its children and families. Functioning as an extension of community, government—local, regional, and national—becomes the agent responsive to the will and opinion of the people, entrusted with safeguarding children and securing a bright future. Within the United States, the federal government through the Social Security Act (SSA) has established and supported such a positive infrastructure, primarily through the Title V program, but also through other components of the SSA as well.

Sustaining and improving the health status of mothers, infants, children, and adolescents is a major priority for the health and human services establishment in this country. The traditional emphasis of maternal and child health has been on issues such as prenatal care, proper nutrition, infant and maternal mortality and morbidity, breastfeeding, and services to children with special health needs (handicapping conditions). In recent years, however, the focus has been broadened considerably to reflect the variety of emerging complex public health issues that are facing the nation. Important contemporary issues include: adolescent health, injury prevention, HIV/AIDS, genetics, maternal substance abuse, services to incarcerated youth, to mention just a few. In addressing maternal and child health issues it is necessary also to view them within the context of other related issues such as women's health, family planning, and social welfare.

DEVELOPMENT OF MCH SERVICES UNDER FEDERAL LEADERSHIP

Maternal and child health services in the United States have historically been linked directly with the federally supported programming that began with the creation of the Children's Bureau in the Department of Labor in 1912. The primary role of the Children's Bureau initially was to define the scope of the problem of infant mortality and disseminate information to states regarding successful interventions to address the problem. Major early accomplishments of the Bureau included the development of a U.S. Birth and Death Registry and the passage of laws regarding child labor, juvenile courts, mother's pensions, illegal transportation of children, and sex offenses against children (Magee and Pratt, 1985).

The success of the Children's Bureau provided much of the impetus for the Sheppard-Towner Maternity and Infancy Act, passed in 1921. This Act created the first national maternal and child health program that involved federal grants in aid to states. During the period 1921–29 when this act was in place, the number of state child hygiene programs and the number of permanent maternal and child health centers increased greatly, and there was a widespread expansion of public health nursing services. Ultimately, this legislation laid the groundwork "for the development of nationwide maternal and child health programs administered by the states and set the precedent for later federal–state relationships" (Insley, 1977).

The present federally supported program grew directly out of the Social Security Act of 1935. During the period following the termination of Sheppard-Towner, the states' ability to promote health care and nutrition gradually eroded, and by 1933 the infant mortality rate once again began to increase (Magee and Pratt, 1985). Title V of the Social Security Act was designed to address these and other health problems through the creation of a coordinated system based on federal–state partnership. Under Title V the Maternal and Child Health (MCH), the Crippled Children's (CCS), and the Child Welfare Services (CWS) programs were created. "The Act made it very clear that it was not intended to simply pay for services . . . (but) was to extend and improve services available in each state . . . , especially in rural areas and in areas suffering from severe economic distress" (Magee and Pratt, 1985). Under the MCH component of the program funds were typically used "for prenatal care, well baby clinics, school health services, immunization, public health nursing and nutrition services, and health education" (Lesser, 1985).

In regard to CCS, the states were instructed to "insure services for locating crippled children as well as providing services and facilities for diagnosis, hospitalization and aftercare." Additionally, states were to "provide for cooperation with medical, health, nursing and welfare groups, and organizations, and with the state vocational agency" (Lesser, 1985). The CWS program was designed to assist states in establishing and expanding systems for the protection and care of homeless, dependent, and neglected children, and children in danger of becoming delinquent (Magee and Pratt, 1985).

The new Title V program was administered under the auspices of the Children' Bureau. Although the evolution of the federal program since 1935 has been extensive, the Bureau's philosophy of targeting the underserved; prevention;

systems improvement; and multidisciplinary, coordinated services continues to remain as the primary underpinning of the present federally supported maternal and child health program.

In 1953 the Children's Bureau was moved into the newly created federal Department of Health, Education, and Welfare (DHEW). In 1963 the Bureau was shifted to the Welfare Administration of DHEW. In 1969 an important and long-awaited change occurred. The Medical Services component of the Children's Bureau (including the Maternal and Child Health and Crippled Children's Services), which was responsible for medical and public health programs for mothers and children, was placed under the administration of the U.S. Public Health Service, where primary responsibility remains today. The Child Welfare Services Program remained under DHEW.

The Title V program has been amended on numerous occasions. The changes between 1969 and 1981 granted considerable flexibility to the states in the use of their federal allocation. In 1981 the Title V funds were combined into the present maternal and child health block-grant structure under the Omnibus Budget Reconciliation Act (OBRA). The block-grant process was designed to shift program planning, control, and accountability away from the federal government to states and local jurisdictions. The process has been expanded and streamlined through subsequent amendments, the most significant adjustment being made under OBRA in 1989.

PRESENT FEDERAL ROLE IN MATERNAL AND CHILD HEALTH PROGRAMS UNDER TITLE V

The Maternal and Child Health Bureau (MCHB) in the Health Resources and services Administration in the U.S. Public Health Service is the administrative unit that "provides leadership to both the public and private sector to build the infrastructure for the delivery of health care services (and preventive programs) to all mothers and children in the nation" (U.S. MCHB, 1993). The Bureau administers four major programs: the Maternal & Child Health Services Block Grant, the Healthy Start Initiative, the Emergency Medical Services for Children Program, and the Abstinence Education program.

The primary statutory responsibility of the Bureau is the administration of the Maternal and Child Health Services Block Grant ($700 M in 1999) under Title V of the Social Security Act. Congress annually authorizes the levels of appropriation for Title V and approximately 85% of the funds are distributed via the block grant to states and other federal jurisdictions using a formula based on the percentage of low-income children living in each state. States are presently required to match every $4 of federal dollars with $3 in cash or in kind. States and in some cases local health departments (designated as Title V agencies) are required to develop and submit an annual block-grant application and plan. The goals of the block-grant program (U.S. MCHB, 1993) include:

- Reduce infant mortality and the incidence of handicapping conditions among children

- Increase the number of children immunized against disease
- Increase the number of low-income children receiving health assessments and follow-up diagnostic and treatment services
- Provide and assure access to comprehensive prenatal care for women
- Provide and assure access to preventive and primary child care services
- Provide and assure access to comprehensive care, including long-term care services, for children with special health care needs
- Provide and assure access to rehabilitation services for blind and disabled children under 16 years of age who are Supplemental Social Security eligible
- Facilitate the development of comprehensive, family-centered, community-based, culturally competent, coordinated care systems of services for children with special health care needs and their families

Under the Title V requirements, states must allocate at least 30% of the block-grant funds to services for children with special health care needs, at least 30% to support primary and preventive care, and less than 10% can be used for administrative purposes. The combination of federal and state resources resulted in nearly $2.7 billion being used for service and program development in FY97 (MCHB, 2001).

The Maternal and Child Health Bureau also administers a program of discretionary grants, Special Programs of Regional and National Significance (SPRANS), which comprise the remaining 15% of the Title V appropriation. Under this category, research, training, genetics, hemophilia, and other projects and programs are supported.

LOCAL AND STATE MCH STRUCTURES

Each state health department has an administrative unit on maternal and child health that is responsible for the Title V application and for the administration of federal block-grant funds (and state and local match). This MCH unit is responsible for needs assessment and planning statewide, and for developing and monitoring standards and protocols of health care relating to mothers, infants, and children. Data collection, information tracking, and evaluation are also major functions of this unit.

Other responsibilities include: developing special services for high-risk mothers, infants, children, and adolescents; promoting the development of regional perinatal care, genetics diagnosis, counseling and treatment services; promoting the development of special laboratory services, providing advice and consultation to local communities to develop MCH services; promoting statewide immunization programs; promoting adolescent health services, including those to prevent and care for pregnancy in teenagers; promoting the development of child abuse and neglect prevention, early intervention and treatment services; developing and consulting with school health services; and improving the nutritional status of mothers, children, and youth. The unit also has responsibility for coordinating planning and program implementation with other state agencies such as welfare, education, mental health, and others (Wallace, 1988). In many states the MCH unit under the state health department provides extensive direct services, including public health social work services, to mothers, children, and families. In other states, minimal services are provided directly, and the MCH unit acts more in a planning and coordinating role.

An increasing number of counties and cities also have public health departments that have an MCH unit of some type. This unit may range from an individual in charge, to an extensive system for planning, assessment, and service delivery. This local MCH unit should serve as an advocate for improvement of the health of mothers and children in the local community. In many cases it delivers some direct services to mothers and children, often in partnership with local hospitals and clinics. The MCH unit works in collaboration with a variety of community-based programs, including health centers, mental health agencies, child protective services and with schools, day care, juvenile justice, housing, and rehabilitation services. In addition, it works closely with neighborhood organizations, advocacy groups, professional societies, and other voluntary organizations. These jurisdictions are responsible for planning at the local level and in certain circumstances may develop formal Title V applications for their service area.

OTHER CHILD AND FAMILY HEALTH ACTIVITIES UNDER THE SOCIAL SECURITY ACT

Although Title V of the SSA is typically thought of as the primary vehicle to support MCH services, several other SSA Titles are extremely important in terms of their influence on the health and welfare of mothers, children, and families. Many of these Titles under SSA are described and discussed in greater detail in other chapters of this publication. Title IV of SSA provides for support of the Temporary Assistance for Needy Families program (enacted in 1996 and which replaced the Aid to Families with Dependent Children program under Title IV) as well as for a range of programs supporting state and local child welfare programs. The two major health care insurance programs affecting children and families in poverty [Medicaid (Title XIX), and the State Child Health Insurance program (Title XXI)] are also enabled under the amended SSA. In addition, the Social Services Block Grant (Title XX), administered by the Administration for Children and Families (ACF) in the Department of Health and Human Services (DHHS), authorizes the provision of nearly $2 billion to states to fund social service programs to "achieve economic self-sufficiency; to prevent or remedy neglect, abuse or exploitation of children . . . ; to avoid or reduce inappropriate institutionalization; and to provide appropriate referral for institutional care . . . ". Under the SSBG, states have considerable flexibility in how they structure these family support programs (ACF, DHHS, 2001).

Many families with children also benefit greatly from programs and services authorized under the Supplemental Security Income (Title XVI) program. Survivor benefits are being paid to 7.2 million people, including 2 million children (National Organization for Women, 2001). And finally, the provisions with which SSA is most typically identified—old age and disability—also have major importance for families with children. Four million disabled workers and 1.6 million dependents receive cash benefits, and in many cases elderly relatives are part of the family unit and their income dramatically affects the economic status of the household.

THE STRUGGLE FOR COMPREHENSIVE HEALTH INSURANCE FOR CHILDREN AND FAMILIES

An important facet of the funding of preventive, diagnostic, and treatment services for children and youth is the availability of insurance coverage, whether it be private or public. Although a variety of health insurance programs are supported through various titles of the Social Security Act, through other government sources (i.e., CHAMPUS, Indian Health Services, and various state initiatives), and through private insurance carriers, this translates in practice to an uncoordinated patchwork of disparate programs. It does not support the concept of a "health home," an ideal advocated by the American Academy of Pediatrics and others. The expanding SCHIP program in conjunction with Medicaid, has created an effective insurance safety net for many children, but this coverage is not available to all children. Many uninsured or underinsured children are not enrolled in these programs, and if eligible, many do not take advantage of them. Even in cases in which children are covered, too often their parents and other adults in the home lack any kind of health insurance. Still lacking in the United States is a comprehensive strategy to weave all of these elements into a coherent system to provide health coverage for all children, and hopefully in the future for their families as well. (See the article by Hung et al. in this publication for a discussion of health insurance issues in greater depth.)

PROSPECTS FOR THE FUTURE

In summary, as maternal and child health professionals, we typically look to the Title V of the SSA as of primary importance to the health and welfare of mothers and children. But it must be recognized that the SSA is much more than Title V. It stands as perhaps the major symbol of the federal commitment to, and support for, families across the life span. It represents our closest effort to creating a comprehensive national plan to support health care coverage for children and families. Much remains, however, to be done to create such a workable system that is grounded in, and is supported on the principles of equity and social justice.

One of the realities of the SSA is that it continues to evolve. Amendments are constantly being made and these amendments dramatically affect the immediate and long-term health and welfare of families. It is therefore necessary for the programs supported through the SSA be constantly monitored, evaluated, and reviewed to assure that they continue to address the changing needs of children and families throughout the United States. It is through this process of continuous adjustment and improvement that the United States has the opportunity to build upon the Social Security Act to create a comprehensive national health insurance approach with the potential for ultimately eliminating the health disparities that remain so persistent in this nation.

REFERENCES

Administration for Children and Families, Dept. of Health and Human Services. (2001). *About ACF.* Washington, DC.

Insley, V. (1977). Health services: Maternal and child health. In R. Morris (ed.), *Encyclopedia of social work* (vol. 1, pp. 552–560). Washington, DC: National Association of Social Workers.

Lesser, A.J. (1985). The origin and development of maternal and child health programs in the United States. *American Journal of Public Health,* 75, 6, 590–598.

Magee, E.M. and Pratt, M.W. (1985). 1935–1985: *50 Years of U.S. Federal Support to Promote the Health of Mothers, Children and Handicapped Children in America.* Vienna, VA: Information Sciences Research Institute.

National Organization for Women. Website. (2001). Available at http://www.now.org/

U.S. Maternal and Child Health Bureau, Dept. of Health and Human Services. (1993). *MCHB Fact Sheets.* Rockville, MD: U.S. Public Health Service.

U.S. Maternal and Child Health Bureau, Dept. of Health and Human Services. (2001). *MCHB Fact Sheets.* Rockville, MD: U.S. Public Health Service.

Wallace, H.M. (1988). Organization and provision of major public programs for mothers, infants, children and youth and their families. In H.M. Wallace, G.M. Ryan, and A.C. Oglesby (eds.), *Maternal and Child Health Practices* (3rd Edition). Oakland, CA: Third Party.

Article 5

The Child Care System in the United States

Robert C. Fellmeth

CHILD CARE DEMOGRAPHICS IN THE 21ST CENTURY

Demand

Child care is divided into two markets: full-time child care for children under five years of age, and part-time (usually after school) care for older children. Full-time child care is in turn divided into two submarkets: full-day infant care and full-day toddler care.

U.S. Full-Day Infant and Toddler Care. Of the 21 million children in the United States under 6 years of age, 13 million are in child care. Among children under the age of 1, 45% received regular child care.[1] Child care demand has been driven traditionally by numbers of women in the work force. That demand increasingly includes the parents of very young children. In 1998, 61.9% of women in the United States with children under age 3 were working.[2] And the trend is expected to continue: In 1992, 75% of all women between the ages of 25 and 54 were working; the Bureau of Labor Statistics projects that proportion to increase to 83% by 2005.[3] In 2000, 78.5% of families maintained by women (no spouse present) included an employed person; this figure was 0.9% higher than in 1999 and about 9% higher than in 1994.[4] Also in 2000, both parents were employed in 64.2% of married couple families with children under 18.[5]

Surveys of the important preschool (full-day) market reveal the identities of current child care providers. Where mothers are employed, almost 39% of children under the age of 5 are now cared for in another's home; another 25.8% are cared for in organized child care facilities. A 1996 Census Bureau population report found 30% of preschoolers in organized child care facilities (centers), 21% with nonrelative child care providers (family day care or in-home babysitters), 17% with grandparents, 16% with their fathers, 9% with other relatives, and 7% whose mother worked at home or in other miscellaneous arrangements.[6] Care by relatives is substantially higher where family income is below the poverty line, with 60% placed with relatives, compared to 46% of children in higher-income families.[7]

A 1999 national survey of three- to five-year-olds who were cared for outside the home found a somewhat similar breakdown, with 59.1% in a center-based program, 15.9% in "nonrelative" care (either licensed family child care, or with neighbors or friends), and 23.3% with relatives. The ethnic breakdown indicates substantial differences, with Whites using center-based programs at 59.4%, non-relative care 19.3%, and relative care a low 18.8%. Black children of the same age are predominantly in a center-based program at 72.5% (reflecting the use of Head Start), with 36% in relative care and very few (8%) in nonrelative care.[8] Hispanic preschool children have the least center-based contact, at 44.4%, slightly more nonrelative care at 12.7% and relative care halfway between the White and Black rates at 25.9%.[9] The numbers confirm the thesis of advocates that nonrelative family child care remains either unaffordable or is unavailable for minority parents (e.g., not located in urban low-income neighborhoods), that Head Start has yet to be embraced by or is unavailable to Hispanic parents, and that relatives of minority children bear a substantial child care burden.

A recent report by the Urban Institute examined the child care patterns of children under age 3 of working mothers in the United States. The report estimated that 73% of infants and toddlers of employed mothers are primarily cared for by someone other than a parent while their mother is working; 27% are cared for by relatives; 22% are cared for in centers; 17% are cared for in family child care settings; and 7% are in the care of nannies or babysitters. The report further noted that 39% of infants and toddlers of employed mothers are in care full-time. The average time in nonparental care per week for infants and toddlers of employed mothers is 25 hours. Finally, 34% of infants and toddlers of working mothers are in two or more nonparental child care arrangements.[10]

U.S. Part-Time Care for Children 5 to 14 Years of Age. Part-time child care for children in school is also driven by maternal employment. Of the 38.8 million U.S. children between 5 and 14 years of age, only 14.4 million have a parent at home who is not either working or in school.[11] Public schools provide some 18,000 after-school care programs nationally. However, 70% of U.S. public schools fail to offer significant services.[12] Accordingly, experts estimate that 5 million school-age children spend substantial time in "latchkey" status—home alone without adult supervision.[13]

New Demand from Federal Welfare Reform. In addition to the current child care demand created by households in which both parents work outside the home, additional demand comes from unemployed parents who live below the poverty line and who would require child care in order to work. Welfare reform pursuant to federal welfare reform (the Personal Responsibility and Work Opportunity Reconciliation Act of 1996 PRWORA) required such employment by large number of parents now receiving Temporary Assistance to Needy Families (TANF), formerly Aid to Families with Dependent Children (AFDC).[14]

The PRWORA included a two-year maximum period (starting from January 1998) before just under 80% of those receiving TANF must be in a "work activity." For the vast majority of parents receiving aid, such activity will require child care, which the PRA requires states to provide (see discussion below). Literal compliance with the law will require an extraordinary bolus of child care capacity and subsidy after 2001, particularly if an economic downturn increases unemployment and reinflates TANF rolls.

Distribution of Supply

The distribution of supply versus demand is another concern. A study of licensed child care supply in Los Angeles County found the most affluent quarter of communities (by zip code) had more than twice the available spaces of the poorest quarter.[15] In poor areas of Los Angeles, where over one-third of the children live in TANF-receiving homes, there are 10 to 20 children under 6 years of age for every available licensed child care space.[16]

The shortage of licensed spaces is most severe in minority neighborhoods. In a recent examination of one such neighborhood—with a 59% Latino population—a Los Angeles Times investigation found "six slots in licensed day-care centers for every 100 children under 6 years of age," about one-fifth the rate of spaces/child extant in Burbank or Pasadena, with a middle class population and the Latino percentage at a more typical 22%.[17]

In October of 2000 the Human Services Alliance released a report on the current undersupply of child care slots in Los Angeles. The Report surveyed 500 low-income parents and put a human face on the numbers. Virtually all of those surveyed qualify for child care subsidies, but supply does not exist for their use. Alarmingly, 52% reported that a lack of child care caused them to lose a job, and 68% reported that it impeded them from attempting employment. One-half of those surveyed did not have a provider outside the family of any type, although 87% of those without placement were actively seeking it. As the data for California indicates, parents stay home and eschew employment (now required for safety-net assistance), count on family or friends, or latchkey their children at home alone.[18]

Child Care Costs

Table 1 presents approximate ranges of the average weekly cost of child care in California for 1997, which have increased slightly to 2000 and which are within the range of typical current national costs given the consistency of low child care compensation across the 50 states. The precise charge varies by facility, but the averages and price ranges represented apply to the vast majority of families. A typical family with one two-year-old child and one four-year-old child will incur approximately $10,000 per annum for child care costs. The benchmark family of one mother and those two children will earn, after social security and other deductions, approximately her child care costs. One infant at average cost will leave her with about $3,500 in net cash for rent and food.

A single parent earning minimum wage, with one child in full-time child care, would be expected to pay approximately 47% of her wages for licensed child care.[19] A family of one mother working full-time at minimum wage with two children under five (infants or preschool) will earn—after Social Security and other deductions—about the same amount as her child care will cost. One infant will cost 75% of the mother's take-home pay; two children over six will leave her with $3,000 per year in net earned income.

TABLE 1 CALIFORNIA RANGE OF AVERAGE ANNUAL CHILD CARE COSTS, 1997[20]

	Family Day Care	Day Care Center
Infant	$4,108–$7,020	$6,552–$9,412
Preschooler (2–5)	$3,900–$6,656	$4,888–$6,136
School Age	$3,536–$5,980	$4,472–$5,824

California Resource and Referral Network (CRRN) 1999 data finds infant care at $577 per month at centers and $432 per month in licensed family child care homes. Preschoolers up to 5 years of age cost an average of $420 at centers and $422 in family child care.[21] The CRRN 1999 survey found that even for the median household income of $38,979, and before deductions, the cost of one infant and one preschooler would consume 30% of total income.[22]

THE SPECIAL PROBLEM OF CHILD CARE FOR IMPOVERISHED CHILDREN

Media coverage of welfare reform has not focused on child-related impacts. One survey in the late 1990s found only 6% of coverage of the PRWORA or welfare reform focused on children. Over two-thirds of the articles did not mention children in their coverage.[23] The inattention to realities impacting children is exacerbated by the lack of a ready "handle" for public attention. Subject matter that is gradual and pervasive (such as latchkeyed children, child poverty, nutritional shortfall) does not qualify for coverage *ipso facto*. It generally requires an element recognized by the media subculture as a "story" (i.e., a petty irony (boy bites dog), a contest or a ranking, the setting of a record, sex, violence, cute animals, dramatic pathos, or celebrity association).

The situation facing impoverished families does not often lend itself to such attention. In contrast, the public has been given a somewhat distorted picture of welfare families, demonized by opportunistic politicians, and colored by a parade of afternoon talk-show misfits such as the "welfare queen"—a minority, unmarried teen, demanding a right to motherhood at public expense, producing fatherless children who replicate the dependency pattern in ever larger numbers, and whose children constitute gangs, increase crime, and incur imprisonment costs for society.

There is a subset of TANF families corresponding to this abusive picture, but a study of the recipients in the largest state of California reveals disparities between that popular picture and the reality. The TANF parent's average age is 31; unmarried mothers under 19 make up but 2% of families receiving aid; the average number of children among single parent recipients is 1.9; the average child support received for children from absent fathers nationally is about $45 per child per month. Fewer of the poor were receiving AFDC, and at substantially reduced grant levels, in 1996 than in the 1970s or 1980s. The federal TANF account makes up less than 1.5% of the budget; 70% of the recipients are children.[24]

Although a large number of recipients have married and responsibly planned their children, intending to provide for their care, those recipients representing irresponsible decisions by females or predatory behavior by males, have clearly increased, at least to the late 1990s. The growth in single parent births—not just by teens, but more substantially by older women—forms a substantial portion of the new child care need.

The Child Care Conundrum from Impoverished Families

A Critical Factor: Unwed Births. Table 2 presents 1995 national census data comparing the income of two-parent married households with children with that of single female parent households with children for all races. The numbers indicate a stark disparity between the two groups, with children in single female parent families living below the poverty line at five times the rate of children of married couples.

TABLE 2 PERCENTAGE OF PERSONS IN POVERTY BY DEFINITION OF INCOME AND SELECTED CHARACTERISTICS, 1995

Income Counted	Married Couples w/Children	Female Householder, No Husband Present, w/Children
Income before taxes less gov't transfers	11.0%	51.7%
Income before taxes plus health insurance supplement	10.2	49.6
Income less federal income taxes	11.2	51.4
Income after taxes plus Earned Income Tax Credit	9.6	47.4

Table 3 presents the census data looking more closely at the degree of disparity where there are multiple children. The 1992 data providing this breakdown by numbers of children and age groupings has not been updated, but other data presented below indicates that the correlations hold true in 1999–2000. In

1992 dollars, households with one child under six years old living with a single female parent had a median family income of $11,243 and two persons to clothe, house, and feed. Single-parent households with two or more children under six years old had a median annual income of $6,948, and three or more persons to provide for.

Children living in two-parent families consistently have median household incomes three to five times the amount in female-headed single-parent households. The disparity holds for all ethnic groups.[25] The median income of a married couple with children exceeds that of childless couples (partly reflecting couples waiting to have children a number of years after marriage and as incomes begin to rise).[26] The data indicates poverty for a large proportion of children in single-parent households, and in extreme poverty (generally defined as below one-half of the poverty line) for most of those single-parent households with more than one young child.

TABLE 3 U.S. INCOME OF FAMILIES WITH CHILDREN: MARRIED VS. SINGLE PARENTS

	Median Income	
All Races	Married Parent	Female Single Parents
One child, under 6	$40,938	$11,243
One child, 6–17	48,869	18,050
Two or more children, all under 6	40,952	6,948
Two or more children, some under 6, some 6–17	40,815	9,742
Two or more children, all 6–17	47,429	16,330
No children	39,766	27,495

The usually understated Census Bureau Current Population Report recently concluded: "Across all racial and ethnic groups, female-householder families contrasted most starkly with married-couple families. Families with a female householder, no husband present had the highest poverty rate [1998: 30%] and comprised the majority of poor families [1998: 53%]. Married-couple families, by contrast, had the lowest poverty rate [1998: 5%]."[27] Where the census data isolates families with children, the disparity increases further, as Table 4 indicates.

TABLE 4 PERCENT OF FAMILIES BELOW POVERTY LINE—1998[28]

	Married Couple with Children	Single Females with Children
White	8.4%	40.0%
African American	12.1	54.7
Hispanic	23.3	59.6

The percentages of those living below the poverty line go up further where numbers of children living in single-parent versus married-couple families are counted (rather than counting numbers of parents or families). Recent 1998 national data[29] finds 48.6 million children living with two parents at a median income of $52,553. Another 16.2 million children are living with only their mother and another 3.1 million are living only with their father. Both single parent levels are record highs. The median income of children's families where only fathers were present is $29,313. The median income of children's families with only mothers present is $16,236. As Table 4 indicates, the most recent data reveals a poverty incidence among single females with children three to five times that of married couples with children.

In its recent year 2000 and 2001 publications, the National Center for Children in Poverty has identified "single parenthood" as the most significant single "determinant of young child poverty." The Center notes: "In 1997, children under age six living with single mothers were five times as likely to be poor (56%) as those living with two parents (11%)."[30]

Exacerbating Factors: Multiple Children, Young Children. Looking within the single-parent population allows us to see which factors most correlate with extreme child poverty. Within the 16.2 million children in mother-only homes, 5.7 million live with mothers who are divorced (at a $21,316 median), 3.6 million with mothers who are married but the father is "absent" (at a $15,297 median), and a record 6.7 million (up 300,000 since 1996) with mothers who never married (at a median of $12,064, about 12% below the poverty line for the benchmark family of three persons). Of particular concern, the 1998 data measuring numbers of children (rather than parents or families) finds 57.8% of children living with unwed mothers to be living below the poverty line, and two-thirds are below 125% of the line.[31]

The breakdown by age of child indicates that youngest children—in greatest need of adequate nutrition for developing brains—fare the worst. The median income of unwed single mothers with children under 6 years of age sinks further to $11,687.[32] And, as noted above, the number goes down further where there are two or more younger children in such families—to a median of just over $9,000 per year, to be divided between those additional children. The most recent U.S. Census Bureau Population Report, covering data through 1998 concluded: "children under 6 remained particularly vulnerable in 1998, the overall poverty rate . . . was 20.6%, statistically unchanged from 1997. Even more striking, related children under age 6 living in families with a female householder, no husband present, had a poverty rate (54.8%) that was more than five times the rate for their counterparts in married-couple families (10.1%)."[33]

The close correlation between unwed births and child poverty holds true for all ethnic groups. The poverty rate of white children of single mothers is 40%, and for children under 6 the percentage grows to 50.4%. Among African American children of unwed mothers, 55% live under the poverty line, and 60% of those under 6 years of age are below the line. Among Hispanic children living with single mothers, 60% live below the poverty line, and 67% of those under 6 years of age live in impoverished conditions.[34]

National income trends since 1969 show that income in constant dollars is up 10% for single mothers with children, down 8% for single fathers with children, and up a remarkable 25% for married couples with children—much of it driven by increased work participation of married women.[35]

Trends in Single Parent Incidence. Despite the strong correlation between child poverty and single parenthood, the number of parents choosing single parenthood has grown substantially throughout the nation. The percentage of first births to unmarried women was static at 8% to 10% of all births from the 1930s through the 1960s. However, as Table 5 indicates, the percentage of mothers giving birth to their first child without marriage then almost doubled to 18% by the early 1970s, and over the subsequent twenty years, has more than doubled again, to 40.5% in the surveyed 1990–94 period.[36] These percentages count premarital births; another relatively constant 10% to 12% of births come from sexual acts conceiving children that occur prior to marriage.[37] As of the mid-1990s, for perhaps the first time in the nation's history, the majority of mothers having sex leading to their first children did so prior to marriage.[38]

Parents choosing to have children without a second parent, divorcing, or parenting alone for other reasons more than doubled from 1974 to 1994. Whereas one in seven families with children were headed by a single parent in 1970, by 1998 that number had increased to 28.8%; 40.4% of these were never married and 21.4% had been married but the spouse was absent from the home without a divorce. Only 34% derive from traditional divorces with court-ordered child support and visitation rights defining paternal involvement.[39]

Marriage, traditionally representing a formalized commitment to family, now has markedly lower incidence: in 1970, 71.7% of all adults (over 18) were married; in 1996 the percentage had declined to 60.3%—with the decrease attributable to roughly equal increases in divorce and in decisions not to marry at all.[40] However, the decision not to marry has not influenced substantially the decision to have children—with the incidence of childbirth outside of marriage growing markedly. In 1970, 40.3% of all households consisted of a married couple with children; by 1996 that percentage had dropped to 25%.[41] The Bureau of the Census projections for the coming decade estimate an increase of single-parent households with children from 24% to 28%—from 8 million such families to 9 million, including the addition of 800,000 more female single-parent families (from 6.4 to 7.2 million). Two-parent families are projected to decline yet further, from 24.8 million in 1998 to 23.1 million by 2010.[42]

Not Just Teens, Mostly Adult Women. The distribution of unwed births by age indicates the prevalence to mothers from 20 to 35 years of age. Table 5 presents the not-atypical California detailed count. The state's teen birth rates are close enough to the national mean to indicate that this distribution is a reasonable estimation of the national age breakdown for unwed births.

TABLE 5 GROUPINGS OF UNWED MOTHERS[43]

Age	Number of Births (1995)
under 15	1,259
15–19	42,537
20–24	55,269
25–29	37,908
30–34	24,776
35–39	12,078
over 40	2,901

The most recent count of California families with children receiving TANF welfare support revealed that only .2% are headed by a mother under 18, another 1.3% are 18 years of age and 1.8% are 19 years of age. A total of 96.6% of its TANF parents are over 19 years of age, and one-quarter of these are married.[44] A somewhat larger percentage receiving support may have had their first child as a teen, thus placing themselves in economic jeopardy for later TANF need, particularly where they have additional children. California's count of the "age of mother at birth of oldest child in assistance unit" reveals that a somewhat higher 23.4% of current parent recipients were under 19 when their first children were born, while 58% were over 21 years of age or older.[45] National TANF surveys breaking down age of mother at first birth find substantially more African American and Hispanic women having their first babies at an earlier maternal age, with 40% of African American women under 20 years of age when giving birth to their first child, and 33.7% of Hispanic women.[46] But women in all groups are giving birth in substantial numbers to their first children, as well as subsequent children, without husbands or other paternal commitment across the spectrum of their childbearing years.

The most recent Centers for Disease Control and Prevention study "Nonmarital Childbearing in the United States, 1940–99" concluded: "Because of steep increases in birth rates for unmarried women aged 20 years and over and in the number of these women . . . the proportion of all nonmarital births that are to teenagers has dropped considerably."[47]

Child Support and Paternal Commitment

Related to child poverty and child care demand is the commitment of a parent absent from the family. Child care collection has accelerated nationally since 1995. Nevertheless, the federal Office of Child Support Enforcement (OCSE) reported total national support collection of $17.9 billion in the year 2000 covering a caseload of 17.4 million and involving just over 19 million children.[48] This total amounts to $78.50 per month per child due child support from an absent parent, of which about $45 per month is received by the family for the benefit of the children. The remainder recompenses federal and state jurisdictions for (TANF) welfare costs paid for affected children.

The lack of support from the absent parent means that single mothers must obtain child care and work, or rely on TANF assistance.

Welfare Reform, Child Poverty, and Child Care

Historical Program Line-Up. Consistent with rapid growth in demand and supply, public subsidies for special populations needing assistance have increased as well. The General Accounting Office has identified more than 90 federal funding programs for child care, administered by 11 agencies. Most are specialized programs serving circumscribed populations: military, disabled respite care, college students, and others. Child care complexity is further exacerbated by state programs supplementing their federal counterparts, particularly state-funded preschool programs, or general child care subsidies separate and apart from federal funding streams.

Federally originated programs, which contribute federal funds to state agencies for state administration, have traditionally focused on the AFDC (TANF) program and are largely intended to facilitate the employment of parents on welfare. Historically, these programs have included child care under the federal "JOBS" program—combining job training, placement, and child care for TANF parents. Realizing that when these parents obtain jobs, they are unable to continue where lacking child care support, the federal government advanced "Transitional Child Care" for up to one year to those who were newly employed. Then the federal government, eventually acceding to the obvious, developed "at-risk" child care directed at those who are working but are likely to regress into welfare dependency without child care assistance. Unfortunately, each of these programs (and others) have separate rules, application procedures, and administrative costs—with many parents forced out of employment as they fell between or outside the discrete and separate programs. And they have historically been administered by state departments of social services, separately from the extensive state child care programs often run by state departments of education.

Many of the federal and state programs became indirectly coordinated through the evolution of "resource and referral" (R&R) agencies in most states. These agencies have served very successfully as a "marketplace" for child care—both privately paid and publicly subsidized. Very simply, family child care providers and child care centers notify their local R&R agency when they have slots available, and provide information to the R&R about their facilities. The R&R agency also helps on the supply side by assisting new providers with state licensure. Each R&R agency has a widely publicized local "hotline" number. When a parent needs child care, the line is called and an expert discusses available slots, their location, and features. Importantly, the R&R agency also has expertise in available subsidies and can determine whether a parent may qualify and help with the paperwork.

Head Start and Tax Expenditures. Head Start programs are structurally distinct. Unlike most federal participation in the states, it does not occur by way of funding through state agencies, but is operated directly by the federal government.

In addition to federal assistance to state programs, separate state programs, and the stand-alone Head Start program, both federal and state jurisdictions sometimes enact tax expenditures. These are usually tax credits to pick up part of child care expenses through tax forbearance, or credits to businesses who provide child care facilities or services. The major existing subsidy is a federal child care credit. A family whose income is less than $10,000 annually may claim 30% of their child care costs as a tax credit; a family whose income is over $28,000 annually may claim 20%. The maximum cost for which a credit may be claimed is $2,400 for one child and $4,800 for two or more children.[49] Studies of the federal system indicate that the credit benefits some poor families, but also tends to extend to the middle class more than do the direct subsidy programs.[50]

PRA Child Care Changes and Provisions. The Personal Responsibility and Work Opportunity Reconciliation Act of 1996 (PRWORA) includes a list of new requirements on those receiving TANF aid. Most germane to child care is the work requirement. There is a statutory 60-month absolute limit on TANF grant assistance, increasing percentages of those receiving aid must be employed full-time upon pain of federal funding penalties, and states may require employment of TANF parents at earlier intervals. Many jurisdictions are implementing cutoffs of TANF at the two-year mark for those who have not obtained employment. Many states are following the disingenuous pattern of cutting off "the parent's share," as if reducing grants for the benchmark family of three from $630 to $420 holds children harmless because the subtraction is not designated as coming from the child.

The federal statute does require states to provide those who must work "adequate child care." Child advocates have demanded compliance with this requirement at state and local levels. However, the supply is so inadequate in the impoverished neighborhoods where welfare reform has major application that states and local authorities grant permission for relatives and other "informal" arrangements to provide care.

The PRWORA led to a new "Child Care and Development Fund" (CCDF). This fund absorbed both the "transitional" and the "at-risk" programs previously extant, and included as well the old Child Care and Development Block Grant (CCDBG)—creating a single "super child care block grant." Under this new "capped entitlement" funding scheme, states receive a mandatory base amount at the level each previously received under Title IV-A in 1992–94, 1994 alone, or 1995 alone, whichever is highest. These funds are sent as a block grant without any required state match—unlike the previous programs they absorbed. The Congress then appropriated $7.2 billion in total for the grant over six years.

A state may obtain additional funds beyond this block grant on a matching basis *if* the state (1) obligates all of the block grant money allocated to it for the fiscal year it seeks new money, and (2) spends at least as much as it has been spending from its own resources in matching federal funds or in providing its own child care. In other words, more money is available beyond the block grant on a matching basis, so long as the state is spending above and beyond what it previously spent on child care and is not diverting previous state commitment so it can be "supplanted" with federal funds.[51] If the state so complies, it can get its share (based on its percentage of the nation's children under 13 years of age) of another $3.5 billion in federal capped entitlement funds at fiscal year 1995 rates. *This* funding the state must match 50/50.

States must spend at least 70% of all of these funds on TANF recipients, those leaving TANF, or those in danger of falling back onto TANF (see the three federal programs described above and now within the block grant).

As noted, this Child Care and Development Fund also includes the previous Child Care and Development Block Grant which had financed the resource and referral agencies described above, given grants for quality improvement (monitoring, training, technical assistance), and expended 78% of its funds on direct services to purchase child care with certificates, contracts, grants, or as part of before and after school care—mostly for the working poor.[52] This CCDBG continues within the Fund at $6 billion nationally over the next six years—but is subject to annual appropriations approval. Money not obligated by the state by the end of the fiscal year reverts to the federal government for redistribution to other states.

Current Problems and Prospects for Impoverished Children. The realistic forecast of problems attending the PRWORA and related policy shifts is not sanguine. Although the amounts devoted to child care have increased facially, the Congressional Budget Office has estimated that if states simply maintain current spending for the working poor so they can remain on the job and meet the minimum work requirements of TANF recipients, the spending is $1.4 billion short over its six-year period.[53] But even if increases occur, two serious problems remain. First, quality child care is not available in the areas where the PRWORA creates the demand. Accordingly, the work requirement is imposed without the assurance of "adequate child care" notwithstanding the theoretical appropriation of funds. As the data shows, impoverished parents use relatives and neighbors, and latchkey their children. Beyond the latchkeying of children from toddlers to teens are recent studies showing lack of parental supervision over teen youth by now-working TANF parents. The "adequate child care" assurance has not been extended in most states for children over 12 years of age.

The second problem is the actual diminution of child care for the working poor. In some states, child care is divided into 3 stages: stage 1 is 6 months of child care while a parent is in training for employment, stage 2 covers those who have obtained work and are transitioning off aid. Stage 3 consists of those who have been employed more than one year (more than 2 years in some states). Child care subsidy is provided in theory to meet the full need (assuming availability as noted above) for stages 1 and 2. But stage 3 child care is excluded from assured provision.

What this means is that the working poor, who have never sought assistance, are disadvantaged and are simply not able to pay current child care costs at current typical wage levels. They are relegated to relatives, neighbors, and latchkey arrangements. Moreover, even for the TANF recipients, they do not achieve a sudden pay raise of $4,000 to $10,000 in net pay at the one- or two-year mark of employment. But under current plans most will be cut off. Such parents then face a Hobson's choice: latchkey their children (or entrust them to uncertain care) or quit employment to care for them. If the last choice is made, they then face possible penalties and the certain 60-month final cut-off of TANF assistance.

THE WORKING POOR AND THE GOAL OF SELF-SUFFICIENCY

The plight of the working poor is central to the long-range goal of self-sufficiency and elevation of children to above the poverty line through work. The poor are largely excluded from child care assistance outside of removal from TANF rolls and federal Head Start (and some state counterparts) focusing on school preparation of four-year-olds. Those who work face the conundrum discussed above. Federal and state policies impede the aspirational progression of such families by failing to provide the obvious solution: a child care subsidy for those who work, on a sliding scale that decreases gradually as income increases.

The federal minimum wage increase to $5.15 per hour produces $10,753 for full-time work. After subtracting payroll deductions and adding on the maximum earned income tax credit, a mother and two children will remain below the poverty line. Some states specify slightly higher minimum wage levels, but even the most generous states will barely allow full-time work to yield net income above the poverty line.[54] If we were to hold even the 1968 minimum wage in constant dollars, the level as of 2001 would be $8.37 per hour.[55]

Apart from the minimum wage, average hourly wages of females from 15 to 24 years of age who have not completed high school or who have only a high school diploma have dropped 16% between 1979 and 1993 in constant dollars. In 1979, 18.5% of all households headed by females from 15–24 years old lived below the poverty line; by 1993, the proportion climbed to 38.1% for all races, and to 63% for young African American women.[56]

Table 6 indicates the income needed by a single-parent family with two children (one infant and one preschool age) to be economically self-sufficient in Los Angeles and Tulare Counties, representing high-cost urban and moderate-cost rural settings, respectively. The amounts shown, based on a series of economic studies, are based on minimum housing/nutrition needs in and assume no subsidies.[57]

Under the Bureau of the Census' official poverty thresholds, the study's urban family requiring $34,296 annually or the rural family needing $22,296 would not be considered poor unless income for a parent and two children is below $14,630 as of 2001.

For those who are able to obtain work, the EITC and higher minimum wage promise to move large numbers of parents and families to the area of $1,000–$1,400 per month in take-home income. But the various subsidies for impoverished parents—some designed to protect children—here interact to make it more difficult for families to move from the poverty line to this "liveable wage," which would allow modest shelter, adequate nutrition, and child care without public subsidy.

TABLE 6 WAGES NECESSARY TO ACHIEVE SELF-SUFFICIENCY[58]

For Family W/One Adult, One Infant, One Preschooler	Los Angeles-Long Beach, CA	Tulare County, CA
Housing	$855.00	$480.00
Child care	759.75	571.45
Food	281.40	281.40
Transportation	117.81	117.81
Medical care	176.79	176.79
Miscellaneous	219.07	162.74
Total Taxes (minus EITC and CCTC)	448.62	268.77
Earned Income Tax Credit (−)	0.00	($108.75)
Child Care Tax Credit (−)	($80.00)	($92.00)
Self-sufficiency wage (monthly)	$2,858.44	$1,858.56
Self-sufficiency wage (hourly)	$16.24	$10.56

As a single mother of two passes $1,000 per month, she sequentially loses TANF, begins to pick up federal (and some state) tax liability, loses food stamps, progressively loses the EITC, loses eligibility for subsidized school lunches, loses priority for subsidized child care (if available), and loses medicaid.[59] Private-sector child care and medical coverage for dependents are increasingly rare.[60] The rate of fall-off of this assistance places many parents in a quandary—additional earnings can reduce net benefits available for the family.

The two major costs impeding self-sufficiency as subsidies drop off at the poverty line are housing and child care. Child care costs are critical: It is the single largest expense for working parents with more than two children, or with two children under 5, or with two children outside high-rent urban settings.

CHILD CARE QUALITY

Safety

Increasingly, parents entrust their children for most of the day to care and facilities of strangers, either in a commercial center context, or in the home of a day care provider. Safety issues are of particular importance given the tendency of young children to test their environment, and the increase in allowable children per facility discussed above. In January 2000, the General Accounting Office released a national review of state child care safety and health regulation using 1999 data. The results indicated the inspections are not generally assured often and that caseloads are high.[61]

Quality of Care

Both adequacy and quality of child care have become a subject of scholarship and commentary. Over the last three years, more than twenty major reports, studies, and surveys have covered basic child care issues, particularly in light of welfare reform. Studies generally conclude that attention in the early developmental years is important and has lasting impact. Even with substantial increases, the supply of subsidized child care is inadequate given PRWORA-generated demand; the working poor are driven back onto TANF because of their lack of access to care for their children, and the quality of child care is uneven and disappointing.[62]

A four-state study of quality in child care centers found that only 14% could be rated as high in quality.[63] The Packard Foundation's Center for the Future of Children concluded that "(1) the quality of services is mediocre, on average; (2) the cost of full-time care is high; (3) at the present time, the cost of increasing quality from mediocre to good is not great, about 10%; [and] (4) good child care is dependent on professionally approved staffing ratios, well-educated staff, low staff turnover. . . . [64] One of the leading authorities in the field concludes that the state of child care "reflect[s] the low priority given to children's care and women's work in American society."[65]

Other recent studies have raised serious questions about the impact of low-quality child care on children, particularly given the sacrifice of parental time and attention often implicated. The reported problems with older children of TANF parents now forced to work and hence lose substantial parental monitoring are here underlined by data showing low levels of parental or other adult supervision for children over the age of 10. These children are increasingly latchkeyed home alone, or are sometimes relied upon themselves to care for younger siblings. An increasing number lack direct paternal impact and often lack male models. The popular culture tends to fill that vacuum with regrettable messages about laudable male qualities: being decisive, forceful, tough, threatening, violent. Although such caveats are discounted by many child care advocates, the implications of enhanced peer group influence, or reliance on popular culture, are not a source of comfort.

The concerns of many were heightened by some preliminary findings released in April of 2001 from the substantial longitudinal study of child care consequences conducted to date. Financed by the National Institute of Child Health and Human Development, the study started in 1991, with 1,364 children from 10 cities undergoing detailed surveys, and follow-up study—including observation of classroom and social behavior. Three preliminary findings have emerged from the first seven years of observation: (1) 17% of kindergartners who had been in child care showed more assertive and aggressive behaviors; (2) family relationships correlate more closely with measures of aggression than does child care; (3) higher-quality child care correlates with academic success in early school years.

The first finding produced great controversy because of the political ramifications implicit in a message that child care was not beneficial to children. Although the degree of aggression increase is not severe, it is statistically significant and not appropriately rejected based on notions of political correctness. Rather than view such findings as an assault on parental prerogative, it should trigger active further inquiry. What are the implications of the aggression measured? What is their relation to delinquency? What are the detailed characteristics of child care provided that correlate with such aggression, e.g., age of child, extent of adult supervision, degree of cognitive stimulation?

However, a full-time parent is not an option for millions of children, and the findings of this and other studies confirm the advantages of high-quality child care where it is provided, with this study confirming: "The quality of child care over the first three years of life is consistently but modestly associated with children's cognitive and language development. The higher the quality of child care (more positive language stimulation and interaction between the child and provider), the greater the child's language abilities at 15, 24, and 36 months, the better the child's cognitive development at age two, and the more school readiness the child showed at age three." The study also acknowledged that other variables were more influential, including family income, maternal vocabulary, home environment, and maternal cognitive stimulation.[66]

Recent additional evidence has been presented during 1999–2001 concerning the deleterious consequences of latchkeying children and the advantages of high-quality child care. In addition to four studies,[67] the *Journal of the American Medical Association* published a peer reviewed article on May 8, 2001, that involved a long-term (17-year) study of 1,539 low-income children enrolled as 3- and 4-year-olds in Chicago Public Schools' Child-Parent Centers, with half-day care similar to Head Start, and some school-age services linked to elementary schools at ages 6 to 9. The results were more decisive than the NICHHD study discussed above, with those admitted in the program 33% less likely to be arrested and 41% less likely to be arrested for a violent crime, and 20% more likely to finish high school as compared to control groups. The study conclusion: "Participation in an established early childhood intervention for low-income children was associated with better educational and social outcomes up to age 20 years."[68]

Quality is compromised by three factors: (1) a general lack of any certification or other system to provide enhanced status to providers as a positive incentive to learn and improve;[69] (2) high staff turnover (now at 20% to 30% per annum); and (3) low pay. The last factor is of particular importance, and influences the first two. Some family day care workers do not earn minimum wage. Current compensation allows a full-time child care worker providing for a 6-year-old to receive $3.57 up to $527 per month. These workers, in whose hands children are placed, generally live below the poverty line themselves.[70] At the higher end for child care, the average salary of a preschool teacher in California is about $24,600 for 12 months of work. An elementary school teacher *starts* at $24,835 for a ten-month year with a realistic career track to earn $50,000.[71]

On April 29, 2001, a University of California at Berkeley study focusing on California reported that salaries for child care teachers have fallen over the last six years in relation to inflation. The study focuses on child care centers in Santa Cruz, Santa Clara, and San Mateo counties, but its results appear to be fairly generalized. In examining centers, the study overstates income because of the much smaller compensation (generally close to minimum wage) available for licensed family day care providers. But the study found that "just 24% of teaching staff employed in 1996 were still on the job in 2000, more than half of the centers reporting turnover last year had not replaced the staff they lost, when teachers leave a center about one-half leave child care provision entirely, and wages for teachers decreased 6% adjusted for inflation since 1994."[72] The study found "the presence of a greater proportion of highly trained teaching staff in 2000 is the strongest predictor of whether a center can sustain quality improvements over time. Wages is also a significant predictor."[73]

CHILD CARE ASPIRATIONS FOR THE NEW MILLENNIUM

Adequate Supply

The first requirement must be an adequate supply of spaces where acceptable relative care is unavailable, and for adequate subsidy to allow parents to work. The latter requirement is essential where parents suffer TANF cut-offs if not employed.

If the national policy to restrict the safety-net protection of children continues, adults and not children must face the consequences. The current paradigm is a game of musical chairs for millions of children, with the TANF parents of over three million children certain to be left standing when the music stops and unemployment continues. Those children are then in a catch-22 that no civilized society can countenance: parents are cut-off from basic safety net support and their children must either go without essentials, or suffer surrender by otherwise loving and competent parents to whom they have bonded into state foster care (at a public cost substantially above TANF). If we have decided to inhibit decisions to have children without ability to provide for them privately, required public service work provides such a disincentive. It or some other alternative is ethically compelled short of the current disincentive—reliance on the misery of children.

Where public service employment is provided (or if the unrealistic projections of full employment of PRWORA sponsors were to prove accurate), child care supply will have to be increased many times the proposed funding in the President's plan, in addition to the costs of public service employment itself. For a somewhat different alternative, see the Prevention recommendation below.

Rational, Efficient, Comprehensible

The historical pattern of child care subsidies is a patchwork of federal and state programs to meet the needs of narrow populations, or to facilitate removal of parents from welfare roles. The predictable result has been fragmentation, confusion, inefficiency, barriers to care, and administrative costs. These problems are exacerbated for parents cut-off from TANF. Such a cut-off deprives parents of the single social worker who historically arranges for child care (and medicaid) options.

It is part of the holy grail of child advocates that children need a seamless system of child care, based on the needs of the children involved. As most of Europe has already done, it is time to create a universal sliding scale of child care subsidy, based on income and number and age of children. In the alternative, those needing government services should be able to avail themselves of the same technological advances used in the private sector to rationalize confusing alternatives. A "social service" card could be issued to all impoverished or otherwise eligible parents, with a magnetic coded strip updated periodically for income, family size, child disabilities, and other qualifying facts. Swiping such a card through a machine could array all available programs, giving a parent the efficiency of a shopper's choice, and the same card would qualify for services chosen without endless forms, trips across town, lines, and interviews for each service each eligible child needs. Either a child needs and deserves a public investment for the benefit of all of us, or not. If so, barriers to its provision should be bureaucratically minimal and technologically facilitated.

Safe and Enriching

In addition to adequate child care supply, quality is important. Recent research indicates that child care and preschool programs can contribute meaningfully to the cognitive development of a child, and assist in his or her socialization. Parental roles remain primary, but attentive and stimulating child care can be a benefit. Unfortunately, the child care industry pays those to whom our children are entrusted low wages, among the lowest in the nation. As discussed above, the political trend remains focused on warehousing children in the lowest-cost arrangement so parents can work and move off welfare.

In the 21st century, four areas of improvement can lead to fruitful investment in the future of children. First, control over child care should pass from departments of social services concerned about adult welfare accounts, to state departments of education, concerned about child development.

Second, child care must be intelligently regulated through a licensing system specifying the number and qualifications of providers, insuring background checks on employees, subject to facility spot inspections, and subject to a flexible system of civil penalties for violations—high and certain enough to get the attention of providers, low enough to maintain the incentive to provide adequate supply.

Third, the increased number of impoverished children in child care gives us the chance to assure immunization coverage, health checks, and nutritional assurance. The last is currently addressed through the Child and Adult Care Food

Program (CACFP), and those young children in child care with parents hovering near the poverty line are especially vulnerable to nutritional shortfall—particularly given food stamp benefit reductions. Moreover, infant and pre-school settings reach children during the period from 0 to 5 years of age, when brain development makes adequate nutrition a particularly important investment.

Finally, the 21st century should yield creative use of public- and marketplace-based incentives to upgrade educational quality: scholarships, certification standards, tax credits for computer, educational telecommunications, and other capital enhancements, higher recompense (including public subsidy premiums) for enhanced quality. A variety of marketplace strategies and rewards, together with public subsidies, can be arranged to direct care providers into further enrichment of the children in their charge, rather than toward higher volume and minimum interaction.

Financing

Public subsidies required may be financed from a wide variety of possible sources. The Ewing Marion Kauffman Foundation and the Pew Charitable Trusts have published a compendium of current financial sources.[74] Current sources of child care financing currently include: children's services special (property) taxing districts (Florida), a special Families and Education Levy (Washington state); allocation of a minimum percentage of the budget for children's education or services (California Proposition 98, San Francisco Proposition J), a dedicated sales tax (Aspen, Colorado), a local-option sales tax (Ames, Iowa), a voluntary income tax check-off for child care (Colorado), various state child care and employer tax credits (22 states), enterprise zone tax credits (Colorado), property tax abatement for child care facilities (Travis County, Texas), child care licensing fees, vanity license plate revenues (Kid's plates in California and Massachusetts), lottery revenue (Georgia, Florida), tax exempt bonds (Illinois), state loan guarantees (Maryland), public grants (New York), and others.

The 1980s and '90s have been a period of "looking out for No. 1." A long national tradition of sacrifice and investment in our children, to give them more than we had, has been violated. A study of California public spending on children since 1989 created a private and public adult "selfishness index." The former measured maternal unwed birth rates and paternal child support contribution rates, adjusted for inflation. The latter measured almost all public spending for children per child in poverty, as a percentage of adult personal income. Both indices have fallen markedly since 1989, with 1999 representing record levels of adult private and public commitment to themselves over their children.[75] This self-destructive trend is reflected in the disproportionate political power of the elderly, now with a poverty rate one-third the level extant for their grandchildren. Senior citizens, deserving of respect and assistance, receive publicly arranged financial and medical security substantially beyond either provided for the nation's children.

A Path to Self-Sufficiency

Child care is the doorway out of welfare and poverty for the children of single parents. Even with one young child, blue-collar single parents cannot work and surmount the poverty line without child care help. It makes little sense to a responsible parent to work full-time to pay someone else to care for your children, and take home virtually no net pay to house and feed them. The result of insufficient assistance is TANF dependency. With TANF timelines, cut-downs to token TANF grants, and reduced food stamps will come increased homelessness and undernutrition.

The plight of single-parent households is particularly stark. There is a low ceiling, and with welfare reform, little floor. Successful child care can do more than provide a safety net stop gap to allow initial employment. In combination with an enhanced Earned Income Tax Credit, it can bridge the gap from the $1,000 to $1,400 per month barrier to eventual self-sufficiency. Without sliding-scale assistance well beyond that currently provided, millions of parents are vulnerable to a slide back well below the poverty line, often without a TANF safety net for their children where their previous allocation or state policies preclude it. The goal of a safety net should be a hand up toward self-sufficiency, with the incentive from work always present in the form of incremental financial gain.

Given the dominant role of child care costs in the personal budgets of working parents, it is the critical mechanism (in combination with the EITC) to provide a bridge. Child care subsidies should remain 100% up to 125% of the poverty line, and then decline gradually and incrementally as family income increases above that level.

Prevention

Underlying all of recommendations for child care for the 21st century is a new contract for our children. Currently, children are most often an unintended byproduct of adult sex. Many adults treat conception as a form of divine intervention. Intellectually, we all know that it is substantially controllable—and that control must be discussed as mature adults.

A covenant can be agreed upon, made a part of our education and culture, that children deserve a *bona fide* attempt by two married parents to prepare for them, and to provide for their needs. If such an ethic were to take hold, much would follow. One consequence would be increased political backing for strong safety net support. Where the cause of child poverty is layoff, illness, divorce, or trauma affecting parents, public support for child safety net support would be strong and reliable. That support would allow much more to be expended on enriched child care for the smaller number of children then in need. And substantial resources would remain to begin the important work of improving child care quality for all children.

REFERENCES

1. The White House, Office of the Press Secretary, *Child Care: A Challenge for America's Working Families* (Washington, D.C.; January 7, 1998) (available from the White House Virtual Library at http://www. whitehouse.gov/cgi) (citing data from the U.S. Department of Education's National Center for Education Statistics).

2. Bureau of Labor Statistics, *Employment Status of Mothers With Own Children Under Three Years Old by Age of Youngest Child, and Marital Status, 1997–98 Annual Averages* (Washington, D.C.; 2000) at Table 6 (available at http://stats.bls.gov/news.release/famee. t06.htm).

3. Bureau of Labor Statistics, *Bulletin 2452* (Washington, D.C.; April 1994) at Table A-1.

4. Bureau of Labor Statistics, *Employment Characteristics of Families Summary* (April 19, 2001) (available at http://stats.bls.gov/newsrels.htm).

5. Ibid.

6. Lynne M. Casper, U.S. Department of Commerce, Economics and Statistics Administration, Bureau of the Census, *Who's Minding Our Preschoolers?* (Current Population Reports No. P70-53) (Washington, D.C.; March 1996) at 1. See op. cit. at 2 (Table 1) for a breakdown by employment status of mothers (full-time, part-time, night shift, day shift) and identifying who provides care in the child's home or in the provider's home (relative, nonrelative, and others).

7. Ibid. at 5 (Figure 4).

8. The total percentages add up to over 100%, particularly for the Black population because of the mix of more than one care arrangement for many children and partly reflecting the part-day four-day-a-week structure of Head Start; see discussion below.

9. U.S. Department of Education, National Center for Education Statistics, *Digest of Education Statistics 2000* (Washington, D.C.; 2001) at Table 48.

10. The Urban Institute (Jennifer Ehrle, Gina Adams) and Child Trends (Kathryn Tout), *Who's Caring for Our Youngest Children? Child Care Patterns of Infants and Toddlers,* (Washington, D.C.; January 2001) at viii.

11. Based on 1997 data, see Administration for Children and Families, Department of Health and Human Services' Child Care Bureau, *Out-of-School Time School-Age Care* (available at www.acf.dhhs.gov/programs/ccb/faq/school.htm).

12. Ibid.

13. Ibid.

14. See discussion below.

15. Bruce Fuller and Casey Connerty, PACE Center, University of California, Berkeley; Fran Kipnix, California Child Care Resource & Referral Network; Yvonne Choong, University of Chicago, *An Unfair Head Start: California Families Face Gaps in Preschool and Child Care Availability* (1997).

16. Little Hoover Commission, *Caring for Our Children: Our Most Precious Investment* (Sacramento, CA; September 1998), at 41.

17. Melissa Healy, *Latinos at Center of Chicken-Egg Debate Over Child-Care Funds,* LOS ANGELES TIMES (September 29, 1998) "Community Section" at 1.

18. Sam Mistrano, *Transforming Child Care from the Ground Up*, Human Services Alliance (Los Angeles, CA; October 2000), passim.

19. California Attorney General's Office, *Women's Rights Handbook* (Sacramento, CA; 1998) at 224.

20. California Child Care Resource & Referral Network, *Regional Market Rate Ceilings for California Child Care Providers* (San Francisco, CA; July 1997) at Figure 2 and Figure 3; the weekly figures are expressed in annual terms.

21. Urban Institute, *Child Care in California: A Short Report on Subsidies, Affordability and Supply*, 2001, Figure 2, at 2.

22. California Child Care Resource & Referral Network, *The California Child Care Portfolio 1999* (San Francisco, CA, 2000) at 3–5, see www.rrnetwork.org/99folio.html. One study found that child care costs account for 24%–31% of the budget of the working poor, but only 6% of the budget of upper-middle-class taxpayers. See D. A. Phillips, ed., *Child Care of Low-Income Families: Summary of Two Workshops* (Washington, D.C.; National Academy Press, 1995) at 12.

23. *Children Now, Children & Welfare Reform: High Stakes, Low Coverage* (Oakland, CA, January 15, 1998). The survey covered 680 articles dealing with welfare reform during 1996-1997 in the nation's major substantive news press sources: Washington Post, New York Times, Los Angeles Times, Wall Street Journal, Newsweek, Time, and others.

24. See Robert C. Fellmeth, *California Children's Budget 1997–98* (Children's Advocacy Institute, 1997), Chapter 2, at 2-12 to 2-17 and citations therein.

25. U.S. Department of Commerce, Bureau of the Census; *Money Income of Households, Families, and Persons in the United States: 1992* (Current Population Reports, Consumer Income, Series P60-184) (Washington, D.C.; 1993) Table 18 at 68–76; see also http://www.census.gov/hhes/www/income99.html.

26. This is partly a reflection of length of time working, because younger couples who have not yet had children are closer statistically to initial entry into the workforce. It also suggests enhanced resources for children where there is such a delay.

27. U.S. Department of Commerce, Bureau of the Census, *Money Income in the United States: 1997* (Current Population Reports P60-200, Washington D.C.; September 1998) at viii. Note that the updated 1998 numbers are in brackets; source: U.S. Department of Commerce, Bureau of the Census; *Poverty in the United States 1998* (Current Population Reports, Consumer Income, Series P60-207) (Washington, D.C.; 9-99) at Table 2 (hereinafter *"Poverty in the United States 1998"*); see also updated information at http://www.census.gov/hhes/www/income99.html.

28. U.S. Department of Commerce, Bureau of the Census; *Consumer Income 1998* (Current Population Reports, Consumer Income, Series P60-206) (Washington, D.C.; 2000) at Table A, see also http://www.census.gov/hhes/www/income99.html.

29. Terry Lugaila, *Marital Status and Living Arrangements: March 1998 (Update)*, Current Population Report P20-514, Bureau of the Census, Department of Commerce, Washington, D.C., December 1998, Table 6 at 36 (hereinafter *"Marital Status: March 1998"*).

30. National Center for Children in Poverty, *Children in Poverty—A Statistical Update*, Mailman School of Public Health at Columbia University, June 1999 at 6.

31. Ibid. at Table 6.

32. Ibid.

33. U.S. Department of Commerce, Bureau of the Census; *Consumer Income 1998* (Current Population Reports, Consumer Income, Series P60-206) (Washington, D.C.; 2000) at viii, Table A; see also http://www.census.gov/hhes/www/povty99.html.

34. *Poverty in the United States 1998, supra* note 27, at Table 2; see also http://www.census.gov/hhes/www/povty99.html.

35. See John McNeil, *Changes in Median Household Income: 1969 to 1996* (Current Population Report Special Study P23-196, Bureau of the Census, U.S. Department of Commerce, Washington, D.C., July 1998) at 2-4. This study used data from the Survey of Current Business of August 1997.

36. U.S. Department of Commerce, Bureau of the Census, *Trends in Premarital Childbearing 1930 to 1994* (Current Population Reports P23-197, Washington, D.C.; October 1999), Table 1, column 3, at 2 (hereinafter *"Premarital Trends, 1930 to 1994"*).

37. Ibid. at Table 1, column 4, at 2.

38. See the 47.2% of "post maritally conceived first births" counted in 1990–94; ibid. at Table 1, column 5, at 2.

39. *Marital Status: March 1998, supra* note 29, at 36, Table 6. Note that the summary on page one does not correspond precisely to the data gathered and arrayed in the tables, which we have relied on for our percentages. Note also that the percentages do not total 100% because of approximately 4% of single parent households with children deriving from the death of a spouse. Where this occurs, median income for widows with children is $23,192, and for male widowers it is $43,575.

40. Ibid., at 1.

41. *1997 Population Profile of the United States*, Current Population Report Special Study P23-194, Population Division, Bureau of the Census, Department of Commerce, Washington, D.C., at 24.

42. Jennifer Cheeseman Day, *Projections of the Number of Households and Families in the United States: 1995 to 2010*, Current Population Report P25-1129, Bureau of the Census, Department of Commerce, Washington, D.C., 1996, at 13.

43. See California Department of Health Services, Center for Health Statistics, *Health Data and Statistics* (Sacramento, CA; 1997) at Table 2-4. Data correlating marital status of birth mothers with age has not been published since 1995. A new state law effective in 1999 requires marital status information to be gathered at point of birth for statistical purposes which should facilitate the updating of this information in future years (see new Health and Safety Code § 102426).

44. California Department of Social Services, *TANF Characteristics Survey 1998*, 1999, Tables 18 and 19, at 34.

45. Ibid., Table N at 15.

46. U.S. Department of the Commerce, Bureau of the Census, Current Population Reports: *Births and Deaths: 1997*, 1999, percentages calculated from data presented in Table 2 at 11.

47. Stephanie Ventura and Christine Bachrach, *Nonmarital Childbearing in the United States, 1940–99* Centers for Disease Control and Prevention, National Vital Statistics Report, Volume 48, Number 16, October 18, 2000 at 7.

48. See http://www.acf.dhhs.gov/programs/cse/pubs/2000/datareport/ch01.html.

49. A separate federal "Wee Tot" Earned Income Tax Credit (EITC) Supplement allowed a credit of 5% of earned income up to $388 for a parent who stays home to care for a newborn and in so doing loses eligibility for straight earned income tax credit benefits. That credit was repealed in 1994.

50. A study by Harvard University's Professor Bruce Fuller surveyed 1,800 child care centers in 36 states and concluded that families with annual incomes over $50,000 pay just 6% of their incomes for child care, while families earning under $15,000 devote 23% of their income for child care. The tax credits provide a tax expenditure of $4 billion annually. One-third of the credit goes to families with incomes above $50,000 per year. For a discussion, *see* Diego Ribadeneira, *Day Care Credits Said to Favor Well Off*, BOSTON GLOBE, Sept. 18, 1992, at 3.

51. Such a supplantation danger is an endemic problem in federal-state and state-county relations; the larger jurisdiction wishes to subsidize an increase in resources in an area, which is frustrated when the new money is taken and an equivalent amount previously spent by the receiving jurisdiction for the subsidized purpose is then subtracted and diverted elsewhere or "supplanted." To discourage these diversions, the donor jurisdiction often requires that there be a "maintenance of effort" (MOE) by agencies receiving funds—to ensure that it maintain the same spending it had been committing and treat new money as a genuine "add-on."

52. Most of its clients were the working poor—with 67% earning below the poverty line, and 90% below 150% of the line. Essentially, it funded parents who were "at-risk" of falling back onto AFDC (TANF), but had not been on AFDC previously and therefor would not be eligible for the "at-risk" program.

53. See Shelley Smith, Mary Fairchild, and Scott Groginsky, National Conference of State Legislatures, *Early Childhood Care and Education: An Investment that Works* (Washington, D.C.; January 1997) at 68, citing an August 14, 1996, Congressional Budget Office memorandum.

54. For example, in March 1998, California's minimum wage was raised to $5.75 per hour. On October 24, 2000, the state's Industrial Welfare Commission increased the state minimum wage to $6.25 effective January 1, 2001, and to $6.75 per hour on January 1, 2002.

55. See data and discussion in California Budget Project, *California's Recent Minimum Wage Increases: Real Wage Gains with No Loss of Jobs, Minimum Wage Remains Inadequate to Meet California's Cost of Living*, Budget Brief (June 2000) at 4 (hereinafter *"California's Recent Minimum Wage"*). See www.cbp.org.

56. Richard May, Center on Budget and Policy Priorities, *1993 Poverty and Income Trends* (Washington, D.C.; March 1993) at 19–20, 61; note that over the same 1979–93 period, the top 5% of all income earners increased their income 35% in constant dollars, from $89,000 to $121,000. *Id.*

57. Diane Pearce, Wider Opportunities for Women, *The Self Sufficiency Standard for California* (1996) at 5.

58. The standard is calculated using U.S. Department of Housing and Urban Development annual Fair Market Rents; State Market Surveys of Child Care, U.S. Department of Agriculture, Low-Cost Food Plan; average costs of commuting using public transportation if available or ownership of a six-year-old car where public transportation is not available; medical costs based on full-time work with employer-provided health coverage, estimated costs from Families USA, National Medical Expenditure Survey; miscellaneous expenses of 10% of all other costs; taxes include sales tax, state income tax, payroll tax, and federal income tax.

59. 1997 federal legislation allocates new tobacco tax funds for child health, allowing medicaid expansion to 200% or more of the poverty line. Many states are using these funds for private medical care add-on programs that require substantial co-payments, both per visit, and on a monthly basis. Parents are not covered as to their own expenses, and children are relatively inexpensive medicaid beneficiaries compared with adults and particularly the elderly. The new funding may allow a reduction of up to $80 per month in the projected $176 per month medical costs of Table D.

60. See discussion and citations in *California Children's Budget 2001-02*, CAI, 2000, Chapters 4 and 6.

61. General Accounting Office, Child Care: State Efforts to Enforce Safety and Health Requirements, GAO/HEHS-00-28 (January 2000) at 19, 28, 37.

62. See, e.g., David Illig, California Research Bureau, *Birth to Kindergarten: The Importance of the Early Years* (Sacramento, CA; February 1998) (conducted by request of Senator Dede Alpert); Jane Knitzer and Stephen Page, Columbia University National Center for Children in Poverty, *Map and Track: State Initiatives for Young Children and Families* (New York; NY; 1998); Anne Mitchell, Louise Stoney, and Harriet Dichter, *Financing Child Care in the United States,* Ewing Marion Kauffman Foundation and The Pew Charitable Trusts (1997); Sharon L. Kagan and Nancy E. Cohen, Yale University, The Bush Center in Child Development and Social Policy, *Not By Chance: Creating an Early Care and Education System for America's Children* (New Haven, CT; 1997); Mary L. Culkin, Scott Groginsky, and Steve Christian, National Conference of State Legislatures, *Building Blocks: A Legislator's Guide to Child Care Policy* (Washington, D.C.; 1997); Children's Defense Fund, *Study Reveals Working Families Are Locked Out of Child Care,* 19:4/5 CDF REPORTS 1 (Washington, D.C.; April/May 1998); U.S. General Accounting Office, *Welfare Reform: Implications of Increased Work Participation for Child Care* (GAO/HEHS-97-75) (Washington, D.C.; 1997); Mark H. Greenberg, Center for Law and Social Policy, *The Child Care Protection Under TANF* (Washington, D.C.; 1998); U.S. General Accounting Office, *Welfare Reform: States' Efforts to Expand Child Care Programs* (GAO/HEHS-98-21) (Washington, D.C.; 1998); Center for the Future of Children, The David and Lucile Packard Foundation, THE FUTURE OF

CHILDREN: FINANCING CHILD CARE (Richard E. Behrman, M.D., ed.) (Los Angeles, CA; Summer/Fall 1996).

63. Suzanne W. Helburn, ed., University of Colorado, Center for Research in Economic and Social Policy, *Cost, Quality, and Child Outcomes in Child Care Centers: Technical Report* (Denver, CO; 1995).

64. Suzanne W. Helburn and Carollee Howes, Center for the Future of Children, The David and Lucile Packard Foundation, *Child Care Cost and Quality*, 6:2 THE FUTURE OF CHILDREN: FINANCING CHILD CARE (Richard E. Behrman, M.D., ed.) (Los Angeles, CA; Summer/Fall 1996) at 79–80.

65. Ibid., at 80.

66. See Robin Peth-Pierce, *Early Child Care: About the NICHD Study of Early Child Care* (2001) at 10.

67. *Child Care Outcomes When Center Classes Meet Recommended Standards for Quality*, American Journal of Public Health, 1999; National Center for Early Development and Learning, *The Children of the Cost, Quality, and Outcomes Study Go to School*, 1999; Nancy Kerrebrock, Eugene Lewitt, *Children in Self-Care*, The Future of Children 9(2), Packard Foundation, 1999, at 151-160; Jill Posner and Deborah Candell, *After-school Activities and the Development of Low-Income Urban Children: A Longitudinal Study*, Developmental Psychology 35(3): 868-879.

68. Arthur J. Reynolds, PhD, Judy A. Temple, PhD, Dylan L. Robertson, Emily A. Mann MSSW, *Long-term Effects of an Early Childhood Intervention on Educational Achievement and Juvenile Arrest: A 15-Year Follow-up of Low-Income Children in Public Schools*, 285 JOURNAL OF THE AMERICAN MEDICAL ASSOCIATION 2339–2346, May 9, 2001; see www.jama.com.

69. See the interesting study by William T. Gormley, Jr., and Jessica Lucas, *Money, Accreditation and Child Care Center Quality*, Foundation for Child Development, Working Paper Series (August 2000) passim (see www.ffcd.org). The study cites 18 states providing certification to assure and demonstrate enhanced child care quality, and which also triggers enhanced compensation. Evidence is compelling that this incentive driven technique for enhancing quality works.

70. For a discussion of labor commissioner protests by workers and rate levels extant, see Carla Rivera, *Day-Care Providers Say State Reimbursements Fail to Pay a Living Wage.*, LOS ANGELES TIMES (May 19, 2000) at B-3.

71. *The California Child Care Portfolio 1999*, *supra* note 22, at 2–5.

72. See Marcy Whitebrook, Laura Sakai, Emily Gerber, Carollee Howes, *Then & Now: Changes in Child Care Staffing, 1994–2000*, Institute of Industrial Relations (Berkeley, CA; April 2001) *passim*.

73. Ibid., summary at 4.

74. See *Financing Child Care in the United States: An Illustrative Catalog of Current Strategies*, Ewing Marion Kauffman Foundation and Pew Charitable Trusts, January 13, 1998, see http://www.pewtrusts.com/docs/childcare/index.htm.

75. See *California Children's Budget 2000-01*, CAI, June 2000, Chapter 1.

ARTICLE 6

CHILDREN IN FOSTER CARE: CHALLENGES IN MEETING THEIR HEALTH CARE NEEDS THROUGH MEDICAID

Margo Rosenbach, Kimball Lewis, and Brian Quinn

INTRODUCTION

Children in foster care are of special interest to policymakers because they are a particularly vulnerable group. Many have physical, emotional, or developmental problems, sometimes resulting from abuse or neglect they have suffered. Yet there have been ongoing concerns about the adequacy of the health care services they receive. These concerns have grown as managed care has become a more dominant form of health care delivery for this group.

To complicate matters, existing data provide only a limited snapshot of these children's health-related characteristics. To address problems related to the health care of children in foster care, policymakers must have detailed information about health status, health care utilization, and expenditures.

This publication summarizes a study Mathematica Policy Research, Inc., conducted for the Office of the Assistant Secretary for Planning and Evaluation in the U.S. Department of Health and Human Services. The data source is the State Medicaid Research Files (SMRF), a series of analytic files maintained by the Health Care Financing Administration (HCFA) containing Medicaid eligibility and claims data. Three states—California, Florida, and Pennsylvania—were selected for this study based on the following criteria: (1) the availability of Medicaid claims and enrollment data in the SMRF files, (2) the ability to identify foster care children in the SMRF files, (3) an identifiable foster care population of at least 10,000 children, (4) the degree to which children were enrolled in Medicaid managed care, and (5) variation in features of state foster care systems.

The study period for California and Florida was 1994 and 1995; for Pennsylvania, it was 1993 and 1994 (representing the most recent years of data available in each state). The study population was made up of children under age 19 with a foster care placement during the year. The three comparison groups

197

included children under age 19 who received adoption assistance, Aid to Families with Dependent Children (AFDC), or Supplemental Security Income (SSI) benefits because of disability. The study captures only health care utilization and expenditures that were paid by Medicaid. Foster care children may have received health care that was not billed to Medicaid or that was paid by other sources. As a result, the study understates the total amount and cost of health care services provided to children in foster care.

FINDINGS IN BRIEF

The main findings from the study include:

- Children in foster care represent between 1 and 3 percent of Medicaid children but between 4 and 8 percent of Medicaid expenditures.
- Most children were enrolled in Medicaid before they entered foster care, but between one-third and one-half lost their Medicaid coverage when they left foster care.
- Children in foster care were more likely than other groups of Medicaid children to have a mental health or substance abuse condition.
- Health care utilization varied considerably across the three states studied.

DISPROPORTIONATELY LARGE MEDICAID EXPENDITURES

Medicaid expenditures for children in foster care were disproportionately large, relative to their share of Medicaid enrollment. Although they made up between 1 and 3 percent of the children enrolled in Medicaid in 1994, they accounted for 4 to 8 percent of Medicaid expenditures. Yet, children receiving SSI, who made up between 2 and 5 percent of those enrolled in Medicaid, were responsible for 15 to 27 percent of total expenditures. Although AFDC children represented the largest share (51 to 58 percent), their share of expenditures was smaller (38 to 50 percent).

COVERAGE DISRUPTIONS

Research has shown that continuous, year-round health insurance coverage is related to improved access to care (Figure 1). Children in foster care had less continuous Medicaid coverage than children receiving SSI benefits and children in families receiving adoption assistance. Only 7 in 10 foster care children were enrolled continuously in Medicaid for all of 1994.

FIGURE 1

Medicaid coverage before and after enrollment in foster care, 1994–1995

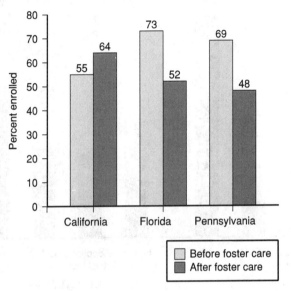

Source: HCFA State Medicaid Research Files.

Although the majority of children were enrolled in Medicaid before they entered foster care, one-third to one-half were not enrolled in Medicaid during the month after their foster care eligibility ended.

In all three states, significant numbers of children lost Medicaid in the month they left foster care. Only California had more children enrolled in Medicaid after foster care, compared with the number enrolled before foster care.

Children receiving SSI or adoption assistance had more continuous Medicaid coverage than children in foster care (80 to 90 percent were covered for the entire year). In general, foster care children and AFDC children had similar patterns of continuity in Medicaid coverage, except in Florida, where turnover for AFDC children was much higher (only 56 percent were enrolled the full year).

HIGH RATES OF MENTAL HEALTH AND SUBSTANCE ABUSE CONDITIONS

Children in foster care were more likely than other groups of Medicaid children to have a mental health or substance abuse condition—either alone or in combination with a physical condition. They also had a higher likelihood of co-morbidities than AFDC and adoption assistance children, but they were less likely than SSI children to have multiple diagnoses (Figure 2).

FIGURE 2

Frequency of chronic illness and disability, 1994

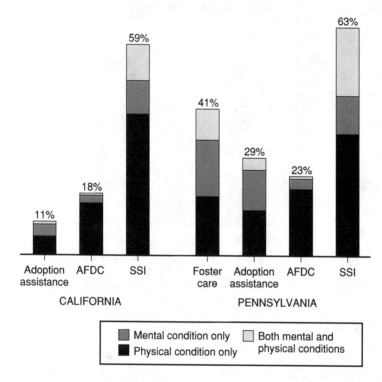

Source: HCFA State Medicaid Research Files.

We used the Chronic Illness and Disability Payment System (CIDPS), developed by Richard Kronick and colleagues at the University of California at San Diego, to identify children with physical or mental conditions, based on diagnoses in Medicaid claims data (Kronick et al. 2000). These data were not available for Florida, since diagnoses were not listed on outpatient claims.

About one in three foster care children in California had a CIDPS condition (32 percent), versus two in five in Pennsylvania (41 percent). The most common conditions in the foster care population were mental conditions (18 percent in California; 24 percent in Pennsylvania). The most common physical conditions were those associated with the central nervous system (5 percent) and pulmonary conditions (6.5 percent).

SSI children were more likely than foster care children to have a CIDPS condition, because of the higher rate of physical conditions among SSI children. The rate of physical conditions was two to three times higher for SSI children than foster care children. On the other hand, the rate of mental health conditions was slightly higher for foster care children.

AFDC children were less likely than foster care children to have a CDPS condition, on the order of about one-half the rate. This was entirely due to lower rates of mental health conditions.

Children receiving adoption assistance were less likely than foster care children to have a CDPS condition (11 percent in California; 29 percent in Pennsylvania). This could be a function of either risk selection in the adoption process (that is, healthier children are adopted) or the more stable risk profile of children who have been in adoptive families for several years.

VARYING UTILIZATION ACROSS STATES; INADEQUATE PREVENTIVE CARE

Health care utilization patterns varied considerably across states. In general, foster care children in California were less likely to receive health care services than children in the other two states. Over 80 percent of the foster care children in Florida and Pennsylvania had at least one provider visit in 1994, compared to 65 percent in California (Figure 3).

FIGURE 3

Foster care children's receipt of selected types of health care, 1994

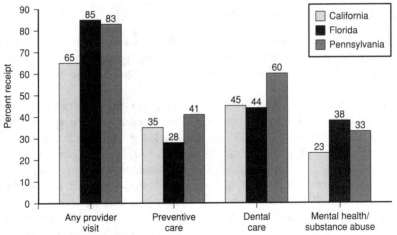

Source: HCFA State Medicaid Research Files.

In California, foster care children also were less likely than AFDC and SSI children to see a provider during the year. In the other two states, foster care children were more likely than AFDC children to see a provider. In Florida, they were also more likely than the SSI population to see a provider during the year.

The likelihood that foster care children received a preventive check-up during 1994 ranged from 28 percent in Florida to 41 percent in Pennsylvania. In

California and Pennsylvania, foster care children were more likely than other Medicaid children to have a preventive check-up during the year. Nevertheless, many foster care children did not receive routine check-ups, despite recommendations for an annual physical and mental health assessment each year. In addition, very few received an assessment during the first two months of a foster care placement. Interestingly, children with no prior Medicaid coverage received early assessments more often, suggesting that providers were more likely to perform assessments on those who were newly enrolled in Medicaid.

Foster care children were far more likely to receive dental care than other groups of Medicaid children. Sixty percent of foster care children in Pennsylvania and 44 to 45 percent in California and Florida had at least one dental visit in 1994, compared with 28 to 38 percent of the AFDC population and 31 to 35 percent of the SSI population.

The likelihood of foster care children receiving mental health or substance abuse treatment services varied substantially across states, from 23 percent in California to 38 percent in Florida. Foster care children were more likely than other groups of Medicaid children—including those receiving SSI—to receive mental health or substance abuse services. Most received treatment on an outpatient basis. The average number of outpatient visits per user varied widely (6 in California; 18 in Florida; 22 in Pennsylvania).

WIDE RANGE OF MEDICAID EXPENDITURES

Average Medicaid expenditures varied widely across states but were lowest in California, consistent with the lower utilization in that state. In general, expenditures were highest for the SSI population and second-highest for foster care children.

Average monthly Medicaid expenditures for foster care children ranged more than twofold, from $154 in California to $375 in Florida, with Pennsylvania averaging $293 (Figure 4). Medicaid spending for foster care children was two or more times higher than the average for all Medicaid children. Average monthly Medicaid expenditures for SSI children were between four and seven times higher than expenditures for all Medicaid children. Medicaid expenditures for AFDC children were well below the average for all Medicaid children.

Infants in foster care had by far the highest average monthly expenditures, driven primarily by high inpatient costs. Spending also varied by health condition. Compared to spending for foster care children with no CDPS condition, spending was 10 to 12 times higher for those with both physical and mental conditions, and 5 to 7 times higher for those with either a physical or mental condition.

FIGURE 4

Monthly Medicaid expenditures
by type of health condition, 1994

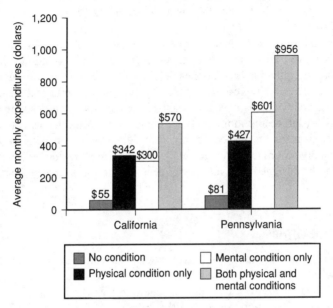

Source: HCFA State Medicaid Research Files.

THE POLICY PICTURE

These findings provide important guidance for policy and practice—to improve the delivery of health care services to children in foster care, especially in the changing health care environment. Four main implications emerge from this study:

- *Continuity of coverage is important.* Discontinuities in health insurance coverage can have an adverse effect on access to care. Policymakers should focus on ways to improve continuity of health insurance coverage for children in foster care.
- *Medicaid may be underutilized as a funding source.* States have considerable flexibility in how they use Medicaid to pay for services for children in foster care. Medicaid can fund a comprehensive continuum of care, ranging from screening and assessment to follow-up treatment and ongoing therapies. Evidence of state-level variation in Medicaid expenditures suggests that states differ in the use of Medicaid to serve children in foster care.
- *A broad-based concept of care coordination is needed.* The low level of compliance with screening and assessment protocols underscores the

importance of care coordination as a vehicle for overcoming structural barriers to care, especially fragmentation between the child welfare and health care systems. A broad-based concept of care coordination is especially relevant for foster care families, whose needs may involve multiple systems of care, such as public health, child welfare, mental health, schools, and juvenile justice.

- *The structure of managed care systems should recognize foster care children's needs.* This study highlights the foster care population's special needs, especially the need for behavioral health care services. Because children in foster care represent only 1 to 3 percent of the child Medicaid population, policymakers may lose sight of their needs when designing programs for larger and more visible groups. Payment mechanisms (such as risk adjustment or risk corridors), provider networks, benefit packages (especially coverage of mental health services), and provider education all need to be designed with the special needs of the foster care population in mind.

FOCUS ON THE FUTURE

Like all research studies, this one raised questions that could be explored in future studies. The first involves state-level variation—what accounts for the significant variation in diagnoses, utilization, and expenditure patterns across states? This study has taken a first step to document the differences. Further work is needed to explain them. Possible factors include the role of child welfare and health agencies in coordinating and advocating for health care services for children in foster care; the role of the courts in mandating health care for children in foster care; characteristics of state programs (such as the use of health passports, level of staff caseload, and availability of transportation services); variations in the Medicaid benefit package; availability of providers to serve the population; provider knowledge concerning services needed by the population; generosity of reimbursement rates; differences in case mix; and level of stigma about accessing services.

Another question raised by the study involves the extent of unmet need. We cannot tell from claims data whether variations in utilization levels are the result of overutilization in some groups or underutilization in others. Without external benchmarks against which to evaluate patterns of care, coupled with more detailed clinical assessments, we cannot tell whether lower rates of utilization are indicative of access barriers or simply lower health care needs. To gain a better understanding of unmet needs in the foster care population, policymakers and researchers could perform a medical records review or conduct a survey of foster care families and caseworkers.

STUDY LIMITATIONS

Although this study has shed light on patterns of diagnoses, utilization, and expenditures for children in foster care, the generalizability of the results may be limited for several reasons:

- *The data are for three states.* Although this is an improvement over previous studies that focused on a single state, the results cannot be generalized to all states or to the nation as a whole. Using multiple states demonstrates the extent of variation and can provide useful comparisons to other states.
- *The data were from the mid-1990s.* We used the most recent data available at the time, but more recent data would be desirable to ascertain whether patterns have changed.
- *The analyses of diagnosed conditions, expenditures, and utilization exclude children enrolled in managed care.* The SMRF did not gather encounter data for capitated services, so children enrolled in managed care were excluded from this study. To the extent that utilization patterns differ systematically for children in foster care who are enrolled in managed care, the differences will not be captured in the analysis.

Using the SMRF for research purposes has some other limitations. The file has no provider specialty, which precluded us from looking at this aspect of continuity of care, or specialty referral patterns. In addition, not all states report such basic data as diagnoses, but to our knowledge there is no central database that indicates which SMRF files contain specific data elements and with what degree of completeness. Many states also use state-specific procedure codes, but the definitions are not uniformly available to researchers. States can also differ in the way they code type-of-service categories, especially for mental health. Furthermore, the SMRF contains only a single eligibility category each month, hampering our efforts to identify children receiving SSI benefits who were placed in foster care. Finally, it is unclear whether the date of foster care placement on the eligibility file is accurate. This affects all analyses of pre- and post-placement utilization.

WHAT'S NEXT?

As the health care needs of children in foster care have garnered increasing attention, interest has grown in developing performance measures to track the effectiveness of child welfare services. This study shows how utilization and expenditure measures can be operationalized using Medicaid data. Additional analyses, based on more recent data, would help portray how children in foster care are faring in the new millennium—including whether they are receiving more continuous coverage and more comprehensive care as a result of state efforts to improve their health care.

ARTICLE 7

THE HEAD START PROGRAM: PAST, PRESENT, AND FUTURE

Anne Cohn Donnelly and Frederick Green

THE HISTORY AND INTENT OF HEAD START

As recounted by Ed Zigler,[1-3] one of the founders and later steward of Head Start, the federal Head Start program began in 1965 with very high expectations and high hopes; this is most likely what made its launching possible. The hopes and expectations were that Head Start would significantly improve the chances that poor children would succeed in life. The idea was hatched during the great "War on Poverty" in response to one simple statistic in 1964—nearly half of the nation's poor people were children and most were under age 12. Program designers understood that a war on poverty must address the needs and conditions of these poor children; they also knew that a war on poverty that would benefit children was a war most of the public would support. Head Start was the only weapon in the war targeting children; most of the war's programs were for adults and older teens.

In its conception, and from its inception, Head Start was seen as a comprehensive program: a child care and education facility for preschoolers, which would address the need for systematic evaluation of the health status of children through episodic screening for hearing and eye care, proper nutrition, the provision of immunization and other facets of young children's physical and mental health. It would also focus on motivating children and creating a climate that would help in the development of children's mental processes and skills. In other words, it would address all facets of child development. At the same time it would involve parents as integral parts of the children's lives and education for their children's benefit as well as their own. An emphasis would be placed on employing the parents and other poor people, in the program.

In its inception, Head Start was to be a summer-only program with the plan that poor preschool children from low-income families would be ready to begin kindergarten or first grade. Communities would use otherwise closed school facilities and provide summer jobs to teachers. It did not take long to see the benefits of year-round support for these children and the program began to grow to encompass a full year (e.g., 10 months) in its second year, sprouting up in churches, store fronts, and other available community facilities.

The program was to be for all poor children of preschool age. Although handicapped or disabled children were not a part of the earliest design, in response to an understanding that these children have special needs, in time a special focus was established. A set proportion of enrollment (e.g., 10%) would consist of children with disabilities and be served by Head Start centers.

Unlike special initiatives of today, when Head Start began the idea was that it would serve a significant portion of the target population—at least 100,000. It was launched as an "instant" nationwide program. The movers and shakers behind Head Start and the rest of the War on Poverty were ready for action, not pilots and demonstrations and evaluations. Once President Lyndon Johnson's wife Lady Bird signed on as the Honorary Chairperson and a kick-off reception was held at the White House, enthusiasm grew, and in its first year Head Start in fact served over half a million children. This nationwide implementation gave instant visibility to the program and gathered grassroots support virtually across the country or, as some like to point out, in every Congressional district. It was this widespread community support that has stood this federal effort in good stead through repeated bipartisan federal reauthorizations.

Of course, not everyone embraced Head Start. Some segments of some communities saw federally supported child development programs as "contrary to the American ethos." Some felt that childcare programs should impact parents directly by helping them off the welfare rolls rather than targeting children to enhance their developmental potential. Despite competing views, Head Start flourished.

Community enthusiasm for the program was matched by the enthusiasm of volunteers in Washington D.C., and across the country—volunteers to help representatives from poor neighborhoods write proposals, volunteers to help government officials review proposals, volunteers to help set up and operate funded efforts. This enthusiasm was widespread, from spouses of high-ranking government officials to pastors in local churches to all manner of health and education professionals. (For example, doctors and dentists would do free checkups. High visibility national groups such as the American Academy of Pediatrics joined the cause.) To help maintain and promote this volunteerism, part of the 20 percent local match required of grantees could consist of volunteered time. Health and hospital facilities and others were urged to have community advisory committees, a form of community control. This was in contrast to most such community facilities, which were typically governed by non-neighborhood residents.

The original push for substantive parental involvement in Head Start was in many ways revolutionary: The concept was that children would benefit from their parents' direct involvement in the program. The parents could learn about child development and facets of child learning and also fill some staff positions. The concept initially was that parents would not totally control Head Start but that, with 51% membership on the programs' policy councils, parents would have shared control in planning and administration. The roles of parents in program direction and community activism emerged later. (In 1973, for example, the national Head

Start Association was formed by the Head Start directors; a year later, in recognition of the importance of parents, parents were admitted to the Association.)

In order to ensure that there was a cadre of trained caregivers to meet children's development needs and who were more affordable than BA-degreed teachers, Head Start established opportunities for parents and other community people to be trained as Child Development Associates (CDA) so they could provide quality services in Head Start and other childcare programs. This would be the beginning of a career ladder for many people. Over the years there have been many ups and downs in the implementation of this training initiative. (Today it is proposed that centers be required to have at least one teacher in every classroom of 17–18 children with a recognized credential in child development or at least an Associates degree in early childhood education.)

INNOVATIONS IN HEAD START

From the earliest years there have been a number of programmatic innovations in Head Start in addition to efforts to move the program from a part-day summer program to a full-year full-day one. The thought was that there would be flow of children from support in the earliest years through Head Start and thereafter. The three innovations that stand out are: (1) efforts to follow children into elementary school after Head Start; (2) efforts to reach children before they enter Head Start (e.g., from pregnancy or birth); and (3) efforts to reach out to families in their homes as well as through center-based programs.

In 1967, a Follow-Through program was designed and initiated to extend comprehensive services to Head Start children when they entered kindergarten through third grade; efforts like this, which were never fully funded, have continued throughout Head Start's history. As such, in the early years Follow-Through became an experiment to develop and compare the effectiveness of various curriculum models. Today, this effort is embodied in the Head Start Transition Project. Also in 1967, still the early years of Head Start, Parent and Child Centers were set up in several (33) of the Head Start Communities to serve families with young children from birth to age 3. Centers like these, which have continued ever since, are the precursors to Early Head Start. One of Head Start's most successful innovations, which also began in the early years, was Home Start, an effort designed to offer all the benefits of Head Start in the home. This home-based intervention, which was especially well suited to rural areas, has continued ever since as the home-based option to any Head Start program. Today, the home-based component is, in general, as much an integral part of Early Head Start as it is of Head Start.

EARLY HEAD START

By the early 1990s, recognition that children need positive child development experiences starting at birth was widespread.[4] The reauthorization of the Head Start Act in 1994 made it possible for Head Start to include an "early" Head Start component for babies and toddlers. The Early Head Start Program officially began in 1995. The program, which awarded grants competitively, pooled Head Start's existing programs for families with infants and toddlers with the Parent and Child Centers, the Head Start home-based component and the government's Comprehensive Child Development Program. The hope was that Early Head Start would finally establish the beginnings of a full continuum of support for low-income children and their families.

The idea behind Early Head Start was to put resources into supports and services that would build communities while providing healthy child and family development. The concept was to offer a constellation of services (health, social services, early childhood education) to families with newborns through age 3, while maintaining a commitment to training, quality, service coordination, and evaluation. In many ways the specific goals for Early Head Start were no different than Head Start, although there was recognition that support to and education of parents of these very young children was an essential feature. Further, Early Head Start recognized that for infants and toddlers to develop optimally, they must have healthy beginnings and the continuity of responsive and caring relationships with the primary adults in their lives. The program reflects research from the previous three decades that has shown that when programs focus on both the child *and* the parent and family through early high-quality, comprehensive, and intensive services, even the most vulnerable children and families can develop in positive ways.

The Early Head Start program thus was designed with the benefit of 30 years of experience with the Head Start program. Early Head Start was at its inception founded on a set of principles that matured slowly for its parent program:

- A commitment to excellence
- A focus on prevention and promotion
- A commitment to developing strong, caring continuous relationships
- Strong involvement of parents
- The inclusion of children with disabilities, and their families
- Comprehensive, flexible, responsive, and intensive services
- A smooth transition from Early Head Start to Head Start of other high-quality preschool programs
- Collaboration with other community providers and institutions that touch children and their families

To meet these commitments, Early Head Start efforts are concerned with the development of the child, the family, the staff, and the community. In its first year, 143 Early Head Start projects were supported, serving 22,000 children under the age of 3. And, by the year 2000, nearly 600 projects, in all 50 states and the District of Columbia and Puerto Rico, served 45,100 children under the age of 3, or 6 percent of the overall Head Start enrollment.

VARIATION ACROSS HEAD START PROGRAMS: A QUESTION ABOUT QUALITY

In recognition that the poor were not a homogeneous group and that poor communities each has their own culture, at the outset Head Start was not a precisely defined program. There was not a proscribed curriculum. Rather, each grantee was given latitude in shaping the form of the program. As a result, Head Start programs early on varied significantly; the lack of a consistent set of standards and also the lack of a specific set of beliefs about early childhood contributed to this variability. In part this variability was due to the variety of models suggested in the early years. There were differences in selecting and hiring of teachers and a general lack of trained teachers in some communities.

Variability across Head Start sites was seen over time, and questions about quality were raised. Certainly the uneven training of teachers and the low pay contributed to these concerns. But other issues surfaced as well. The class size in Head Start rooms was variable. The delivery of health services to children was not consistent. The services offered to families identified with multiple problems were not always comprehensive. Even the facilities within which Head Start programs found themselves were varied—many were temporary and not all met codes for safety. As a result, over time standards were set and imposed on Head Start grantees; over time programs began to look more comparable and began to address issues of quality.

WHAT HEAD START HAS ACCOMPLISHED

The story of Head Start's accomplishments can be told in two ways—through numbers and through measured outcomes. The numbers alone are impressive.

The Numbers

Since Head Start's inception in 1965, when it was launched as a summer-only program, through the year 2000, over 19 million children and their families have been served (Table 1). It is important to note that enrollment dropped dramatically after the first year; Head Start achieved the 1965 enrollment size again in 1991. By 2000, federal spending grew from $96 million to over six billion dollars. In contract to this growth in dollars, in 1965, 561,000 children were served during the summer; in 2000, the number was just over 857,000 for year-round services, with a significant number now receiving full-day services year round, an important development in light of welfare reforms during the 1990s.

A profile of the children served in 2000 tells an important story (Table 2). The program serves a diverse population with a significant representation of pre-kindergarten children. Children 4 years old made up 56% of the Head Start population and 3-year-olds made up 33% of the children served. These children were served in 18,200 Centers which in turn were supported through 1,525 grantees. There were over 180,400 paid staff supported by over 1,252,000 volunteers. Of the paid staff, 32% were parents of current or former Head Start children. And, according to the Head Start Bureau, 75% of the volunteers were parents. Of the children enrolled in Head Start, 12.7% had defined disabilities and 59% were enrolled in compatible community programs that provided their medical and dental care, such as Medicaid and early periodic screening and detection programs.

In terms of raw numbers, the program has touched literally millions and millions of lives. Yet, today, with these large numbers, only about one-third of the eligible poor children are served by the program.

TABLE 1 HEAD START ENROLLMENT AND APPROPRIATION HISTORY

Year	Enrollment	Congressional Fiscal Appropriation
1965 (Summer Only)	561,000	$96,400,000
1966	733,000	198,900,000
1967	681,400	349,200,000
1968	693,900	316,200,000
1969	663,600	333,900,000
1970	477,400	325,700,000
1971	397,500	360,000,000
1972	379,000	376,300,000
1973	379,000	400,700,000
1974	352,800	403,900,000
1975	349,000	403,900,000
1976	349,000	441,000,000
1977	333,000	475,000,000
1978	391,400	625,000,000
1979	387,500	680,000,000
1980	376,300	735,000,000
1981	387,300	818,700,000
1982	395,800	911,700,000
1983	414,950	912,000,000
1984	442,140	995,750,000
1985	452,080	1,075,059,000
1986	451,732	1,040,315,000
1987	446,523	1,130,542,000
1988	448,464	1,206,324,000
1989	450,970	1,235,000,000
1990	540,930	1,552,000,000
1991	583,471	1,951,800,000
1992	621,078	2,201,800,000
1993	713,903	2,776,286,000
1994	740,493	3,325,728,000
1995	750,696	3,534,128,000
1996	752,077	3,569,329,000
1997	793,809	3,980,546,000
1998	822,316	4,347,433,000
1999	826,016	4,658,151,448
2000	857,664	5,267,000,000

Note: A total of 19,397,000 children have been served by the program since it began in 1965.

Source: Head Start Bureau, Department of Health and Human Services, Washington, D.C. 2001.

TABLE 2 THE HEAD START CHILD IN 2000

Ages	Percentage of Head Start Enrollment
5-year-olds and older	5%
4-year-olds	56%
3-year-olds	33%
Under 3 years of age	6%

Income*	
Less than $9,000 per year	61%
Less than $12,000 per year	78%

*Data from 1997.

Racial/Ethnic Composition	
American Indian	3.3%
Hispanic	28.7%
Black	34.5%
White	30.4%
Asian	2.0%
Hawaiian/Pacific Islanders	1.0%

Total enrollment in 2000 was 857,664.
Source: Head Start Bureau, Department of Health and Human Services, Washington, D.C. 2000.

The Outcomes

Evaluation of outcome data was recognized from the very outset of Head Start as important. Also most would agree that the hasty evaluation of the first summer's program was of little value. In fact, the evaluations in the earliest years were problematic because of their narrow scope. Early political supporters had believed (and promised) that Head Start would improve children's IQ, and early evaluations studied whether or not it had, rather than the broader issues of child development Head Start was really intended to address. More recent evaluations have addressed these broader issues.

What did the studies find? The early evaluations studies did demonstrate gains in IQ, but the gains were only temporary. Initial IQ gains decayed over time and Head Start in those early years was found to have no measurable impacts on school achievement or performance after third grade. (These early studies, coupled with the political climate, help explain years of shrinkage or at least no or minimal growth in the program size as shown in Table 1.)

Later studies, which looked at child development more globally and at Head Start *and* comparable programs, resulted in findings that supported the ability of intensive, carefully implemented interventions to produce important changes. Findings showed children being less likely to be held back in school and less likely to require remedial education. Overall, Head Start studies and Head Start children had better health, immunization rates, and nutrition as well as enhanced socio-emotional traits and family relationships. Individual parents reported improved relationships with their children. Further, studies of comparable programs documented cost savings: for every dollar spent on preschool programs like Head Start, taxpayers save up to $7.

Thus, overall the findings about Head Start are positive. They show a variety of salutary effects for families, children, and communities. Head Start advocates have used these findings to support the continuation of the program, to promote Early Head Start and the follow through program, *and* to leverage support to strengthen and tighten the standards for all Head Start programs.

HEAD START'S FUTURE

The environment in which Head Start operates certainly helps to define the future needs of Head Start. For example, of the many social, economic, and political changes over Head Start's 35-year history, many look to recent reforms in the welfare system as pivotal for changes in the need for Head Start's services. As more and more parents of preschool children rotated off the welfare rolls to work, the need for child care—and for the unique assistance of Head Start—grew. Now, as the extended period of prosperity in the country appears to be on the wane and economic distress extends to a larger proportion of the population, the number of children eligible for Head Start services could increase. As one looks to the future of the Head Start program certain challenges remain evident:

1. *There will undoubtedly be a need to expand the size of the program.* There was major growth in Head Start in the 1990s. At the end of the 90s, the nation's governors established as the top national educational goal for the year 2000 that all children will be ready to learn when they enter school. During the 90s, the nation's welfare system was reformed. The growth in Head Start since the early 1990s in no way meets the need. Today, about one-third of the eligible population is served. With the changing economic climate, that population will undoubtedly change.

2. *There is a need to find a way to care for more of our youngest children.* The advent of Early Head Start opened the door for serving this population; research continues to show that these earliest years are a time when Head Start may be able to have its biggest impact. Yet, a tiny percentage of that population today is served through the Early Head Start program. There is a need to give local communities the flexibility to spend as many of their Head Start expansion funds on infants and toddlers as they need to. The more discretion local programs have in allocating their dollars by age group, the more able they will be to respond to local need.

3. *There is a need to maintain vigilance over the quality of all Head Start services and most especially the training of its teachers.* Uneven quality has plagued the program from the beginning. As with most any preschool (or school) program, the individual site may only be as good as the teachers at that site. Qualified teachers need to be trained to do their jobs; they also need to be individuals with the warmth, compassion, and understanding to work with young children and their families. Because of the low wages paid to Head Start workers, it has been hard to attract and retain such qualified teachers. The future success of the program depends upon finding innovative ways to meet this challenge. These innovations may focus on the parents themselves.

In addition to these three issues, and as more and more parents are working and/or are facing economic distress, it may well be time to consider the benefits to society of changing the eligibility requirements for Head Start so that more than just the very poor can benefit from the program.

CONCLUSIONS

Since its inception, Head Start has had the constant support of people involved in the program within the community. Despite the fact that Head Start has fallen in and out of favor with policymakers—in some large measure because of evaluation studies with designs too narrow to capture the comprehensive nature of the program—the program today thrives, maintains bipartisan support, and appears to have important impacts on the vast majority of population served. It can be argued that with a changing economic climate and increased understanding about the needs of children in their earliest years of life, it is now time to increase the scale of Head Start and programs like it, so the benefits of this comprehensive child development program can universally reach all of Americans youngest citizens.

REFERENCES

1. Zigler, E. & S. Muenchow, 1992. Head Start: *The Inside Story of America's Most Successful Educational Experiment.* New York. Basic Books.

2. Zigler, E. & S. J. Styfco, 1993. *Head Start and Beyond: A National Plan for Extended Childhood Intervention.* New Haven. Yale University Press.

3. Zigler, E. & J. Valentine, editors. 1997. *Project Head Start: A Legacy of the War on Poverty.* Second Edition. Alexandria. The National Head Start Association.

4. *The Statement of the Advisory Committee on Services for Families With Infants and Toddlers.* 1994. Washington D.C. U.S. Department of Health and Human Services.

ARTICLE 8

COMMUNITY-BASED COALITIONS: THE HEALTHY START INITIATIVE

David S. de la Cruz, and Maribeth Badura

INTRODUCTION

Giving people a voice in the systems that affect their lives can be very powerful. When a community is able to redesign its health and social service systems, both the community and its members are transformed. But community participation in reshaping systems does not just happen by itself. If members of a community are truly to have an impact, they must have an organized voice. Collaborative efforts, including coalitions, are becoming that voice.

OVERVIEW OF COALITIONS

A coalition is a union of people and organizations working to influence outcomes on a specific problem.[1] Coalitions are useful for accomplishing a broad range of goals that reach beyond the capacity of any individual member organization. These goals range from information sharing to coordination or services, from community education to advocacy for major environmental or policy changes.[2,3]

Coalitions offer numerous potential advantages over individuals or organizations working independently.[1] The broader purpose and breadth of coalitions give them more credibility than individual organizations and can reduce the suspicion of self-interest. Among the many benefits of coalitions are the following. They can:

- Conserve resources, which continue to be limited
- Reach more people within a community than is possible with a single organization
- Accomplish objectives beyond the scope of any single organization
- Have greater credibility than an individual organization
- Provide a forum for sharing information

- Provide a range of advice and perspectives to the lead agency
- Foster personal satisfaction and help members understand their jobs within a broader perspective
- Foster cooperation among grassroots organizations, community members, and diverse sectors of a large organization
- Build trust and consensus among people and organizations that have similar responsibilities and concerns within a community

However, a coalition is not appropriate in every situation and is only one of a variety of tools for accomplishing organizational goals.[1,4] A lead agency should carefully consider the responsibilities of developing and coordinating a coalition. The success of a coalition is usually uncertain. In addition, lead agencies tend to underestimate the requirements needed to keep coalitions functioning well, especially the commitment of substantial staffing resources. Coalitions also require significant commitment from the members, who frequently must weigh coalition membership against other important work. Potential results of coalition efforts often diverge from the initial expectations of the organizations that created them. Furthermore, some tasks are inappropriate for coalitions because they may require an intensity of focus that is difficult to attain with a large group.[3,5]

Also, before initiating a coalition, it is important for the lead organizations to determine whether related groups already exist within the community.[6,7] At times, it will be far more effective to participate in an already existing group with compatible goals than to form a new coalition. Finally, people and organizations often define terms differently. It is important to clearly define the type of group that will be formed, including its mission, membership, and structure, and to make sure that all participants understand and agree with this information.

There are eight steps to building an effective coalition:[1,8]

1. Analyze the program's objectives and determine whether to form a coalition
2. Recruit the right people for coalition membership
3. Devise a set of preliminary objectives and activities
4. Convene the coalition
5. Anticipate the necessary resources
6. Define elements of a successful coalition structure
7. Maintain coalition vitality
8. Make improvements through evaluation

Healthy Start is a federally funded community-based initiative that uses coalitions and community collaboration to successfully implement its activities. The following description of the Healthy Start Initiative (HSI) includes ways in which coalitions have been used.

OVERVIEW OF THE HEALTHY START INITIATIVE

For many years, infant mortality has been used as a key indicator of a society's health status. The fact that in 1989 the United States ranked 21st among industrialized nations in infant mortality rates challenged maternal and child health experts. This alarming rate led the White House Task Force to Reduce Infant Mortality to convene and make recommendations that were adapted by the Interagency Committee on Infant Mortality in 1990. This targeted approach to reduce infant mortality was one of the most recent efforts, among many through the years, of tackling a problem that, although showing signs of some improvements, still required attention.

Despite recent gains in reducing infant deaths, infant mortality remains a serious and tragic problem that can be solved only if all stakeholders—community members (including its leaders), businesses, health care professionals, and policymakers—work together to find answers. To help find these solutions and put them into practice across the country, the Healthy Start Initiative was initially established as a demonstration program in 1991. HSI was founded on the premise that community-driven strategies were needed to attack the causes of infant mortality and low birth weight, especially among high-risk populations.

The principles guiding the planning and operation of the initiative are innovation, community commitment and involvement, increased access to services, service integration, and personal responsibility. A unique hallmark of the initiative is the development and mobilization of strong community coalitions of consumers, local and state governments, the private sector, schools, providers and neighborhood organizations to improve perinatal health care and birth outcomes for women and infants. This is accomplished by promoting healthy behaviors and combating the causes of maternal and infant mortality and morbidity.

Healthy Start is an initiative mandated to reduce the rate of infant mortality and improve perinatal outcomes through grants to project areas with high annual rates of infant mortality. Therefore, the HSI focuses on the contributing factors that research shows are influencing the perinatal trends in high-risk communities. Specifically, Healthy Start:

- Is committed to implementing evidenced-based practices and innovative community-based interventions to support and improve perinatal delivery systems in project communities
- Is focused primarily on perinatal and infant clients and their families
- Strives to assure that every participating woman and infant gains access to the health delivery system and is followed through the continuum of care
- Provides strong linkages with the state and local perinatal system

During its demonstration phase, which ended in 1997, there were 22 HSI demonstration projects that developed and implemented community-based strategies to reduce infant mortality in areas with a high incidence of infant mortality. These strategies affected all aspects of the continuum of perinatal care. The primary mission of HSI during the demonstration phase was to identify and implement a broad range of community-based strategies for significantly reducing infant mortality in communities with a very high rate of infant mortality. Nine categories of community-driven infant mortality reduction strategies emerged from the HSI demonstration phase, including one organizational category and eight service-intervention categories. These nine categories were:

- Community-based consortia

- Care coordination/Case management
- Outreach and client recruitment
- Enhanced clinical services
- Family resource centers
- Risk prevention and reduction
- Facilitating services
- Training and education
- Adolescent programs

Since 1997, HSI broadened its primary mission to reduce contributing factors to infant mortality and improve perinatal outcomes by initiating support to additional communities seeking to adapt or replicate successful Healthy Start strategies. In keeping with the commitment to community-based strategies, all HSI projects funded since 1997 were required to have an ongoing working relationship with a community-based consortium that has both: (1) active involvement in the proposed project area, and (2) experience with implementing maternal and child health strategies in the proposed project area.

More recently, in October 2000 President Clinton signed into law the Children's Health Act of 2000 (P.L.106-310), which included HSI authorization in the section: "Title XV- Healthy Start Initiative." Under this legislation, the HSI continues to be defined as: "an initiative to reduce the rate of infant mortality and improve perinatal outcomes, makes grants for project areas with high annual rates of infant mortality." The Healthy Start Initiative requires all funded projects to have or to "establish, for project areas under this subsection, community-based consortia of individuals and organizations (including agencies responsible for administering block-grant programs under Title V of the Social Security Act, consumers of project services, public health departments, hospitals, health centers under Section 330, and other significant sources of health care services) that are appropriate for participation in projects under subsection (a)."

The HSI has federal authorization through FY 2005. The legislation also requires future HSI grantees to coordinate their HSI-funded services and activities with the state agency or agencies that administer the Maternal and Child Health (MCH) block-grant programs under Title V of the Social Security Act. The purpose of this coordination is to promote cooperation, integration, and dissemination of information with statewide systems and with other community services funded under the Maternal and Child Health block grant. The Healthy Start Initiative continues to directly address the Healthy People 2010 goal related to eliminating health disparities, and in particular, the objectives related to maternal and infant health.

The current phase of HSI began July 1, 2001, and will continue to May 31, 2005. Communities in 34 states and the District of Columbia will share $75.4 million in new grants intended to reduce high infant mortality rates and other health problems related to pregnancy and women's health. The 74 communities will join 11 other Healthy Start communities that received funds in Budget Year 2000 to improve perinatal health while reducing racial disparities.

Utilizing HSI funds, existing programs, or other resources available, every HSI-funded project assures the availability of a core set of services and activities to the perinatal population in the project area. The communities that received Healthy Start awards will extend the following core services from prenatal care through the baby's second year for the mother and the infant:

- A community-based consortium of families, local leaders, and public and private health organizations
- Case management and links to health care and other services for the mother and her infant(s) (e.g., ensuring that the mother and infant both have a medical/health home and are receiving all needed developmental and specialty care)
- Direct outreach from trained community members
- Health education to address risk factors
- A plan that mobilizes community-based organizations and local, state, public, and private providers to identify and address barriers to quality, family-centered services

As needed, projects also support an expansion of clinical services and enabling services such as transportation and child care, to facilitate families timely receipt of all necessary services.

With the funding made available in July 2001, HSI focuses its Fiscal Year 2001 funds into four areas:

- Eliminating Disparities in Perinatal Health (General)
- Interconceptional Care for High-Risk Women and Their Infants
- Improving Women's Health through Screening and Intervention for Depression during and around the Time of Pregnancy
- Eliminating Disparities in Perinatal Health (Border Health)

Eliminating Disparities in Perinatal Health (General)

The goal of the Eliminating Disparities in Perinatal Health grant is to enhance a community's service system to address significant disparities in infant mortality and other perinatal health indicators by enhancing a community's service system. Disparities include those based on race/ethnicity, immigrant status, education, income, disability, and geography. To address the identified disparity and the factors contributing to it, the scope of project services must cover pregnancy and interconceptional phases for women and infants residing in the proposed project area. To promote healthier women and infants, services are given to both mother and infant up to the infant's second birthday.

Interconceptional Care for High-Risk Women and Their Infants

The purpose of this program is to improve the health of high-risk women and high-risk infants and to avoid future adverse pregnancy outcomes. This grant funding will support communities to enroll high-risk infants and pregnant and postpartum women identified as high-risk during an antepartum hospitalization or at the time of delivery. These high-risk women/ infants will be followed for two years or through the next pregnancy, ensuring they are enrolled in the health care system for appropriate care and follow-up. Projects also target in the immediate postpartum period, women who sustained a fetal loss, or delivered without receipt of an appropriate level of prenatal care.

Improving Women's Health through Screening and Intervention for Depression during and around the Time of Pregnancy

The purpose of this program is to promote systems of care that address gaps in routine screening and skilled assessment for depression during or around the time of pregnancy and to enhance linkages to community-based intervention services for depression, which are age and culturally specific for women of reproductive age. Projects funded under this competition must establish an infrastructure network of community prenatal, family planning, and mental health service providers that will lead to early identification and increased capacity to effectively screen, perform skilled assessment, and successfully engage pregnant and postpartum women who are experiencing depression into appropriate mental health services.

Eliminating Disparities in Perinatal Health (Border Health)

Similar to the competition for the general population, the purpose of this competition is to enhance a border community's (selected communities must be within 62 miles of the U.S.-Mexican border, and have a high incidence of poor perinatal indicators) perinatal service system to address significant disparities in perinatal health. To address these factors, the proposed project services should cover pregnancy, perinatal, and interconceptional phases for women and infants residing in the proposed project area. To promote healthier women and infants, services are to be given to both mother and infant up to the infant's second birthday.

As more communities try to improve their health and social systems to make them more responsive to the needs of the community members, collaborative efforts are becoming recognized as effective vehicles for change.[9,10] The federal Healthy Start Initiative has recognized that power and has placed collaboration, in the form of community-based coalitions and consortiums, at the center of its efforts. A key component of the Healthy Start Initiative is to reduce infant mortality by helping communities assess their own needs and decide which interventions work best to meet their individual and unique needs.

Although Healthy Start focuses on reducing infant mortality, its efforts to involve the community in collaboration can be replicated to tackle other public health problems. As the health care system in the United States continues to evolve, the benefit of collaboration becomes even more relevant: As a community transforms its systems to meet its needs, the community is empowered.

By emphasizing the consortium model, The Healthy Start Initiative focuses the power of collaboration on the problem of infant mortality. A well-organized community can lead to benefits that ultimately reduce maternal and infant mortality and morbidity rates. These benefits include increasing the public's understanding of the problem, strengthening the public's commitment to deal realistically with the problem, using existing resources more efficiently and effectively, and mobilizing additional resources.

THE HEALTHY START INITIATIVE

At the heart of the Healthy Start Initiative is the belief that the community, guided by a consortium of individuals and organizations from many sectors, can best design and implement the services needed by the women, children, and families in that community. Programs designed by local communities will best address their unique needs and mobilize their resources. Advised by consortia, Healthy Start communities can focus the power of collaboration on the problem of infant mortality. The key reason that collaboration is essential to fighting infant mortality is found in the complexity of the problem itself. Because infant mortality is affected by socio-economic conditions such as poverty, inadequate housing, unemployment, racism, and violence, no one single organization can solve the problem. A collaborative, multidisciplinary approach within the community can create the long-term vision needed to attack the problem from a variety of angles.

Healthy Start Community Project Case Examples

The following are case examples from Healthy Start-funded communities. These examples are meant to demonstrate how the different communities use their consortium to collaborate and build coalitions that help them in their fight against infant mortality.

The Boston Healthy Start Initiative. The Boston Healthy Start Initiative is a partnership between the Boston Department of Health and Hospitals and a consortium of community residents and service providers. This structure places the power for change directly in the hands of families and communities. Consumers are involved in Boston Healthy Start Initiative policy development, implementation, and evaluation of all activities through their participation in the consortium, focus groups, public information forums, and a number of other community-based activities.

Consumers and residents make up over 60 percent of the consortia membership and are well represented on all of its committees. These committees play a major role in planning as well as monitoring project activities and progress. The Evaluation Committee, for instance, receives regular reports from administrative staff as well as the Management Information System and Infant Mortality Review, and recommends modifications of current programs and activities. The Transition Committee develops proposals for new programs. The Executive Committee and Core Group Committees receive recommendations and information from other committees, and establish overall policy. The Finance Committee reviews the budget and monitors financial performance.

In addition to guiding the internal work of the Boston Healthy Start Initiative, the consortium develops relationships with other collaboratives and organizations, such as the March of Dimes, the Boston Housing Authority, the Massachusetts Department of Public Health, the Latino Health Institute, the Alliance for Young Families, and Community Health Education Centers.

Healthy Start/New York City. Healthy Start/New York City has a project-wide consortium and one consortium in each of its three service areas. This structure has been formalized through the development of by-laws that define the roles and responsibilities of each of the principals, including the grantee, subcontractor agencies, and project committees. Creation of these by-laws, through a group process at the inception of the project, has helped establish a team approach in New York City and limited turf and control issues among key stakeholders. In addition, the four consortia have provided an important vehicle for collaboration among disparate organizations, including grassroots and well-established public and private sector organizations, as well as providers and local residents within a large city with a complex service infrastructure.

The administrative and management structure of the New York City Healthy Start consortia has been important. The consortia have been used to empower project area residents and clients by involving them in the design and implementation of activities, thereby heightening community awareness of the vital need for local maternal and child health-related services.

The goals of the consortia are to empower project area residents and clients and to ensure that all clients have access to a wide variety of services to meet their health care and social support needs. The consortia's objectives are to maintain the proportion of consumers who actively participate in consortium activities, particularly in leadership positions, and increase the knowledge and skills of consortium members through a variety of training and educational opportunities.

The primary purpose of each consortium is to guide the project on matters related to policy and program. Each consortium builds effective, community-driven partnerships that address the risk factors for infant mortality and morbidity. This mission—coupled with a strong collaborative process—unifies the project across its broad geographic, cultural, and linguistic scope. Unity is achieved and maintained via collaborative community needs assessments, program planning, and the tracking and monitoring of progress.

The project-wide guiding principles for the Healthy Start/New York City are to:

- Greatly increase access to social and health services networks for women at risk of infant mortality and for their families
- Ensure that every pregnant client has access to prompt, sensitive, and affordable prenatal care
- Inspire and sustain awareness of infant mortality within the project's service area
- Strengthen provider linkages and involvement in the project's activities

- Encourage interventions focused on men's interests and needs, to support their role in stabilizing their families
- Focus attention on community development, and establish interventions that address social and economic problems
- Involve the community at all levels of program planning, development, and implementation

Dallas Healthy Start. To minimize duplication of services and to promote collaboration, the Dallas Healthy Start consortium focuses on organizing and coordinating existing services of agencies such as the Greater Dallas Community of Churches; Visiting Nurses Association; Girls, Inc.; the YMCA and YWCA; Dallas Housing Authority; and the Boys and Girls Clubs. These agencies provide services and education for nutrition, parenting, smoking cessation, male mentoring, early childhood development, and other topics relevant to reducing infant mortality. This community-based approach also mobilizes local community residents, helping them design and implement successful programs.

Pittsburgh/Allegheny County Healthy Start. Throughout its 10-year history, the Pittsburgh/Allegheny County Healthy Start consortium has come to represent success in removing the "wall of isolation" through enhanced community involvement, individual sensitivity, and a commitment to the quality of life. By encouraging community commitment and involvement as well as forming collaborative relationships between traditional and nontraditional parts of the community, the Healthy Start community-based consortium model has been central to the project's success in Pittsburgh/Allegheny County.

The Pittsburgh/Allegheny County Healthy Start project area comprises six separate and geographic service areas. Community representation from these areas is an important factor in achieving credibility among the target population. Service-area consortia, made up of broadly-based representation of the community, connect the project to each of the six targeted service regions. Each of the six service-area consortia is comprised of 18 to 25 members, including Healthy Start participants, clients, and consumers, neighborhood organizations, and, city, county, and state legislators. Each member brings a different set of human resources and skills to the project. Membership involvement was formalized through by-laws and conflict of interest procedures that were developed with membership input, thereby enhancing the consortia's capacity building abilities.

Supporting the "bottom-up" approach, the organizational framework for the project is designed to support the comprehensive participant-driven approach of the project. Pittsburgh/Allegheny County Healthy Start maintains community representation at all levels of planning and implementation. Community members also give insight regarding effective program implementation strategies. The consortium structure is aligned to ensure that all management and program initiatives are responsive to the needs and realties of the at-risk participant.

The essence of the project's consortium organizational model focuses on community involvement and inclusion, new approaches to issues, and a creative structure that lends itself to flexibility. These consortia identify gaps in services, monitor program implementation, and assist with community education and advocacy efforts.

The consortium provides responsibility for:

- Planning and implementing a regional health fair and six community baby showers
- Consumer participation in evaluation of services
- Increasing provider responsibility in maintaining consumer participation in the system
- Improving sensitivity of providers to the community's cultural, linguistic, and gender needs
- Increasing the efficiency of agency data systems
- Sharing of data across providers (within confidentiality limitations)
- Establishing a community group structure to assist with ongoing project activities

In their advisory capacity, the consortia work with the community liaison and outreach teams to monitor program implementation and recommend changes for any modifications that may be necessary. Finally, in addition to their advisory role, the consortia serve as a central line between the Pittsburgh/Allegheny County Healthy Start project and the community, acting as regional advocates for the project's initiatives. Maintained throughout the lifetime of the project, these collective bodies continue to provide a community voice and governance structure that ensures a service system that is responsive to, and reflective of, local needs, preferences, and social composition.

Great Expectations of New Orleans. To address the city's fragmentation of maternal and child health services, Great Expectations Healthy Start of New Orleans is building relationships among communities, churches, health care advocates, providers, and government agencies. The Great Expectations' strategy is to organize Service Area Advisory Councils (SAAC) in each community and provide them with staff support and technical assistance. SAAC members identify their own community agendas for reducing the city's infant mortality rate. The consortium committee provides local oversight and ideas necessary to make the program responsive to client needs and helps agencies, contractors, and staff to monitor progress, coordinate work, and plan and evaluate services. Great Expectations relies upon the knowledge, commitment, and experience of its consortium members to help design future programs and services.

CONCLUSIONS AND RECOMMENDATIONS

Based on the national Healthy Start experience—several actions to foster collaborations have been identified. Although the following actions are a result of lessons learned by the Healthy Start Initiative, they are also applicable to any agency or organization involved with consortium development:

- *Bring together all those involved in Healthy Start programs that are working on developing the consortium and the local councils as parties to a community summit meeting.* At the very least, those already working on these issues in the various communities should be brought together to discuss their concerns and strategies. Consumers and activists need to be part of that discussion—they are the individuals involved in the front line of community organizing.

- *Provide information on other efforts in collaboration and community organizing.* There are many other collaborative efforts occurring around the country that might have lessons for the Healthy Start Initiative. Disseminating this information on a regular basis would be helpful. It would be even more valuable if opportunities were created for Healthy Start program staff to meet with some of the leaders of these other efforts, either through visits to their communities or through attendance at national conferences that deal with these issues.

- *Provide help for training staff and community members in coalition/consortium building and community organizing.* Healthy Start program staff and consumers need training in building coalitions and organizing their communities. Staff and consortium members at all levels should be involved. Leaders of the local councils as well as leaders of the project consortium could benefit from training. Consumers also need to be part of the training.

- *Obtain support and guidance from the federal Healthy Start Office staff, who, in turn, should continue to be receptive and understanding to the unique needs of each community.* The Healthy Start Branch of the Division of Perinatal Systems and Women's Health should continue to strive to be receptive to comments and suggestions from the Healthy Start project sites. Open communication and dialogue are necessary to support the consortium development effort.

Many diverse factors contribute to our national infant mortality rate. Considerable progress has been made in identifying these factors and meeting the challenges they present, but much more work still needs to be done. Through the years of the Healthy Start Initiative, disparities—racial, economic, and geographic—in access to early prenatal care have been reduced, resulting in a trend toward healthier birth outcomes. But the work must continue. The Healthy Start communities have identified community-based strategies that can significantly and effectively reduce infant mortality, thereby increasing our knowledge of successful approaches to guarding the health of both mother and infant.

The importance that the Healthy Start Initiative invests in collaboration can be summarized by an excerpt of the remarks presented by Kevin L. Thurm, former Deputy Secretary U.S. Department of Health and Human Services at a Healthy Start conference:

> *From community leaders to clergy, from parents to teachers,*
> *from health care providers to corporations, it will take all of us*
> *working together to do right by our children and our families,*
> *to reach parents where they read, work, and live, to reach them*
> *in their homes and at their jobs, on buses and in the streets, to*

reach across boundaries of culture and geography, race and income, providing hope and healing for all parents, all families, all Americans.

If we continue to stand together and work together, we can win the fight against infant mortality—the fight for the future of our children and our country.[11]

ACKNOWLEDGMENT

The authors wish to acknowledge and thank Thurma McCann Goldman, MD, for her help and assistance in the preparation of this document.

REFERENCES

1. Cohen, L., Baer, N., and Satterwhite, P. Developing effective coalitions: An eight-step guide. *Injury Awareness and Prevention Centre News.* 1994; 4 (10).

2. Butterfoss, F.D. Coalitions for alcohol and other drug abuse: Factors predicting effectiveness (unpublished doctoral dissertation). School of Public Health, University of South Carolina, 1993.

3. Goodman, R.M., Wandersman, A., Chinman, M., Imm, P., and Morrisey, E. An ecological assessment of community-based interventions for prevention and health promotion: Approaches to measuring community coalitions. *American Journal of Community Psychology.* 1996; 24 (1).

4. Chinman, M.J. *Benefits, costs and empowerment in community coalitions* (unpublished doctoral dissertation). Clinical/Community Psychology Program, University of South Carolina, 1995.

5. Wandersman, A. and Florin, P. Careful community research and action. *The Community Psychologist.* Summer, 1990; 4–5.

6. Amherst H. Wilder Foundation. Factors influencing the success of collaboration. In *Collaboration: What makes it work.* 1992.

7. Butterfoss, F.D., Goodman, R.M., and Wandersman, A. Community coalitions for prevention and health promotion. *Health Education Research.* 1993; 8 (3) 315–330.

8. Wandersman, A., Valois, R., Ochs, L., de la Cruz, D.S., Adkins, E., and Goodman, R.M., Toward a social ecology of community coalitions. *American Journal of Health Promotion.* 1996; 10 (4): 299–307.

9. Bracht, N. and Gleason, J. Strategies and structures for citizen partnerships. In N. Bracht (ed.). *Health promotion at the community level.* Vol. 15. Newbury Park: SAGE Publications, 1990, pp. 109–124.

10. Kumpfer, K.L., Turner, C., Hopkins, R., and Librett, J. Leadership and team effectiveness in community coalitions for the prevention of alcohol and other drug abuse. *Health Education Research.* 1993; 8 (3): 359–374.

11. Thurm, K.L. Presentation at "Winning the Fight Against Infant Mortality: A National Summit on Community and Corporate Initiatives." Washington, D.C., September 1996.

U N I T   3

HEALTH EXPENDITURES AND HEALTH INSURANCE

INTRODUCTION

Most developed countries, including Australia, Canada, Japan, and the countries of western Europe, have some form of universal health insurance coverage, many of them assuring services for women and children. Japan has the lowest reported infant mortality rate in the world, whereas the United States ranks number 27 in the world in its infant mortality rate, down from number 23 in prior years. The infant mortality rate is considered to be broadly indicative of a nation's health status.

Many health experts believe that a major factor contributing to a family's health status is health insurance coverage. Lack of universal health insurance is one likely element in explaining the ranking of the United States in relation to other developed countries. Health status is also determined by broader priorities: Important factors include availability of contraception; accessibility to abortion services; general education and specific sexualilty education; availability of pre-natal care; improved nutrition for women of child-bearing age and infants; the status of girls and women of child-bearing age; and poverty.

Notwithstanding these important factors and those of welfare services and cultural reforms, expenditures for health and health insurance coverage play an essential role in determining the nation's health status. The articles in this unit discuss insurance for children and adolescents; state and federal initiatives; insurance in a managed-care environment; and health spending at the beginning of the century. The unit provides detail and insight into the role of health expenditures and health insurance in improving health in the 21st century.

ARTICLE 1

INFLATION SPURS HEALTH SPENDING IN 2000*

*Katharine Levit, Cynthia Smith, Cathy Cowan,
Helen Lazenby, and Anne Martin*

INTRODUCTION

Health spending totaled $1.3 trillion in 2000, with spending averaging $4,637 per person (Table 1). Nominal health care expenditures increased 6.9 percent in 2000, the third year of accelerating growth (Table 2). The 1.2-percentage-point gain in the rate of spending growth in 2000 primarily reflects an increase in economy-wide inflation and a gain of only 0.3 percentage points in real spending.[1]

Spending growth in 1999 and 2000 slightly outpaced growth in gross domestic product (GDP), the first sign that the nine-year stability in health spending's share of GDP may be coming to an end. The health spending share of GDP increased slightly, from 13.1 percent in 1999 to 13.2 percent in 2000. Available data for 2001 indicate that GDP growth decelerated as health care employment (Figure 1), medical inflation, and premium growth escalated. This suggests a stronger increase in the health spending share of GDP in the near future.[2]

Strong economic growth between 1997 and 2000 and the accompanying tight labor market caused those who are insured through employer-sponsored plans to choose less restrictive, more costly options. This resulted in faster growth in private health care spending than existed between 1993 and 1997, when cost containment strategies and increasing enrollment in managed care plans helped to dampen spending growth.

Expanding budget surpluses supported federal policy initiatives that increased funding for Medicare. Congress passed two major pieces of legislation that added to Medicare funding in 2000: the Balanced Budget Refinement Act (BBRA) and the Medicare, Medicaid, and SCHIP Benefits Improvement and Protection Act (BIPA). After the Balanced Budget Act (BBA) slowed Medicare spending growth to 0.6 percent in 1998 and 1.5 percent in 1999, the effects of the BBRA boosted

*Published by Project Hope, *Inflation Spurs Health Spending in 2000.* Volume 21, Number 1, pp. 172–181, © 2002. *www.healthaffairs.org.*

TABLE 1 NATIONAL HEALTH EXPENDITURES (NHE), AGGREGATE AND PER CAPITA AMOUNTS, AND SHARE OF GROSS DOMESTIC PRODUCT (GDP), SELECTED CALENDAR YEARS 1970–2000

Spending Category	1970	1980	1988	1993	1997	1998	1999	2000
NHE, billions	$73.1	$245.8	$558.1	$888.1	$1,091.2	$1,149.8	$1,215.6	$1,299.5
Health services and supplies	67.3	233.5	535.4	856.3	1,053.9	1,111.5	1,175.0	1,255.5
Personal health care	63.2	214.6	493.3	775.8	959.2	1,009.9	1,062.6	1,130.4
Hospital care	27.6	101.5	209.4	320.0	367.5	379.2	392.2	412.1
Professional services	20.7	67.3	176.3	280.7	352.3	375.7	397.0	422.1
Physician and clinical services	14.0	47.1	127.4	201.2	241.0	256.8	270.2	286.4
Other professional services	0.7	3.6	14.3	24.5	33.4	35.5	36.7	39.0
Dental services	4.7	13.3	27.3	38.9	50.2	53.2	56.4	60.0
Other personal health care	1.3	3.3	7.3	16.1	27.8	30.2	33.7	36.7
Nursing home and home health	4.4	20.1	48.9	87.6	119.6	122.7	121.6	124.7
Home health care[a]	0.2	2.4	8.4	21.9	34.5	33.6	32.3	32.4
Nursing home care[a]	4.2	17.7	40.5	65.7	85.1	89.1	89.3	92.2
Retail outlet sales of medical products	10.5	25.7	58.7	87.5	119.8	132.3	151.8	171.5
Prescription drugs	5.5	12.0	30.6	51.3	75.7	87.2	103.9	121.8
Durable medical equipment	1.6	3.9	8.7	12.8	16.2	16.5	17.6	18.5
Other nondurable medical equipment	3.3	9.8	19.4	23.4	27.9	28.6	30.4	31.2
Program administration and net cost of private health insurance	2.8	12.1	26.6	53.3	59.2	63.7	71.5	80.9
Government public health activities	1.4	6.7	15.5	27.2	35.5	37.9	40.9	44.2
Investment	5.7	12.3	22.7	31.8	37.2	38.3	40.5	43.9
Research[b]	2.0	5.5	10.8	15.6	18.7	20.6	23.1	25.3
Construction	3.8	6.8	11.9	16.2	18.5	17.7	17.5	18.6
NHE per capita	$ 347.6	$1,067	$2,243	$3,381	$4,001	$4,177	$4,377	$4,637
Population (millions)	210.2	230.4	248.9	262.6	272.7	275.2	277.7	280.2
GDP, billions of dollars	$1,039.7	$2,795.6	$5,108.3	$6,642.3	$8,318.4	$8,781.5	$9,268.6	$9,872.9
Real NHE[c]	$251.5	$430.8	$695.7	$944.2	$1,070.3	$1,114.1	$1,161.4	$1,214.0
Chain-weighted GDP index	29.1	57.1	80.2	94.1	102.0	103.2	104.7	107.0
Personal health care deflator[d]	17.7	37.7	68.0	90.3	102.1	104.4	107.3	110.9
NHE as percent of GDP	7.0%	8.8%	10.9%	13.4%	13.1%	13.1%	13.1%	13.2%

Sources: Centers for Medicare and Medicaid Services, Office of the Actuary, National Health Statistics Group; U.S. Department of Commerce, Bureau of Economic Analysis; and U.S. Bureau of the Census.

[a]Freestanding facilities only. Additional services of this type are provided in hospital-based facilities and counted as hospital care.

[b]Research and development expenditures of drug companies and other manufacturers and providers of medical equipment and supplies are excluded from "research expenditures" but are included in the expenditure class in which the product falls.

[c]Deflated using GDP chain-type price index (1996 = 100.0).

[d]Personal health care (PHC) chain-type index is constructed from the Producer Price Index for hospital care, Nursing Home Input Price Index for nursing home care, and Consumer Price Indices specific to each of the remaining PHC components.

TABLE 2 NATIONAL HEALTH EXPENDITURES (NHE), AVERAGE ANNUAL
PERCENTAGE GROWTH FROM PRIOR YEAR SHOWN, SELECTED
CALENDAR YEARS 1970–2000

Spending Category	1970[a]	1980	1988	1993	1997	1998	1999	2000
NHE	10.6%	12.9%	10.8%	9.7%	5.3%	5.4%	5.7%	6.9%
Health services and supplies	10.4	13.2	10.9	9.8	5.3	5.5	5.7	6.9
Personal health care	10.5	13.0	11.0	9.5	5.5	5.3	5.2	6.4
Hospital care	11.7	13.9	9.5	8.8	3.5	3.2	3.4	5.1
Professional services	9.5	12.5	12.8	9.8	5.8	6.7	5.7	6.3
Physician and clinical services	10.1	12.9	13.2	9.6	4.6	6.6	5.2	6.0
Other professional services	6.6	17.1	18.8	11.4	8.1	6.4	3.3	6.3
Dental services	9.1	11.1	9.4	7.3	6.6	6.0	6.1	6.3
Other personal health care	7.2	10.0	10.5	17.2	14.5	8.8	11.7	8.9
Nursing home and home health	17.2	16.3	11.8	12.4	8.1	2.6	–0.9	2.5
Home health care[b]	14.5	26.9	17.1	21.0	12.1	–2.8	–3.7	0.3
Nursing home care[b]	17.4	15.4	10.9	10.2	6.7	4.7	0.2	3.3
Retail outlet sales of medical products	7.8	9.4	10.9	8.3	8.2	10.4	14.8	13.0
Prescription drugs	7.5	8.2	12.4	10.8	10.3	15.1	19.2	17.3
Durable medical equipment	9.7	8.9	10.7	8.0	6.0	2.3	6.3	5.4
Other nondurable medical equipment	7.4	11.4	8.9	3.9	4.4	2.6	6.3	2.7
Program administration and net cost of private health insurance	8.6	15.9	10.3	15.0	2.7	7.5	12.3	13.1
Government public health activities	13.2	17.4	11.0	11.9	6.9	6.8	7.8	8.3
Investment	12.9	7.9	8.0	7.0	4.0	2.9	5.8	8.4
Research[c]	10.9	10.8	8.9	7.6	4.7	10.1	11.9	10.0
Construction	14.1	6.1	7.2	6.4	3.4	–4.4	–1.3	6.4
NHE per capita	9.3	11.9	9.7	8.6	4.3	4.4	4.8	6.0
Population	1.2	0.9	1.0	1.1	0.9	0.9	0.9	0.9
Gross domestic product (GDP)	7.0	10.4	7.8	5.4	5.8	5.6	5.5	6.5
Real NHE[d]	7.7	5.5	6.2	6.3	3.2	4.1	4.2	4.5
Chain-weighted GDP index	2.7	7.0	4.4	3.2	2.0	1.2	1.4	2.3
Personal health care deflator[e]	3.9	7.9	7.6	5.8	3.1	2.2	2.8	3.4

Sources: Centers for Medicare and Medicaid Services, Office of the Actuary, National Health Statistics Group;
U.S. Department of Commerce, Bureau of Economic Analysis; and U.S. Bureau of the Census.

[a]Average annual growth in 1960–1970.

[b]Freestanding facilities only. Additional services of this type are provided in hospital-based facilities and counted
as hospital care.

[c]Research and development expenditures of drug companies and other manufacturers and providers of medical
equipment and supplies are excluded from "research expenditures" but are included in the expenditure class in
which the product falls.

[d]Deflated using GDP chain-type price index (1996 = 100.0).

[e]Personal health care (PHC) chain-type index is constructed from the Producer Price Index for hospital care,
Nursing Home Input Price Index for nursing home care, and Consumer Price Indices specific to each of the
remaining PHC components.

Medicare spending to 5.6 percent in 2000. The full effects of BIPA will not be felt until 2002.

Because spending for services in both the private and public sectors increased at similar rates in 2000 (6.9 and 7.0 percent, respectively), there was little change in the public share of health spending (Table 3). Public spending in 2000 accounted for 45 percent of all national health expenditures, and private spending, the remainder.

FIGURE 1

Growth in total and health services employment, January 1999–August 2001

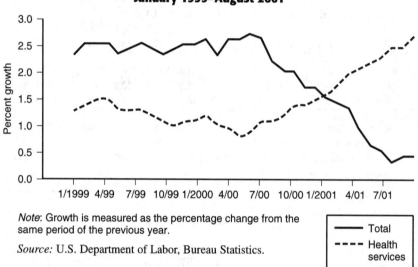

Note: Growth is measured as the percentage change from the same period of the previous year.

Source: U.S. Department of Labor, Bureau Statistics.

—— Total

---- Health services

SYSTEMIC CHANGES IN THE PUBLIC SECTOR

Public policymakers have two conflicting goals: providing greater access to services, and limiting cost growth. A series of adjustments introduced by the BBA along with more intensive fraud-and-abuse investigation strengthened the solvency of Medicare, causing an abrupt slowdown of payments in 1998 and into 1999. State and federal policymakers also attempted to improve insurance coverage in the midst of the longest economic expansion in U.S. history. New policies primarily benefited uninsured children and teens.

SCHIP

The State Children's Health Insurance Program (SCHIP) was created in the BBA to provide additional health care coverage for low-income children. SCHIP is a joint state–federal program under which states may cover eligible children, either through state-specific programs or through Medicaid expansions. SCHIP enrollment grew approximately 70 percent in fiscal year 2000, from 1.9 million to 3.3 million.[3] Total SCHIP spending ($1.8 billion in 1999) increased to $2.8 billion in

TABLE 3 NATIONAL HEALTH EXPENDITURES (NHE), AMOUNTS AND AVERAGE
ANNUAL PERCENTAGE GROWTH, BY SOURCE OF FUNDS, SELECTED
CALENDAR YEARS 1970–2000

Source of Funds	1970[a]	1980	1988	1993	1997	1998	1999	2000
NHE, billions	$73.1	$245.8	$558.1	$888.1	$1,091.2	$1,149.8	$1,215.6	$1,299.5
Private funds	45.4	140.9	331.7	497.7	588.8	628.8	666.5	712.3
Consumer payments	40.6	126.4	293.8	445.0	521.8	557.7	593.8	638.4
Out-of-pocket payments	25.1	58.2	118.9	146.9	162.3	174.5	184.4	194.5
Private health insurance	15.5	68.2	174.9	298.1	359.4	383.2	409.4	443.9
Other private funds	4.8	14.5	37.9	52.7	67.0	71.1	72.7	73.8
Public funds	27.6	104.8	226.4	390.4	502.4	520.9	549.0	587.2
Federal	17.6	71.3	154.1	274.4	358.8	367.7	384.8	411.5
Medicare	7.7	37.4	89.0	148.3	208.2	209.5	212.6	224.4
Medicaid[b]	2.8	14.5	31.0	76.8	94.9	99.6	108.4	118.4
Other federal[c]	7.1	19.4	34.1	49.3	55.8	58.6	63.8	68.7
State and local	10.0	33.5	72.3	116.0	143.6	153.3	164.2	175.7
Medicaid[b]	2.4	11.5	24.1	44.8	64.8	71.8	78.3	84.3
Other state and local[c]	7.6	22.0	48.2	71.1	78.8	81.5	85.9	91.4
Average annual growth in NHE from prior year shown	10.6%	12.9%	10.8%	9.7%	5.3%	5.4%	5.7%	6.9%
Private funds	8.5	12.0	11.3	8.5	4.3	6.8	6.0	6.9
Consumer payments	8.0	12.0	11.1	8.7	4.1	6.9	6.5	7.5
Out-of-pocket payments	6.9	8.8	9.3	4.3	2.5	7.5	5.7	5.5
Private health insurance	10.2	15.9	12.5	11.3	4.8	6.6	6.8	8.4
Other private funds	14.0	11.6	12.8	6.8	6.2	6.1	2.3	1.5
Public funds	15.4	14.3	10.1	11.5	6.5	3.7	5.4	7.0
Federal	20.1	15.0	10.1	12.2	6.9	2.5	4.7	6.9
Medicare	–[d]	17.2	11.4	10.8	8.8	0.6	1.5	5.6
Medicaid[b]	–[d]	17.7	10.0	19.9	5.4	5.0	8.8	9.2
Other federal[c]	9.6	10.6	7.3	7.7	3.1	5.0	8.9	7.7
State and local	10.2	12.8	10.1	9.9	5.5	6.8	7.1	7.0
Medicaid[b]	–[d]	16.8	9.6	13.3	9.6	10.9	9.1	7.7
Other state and local[c]	7.2	11.2	10.3	8.1	2.6	3.4	5.4	6.4

Source: Centers for Medicare and Medicaid Services, Office of the Actuary, National Health Statistics Group.

Note: Numbers may not add to totals because of rounding.

[a]Average annual growth in 1960–1970.

[b]Includes State Children's Health Insurance Program (SCHIP) expansion (Title XIX).

[c]Includes SCHIP (Title XXI).

[d]Not applicable; Medicare and Medicaid became effective in July 1966.

2000. Outreach efforts related to SCHIP campaigns boosted Medicaid enrollment in 1999 and 2000, providing increased coverage for the low-income population.[4]

Medicaid

Although rising Medicaid enrollment has contributed to rising expenditures, public spending would have been even greater had state Medicaid expenditures not been adjusted for states' use of creative and controversial financing arrangements, including disproportionate-share hospital (DSH) payments and upper payment limit (UPL) enhanced payments for both hospitals and nursing homes. States used a large portion of these increased payments for nursing homes for other purposes, whereas hospitals generally retained UPL funds.[5] UPL and DSH provide loopholes that some states have used to boost revenues. Medicaid DSH payments were curbed in the late 1990s, causing a drop in Medicaid hospital spending growth, but UPL payment controls are only now being phased in. State Medicaid hospital and nursing home spending was adjusted to remove estimated amounts retained by the states. After adjustments, total Medicaid spending increased 8.3 percent in 2000.

Legislative Changes

Other systemic changes are related to new Medicare payment policies introduced in 1997–1998 and eased in 1999–2000. Rapid growth in Medicare spending for certain services in the mid-1990s prompted additional scrutiny of public payments. After adjusting for enrollment increases, high rates of Medicare spending growth in 1993–1997 stood in contrast against the deceleration in spending that occurred as managed care enrollment surged and cost growth was constrained in the private sector. Growth in public expenditures prompted renewed fraud-and-abuse investigation of Medicare and led to enactment of the BBA, which slowed growth in hospital, home health, and nursing home payments. As the brunt of the BBA adjustments and fraud-and-abuse enforcement was felt in 1998, average per enrollee Medicare benefit spending fell 0.4 percent and in 1999 increased by a mere 0.1 percent. Concerned about the impact of the BBA, Congress enacted the BBRA in November 1999 to increase payments or delay payment reductions. This caused Medicare per enrollee spending to grow in 2000 (4.7 percent) at a rate slightly slower than per enrollee private health insurance (5.2 percent). Part of the reason for private health insurance's slightly faster growth is its coverage of outpatient prescription drugs, which are not covered by Medicare.

Effects on Nursing Homes

Spending growth for freestanding nursing homes decelerated from 9.1 percent in 1995 to 0.2 percent in 1999 and then rebounded to 3.3 percent in 2000, with spending of $92.2 billion. This industry, facing increased quality-of-care scrutiny, remains heavily dependent on public funding to pay for services.[6] Public

TABLE 4 EXPENDITURES FOR HEALTH SERVICES AND SUPPLIES, BY TYPE OF
SERVICE AND SOURCE OF FUNDS, CALENDAR YEAR 2000

		Private Funds			Public Funds			
Spending Category	Total	Total[a]	Out-of Pocket	Private Health Insurance	Total	Medicare	Federal and State Medicaid[b]	Other Public
Health services and supplies (billions)	$1,255.5	$695.6	$194.5	$443.9	$559.9	$224.4	$202.7	$132.9
Personal health care	1,130.4	641.4	194.5	390.7	489.0	217.0	188.5	83.4
Hospital care	412.1	168.9	13.0	133.9	243.2	125.7	70.1	47.4
Professional services	422.1	282.3	71.8	181.8	139.8	64.4	47.1	28.4
Physician and clinical services	286.4	191.3	33.2	136.7	95.2	59.6	19.1	16.5
Other professional Services	39.0	29.6	11.7	15.0	9.4	4.7	1.5	3.1
Dental services	60.0	57.2	26.9	30.1	2.8	0.1	2.5	0.2
Other personal health care	36.7	4.2	_d	_d	32.5	_d	23.9	8.6
Nursing home and home health	124.7	51.8	31.2	15.1	72.8	18.7	50.4	3.7
Home health care[c]	32.4	15.5	6.4	7.6	16.9	9.2	6.0	1.7
Nursing home care[c]	92.2	36.3	24.9	7.4	55.9	9.5	44.4	2.0
Retail outlet sales of medical products	171.5	138.4	78.5	59.9	33.1	8.2	21.0	3.9
Prescription drugs	121.8	95.3	39.0	56.3	26.5	2.3	21.0	3.2
Durable medical equipment	18.5	13.3	9.6	3.6	5.3	4.6	_d	0.7
Other nondurable medical products	31.2	29.8	29.8	_d	1.3	1.3	_d	_d
Program administration and net cost of private health insurance	80.9	54.2	_d	53.1	26.7	7.3	14.2	5.2
Government public health activities	44.2	_d	_d	_d	44.2	_d	_d	44.2

Source: Centers for Medicare and Medicaid Services, Office of the Actuary, National Health
Statistics Group.

Note: Numbers may not add to totals because of rounding.

[a] Includes other private funds.

[b] Includes Medicaid State Children's Health Insurance Program (SCHIP) expansion (Title XIX).

[c] Freestanding facilities only. Additional services of this type are provided in hospital-based facilities and counted as hospital care.

[d] Not applicable.

spending accounts for 61 percent of all spending, mostly from Medicaid (Table 4). Despite Medicare's small 10 percent share of all nursing home spending, wide swings in Medicare spending growth have affected overall trends in nursing home spending growth. From a high of 45.3 percent in 1994, growth in Medicare spending for skilled nursing facilities plummeted to –18.6 percent in 1999, before rebounding in 2000 with a 13.3 percent increase. This turnaround is attributable to BBRA provisions that raised Medicare payments for some complex patient conditions and for facilities specializing in care for AIDS.

Effects on Home Health

Medicare spending for freestanding home health services declined by 36.8 percent from 1996 to 1999 after years of double-digit growth. This decline resulted from intensified government efforts to detect fraud and abuse, the industry's reaction to increased oversight, greater financial constraints imposed by the BBA, and providers' behavioral responses to the limitations imposed by the BBA provisions.[7]

In November 1999 the BBRA called for a delay in previously mandated BBA Medicare payment reductions to providers and for increased Medicare per beneficiary payment limits for some home health agencies. The Medicare home health agency prospective payment system (PPS), based on per episode payment rates, became effective in October 2000, replacing the interim payment system. Medicare spending rose 0.8 percent in 2000, the first positive growth in four years.

Because it finances a large share of home health services (28 percent in 2000), Medicare influences trends in overall home health spending. The industry had five years of decelerating growth from 1992 through 1997 and actual declines in spending in 1998 and 1999. In 2000 all-payer spending for home health services increased by 0.3 percent. Growth in industry work hours and employment confirmed this turnaround.

A modification in the definition of "home-bound" for Medicare home health coverage in BIPA is expected to increase the number of beneficiaries qualified to receive Medicare home health services in 2001.[8] This will likely contribute to rising spending in the future.

Effects on Hospitals

A deceleration in Medicare hospital spending resulting from the BBA produced a decline of 1.2 percent in 1998 and an increase of only 0.4 percent in 1999. This was partly accomplished by the BBA's slowing of the rate of fee-for-service (FFS) inpatient payment growth for hospitals paid under inpatient PPS. Medicare hospital spending further slowed in 1999 as payments to hospital-based home health agencies (included in these estimates of hospital spending) were reduced.

Medicare hospital spending made a comeback in 2000, similar to that in nursing homes and home health agencies. Its 4.5 percent increase in 2000 was the highest rate of growth since 1997, as the BBRA reduced BBA-mandated Medicare cuts for graduate medical education and lessened reductions in DSH payments for hospitals with a large share of indigent patients. The BBRA also provided for a one-year payment increase to hospitals that are sole providers in their communities, to be implemented in FY 2001.

Two changes in Medicare affect payments for outpatient services. First, changes in Medicare outpatient rules gradually reduced average beneficiary copayments for hospital outpatient services, shifting some spending from beneficiaries to Medicare. Second, starting in July 2000, hospitals receive a prospectively determined fee according to the ambulatory payment classification of services. These two changes contributed to a 10 percent increase in Medicare FFS outpatient spending in 2000. Medicare funds a relatively small share (15 percent) of outpatient services.

Other Changes

Apart from legislative changes, declines in the average complexity of Medicare inpatient services continued for the third consecutive year. Some of these declines in case mix were associated with changes in hospitals' coding of admissions that may be related to investigations of fraud and abuse by the U.S. Department of Justice. Overall, Medicare inpatient spending increased slightly (2.1 percent) in 2000.

PRIVATE-SECTOR SPENDING

Private Health Insurance

As did public spending, the pace of private spending quickened slightly in 2000 to 6.9 percent, up from 6.0 percent in 1999. This uptick is partly the result of accelerating private health insurance premium growth. Premiums ($443.9 billion) rose 8.4 percent in 2000, making this one of the fastest growing health care payer sectors. Premiums increased primarily because benefit costs rose (especially for prescription drugs), insurers sought to restore profitability, enrollment increased, and the mix of plan types shifted to higher cost options. A generally tight labor market also made employers more willing to pay a large share of health premiums, further encouraging plan enrollment.[9] The recent rise in health insurance premium growth may signal the gradual end of what researchers call managed care's one-time impact on slowing spending growth.[10]

For the past two years private insurers have raised premiums more than they have increased the benefits provided. Premiums increased 8.4 percent in 2000, compared with benefit growth of 7.4 percent; in 1999 premiums were up 6.8 percent, compared with benefit increases of 6.2 percent. This produced an upward movement in the net cost ratio (the difference between premiums and benefits divided by premiums)—from 10.6 percent in 1998 to 11.1 percent in 1999 and 12.0 percent in 2000—the second year of an upswing in the underwriting cycle.[11]

Managed Care Backlash

Rising insurance benefit expenses also result from health care providers' taking a stronger stance in negotiating with managed care plans. Physicians' acceptance of health maintenance organization (HMO) capitation is down, with providers citing inability to meet expenses and displeasure with strict management of medical costs by the health plan itself.[12] As a result, some HMOs are abandoning capitation in selected markets for FFS arrangements with physicians and hospitals.[13] The consolidation of hospitals into networks and systems also has increased providers' bargaining power for higher payment from insurers.

Consumers increasingly choose less restrictive forms of managed care, boosting benefit growth per enrollee. The share of workers covered by more restrictive HMOs has remained relatively constant since 1998, while the share covered by preferred provider organizations (PPOs) has risen from 35 percent in 1998 to 41 percent in 2000 at the expense of conventional (FFS) and point-of-service (POS) plans.[14]

Out-of-Pocket Spending

Out-of-pocket expenditures account for 15 percent of national health spending. This share has remained relatively unchanged since 1994, even as managed care plans increased in popularity. Low copayments and smaller deductibles allowed managed care plans to attract enrollees from the previously dominant FFS plans. Consumer spending for prescription drugs in 2000 represented the largest single component—20 percent—of out-of-pocket spending. (Physician and clinical services accounted for 17 percent, and over-the-counter medicines and other medical sundries accounted for another 15 percent.) The large percentage spent by consumers on drugs comes disproportionately from persons age sixty-five and older, many of whom have no third-party coverage for these products.[15]

SPECIFIC HEALTH SERVICES

Growth in spending accelerated for most health care services except for retail sales of medical products and other personal health care services. Although growth in prescription drug spending slowed from 1999 to 2000, it was still the fastest-growing service in 2000.

Drugs: Key Driver of Cost Trends

Growth of prescription drug spending at retail outlets once again exceeded that of other health services by a wide margin, increasing 17.3 percent in 2000, the sixth consecutive year of double-digit growth. Rapidly increasing drug spending accounted for more than a quarter of the total growth in personal health care spending between 1999 and 2000 and raised pharmaceuticals' share of personal health care spending to 10.8 percent in 2000. Rapid growth can be attributed to increased direct-to-consumer advertising, a shift in payment of drugs from consumers to private health insurance companies, and newer therapies and consequent shifts in consumption toward these newer, higher-price drugs.

Factors Driving Growth. The impact of new therapies on spending is related to the number of new drugs, especially blockbusters, entering the market. In 1999 two top-selling drugs, Celebrex and Vioxx, helped to drive spending growth to 19.2 percent. Sales of drugs introduced in 1999 continued to grow rapidly, but none entering the market in 2000 were considered blockbusters, and spending growth slowed to 17.3 percent.

Together with the aging of the population, the introduction of new therapies for chronic conditions gradually adds to the average number of prescriptions purchased. These factors contribute to the rising number of retail prescriptions per capita: 10.5 per person in 2000, from 8.3 in 1995.[16]

Managing the Drug Benefit. Faced with increasing drug benefit spending, insurers established incentives for more efficient drug purchasing using tiered copayment structures that vary copayments depending on the drug purchased.[17] According to the Scott-Levin Managed Care Formulary Drug Audit, the percentage of managed care plans using three-tier benefit structures rose rapidly—from 36 percent in 1998 to 80 percent in spring 2000.[18] Increasing copayments helped to narrow the growth gap between out-of-pocket and total drug spending in recent years.

Some studies show that tiered plans lower health plans' prescription drug spending, as a greater portion of costs is shifted to consumers.[19] Conversely, some researchers believe that the consumption of newer drugs may lower overall health spending by reducing use of more costly services.[20]

Pharmacy benefit managers (PBMs) in 1999 administered 71 percent of third-party payments for drugs, affecting drug selection and prices. On behalf of their clients, PBMs process drug claims, administer benefit plans, and deliver other cost-saving services. One such service is the negotiation of rebates with manufacturers. The rebates are typically shared with insurers, reducing insurers' expenditures. (For this reason, retail sales figures often cited in the trade press are somewhat higher than expenditures included in the National Health Accounts.) Because rebates are negotiated for brand-name products only, PBMs are motivated to boost sales of these drugs by including them in the plan's formulary or preferred status. This preference for brand-name products, along with steady increases in the number of new drugs, contributed to the fact that brand-name drugs' share of retail prescription sales grew to approximately 91 percent of sales in 1999.[21]

Hospitals

Hospital expenditures contributed more to increased spending in 2000 than did prescription drugs, primarily because hospital spending comprises a larger share of total health spending and because hospital spending growth jumped above 4 percent for the first time since 1993. Expenditures rose to $412 billion, an increase of 5.1 percent from 1999. Growth in spending for inpatient services in community hospitals continued to increase at a slow but somewhat accelerated rate—3.4 percent in 2000, up from a 1.9 percent average annual rate in 1993–1999. This corresponds with faster growth in hospital discharges in recent years.[22] The average annual rate of growth in outpatient hospital revenue of 8.3 percent between 1993 and 1999 rose to 8.7 percent in 2000. Faster growth in outpatient revenues than inpatient reflects use of less-invasive technologies.

Hospital revenues grew 1.6 percentage points faster in 2000 than in 1999 but were partly offset by rising expenses.[23] As nonprofit networks and corporate systems consolidated, they were able to negotiate increased payments from private payers.[24] But these gains were tempered by rapidly rising nurses' wages and energy costs. Weekly wages paid to workers in private hospitals increased 4.1 percent in 2000, up from 2.3 percent in 1999.[25] Costs also increased as hospitals hired more-costly temporary staff, provided flexible work arrangements, and offered signing bonuses to meet staffing needs. Although nursing shortages wax and wane, pressures to increase nurses' wages are expected to continue.

CONCLUSIONS

Historical spending trends through 2000 along with historical medical inflation and employment reports for the first half of 2001 indicate that the acceleration in health care costs will likely continue. This stands in stark contrast to recent reports of an increasingly sluggish U.S. economy. Pressure will mount on both public and private payers to finance accelerating health care costs out of decelerating incomes and revenues. Increased job layoffs in the slowing economy will lead to a less competitive job market, reducing private employers' incentive to shoulder rising health care costs, potentially increasing the number of uninsured persons. Competition may force employers to shift a larger share of rising costs to workers, who may no longer be able to afford accelerating out-of-pocket costs. Fewer employers may offer health insurance, and the recently unemployed are often left without coverage. Shrinking tax revenues will likely force government to evaluate health care priorities at a time when the need for coverage is rising. These national health spending estimates may well mark the end of an era of reasonably affordable health care cost growth.

ACKNOWLEDGMENTS

The authors thank the Centers for Medicare and Medicaid Services (CMS) and anonymous peer reviewers for their helpful comments. In addition to the authors, the National Health Accounts team includes Art Sensenig, Pat McDonnell, Lehka Whittle, Carolyn Donham, Anna Long, Madie Stewart, Aaron Catlin, and Mark Zezza. The opinions expressed here are the authors' and do not necessarily represent those of the CMS.

REFERENCES

1. Changes in real spending growth encompass increases in utilization, a changing mix of services, technological impacts, age/sex factors, population growth, and medical inflation in excess of general economywide inflation.

2. Bureau of Economic Analysis, gross domestic product data, <bea.doc.gov/bea/dn1.htm> (11 September 2001); Bureau of Labor Statistics, Consumer Price Index for medical care, <stats.bls.gov/cpihome.htm> (14 September 2001); employment growth for health services, <stats.bls.gov/ceshome.htm> (11 September 2001); and health premiums, Henry J. Kaiser Family Foundation and Health Research and Educational Trust, *Employer Health Benefits, 2001 Annual Survey* (Menlo Park, Calif.: Kaiser/HRET, 2001).

3. Centers for Medicare and Medicaid Services, *State Children's Health Insurance Program (SCHIP) Aggregate Enrollment Statistics for the Fifty States and the District of Columbia for Federal Fiscal Years (FFY) 2000 and 1999,* <hcfa.gov/init/fy99-00.pdf> (6 September 2001). Represents children ever enrolled in SCHIP.

4. Department of Health and Human Services, *State Children's Health Insurance Program Annual Enrollment Report,* <hcfa.gov/init/enroll 99.pdf> (4 September 2001).

5. L. Ku et al., *Medicaid Spending: Rising Again, but Not to Crisis Levels* (Washington: Center on Budget and Policy Priorities, April 2001), 7; and L. Ku, *Limiting Abuses of Medicaid Financing: HCFA's Plan to Regulate the Medicaid Upper Payment Limit* (Washington: CBPP, September 2000).

6. Office of Inspector General, Department of Health and Human Services, *Nursing Home Resident Assessment: Quality of Care*, Pub. no. OEI-02- 99-00040 (Washington: OIG, 2001).

7. U.S. General Accounting Office, *Medicare Home Health Care: Prospective Payment System Could Reverse Recent Declines in Spending*, Pub. no. GAO/HEHS-00- 176 (Washington: GAO, September 2000): 16.

8. The definition was modified to ease the requirement that excursions from the home are made principally for medical treatment. Day trips for psychosocial treatments and religious services are also now permitted. See *2001 Annual Report of the Board of Trustees of the Federal Hospital Insurance Trust Fund*, <hcfa.gov/pubforms/tr> (October 2001). The previous definition can be found in GAO, *Medicare Home Health Care*, 6.

9. Kaiser/HRET, *Employer Health Benefits.*

10. M. Chernew et al., "Managed Care, Medical Technology, and Health Care Cost Growth: A Review of the Evidence," *Medical Care Research and Review* (September 1998): 259–297; and L.C. Baker et al., "HMO Market Penetration and Costs of Employer-Sponsored Health Plans," *Health Affairs* (Sep/Oct 2000): 121–128.

11. C. Hogan, P.B. Ginsburg, and J. Gabel, "Tracking Health Care Costs: Inflation Returns," *Health Affairs* (Nov/Dec 2000): 217–223; and J. Gabel et al., "Tracing the Cycle of Health Insurance," *Health Affairs* (Winter 1991): 48–61.

12. L. Page, "Capitation at the Crossroads: The Trend Is Back to Fee for

Service," *American Medical News*, 5 March 2001.

13. InterStudy *Competitive Edge 11.1, Part II: HMO Industry Report* (St. Paul: InterStudy, April 2001), Executive Summary.

14. Kaiser/HRET, *Employer Health Benefits*.

15. BLS Consumer Expenditure Survey data for 1999 show that 44 percent of out-of-pocket consumer payments come from households headed by people age sixty-five and older; 14 percent of persons covered by the survey are in such households.

16. Calculation of retail prescriptions using IMS National Prescription Audit Retail Prescription Method of Payment Report, and population data from the Bureau of the Census.

17. "Higher Copays: One Way to Control Rising Drug Spending," *Drug Topics* (18 September 2000): 86.

18. Scott-Levin, "Managed Care Copays: Higher and Higher; More HMOs and Pharmacy Benefit Managers Using Three-Tier Cost Control Measures," Press Release, 3 August 2000.

19. Express Scripts, "2000: Top Developments on the Pharmaceutical Landscape," Press Release, 24 May 2001.

20. F.R. Lichtenberg, "Are the Benefits of Newer Drugs Worth Their Cost? Evidence from the 1996 MEPS," *Health Affairs* (Sep/Oct 2001): 241–251. A major portion of savings are from hospital stays, which have become shorter and less expensive partly as a result of using newer medications. See also J.D. Kleinke, "The Price of Progress: Prescription Drugs in the Health Care Market," *Health Affairs* (Sep/Oct 2001): 43–60.

21. IMS Health, "Generics Set for 'Take-Off,' " Press Release, 16 June 2001.

22. J.R. Popovic and M.J. Hall, *Advance Data: 1999 National Hospital Discharge Survey*, Pub. no. 319 (Hyattsville, Md.: National Center for Health Statistics, 24 April 2001). See also Centers for Medicare and Medicaid Services, *Health Care Indicators*, Table 1: Selected Community Hospital Statistics, 1997–2000, <hcfa.gov/stats/ indicatr/tables/t1.htm> (November 2001).

23. CMS, *Health Care Indicators*, Table 10: Quarterly Index Levels and Four-Quarter Moving Average Percent Change in the CMS Prospective Payment System Hospital Input Price Index Using DRI Assumptions, by Expense Category: 1999–2003, <hcfa.gov/stats/indicatr/tables/t10. htm> (November 2001).

24. M. Freudenheim, "Medical Costs Surge as Hospitals Force Insurers to Raise Payments," *New York Times*, 25 May 2001.

25. Bureau of Labor Statistics, average weekly earnings for hospitals, <stats.bls.gov/ceshome.htm> (9 September 2001).

ARTICLE 2

HEALTH INSURANCE OF CHILDREN AND YOUTH

Yun-Yi Hung, Alison Galbraith, Lucy S. Crain,
Sabrina T. Wong, and Paul W. Newacheck

INTRODUCTION

Access to health care is important for the well-being of children and youth. Health insurance coverage plays a key role in providing access to care for children and youth. Children and youth who have insurance coverage are more likely than those who are uninsured to have a regular source of care,[1-4] to have had a physician contact in the past year,[3,5] to be up-to-date on immunizations,[5] and to have fewer unmet health care needs. Further, uninsured children with acute and chronic conditions may be more likely to have poor health outcomes since they utilize fewer inpatient and outpatient services than those with insurance.[1,2,4,6] Uninsured children are also more likely to report financial barriers to having a regular source of care,[5] more likely to be without after-hours care,[4] and more likely to experience long waits and travel times to receive care.[4]

The past two decades have seen dramatic changes in the availability and structure of both private and public health insurance for children.[7] Medicaid expansions, beginning in the 1980s, have increased eligibility for children and led to improvements in access and increased utilization for poor children.[7-9] The establishment of the State Children's Health Insurance Program (SCHIP) under the Balanced Budget Act of 1997 expanded eligibility for insurance to greater numbers of low-income children. Since the late 1980s, the proportion of children with private, employer-based insurance has declined, while public insurance coverage has grown.[10,11] There may be a number of reasons for this shift. Shifts in coverage, specifically the substitution of newly available public insurance for existing employer-based private insurance, has been offered as one explanation, although it is not substantiated.[12,13] The growing number of service-sector jobs and temporary or contracted jobs may be less likely to provide health insurance benefits than did the manufacturing jobs of previous years. With rising medical care costs, employers may be less likely to provide dependent coverage, or may offer coverage with prohibitively high premiums.[1,14,15] However, these trends may be changing in more recent years, as Medicaid coverage rates remain stable while rates of private insurance coverage have shown modest increases.[16]

Even with the Medicaid expansions and SCHIP, not all groups of children and youth have access to health insurance.[2] Poor children continue to be more likely to be uninsured. There are racial/ethnic differences in children's health insurance coverage, with Hispanic children more likely to be uninsured, African American children more likely to have public insurance, and white children more likely to have private insurance.[17] Adolescents are less likely to have health insurance than younger children since they face more restrictive eligibility criteria for Medicaid compared with infants and young children.[17] Insurance rates differ by family structure and parental employment status. Children in families with two employed parents are more likely to be insured, whereas children in one- or two-parent families in which one parent is employed have lower rates of insurance.[1,17] Children living in the South and the West were more likely to be uninsured than children living elsewhere.[2]

Given the recent changes in the health insurance system and the ongoing debate about health care reform, it is important to have updated data on coverage rates and effects on children's access, utilization, and health status. In this article, we present recent data on children's health insurance from the 1998 National Health Interview Survey (NHIS), the most current nationally representative data set available. This chapter will assess health insurance status of children and youth, socio-demographic correlates, and the role that health insurance plays in influencing access to and utilization of health care. These data provide a current, comprehensive profile of health insurance coverage of children and youth that can be used to consider future changes in policy.

Data Source

We used data from the 1998 National Health Interview Survey (NHIS) as the basis for this analysis.[18] The NHIS is a continuing nationwide household survey that is conducted for the National Center for Health Statistics by trained interviewers from the Bureau of the Census. The survey is designed to collect information on the demographic characteristics, health status, and health care use patterns of the U.S. civilian noninstitutionalized population. The survey excludes homeless children and children in institutional facilities. The survey contains three components: the family core, the sample adult core, and the sample child core. The family core includes a short set of questions that are administered for all family members; the sample adult and sample child components include a more in-depth set of questions administered for one adult and one child selected at random in each family.

Health insurance information was collected in the family core. Insurance status was assessed based on responses to a series of questions about who in the family has health insurance and what type of health plan (private or public) he/she was enrolled in at the time of interview. Children were classified as insured if they were reported to have coverage from private insurance, Medicaid, Medicare, public assistance, a state-sponsored health plan, other government programs, or military health plan (includes VA, CHAMPUS, Tricare, and CHAMP-VA). Those children with no reported coverage from any of these sources were classified as uninsured. Following the NHIS conventions, children with Indian Health Service coverage *only* were considered uninsured.

HEALTH INSURANCE STATUS OF CHILDREN AND YOUTH

Data from the NHIS indicate that 87.3% of U.S. children under 18 years old had some kind of health insurance coverage in 1998 (Table 1). Most of these children (68.4%) were covered by private health insurance and about 19.0% were covered through public insurance plans such as Medicaid or CHAMPUS. Nine million children (12.7%) had no health insurance coverage at the time of interview in 1998.

Characteristics of Insured and Uninsured Children

The results shown in Table 1 indicate that there are substantial differences in the likelihood of health insurance coverage based on demographic and socioeconomic characteristics of children and their families. Adolescents (11–17 years) were more likely to be uninsured than young children (0–4 years) (13.6% vs. 11.3%). This difference is primarily attributable to the higher prevalence of public health insurance among young children. There were significant differences related to race and ethnicity. Hispanic children faced the greatest disadvantage; they were twice as likely as blacks (26.2% vs. 13.7%) and almost three times more likely than whites to be uninsured (26.2% vs. 9.0%). Black children were much more likely than white children to have public coverage (38.9% vs. 12.1%) and were about 50% more likely than white children to be uninsured (13.7% vs. 9.0%).

Large differences in coverage according to poverty status are shown in Table 1. Children in poor (below the poverty level) or near-poor (100–199% of the poverty level) families were more than seven times as likely to be uninsured than children in families with incomes above the 300% poverty level (21.6% vs. 2.8% and 22.6% vs. 2.8%, respectively). Also, there were substantial differences in type of coverage by poverty status. Children in families with incomes above the 300% poverty level were five times more likely than poor children to have private health insurance (93.7% vs. 19.0%), while poor children were 17 times more likely to have public health insurance (59.5% vs. 3.4%).

Parental educational attainment and family structure were also related to children's insurance status. In fact, there was a fourfold increase in the likelihood of being uninsured for children in families in which the parent had attained less than a high school education when compared to those in families where the parent had completed at least some college level education (29.9% vs. 7.2%). In addition, children living with one or neither parent were more likely to be uninsured as children living with both parents (15.7% vs. 11.6%). Those living with both parents were far more likely to have private health insurance coverage than children

TABLE 1 Sociodemographic Characteristics of Children under 18 by Type of Coverage: U.S., 1998

Socio-Demographic Characteristics	Population Distribution (in thousands)	Total Covered (N=23,555)	Any Private (N=17,341)	Public Only (N=6,214)	Children without Health Insurance Coverage (%) (N=4,334)
			Type of Coverage †		
All Children	71,710	87.3	68.4	18.9	12.7
Age					
0–4 years	19,691	88.7	64.1	24.6	11.3
5–10 years	24,525	87.2	68.2	19.0	12.8
11–17 years	27,492	86.4	71.6	14.7	13.6
Gender					
Male	36,711	87.3	68.2	19.0	12.7
Female	34,997	87.3	68.5	18.8	12.7
Race and Ethnicity					
White, not Hispanic	46,543	91.0	78.9	12.1	9.0
Black, not Hispanic	10,823	86.3	47.4	38.9	13.7
Hispanic	11,052	73.8	45.3	28.5	26.2
Other	3,290	82.9	65.1	17.8	17.1
Poverty Status*					
Below poverty level	9,990	78.4	19.0	59.5	21.6
100–199% poverty level	12,250	77.4	56.2	21.2	22.6
200–299% poverty level	10,841	90.3	81.6	8.7	9.7
≥ 300% poverty level	23,349	97.2	93.7	3.4	2.8
Parental Educational Level**					
Less than high school	9,005	70.1	25.1	45.0	29.9
High school graduate	17,205	85.0	61.0	24.0	15.0
Some college/college graduate	41,878	92.9	83.0	9.8	7.2
Family Structure					
With both parents	52,170	88.4	77.6	10.8	11.6
With one or no parents	19,450	84.4	43.8	40.5	15.7
Family Size					
1–4 persons	43,172	88.5	71.9	16.7	11.5
5 or more persons	28,534	85.4	63.1	22.3	14.6
Region of Residence					
Northeast	13,253	92.7	74.2	18.4	7.3
Midwest	18,215	91.6	76.5	15.1	8.4
South	24,707	83.7	63.1	20.6	16.3
West	15,534	83.4	62.3	21.1	16.6
Place of Residence					
Metropolitan	56,710	87.8	69.1	18.7	12.2
Nonmetropolitan	14,998	85.2	65.5	19.6	14.8
Self-perceived Health Status					
Excellent, very good, good	70,243	87.4	69.1	18.3	12.6
Fair, poor	1,271	85.0	33.8	51.2	15.0
Disability Status					
Without disability	67,233	87.1	69.3	17.7	13.0
With disability	4,475	90.7	54.7	36.1	9.3

Source: 1998 National Health Interview Survey; original tabulations from public use tapes.

†Private includes all forms of private health insurance. Public includes Medicaid, Medicare, public assistance, a state-sponsored health plan, other government programs, or military health plan (includes VA, CHAMPUS, Tricare, and CHAMP-VA). 233 children had unknown insurance or insurance coverage status and they were excluded.

*Excludes children in families with unknown income.

**If both parents are present, the highest educational level of father or mother is used. If only one parent is present, then the educational level of the parent is used.

living with one or neither parent (77.6% vs. 43.8%), and much less likely to have public health insurance coverage (10.8% vs. 40.5%). Finally, according to this national survey data, there were substantial differences by region of the country. Children living in the South or West were twice as likely as children living in the Northeast or Midwest to be without health insurance coverage in 1998.

Although there was little difference in health insurance coverage by children's reported general health status, there were significant differences by children's disability status. Disability is measured by the presence of a limitation of activity due to chronic conditions. Children with disabilities were more likely to have coverage than children without disabilities (90.7% vs. 87.1%). Also, children with disabilities were more likely to be covered by public insurance programs (36.1% vs. 17.7%).

Multivariate Analysis of Predictors of Insurance Coverage

Many of the demographic and socioeconomic variables presented in Table 1 are highly correlated. This is especially true for the socioeconomic status indicators, such as poverty status and educational attainment. To adjust for such confounding we conducted a multivariate analysis of predictors of insurance coverage among children. All the variables shown in Table 1 were entered into a logistic regression equation predicting presence or absence of insurance coverage.

The results of this analysis are presented in the form of unadjusted and adjusted odds ratios (ORs) in Table 2. The findings indicate that a substantial degree of confounding exists, as indicated by the attenuated odds ratios after adjustment. Both family income and education continued to be powerful independent predictors of the presence of insurance after controlling for other factors. After adjustment, Hispanic children continued to be much less likely to have coverage; however, black children's likelihood of coverage was similar to that of white children. The negative effects of living in a single-parent family or in a family with five or more persons largely disappeared once family income was taken into consideration. The regional differences and the effects of metropolitan and nonmetropolitan residence were still significant. Finally, children with disabilities, or limitation of activity, continued to be more likely to have coverage than children without limitation of activity.

Reasons for Absence of Insurance Coverage

During the interview, families of uninsured children were asked the question *"Which of these are reasons {you/subject name} stopped being covered by health insurance?"* Respondents could indicate more than one reason. As shown in Table 3, two in five respondents indicated that health insurance was too expensive and that they could not afford to purchase it. Almost one in three respondents indicated that a job loss or job change was the primary reason for absence of coverage. Another 18% of respondents indicated reasons associated with loss of Medicaid coverage.

TABLE 2 Odds of Being Without Health Insurance: U.S., 1998

	Unadjusted Odds Ratio (95% CI)	Adjusted Odds Ratio (95% CI)
Age		
0–4 years	1.0	1.0
5–10 years	1.15 (1.04, 1.27)	1.32 (1.16, 1.51)
11–17 years	1.23 (1.11, 1.38)	1.55 (1.35, 1.77)
Gender		
Male	1.0	1.0
Female	1.00 (0.93, 1.08)	0.99 (0.89, 1.10)
Race and Ethnicity		
White, not Hispanic	1.0	1.0
Black, not Hispanic	1.61 (1.36, 1.91)	0.85 (0.68, 1.06)
Hispanic	2.09 (1.47, 2.98)	1.88 (1.21, 2.92)
Other	3.60 (3.21, 4.04)	1.81 (1.52, 2.15)
Poverty Status[*]		
Below poverty level	9.39 (7.52, 11.72)	7.30 (5.33, 9.99)
100–199% poverty level	9.97 (8.14, 12.20)	8.49 (6.63, 10.88)
200–299% poverty level	3.68 (2.90, 4.66)	3.43(2.63, 4.47)
≥ 300% poverty level	1.0	1.0
Parental Educational Level[**]		
Less than high school	5.54 (4.77, 6.44)	2.07 (1.68, 2.55)
High school graduate	2.29 (1.97, 2.66)	1.32 (1.09, 1.60)
Some college/college graduate	1.0	1.0
Family size		
1–4 persons	1.0	1.0
5 or more persons	1.31 (1.18, 1.46)	0.81 (0.70, 0.93)
Family Structure		
With both parents	1.0	1.0
With one or no parents	1.41 (1.26, 1.59)	0.72 (0.60, 0.86)
Region of Residence		
Northeast	1.0	1.0
Midwest	1.17 (0.94, 1.44)	1.17 (0.88, 1.54)
South	2.47 (2.06, 2.96)	1.98 (1.55, 2.53)
West	2.52 (2.09, 3.03)	1.69 (1.31, 2.19)
Place of Residence		
Metropolitan	1.0	1.0
Nonmetropolitan	1.26 (1.08, 1.46)	1.22 (1.02, 1.46)
Self-perceived Health Status		
Excellent, very good, good	1.0	1.0
Fair, poor	1.22 (0.92, 1.62)	0.79 (0.56, 1.12)
Disability Status		
Without disability	1.0	1.0
With disability	0.69 (0.56, 0.84)	0.61 (0.48, 0.77)

Source: 1998 National Health Interview Survey; original tabulations from public use tapes.
[*]Excludes children in families with unknown income.
[**]If both parents are present, the highest educational level of father or mother is used. If only one parent is present, then the educational level of the parent is used.

TABLE 3 MAJOR REASONS FOR LACK OF HEALTH INSURANCE COVERAGE AMONG CHILDREN: U.S., 1998

Reasons[†]	Percent[*]
Cost too high	42.5
Job loss or changed jobs	31.9
Loss of Medicaid coverage	17.8
All other reasons	15.3

Source: 1998 National Health Interview Survey; original tabulations from public use tapes.
[†]Excludes children with unknown coverage status and unknown reasons for absence of coverage.
[*]Percents add to over 100 because respondents can choose more than one reason.

Usual Source of Care

The majority of children (94.1%) had a usual source of care or place to go when they were sick or needed advice about their health in 1998 (Table 4). As expected, insured children were far more likely than uninsured children to have a usual source of care (96.8% vs. 72.8%). Most children with a usual source of care received their care in physicians' offices or HMOs (77.9%). A substantially smaller proportion received their care in health centers and other clinics (19.5%). About 1.5% received their care at hospital outpatient departments and very few children (0.7%) received their usual care in emergency rooms.

There were substantial differences in the distributions of usual sites of care for insured and uninsured children. Insured children were more likely than uninsured children to receive their care in physicians' offices or HMOs (79.8% vs. 57.7%) and much less likely to receive their care in health centers and other clinics (18.2% vs. 34.2%), at hospital outpatient departments (1.4% vs. 3.4%), or at emergency rooms (0.4% vs. 3.8%).

Unmet Needs

The NHIS asked respondents whether there was any time in the past year when children needed medical care, dental care, or prescription medicine but did not get it because their families could not afford it (Table 5). Overall, one in 50 children could not get needed medical care, and 2.1% could not get prescription medicine because their families could not afford it. As might be expected, insured and uninsured children differed substantially in unmet needs. Uninsured children were four times as likely as insured children to have had unmet dental care needs and five times as likely to have had unmet prescription medicine needs (15.9% vs. 3.6% and 7.6% vs. 1.4%, respectively). The gap is even larger for medical care; uninsured children were more than seven times as likely as insured children to have had unmet medical care needs (8.8% vs. 1.2%).

TABLE 4 CHILDREN WITH A USUAL SOURCE OF CARE AND SITE OF CARE, BY INSURANCE STATUS: U.S., 1998

Population Characteristic	Percent with a Usual Source of Care %	Percent Distribution by Site of Usual Source Care*				
		Physician's Office and HMO %	Health Centers and Other Clinics %	Hospital Outpatient Department %	Hospital Emergency Room %	All Other Locations %
Insured children	96.8	79.8	18.2	1.4	0.4	0.4
Uninsured children	72.8	57.7	34.2	3.4	3.8	0.9
All children†	94.1	77.9	19.5	1.5	0.7	0.4

Source: 1998 National Health Interview Survey; original tabulations from public use tapes.
*Percents may not add to 100 due to rounding.
†Includes children with missing insurance information.

TABLE 5 MISSED CARE AMONG CHILDREN, BY INSURANCE STATUS: U.S., 1998

Population Characteristic	Percent who Cannot Afford Needed Medical Care %	Percent who Cannot Afford Needed Dental Care %	Percent who Cannot Afford Needed Prescription Medicine %
Insured children	1.2	3.6	1.4
Uninsured children	8.8	15.9	7.6
All children†	2.1	4.9	2.1

Source: 1998 National Health Interview Survey; original tabulations from public use tapes.
†Includes children with missing insurance information.

Use of Health Services

Table 6 describes the use of health care services for children in 1998. As seen in the table, 87% of children had at least one visit to a health care professional in the past year. Overall, the average number of visits was 4.1 per year. About three-quarters of children had at least one visit to the dentist or had an annual checkup in the past year.

As shown in Table 6, uninsured children used significantly less health care services than insured children. In fact, uninsured children were nearly three times more likely than insured children to not have a visit to a health care professional (30.3% vs. 10.6) and about twice as likely as insured children to not see a dentist or not have a checkup in the past year (54.3% vs. 23.0% and 46.1% vs. 23.8%,

TABLE 6 USE OF HEALTH CARE SERVICES AMONG CHILDREN, BY INSURANCE STATUS: U.S., 1998

Population Characteristic	Average Number of Visits to a Health Care Professional #	Percent with No Visits to a Health Care Professional in the Past Year %	Percent with No Visits to a Dentist in the Past Year %	Percent with No Annual Checkup in the Past Year %
Insured children	4.4	10.6	23.0	23.8
Uninsured children	2.1	30.3	54.3	46.1
All children†	4.1	12.8	26.5	26.3

Source: 1998 National Health Interview Survey; original tabulations from public use tapes.
†Includes children with missing insurance information.

respectively). Finally, insured children had more than twice the number of visits to a health care professional than uninsured children (4.4 vs. 2.1).

POLICY IMPLICATIONS

The information presented above from the 1998 National Health Interview Survey demonstrates the key role health insurance plays as a determinant of access to health care for children. Uninsured children are more likely to lack a usual source of care, to have unmet needs, and to use fewer health care services than insured children. These findings are consistent with the findings of a large body of current literature on health insurance and access to care.[1-6] These findings clearly demonstrate that the best assurance of access to and utilization of health care in the United States is having health insurance.

It is important to note that, while health insurance coverage has been clearly shown to promote access to health care for children, there are nonfinancial barriers that can impede access to care, even for children who have health insurance.[19] Children with Medicaid have been shown to have decreased access compared with children with private insurance.[8,20,21] Even with health insurance coverage, children from racial/ethnic minority groups have decreased access relative to white children.[5,22] Language and cultural barriers can contribute to decreased access for some children, particularly Hispanic children.[22,23] Transportation problems and long wait times also can present barriers, even for insured children.[24]

Health Insurance of Children in the United States

Despite the importance of health insurance, results from the NHIS and other data sources also indicate that insurance is not universal and not evenly distributed. In 1998, 12.7% of children under 18 were without any health insurance coverage. Among those insured, the majority (68.4%) had private health insurance, primarily via their parents' employer-sponsored plan. Another 19.0% were enrolled in public insurance programs, mainly Medicaid, and other programs such as Medicare, public assistance, a state-sponsored health plan, other government programs, or military health plan (includes VA, CHAMPUS, Tricare, and CHAMP-VA).

Private Insurance

The majority of children in the United States obtain their health coverage through their parents' employment. There are great variations in private health insurance practices in terms of premium sharing between employers and employees, benefits coverage, the ways care is delivered, and so on. Employee associations or unions often elect or appoint their representatives to negotiate contracts for insurance products with appropriate benefits for them and their families. In other cases, employers select insurance plans on behalf of employees without consultation. Practices are far from uniform, with the result that there is great variability in private health insurance.

Children's preventive health care needs, including increasingly costly childhood immunizations, can increase the cost of insurance products. Currently, private employers sometimes exclude such preventive services, which are critical components of health care for children. The routinely updated and preferred scope of preventive health benefits for children and youth is that recommended by the American Academy of Pediatrics (AAP) in its Health Maintenance Periodicity Schedule.[25]

In the past, reimbursement under health insurance was based almost exclusively on fee-for-service payment of customary health care charges. Plans paid for services after the policyholder paid an initial deductible and a share of the costs (coinsurance). Because of the use of deductibles and coinsurance, there usually was no co-payment at point of service. Such indemnity insurance products permitted the subscriber almost unlimited choice in selection of physicians and hospital facilities. As health care costs continued to escalate, particularly for hospital care and more recently for pharmaceuticals, the health insurance industry took increasing measures to contain costs. Over the past two decades, cost-containment strategies have focused on shifting families from traditional indemnity coverage to managed care plans. The practice of managed care has resulted in restrictions in access to the choice of health care provider for children and their parents, as well as restrictions in previously covered benefits. The latter is especially true for chronic illness, disabilities, and mental and behavioral health benefits for children and youth. Several localized studies have examined services used by children with chronic and disabling conditions and found that these vulnerable children tend to experience greater difficulty obtaining specialty services in HMOs.[26,27]

Public Insurance

Because their parents are often unemployed or underemployed, children in low-income families rely heavily on public insurance. Historically, children from low-income families receiving public assistance were eligible for Medicaid, the largest public insurance program for low-income families. Over the past two decades public assistance and Medicaid have been de-linked, and now eligibility for Medicaid is generally based on family income and assets and determined by eligibility workers using federal and state guidelines. Guidelines usually reflect adjustment for age, as well as for family size. The de-linking process culminated in 1998 with the replacement of the Aid to Families with Dependent Children (AFDC) program with the Temporary Assistance to Needy Families (TANF) Act, often referred to as "welfare reform."

In 1997, in response to increasing numbers of uninsured children in working poor families, the State Children's Health Insurance Program (SCHIP) was enacted by the Congress. SCHIP provides a state-determined benefit package for children in low-income families who do not qualify for Medicaid because their family incomes exceed Medicaid eligibility thresholds. This population is often described as children of the working poor. The program was specifically designed for children who were not eligible for Medicaid, but whose parents had no employer-sponsored health insurance and could not afford to purchase commercial health insurance. In addition to covering children, a few states have begun to include financially eligible parents under this program. A recent study found that states that extended eligibility to parents above poverty had nearly half the uninsured child rate as states that had not expanded coverage to parents in 1998.[28] In addition, a series of recent reports have commented on other implementation issues for this new program, and may be of interest to the reader.[29–32]

Children with disabilities or special health care needs may be eligible for special public programs. These special programs are offered by state and federal Maternal and Child Health programs and provide coverage for specialized services needed by chronically ill children. Children and youth who are permanently blind and those who have severe, permanent disabilities deeming them eligible for Supplemental Security Income (SSI) coverage are automatically eligible for Medicaid. Other special populations eligible for Medicaid coverage include children in out-of-home placement for a variety of reasons, including the juvenile justice system, foster care, and state residential institutions for the developmentally disabled or emotionally disordered.

Uninsured Children

Families with limited incomes experience a disproportionate share of cost for their health insurance and health care. Although SCHIP has partially addressed the needs of this population, insurance premiums required by many states (although as little as $4.00 to $9.00 per month) and complex application processes can provide effective deterrents to enrollment in SCHIP. Perhaps as a consequence, after a few years of growing experience with SCHIP, many states report only modest changes in the percentages of uninsured children, although data on the effect of SCHIP on uninsured rates are limited thus far.[33]

As noted in the 1998 NHIS data discussed above, uninsured children in the United States are disproportionately Hispanic and poor. They often have unmet health care needs. As the most rapidly growing component of the nation's homeless population is women, children, and youth, these are additional members of the uninsured. Unfortunately, much is unknown about these vulnerable populations, as they are not represented in the NHIS.

CONCLUSIONS

Clearly, more work is needed to ensure that all children and youth are enrolled in health insurance programs that meet their health needs. Many private health insurance plans fail to cover the full range of preventive and developmental services needed by children. More generally, the emphasis on cost containment under many private and public health plans creates barriers to receipt of needed services. Lack of strong federal and state oversight of insurance and managed care practice and their assurance of access to needed health services for children and youth can also be problematic. Furthermore, unregulated private and public market competition among health insurance companies is not necessarily in the best interest of children. Cost-saving provisions of today's insurance plans can delay needed care with resulting long term consequences for developing children and youth.

A comprehensive strategy is needed to ensure that comprehensive health insurance is available to children. Concurrence on the parts of state and federal maternal and child health leaders, private and public insurers, professional societies, families and other child advocates is needed before an entitlement program providing universal health insurance for all American children and youth can be enacted. Organizations such as the American Academy of Pediatrics, in concert with other health advocates and Congressional leaders, have repeatedly introduced such proposals. Only a concerted national effort will allow these proposals to become reality.

REFERENCES

1. Monheit A, Cunningham P. Children without health insurance. *Future Child* 1992;2(2):154–70.

2. Holl JL, Szilagyi PG, Rodewald LE, Byrd RS, Weitzman ML. Profile of uninsured children in the United States. *Arch Pediatr Adolesc Med* 1995;149:398–406.

3. Newacheck PW, Stoddard JJ, Hughes DC, Pearl M. Health insurance and access to primary care for children. *N Engl J Med* 1998;338:513–9.

4. Newacheck PW, Hughes DC, Stoddard J. Children's access to primary care: Differences by race, income, and insurance status. *Pediatrics* 1996;97:26–32.

5. Wood DL, Hayward RA, Corey CR, Freeman HE, Shapiro MF. Access to medical care for children and adolescents in the United States. *Pediatrics* 1990;86:666–73.

6. Stoddard JJ, St Peter RF, Newacheck PW. Health insurance status and ambulatory care for children. *N Engl J Med* 1994;330:1421–5.

7. Hakim RB, Boben P, Bonney J. Medicaid and the health of children. *Health Care Financ Rev* 2000;22(1):133–40.

8. Newacheck PW, Pearl M, Hughes DC, Halfon N. The role of Medicaid in ensuring children's access to care. *JAMA* 1998;280:1789–93.

9. Hill I. The role of Medicaid and other government programs in providing medical care for children and pregnant women. *Future Child* 1992;winter:134–53.

10. Newacheck PW, Hughes DC, Cisternas M. Children and health insurance: An overview of recent trends. *Health Aff (Millwood)* 1995;14:244–54.

11. Yudkowsky BK, Tang SF. Children at risk: Their health insurance status by state. *Pediatrics* 1997;99:E2.

12. Cutler D, Gruber J. Medicaid and private insurance: Evidence and implications. *Health Aff (Millwood)* 1997;16:194–200.

13. Swartz K. Medicaid crowd out and the inverse Truman bind. *Inquiry* 1996;33:5–8.

14. Newacheck PW, Brindis C, Cart C, Marchi K, Irwin C. Adolescent health insurance coverage: Recent changes and access to care. *Pediatrics* 1999;104:195–202.

15. Kronick R. Health insurance, 1979-1989: The frayed connection between employment and insurance. *Inquiry* 1991;28:318–32.

16. Mills R. *Current Population Reports: Health insurance coverage, 1999.* Series P60-211. Washington, DC: United States Bureau of the Census; 2000.

17. Weinick R, Weigers M, Cohen J. Children's health insurance, access to care, and health status: New findings. *Health Affairs* 1998;17:127–36.

18. National Center for Health Statistics. Data File Documentation, National Health Interview Survey, 1998 (machine-readable data file and documentation): National Center for Health Statistics, Hyattsville, MD; 2000. Available at http://www.cdc.gov/nchs/nhis.htm.

19. Friedman E. Money isn't everything: Nonfinancial barriers to access. *JAMA* 1994;271(19):1535–38.

20. St. Peter RF, Newacheck PW, Halfon N. Access to care for poor children. Separate and unequal? *JAMA* 1992;267(20):2760–4.

21. American Academy of Pediatrics Division of Health Policy Research. Data raise concerns about Medicaid access. *AAP News*; April 2001. p. 143,49.

22. Weinick RM, Krauss NA. Racial/ethnic differences in children's access to care. *Am J Public Health* 2000;90(11):1771–4.

23. Flores G, Abreu M, Olivar MA, Kastner B. Access barriers to health care for Latino children. *Arch Pediatr Adolesc Med* 1998;152(11):1119–25.

24. Riportella-Muller R, Selby-Harrington ML, Richardson LA, Donat PL, Luchok KJ, Quade D. Barriers to the use of preventive health care services for children. *Public Health Rep* 1996;111(1):71–7.

25. American Academy of Pediatrics Committee on Practice and Ambulatory Medicine. *Recommendations for preventive pediatric health care* (RE9939); 2000. Available at http://www.aap.org/policy/re9939.html.

26. Horwitz S, Stein R. Health maintenance organizations vs. indemnity insurance for children with chronic illness: Trading gaps in coverage. *Am J Dis Child* 1990;144:581–86.

27. Fox H, Wicks L, Newacheck P. Health maintenance organizations and children with specials health care needs: A suitable match? *Am J Dis Child* 1993;147:546–52.

28. Lambrew J. *Health insurance: A family affair*. A national profile and state-by-state analysis of uninsured parents and their children. New York: The Commonwealth Fund; May 2001.

29. Fox H, McManus M, Limb S. *Access to care for S-CHIP children with special health needs*. Washington DC: The Kaiser Commission on Medicaid and the Uninsured; December 2000.

30. McManus M, Fox H. *S-CHIP administration and accountability*. Washington DC: The Kaiser Commission on Medicaid and the Uninsured; December 2000.

31. Fox H, McManus M. *S-CHIP managed care contracting*. Washington DC: The Kaiser Commission on Medicaid and the Uninsured; December 2000.

32. Fox H, McManus M, Limb S. *Access to care for S-CHIP adolescents*. Washington DC: The Kaiser Commission on Medicaid and the Uninsured; December 2000.

33. Rosenbach M, Ellwood M, Czajka J, Irvin C, Coupe W, Quinn B. *Implementation of the State Children's Health Insurance Program: Momentum is increasing after a modest start*. Cambridge, MA: Mathematica Policy Research, Inc; January 2001.

ARTICLE 3

THE STATE CHILDREN'S HEALTH INSURANCE PROGRAM: A PROGRESS REPORT

Shelly Gehshan

INTRODUCTION

The State Children's Health Insurance Program (SCHIP) was established in 1997 with a mission to provide health insurance to low-income uninsured children and with an appropriation of $20.3 billion dollars over five years. In the last four years, all states, territories, and the District of Columbia have put their programs in place and begun enrolling children. States moved forward quickly to enact authorizing legislation, appropriate funds, and secure approval from the Health Care Financing Administration to get their programs established. The program has enjoyed significant political support, not only because the beneficiaries are children, but because states receive federal matching funds that are 30% higher than for Medicaid and have a great deal of flexibility in crafting their plans to meet their specific, unique needs. This paper provides information about the insurance status of our nation's children, explains the basic structure of SCHIP, and gives an update on state implementation of the program.

THE INSURANCE STATUS OF CHILDREN

In the last five years, two policy changes contributed to big shifts in the insurance status of children. The first was the enactment of the Personal Responsibility and Work Opportunities Reconciliation Act in 1996, which radically restructured state welfare programs and de-linked Medicaid and cash assistance. Prior to 1996, families receiving Aid to Families with Dependent Children were automatically eligible for Medicaid. After 1996, a new eligibility category was created in Medicaid to ensure that low-income families would remain eligible, but states needed to create a new process to enroll them since they were no longer reporting to welfare offices to sign up for both cash and medical benefits.

The difficulties in changing systems caused a steep decline in the number of families with children who were enrolled in the Medicaid program. Although most families leaving welfare remained eligible, they were dropped from the rolls, thought they were ineligible for coverage, or did not apply for Medicaid for their children who may have been eligible even if the parents were not. Most states have worked to re-enroll those families who were dropped, and all states have attempted to put in place eligibility processes and public information so that low-income families now apply for and receive coverage. Nevertheless, the percentage of poor children covered by Medicaid declined from 62% to 55.6% between 1995 and 1999.

The second policy change—the enactment of SCHIP—allowed states to build another layer of insurance coverage for people with income levels above those covered by Medicaid. By the end of the third year of the program (September, 2000), SCHIP plans across the country were providing health insurance for 3.3 million children, a meaningful contribution to reducing lack of insurance in this group. SCHIP and other public programs account for 2.3% of insurance among children.

Despite the initial drop in the Medicaid rolls, and considering the net gain of children insured under SCHIP, the uninsured rate among children is the lowest it has been since 1995. Approximately 10 million children, or 14% of the 72 million children who are under 18, were uninsured in 1999. The primary vehicle for providing health insurance for children, as for adults, is employer-sponsored insurance. In 1999, 64% of children were covered through a parent's policy and another 4% were covered through a private policy. The second largest source was Medicaid: As of 1999, 15% of children, or roughly 20 million, were enrolled in the Medicaid program.

SCHIP REQUIREMENTS AND STRUCTURE

Like Medicaid, SCHIP is not a federally mandated program. If states choose to participate, and all currently do, they have the choice of using SCHIP funds to expand Medicaid, implement a state-designed private insurance program, or some combination of the two. Eight states began enrolling children in 1997, 33 states began in 1998, eight states in 1999 and two in 2000. The variation in enrollment dates is due to (1) differences in how quickly state leaders could form a consensus about the best approach, when state legislatures convened since six states have biennial legislatures, (2) whether states had existing programs in place to expand, and (3) how quickly state agencies could perform necessary planning and contracting. Initially, a majority of states implemented Medicaid expansions as the simplest and quickest path to using SCHIP funds. But over time, more and more states are adding private components in addition to the Medicaid expansions. As of April, 2001 the states using Medicaid, SCHIP plans, and combination plans were as follows:

- *Medicaid*—21 states and jurisdictions have expanded Medicaid: Alaska, American Samoa, Arkansas, the Mariana Islands, the District of Columbia,

Guam, Hawaii, Idaho, Louisiana, Minnesota, Missouri, Nebraska, New Mexico, Ohio, Oklahoma, Puerto Rico, Rhode Island, South Carolina, Tennessee, the Virgin Islands, and Wisconsin

• *Private SCHIP plans*—16 states have established separate state-designed insurance programs: Arizona, Colorado, Delaware, Georgia, Kansas, Montana, North Carolina, Nevada, Oregon, Pennsylvania, Utah, Vermont, Virginia, Washington, West Virginia, and Wyoming

• *Combination plans*—19 states have established a combination of Medicaid expansions and private insurance programs: Alabama, California, Connecticut, Florida, Iowa, Illinois, Indiana, Kentucky, Massachusetts, Maryland, Maine, Michigan, Mississippi, North Dakota, New Hampshire, New Jersey, New York, South Dakota, and Texas

SCHIP VERSUS MEDICAID

The first decision states had to make, either to expand Medicaid or establish a private state-designed program, was often an economic one. The central issue in this decision for many states was the nature of Medicaid as an individual entitlement, as well as numerous requirements for states with respect to benefits, reporting, and providers. A state-designed program can be capped so that no additional appropriations are required for a given year, whereas, under federal law, Medicaid must enroll any person who is eligible, even if that means that supplemental appropriations are needed. In an economic downturn, more children would be expected to become eligible for public insurance programs at a time when state tax revenues were low. As a result, some states considered it economically prudent to establish a private program so they could not be faced at some future time with cost overruns they couldn't control.

Another issue governing the choice was that children enrolled in Medicaid must receive early and periodic screening, diagnosis and treatment (EPSDT). Under this provision in Medicaid law, children must receive preventive health screenings according to a schedule established by the American Academy of Pediatrics. The law also requires states to pay for any treatment the provider deems necessary to remedy a condition or illness detected in a screening, even if the service is not normally provided by the state Medicaid plan. Although only a fraction of enrolled children actually receive required screenings, and not many Medicaid beneficiaries are aware of their legal rights to push states to pay for needed services, states have had difficulty with this requirement. To some policymakers, providing benefits similar to those given to state employees or privately insured individuals—as states generally do in private SCHIP plans—is fair and financially predictable, while providing Medicaid benefits for children is like writing a "blank check."

Finally, although Medicaid was established in 1965, it is still a work in progress. There are perennial problems with low reimbursement rates, poor provider participation and distribution, difficulty for beneficiaries in using the services, and a stigma associated with the program that dates back to its link with cash-assistance programs. In addition, Medicaid has been growing steadily and is one of the biggest line items in state budgets. Because of its size and complexity, cost overruns in Medicaid can trigger a state budget crisis with broad ramifications. Many states did not want to expand Medicaid simply because they wanted a chance to establish a new program over which they had more control and that might work better.

AMENDING SCHIP PLANS

One of the key features of SCHIP is that it is easy for states to amend their programs. States need only submit a request to HCFA and answer any potential questions that arise about conformity to legal requirements. As of May 2001, HCFA had approved 86 amendments to state SCHIP plans and six are currently under review. Many states originally expanded Medicaid because it was easier and quicker than crafting a new program. In order to secure federal funding for the first year of the program, states had to have an enacted plan in place before the end of the 1997 fiscal year. Many states made small Medicaid expansions first, often to provide coverage for all teenagers under 100% of the federal poverty level (FPL). Under Medicaid, states are required to cover children born after September 30, 1983, and have been "phasing in" coverage for adolescents and teenagers one year at a time. After this initial expansion, many states then took time to consider their options, craft a private plan, and apply to HCFA for approval of an amendment.

ELIGIBILITY

SCHIP is designed to provide health insurance for children under 200% FPL, or for states already covering children above 150% FPL, up to 50% FPL higher than the current level. Children who are eligible for Medicaid, are undocumented, are children of state employees, and have private insurance or are in a state-run institution are not eligible for SCHIP. In the few states that do not provide subsidies to state employees to purchase insurance for their families, children of state employees are eligible for SCHIP. States can define eligibility based on income and resources, residency, geographic area, age, and disability status. States have used SCHIP to expand beyond the coverage levels mandated under Medicaid.

The SCHIP law also contained two provisions that allow states to change Medicaid eligibility rules for children. States may now use "presumptive eligibility" for children, which allows providers to deliver and be reimbursed for care to a child who appears to be eligible while his or her application is being processed. States can also offer 12 months of continuous eligibility to children, regardless of changes in income. As of September 30, 2000,[1] the expansion of eligibility is as follows:

> *Below 150% of the FPL:* Seven jurisdictions have expanded eligibility to children below 150% FPL: American Samoa, Guam, Northern Mariana Islands, North Dakota, South Dakota, the Virgin Islands, and Wyoming

Between 150% and 199% of the FPL: 15 states have expanded coverage to between 150 percent and 199 percent of the FPL: Colorado, Idaho, Illinois, Iowa, Louisiana,[2] Montana, Nebraska, New York, Ohio, Oklahoma, Oregon, South Carolina, Virginia, West Virginia, and Wisconsin

Between 200% and 235% of the FPL: 25 states, one territory, and the District of Columbia have expanded coverage to between 200% and 235% of FPL: Alabama, Alaska, Arizona, Delaware, the District of Columbia, Florida, Georgia, Hawaii, Indiana, Kansas, Kentucky, Maine, Maryland, Massachusetts, Michigan, Mississippi, Missouri, Nevada, New Mexico, North Carolina, Pennsylvania, Puerto Rico, Tennessee,[3] Texas, and Utah

At or above 250% of the FPL: Eight states have expanded coverage to or above 250% of the FPL: California, Connecticut, Minnesota,[4] New Hampshire, New Jersey, Rhode Island, Vermont, and Washington

Although it appears there is wide variation in the generosity of coverage levels under SCHIP, much of the differences are the result of the history of Medicaid coverage in each state. States started their coverage expansions from different points. Nearly half the states were covering children at the minimum levels mandated by law, although the other half had expanded beyond those levels prior to the enactment of SCHIP.[5] Eight states had expanded coverage significantly to both children and adults who would not otherwise have been eligible through a Medicaid 1115 waiver. Six states were already covering children at or above 200% of the FPL prior to the enactment of SCHIP, so their expansions were generally smaller.[6]

BENEFITS

States were given three options for crafting their benefit packages for SCHIP. The first is to use the Medicaid benefit package, either as a Medicaid expansion or as a private plan. If a state chooses to expand Medicaid, all Medicaid rules apply. The second is to offer one of three benchmark packages: the Federal Employees Blue Cross/Blue Shield PPO plan; the state employee benefit package; or the coverage offered by the HMO with the largest commercial enrollment in the state. The third option is to offer a benefit package that is the actuarial equivalent of a benchmark plan. Several states have sought and received approval for a benefit package that doesn't conform to any of the three standards. Although states may charge premiums and copayments for services in private SCHIP plans, no copayments are allowed for preventive services such as routine physicals or immunizations.

It is clear from examining the benefit packages offered by non-Medicaid SCHIP plans that most resemble commercial insurance plans. By law, all basic services must be included, such as inpatient and outpatient hospital services; physicians' surgical and medical services; laboratory and X-ray services; and well-baby and well-child care, including age-appropriate immunizations. Most state-designed plan benefit packages have limits in duration and scope that would make them sufficient and appropriate for the majority of children who are generally healthy, but, in most states, would pose problems for children with special health care needs. For example, many states do not cover durable medical equipment and supplies, have low limits on home health care, and limits on occupational, physical, and speech therapy that would be quickly exhausted by a child with a chronic illness. Most states with state-designed plans cover mental health and substance abuse treatment, although some have a combined benefit that would be insufficient for an adolescent with a dual diagnosis. Every state except Colorado, Delaware, and one of Florida's three programs covers some dental services for children,[7] although not all cover orthodontics and many require cost sharing.[8]

IMPLEMENTATION ISSUES

Administrative Costs

Under the statute, states are limited to 10% of actual expenditures for administrative costs, outreach, and direct-service delivery initiatives. The cap has posed a problem for states choosing to develop a state-designed program because much more work must be done for a new program than to expand an existing one. In Medicaid programs, which are mature and require much less oversight, planning, and administration, administrative costs average about 7% of expenditures. However, administrative costs to begin a new program such as SCHIP have been higher than 10% in most states, even without outreach costs. States can spend funds over 10% of expenditures on outreach and administration, but they are not matched by the federal government. If states choose to use their SCHIP funds to expand Medicaid, then costs over the 10% cap are matched at 50%, the customary Medicaid match rate for administrative costs. Some states have shifted a portion of administrative functions and costs to managed care organizations (MCOs) who are providing care to SCHIP enrollees. In doing so, states can then reimburse the MCOs for those administrative costs as part of the capitation rate paid to provide services.

Outreach

As states have made a concerted effort to advertise the availability of their SCHIP plans, many children and families who respond actually are eligible for traditional Medicaid and not the new program. In states with state-designed programs, the SCHIP law requires that anyone eligible for Medicaid be enrolled in that program. In some states, this has meant that as many as half of those applying are eligible for Medicaid. Advocates for children hail this as a victory, although some policymakers have expressed concern about rising Medicaid costs. Recent research by the nonpartisan Congressional Budget Office has shown that Medicaid cost increases have been driven largely by overall health care inflation, increased use of health services, and prescription drug costs, whereas only one-tenth of the increase is due to increased enrollment of children.[9] States have struggled with outreach to special populations, such as children who may be citizens but whose immigrant parents may not be. Medicaid required no outreach, so this function is somewhat new to state health departments and Medicaid agencies and has posed challenges. Outreach is more difficult for SCHIP than it was for Medicaid because it is no longer coupled with cash assistance programs, and because it serves higher-income families who may not have been enrolled in government-subsidized programs in the past. Overcoming the stigma of government welfare programs has been a challenge for states.

Retention and Re-enrollment

In working to make their SCHIP programs successful, most states have designed a short, simple application form and all states with combination or state-designed programs have designed an application form that can be used for both Medicaid and SCHIP (see Table 1). The process that families must complete to continue their coverage is generally different from the original application. However, states are required to verify Medicaid eligibility every six months unless they have elected to extend the eligibility period to 12 months regardless of changes in income. SCHIP eligibility also must be checked after one year, unless the state plan includes provisions lengthening the period of coverage. In both programs, states require families to report changes in income.

States are finding that some portion of children do not re-enroll in SCHIP after their initial eligibility has ended. Reasons for disenrollment include obtaining health coverage through a parent's policy at a new job, eligibility for Medicaid, or failure to complete the redetermination process. Given extensive outreach efforts to secure initial enrollment, many states have realized that they needed to streamline the redetermination process to enhance retention in the program of eligible children. Table 1 shows a variety of mechanisms states use to streamline eligibility.

Family Coverage

The SCHIP statute allows states to provide coverage for families rather than just individual children when it is cost-effective to do so and when the coverage will not substitute for private health insurance. Research has shown that when parents are insured, their children are more likely to get the health care they need. States have seen SCHIP as an excellent opportunity to provide insurance to low-income families and thereby reduce the total uninsured population. The primary way states have attempted to do this is to piggy-back on the employer-sponsored insurance (ESI) available to families of eligible children. As of December 30, 2000, Maryland, Massachusetts, Mississippi, New Jersey, Oregon, Rhode Island, and Wisconsin have received approval to use SCHIP funds to pay a portion of the premiums for employer-sponsored insurance available to eligible families. In practice, this has been a difficult program for states to implement. The coverage

TABLE 1 Mechanisms to Enhance Eligibility for SCHIP and Medicaid

State	Use of Joint Application	Eliminated Assets Test	Continuous Eligibility in Months	Presumptive Eligibility	Simplified Procedures for Redetermination
Alabama	√	√	12		√
Alaska	√	√	6		√
Arizona	√	√	12		√
Arkansas	√				
California	√	√	12		√
Colorado			12		√
Connecticut	√	√	12		
Delaware	√	√	12		√
District of Columbia	√	√	12		√
Florida	√	√	6		√
Georgia	√	√			√
Hawaii	√	√			√
Idaho					
Illinois		√	12		
Indiana	√	√	12		√
Iowa	√	√	12		√
Kansas	√	√	12		√
Kentucky[a]	√	√		√	√
Louisiana					
Maine[b]	√	√	6	√	√
Maryland		√			
Massachusetts	√	√		√	√
Michigan[c]	√	√	12	√	√
Minnesota[d]	√	√	24		
Mississippi	√	√	12		√
Missouri	√	√			√
Montana		√	12		
Nebraska		√	12		
Nevada		√			√
New Hampshire[e]	√	√		√	√
New Jersey	√	√	12		√
New Mexico	√	√	12	√	√
New York	√	√	12	√	√
North Carolina	√	√	12		√
North Dakota			12		
Ohio	√	√			√
Oklahoma					√
Oregon		√	6		
Pennsylvania	√	√	12		√
Rhode Island	√	√			√
South Carolina		√			
South Dakota		√			√
Tennessee		√	12		
Texas	√	√	12		
Utah	√	√	12		√
Vermont	√	√			√
Virginia		√			
Washington	√		12		√
West Virginia	√	√	12		√
Wisconsin	√	√			√
Wyoming		√	12		
Totals = 51	35	46	32	8	39

Notes: This table is current as of September 30, 2000.
HCFA defines "simplified procedures for redetermination" as meaning that states have allowed mail-in or fax-in applications, and have established a mechanism for children to move between SCHIP and Medicaid with no lapses in coverage. Arkansas, Nebraska, South Carolina, Texas, and Wyoming also allow mail-in applications.
[a]In Kentucky, continuous eligibility is available for six months to those children enrolled in a managed care plan. Presumptive eligibility is allowed in the SCHIP plan, but has not yet been implemented.
[b]Maine offers presumptive eligibility under their Medicaid-expansion and state-designed program for pregnant women.
[c]MIChild plans have the option of using presumptive eligibility but none have implemented it yet.
[d]Minnesota covers children from birth to age 2.
[e]New Hampshire provides presumptive eligibility for infants birth to age 1 under the Medicaid-expansion.

Sources: SCHIP Chartbook 2000. The National Conference of State Legislatures, Washington, DC, March 2001. SCHIP 1999 Annual Report. The National Conference of State Legislatures and the National Governors' Association, Washington, DC, January 2000. Data compiled from SCHIP plans, amendments, and evaluations submitted to the Health Care Financing Administration (HCFA).

purchased must meet SCHIP requirements, or wrap-around benefits must be made available through SCHIP or Medicaid. The employer contribution to the premiums must be representative of the employer market in the state. In addition, to prevent the substitution of public for private coverage, most states have established waiting periods, during which families must be uninsured. States can establish exceptions to this rule, such as involuntary loss of employment and health coverage or special health care needs. To date, not many families have received health coverage through these mechanisms. In Massachusetts, which has been operating its program since August 1998, 1,400 family policies have been purchased using SCHIP subsidies.

In 2001, HCFA released regulations guiding the use of 1115 research and demonstration waiver programs with SCHIP funds.[10] In general, states can apply for 1115 waivers if they are covering children up to 200% of the FPL and have done at least three of the following five things: (1) use a joint, mail-in application process for Medicaid and SCHIP; (2) eliminate the asset test; (3) offer presumptive eligibility (4) have 12-month continuous eligibility; and (5) have a simplified redetermination process. States have been very interested in applying for these waivers because they give them the opportunity to use SCHIP funds to expand benefits and services, or expanding eligibility to new groups. As of May 2001, seven states—California, Minnesota, New Jersey, New Mexico, Ohio, Rhode Island, and Wisconsin—had submitted Section 1115 waivers. Most of the waivers submitted thus far seek permission to provide SCHIP coverage for parents of enrolled children or to provide additional services.

CONCLUSION

Although the United States has not made a commitment to provide insurance for all uninsured citizens, or all uninsured children, SCHIP has provided a funding stream and a framework for states to insure low-income children. Even before states were allowed to expand to new populations with Section 1115 waivers, states and advocates saw SCHIP as the best opportunity the federal government has made available in decades to provide coverage to uninsured citizens. Members of the 107th Congress agree, and they have expressed interest in expanding the program to allow states to cover more people. Implementation of the program has presented some challenges, but as of this writing, all states are providing insurance and services to children who previously had no other source of care.

REFERENCES

1. Health Care Financing Administration, State Children's Health Insurance Plan activity map, April 26, 2001; www.hcfa.gov/init/chip-map.htm.

2. Louisiana provides coverage to children younger than 6 up to 150% FPL; children ages 6–18 are covered up to 133% FPL.

3. Tennessee covers children up to 200% of the FPL in Medicaid and children of any income in another part of TennCare.

4. Minnesota provides coverage for infants up to age 2 from 275% to 280% of the FPL.

5. States are required to cover children under age 6 up to 133% of the FPL and must cover children over age 6, born after September 30, 1983, up to 100% of the FPL. When SCHIP was enacted, states were required to provide Medicaid to children below 100% of the FPL up to age 14.

6. *State Children's Health Insurance Program 1999 Annual Report*, National Governors' Association and National Conference of State Legislatures, 2000, Washington, DC, pp. 132–137.

7. Florida has a dental pilot project to provide limited dental benefits to Healthy Kids enrollees in two counties. Florida Healthy Kids is a county-administered program; some counties provide preventive dental services.

8. For complete tables of benefits in non-Medicaid SCHIP plans, see *2000 State Children's Health Insurance Program Chartbook*, National Conference of State Legislatures, 2001, Washington, DC, or see the tables on the NCSL website at www.ncsl.org/programs/health/chiphome.htm.

9. Leighton Ku and Jocelyn Guyer, *Medicaid Spending: Rising Again but not to Crisis Levels*, Center on Budget and Policy Priorities, April 20, 2001, Washington, DC.

10. The letter to state officials outlining requirements and uses of 1115 waivers can be found at: http://www.hcfa.gov/init/ch73100.htm.

ARTICLE 4

THE SUPPLEMENTAL SECURITY INCOME PROGRAM FOR CHILDREN

John Reiss, Helen M. Wallace, and Merle McPherson

SSI PROGRAM BACKGROUND

The Supplemental Security Income (SSI) program for children has been an important part of the federal government's social benefits safety net for low-income children with special needs for more than a quarter of a century.[1] SSI is a nationwide program, administered by the Social Security Administration (SSA), that provides monthly cash payments based on the income of the child's family. In December 2000, almost 850,000 blind and disabled children (under age 18) were receiving SSI payments.

The SSI Program Legislation was passed by Congress in 1972 as Title XVI of the Social Security Act to establish a national program to provide supplemental security income to individuals who were 65 or older, or who were blind or disabled. This legislation replaced four separate federally funded, state-administered cash benefits programs for adults. It created a new federal–state partnership that (1) provided cash benefits to disabled children starting at birth and (2) established national eligibility requirements and uniform benefits that served as an income "floor" for individuals who were aged, blind, or had a disability.

As stated in the 1971 House Report regarding the importance of extending SSI benefits to children, "Disabled children who live in low-income households are certainly among the most disadvantaged of all Americans and ... are (therefore) deserving of special assistance in order to help them become self-supporting members of our society."[2] In most states, children who are SSI beneficiaries also qualify for health care services through the Medicaid program.

In 1975 Congress assessed the effectiveness of the SSI program in helping children with disabilities become self-supporting members of society. It was determined that, although SSI child beneficiaries were receiving cash assistance and access to health care services, they were not receiving other needed services and supports. Due to a lack of formal referral procedure for rehabilitative services, children receiving SSI had only a "haphazard" chance of coming in contact with agencies that could provide these needed services.[3] To address this problem, Congress amended the SSI program and created the Supplemental Security Income-Disabled Children's Program (SSI-DCP), which was administered, in most states, by the Title V Maternal and Child Health/Children with Special Health Care Needs[4] agency. This program was an innovative effort to assure that children receiving SSI benefits had the comprehensive care and services they required. Individual service plans, written under the authority of the state Title V agency, were a hallmark of this program. In 1981 the SSI-DCP was integrated into the new Maternal and Child Health Services Block Grant and subsequently most states discontinued distinct "SSI-DCP" activities. However, today, state Title V CSHCN programs[5] remain actively involved with many children receiving SSI benefits. As mandated in the provisions of the Omnibus Budget Reconciliation Act (OBRA) of 1989 (Public Law [PL] 99-272), state Title V CSHCN programs are to provide the following services: (a) receive referrals of SSI beneficiaries who are under the age of 16 years and (b) provide rehabilitation services to these children to the extent these are not provided through Medicaid (Title XIX); [Section 501 (a) (1) (C) of Title V]. Those age 16 or older are referred to the state Vocational Rehabilitation Agency for services.

In the 1990s, the SSI program underwent two major changes. The first of these changes was mandated in February 1990 through the Sullivan v. Zebley U.S. Supreme Court decision.[6] This Supreme Court decision brought about a liberalization of the SSI childhood disability criteria that then allowed an estimated 300,000 additional children to qualify for SSI benefits during the period 1990–1996. The second change was mandated by Congress in 1996, as part of the Personal Responsibility and Work Opportunity Reconciliation Act. This Congressional reform of the SSI program tightened the SSI childhood disability criteria and resulted in about 100,000 SSI child beneficiaries loosing their SSI benefits.

In the Zebley decision, the Supreme Court found that SSA was not implementing the SSI program as intended by Congress. Because the SSI legislation did not make a distinction between child and adult applicants, the Court found that the procedures used by SSA to determine the SSI eligibility of children, which were not comparable to those used with adults, were unconstitutional. For adults, the SSI disability determination process included an assessment of the adult's "functional status"; SSA did not use a comparable assessment of functioning for child applicants. It was this procedure of not assessing a child's "functional status" that the Supreme Court cited as unconstitutional since it discriminated against children (i.e., children had to meet a stricter standard to quality for SSI than did adults who applied for SSI).

As a result of this ruling, SSA took the following steps:

- Contacted the 452,000 children who had been denied benefits between January 1, 1980, and February 11, 1991, based on medical evidence only (termed the "Zebley class"); reevaluated the 339,000 who responded to SSA; and found approximately 135,000 of these eligible for SSI

- Developed methods for assessing the functional status of children, known as the Individualized Functional Assessment (IFA)
- Developed improved methods for working with other public and private agencies that work with disabled children, to gather better information about the medical condition and functional status of child applicants
- Implemented an active outreach program and worked to improve the ways in which parents get information about the program and apply for benefits

Also, in December 1990, SSA issued regulations revising and expanding its medical standards for assessing mental impairments in children by incorporating functional criteria into the standards and adding such impairments as attention deficit hyperactivity disorder (ADHD), mood disorder, and personality disorder. This revision was undertaken in response to the Social Security Disability Benefits Reform Act of 1984 (P.L. 98-460) and was under way prior to the Zebley decision.

As will be discussed in detail below, Congress closely followed the rapid growth in the number of SSI child beneficiaries following the Zebley decision, and the growth in the total cost of the program. In 1996, over $5 billion was paid in SSI benefits to children. Much attention was given to the number of child SSI beneficiaries with mental impairments, especially those eligible because of attention deficit hyperactivity disorder and other disorders that have been broadly characterized as behavior problems.

PROGRAM DESCRIPTION

The SSI program provides an "income supplement" to low-income disabled adults and children. Eligibility for the program is based both on financial status (income and assets), disability status, and citizenship/residence.

Benefits

The maximum federal SSI monthly payment for a child was $531 in 2001. The amount a SSI beneficiary receives is based on income, the SSI cash benefit being reduced as income increases. For children under 18 who live with their parents, the parents' income is considered when calculating the benefit amount. In most cases, for children 18 and over, family income is not considered.

In addition to the federal payment, states have the option of providing a supplemental cash benefit in order to address the special needs of selected SSI beneficiaries and/or in recognition of the variations in the cost of living. All but seven states and the Northern Mariana Islands provide some supplement to some SSI beneficiaries. The amount of supplemental payment ranges from a few dollars (in several states) up to $172 (in California).

In addition, most children who are eligible for SSI are also eligible for Medicaid. In 32 states and the District of Columbia, a child who is found eligible for SSI is automatically enrolled in Medicaid. Seven[7] other states provide

Medicaid to all SSI beneficiaries, but a separate Medicaid application must be completed. The remaining eleven[8] states do not use SSI status as a criteria for qualifying for their Medicaid program, but rather use more restrictive income, resource, or disabilities standards. These states are often referred to as "209(b)" states, the name coming from the section of the law that authorizes states to use the more restrictive guidelines.[9]

Since the income eligibility requirements for SSI are, in general, more liberal than those for Medicaid, the SSI program provides disabled children in 39 states and the District of Columbia access to the health care services through the state Medicaid program, services for which they might not otherwise qualify. In addition, SSI child beneficiaries are referred to the Title V CSHCN program in their state, which, in turn, assists many SSI child beneficiaries to access health and other needed supportive services that may be available through public and private programs.

Extent of Coverage of Disabled Children by SSI

In December 1989, immediately prior to the Zebley decision, approximately 265,000[10] children were receiving SSI benefits. In 1992, the number of SSI beneficiaries under age 18 had almost doubled, to 556,470. In December 1996, enrollment reached its peak, with 955,174 children receiving SSI (more than three times the number of beneficiaries in 1989). Since 1996, there has been a decline in program participation, with 846,784 children receiving SSI benefits in December 2000. Reasons for this decline are discussed below.

In September 1994 the General Accounting Office (GAO) issued a report on the rapid rise of children on the SSI disability roles,[11] comparing the impact that the new Mental Impairments Listings (issued in 1990) to that of the Individualized Functional Assessment (IFA), which was implemented as a result of Zebley. GAO reported that approximately 60% of the growth in child beneficiaries during 1991 and 1992 was attributable to the mental impairments listing, whereas 40% was due to the IFA. The diagnostic categories of blind and disabled children, ages 0 to 17 years, receiving SSI benefits in December 1988 and December 2000 are shown in Table 1. Mental retardation is, by far, the largest diagnostic group, both in 1988 and in 2000 (41% and 34%, respectively).

Eligibility for SSI: Citizenship, Residency, Financial Status

Eligibility for the SSI program is based on citizenship, residency, financial status (income and assets), and disability status. With certain exceptions, in order to be eligible for SSI, a child must be a U.S. citizen or national and reside in one of the 50 states, Washington, DC, or the Northern Mariana Islands.

To determine the financial eligibility of a child under 18 years old, SSA evaluates the child's and the families' income and resources. For a child to qualify for SSI, the monthly income and resources that are available to the child must be less than dollar limits specified in the SSI regulations. When a child turns 18 parental

TABLE 1 DIAGNOSTIC CATEGORIES OF BLIND AND DISABLED CHILDREN,
AGES 0–17 YEARS, RECEIVING SUPPLEMENTAL SECURITY BENEFITS,
DECEMBER 1988 & DECEMBER 2000

Category	1988 (Number)	1988 (%)	1997 (Number)	1997 (%)	2000 (Number)	2000 (%)
Mental Retardation	108,600	41.9	346,770	40.6	261,200	32.8
Diseases of nervous system/sense organs	66,100	25.5	97,200	11.4	93,140	11.7
Mental disorder (other than mental retardation)	16,000	6.2	217,420	25.4	236970	30.7
Neoplasms	6,900	2.7	13,680	1.6	8,680	1.1
All other (e.g., endocrine disorders; blood disorders; conditions of circulatory, respiratory, gastrointestinal, genitourinary, or musculo-skeletal systems; congenital anomalies; injury; infectious diseases; etc.)	37,300	14.4	178,620	21.0	243,010	28.8

income and resources are not counted, so a child who did not qualify financially as a child may qualify after reaching age 18.

The rules and procedures for determining financial eligibility are complicated, so the following example provides only a general idea of the family income criteria.[12] In 2001, a family with two working parents and two children, one who has a disability and another who does not, could earn up to $39,225 and have the disabled child still qualify. The maximum income level is higher in those states that provide supplements.

After SSA determines that the child meets the citizenship and residence requirements and appears to qualify financially, information about the child's disability and a list of additional sources of information are sent to a state Disability Determination Services (DDS) agency. SSA does not make disability determinations directly, but contracts with a state DDS agency to carry out this determination. State DDSs operate under federal regulations and instructions issued by SSA. It is the responsibility of the DDS to decide whether the child has any medically determinable condition(s), and whether the condition(s) produces a disability that is severe enough to make the child eligible for SSI benefits.

Eligibility for SSI: Disability Status

The rules and procedures for determining disability eligibility are also complicated. State Disability Determination Services agencies uses a team made up of a disability examiner and a medical or psychological professional to decide if, based on the written information that is available to them, the child meets SSI disability criteria. Staff of the DDS never examine the child, nor do they meet with the child/family face-to-face. In determining SSI eligibility, the DDS uses the following sequential process.

In Step 1, the examiner determines if the child is engaged in substantial gainful activity (SGA), that is, is working with an income of greater than $740 (in 2001). If the applicant does engage in SGA, then the claim is rejected. If the applicant child does not engage in SGA, the examiner proceeds to Step 2.

In Step 2, based on the available documentation, the examiner determines if the child applicant has a medically determinable impairment or combination of impairments that is severe. Severe, for the purposes of disability determination means "more that a minimal or slight limitation in a child's ability to function in an age-appropriate manner."

In Step 3, the examiner determines if the child's impairment(s) meets the definition of disability. A child (under 18) is considered disabled if "that individual has a medically determinable physical or mental impairment which results in marked and severe functional limitations, and which can be expected to result in death or which has lasted or can be expected to last for a continuous period of not less than 12 months." In applying this definition, the examiner refers to SSA's Listing of Impairments[13] and decides if the child's impairment or combinations of impairments meets or medically equals the requirements of a listing, or whether the functional limitations caused by the impairment(s) are the same as the disabling functional limitations of any listing and, therefore, are functionally equivalent to such listing. The Listing of Impairments, identifies, for each of the major body systems, impairments that, for a child, cause marked and severe functional limitations.

Prior to the passage of the Personal Responsibility and Work Opportunity Reconciliation Act of 1996 (Public Law 104-193), a child was considered disabled for purposes of eligibility for SSI if he or she "suffer[ed] from any medically determinable physical or mental impairment of comparable severity" to an impairment(s) that would make an adult disabled.[14] Following the Zebley decision, "comparable severity" for children was determined through an Individualized Functional Assessment (IFA).

However, Public Law 104-193 repealed the "comparable severity" criterion in the Act, directed SSA to discontinue the use of the IFA in evaluating a child's disability, and directed SSA to eliminate references to maladaptive behavior in the domain of personal/behavioral function in the Listing of Impairments for children. Thus, under the current law, a child's impairment or combination of impairments must cause more serious impairment-related limitations than were required under the old law and prior SSI regulations. These changes to the eligibility criteria have resulted in a decline in program participation, from a high of more than 955,000 in December 1996 to its current level of about 847,000 in December 2000.

The IFA generated much of the controversy about the SSI program because critics alleged that parents coached their children to fake mental and behavioral disorders. These allegations prompted several examinations of the program by SSA, the HHS Office of Inspector General, and the General Accounting Office.[15] Although these program reviews did criticize some aspects of the program, none of these investigations substantiated allegations of widespread fraud. For a discussion of the role that the media played in focusing public and Congressional attention on alleged fraud in the SSI Program, see "A Media Crusade Gone Haywire," Forbes MediaCritic, September, 1995.

Although the IFA has been eliminated, the new SSI disability determination process does take into consideration the impact of an impairment on a child's functioning. Four methods are used in determining whether a child's impairment has the same disabling functional consequences as a listed impairment. These four methods focus on the following:

1. Limitations of specific functions (i.e., walking, talking)

2. Limitations resulting from chronic illness that are characterized by frequent illnesses or attacks or by exacerbations and remissions

3. Limitations resulting from the nature of the treatments required or the effects of medication

4. Broad functional limitations. In regard to the evaluation of "broad functional limitations," the following six areas of functioning may be considered: (1) cognition/communication, (2) motor, (3) social, (4) responsiveness to stimuli, (5) personal, and (6) concentration, persistence, or pace.

Appeals

SSI child applicants whose disability claim is denied have the right to appeal. There are three levels of administrative appeal: reconsideration hearing before an administrative law judge and Appeals Council review. If a child's claim is denied at each of these three steps, then the case can be reviewed in federal court. Historically, approximately one-half of those cases that have gone through the appeals process have ultimately been approved.

Summary

The Supplemental Security Income program for children serves as a critical component of the nation's social service system for low-income children with special needs. Because SSI is a cash-assistance program, parents have the flexibility to decide how to best use the SSI benefits to meet the needs of their child and family: for expenses such as special food, clothing, equipment, transportation, unreimbursed medical expenses, increased cost of utilities, and child care, including care by a parent who cuts back on work in order to provide such care.

In addition, in many states, SSI eligible children are also eligible for needed health care services through the state Medicaid program. Further, because new beneficiaries are referred to state Title V CSHCN programs, the SSI program can serve as mechanism for linking children with special needs and their families to the family-centered, community-based services that they need.

In the following section, additional recent changes to the SSI program are identified, and the implications of these changes on children with special needs are discussed.

IMPACT OF WELFARE REFORM ON CHILDREN WITH SPECIAL NEEDS

The Welfare Reform Act of 1996 brought about marked changes in the SSI Program that significantly impact current SSI beneficiaries and future SSI applicants. In this section, changes to the SSI program and other benefits program, as mandated by the Welfare Reform Act of 1996, are summarized, potential impacts on children with disabilities and their families are identified, and the implications for programs serving this population are defined.

Changed Eligibility

On February 11, 1997,[16] the SSA published interim final rules for determining SSI eligibility for children. These rules eliminated the "comparable severity" standard, removed the Individualized Functional Assessment (IFA) step from the disability determination process for children, and modified the medical listings to eliminate references to "maladaptive behavior" when evaluating personal/behavioral functioning for children with mental impairment.

In addition, SSA was required to redetermine the SSI eligibility of approximately 288,000 children who had been deemed eligible through the IFA process or due to functional limitations associated with "maladaptive behavior." The Welfare Reform legislation stated that no children were to lose their SSI benefits until July 1, 1997, or the date of their redetermination (whichever was later).

Impact Under the New Criteria

It is estimated that that about 188,000 of the 288,000 "SSI redetermination cases" will ultimately be found eligible for SSI under the new criteria, while about 100,000 (about one-third) of these children will lose their SSI benefits. In addition to these children, the Congressional Budget Office (CBO) estimated, that, between 1996 to 2002, about new 267,000 SSI child applicants who would have qualified for SSI under the old eligibility rules, will be found not eligible under the new statute. CBO estimated that about 48,000 of these denials will be as result of eliminating reference to "maladaptive behavior" in the mental impairment listings.

In addition, child advocates suggest that the implementation of more restrictive eligibility criteria will further reduce the number of children receiving SSI benefits because families, who heard about SSI Program changes through the media, would think that the eligibility criteria were exceedingly restrictive, that the chances of their child being found eligible would be very low, and that it was not worth the time and effort required to complete an application and provide necessary financial and medical information.

In the 1980s prior to the Zebley decision, SSA received between 95,000 and 132,000 SSI applications for children annually. Following the Zebley decision, SSA and many child advocacy organizations implemented a variety of public information and outreach efforts to inform potential child beneficiaries and their families about the SSI Program. From 1990 through 1996, the number of applications grew from 163,690 in 1990, to a peak of 541,420 in 1994, with a modest decline to 503,190 in 1995 and 462,780 in 1994. Following implementation of the new restrictive criteria, the number of applications fell to 332,940 in 1997; then rose slightly to 337,640 in 1998 and 350,170 in 1999 (the last year for which data are available). These data give support to the notion that families are less inclined to apply for SSI benefits under the new eligibility criteria and that there may be a significant number of children who would qualify for SSI if they applied.

As noted above, SSI child beneficiaries receive cash benefits and, in many states, are eligible for health care through the Medicaid program. This SSI status provides children with special protections in regard to enrollment in Medicaid managed care arrangements. Although the Balanced Budget Act of 1997 permits states to enroll Medicaid populations in managed care without applying to the Health Care Financing Administration (HCFA) for a waiver, SSI program participants, along with four other categories of children are excluded from mandated enrollment.[17] Those children who lost SSI benefits through the redetermination process, those new child applicants who did not quality under the more restrictive criteria, and those potential new beneficiaries whose families were discouraged from applying are not afforded the additional managed care safeguards that help assure access to all medically necessary services from providers with appropriate training and experience.[18]

Medicaid Benefits: Retained by Children who Lose SSI

Under the provisions of the Welfare Reform Act, SSI and associated benefits (i.e., Medicaid) for those recipients who did not meet the new eligibility criteria would have been terminated beginning in July 1, 1997, or the date of the redetermination, whichever came later. However, this termination of health care benefits was in conflict with efforts of the Clinton Administration and Congress to increase children's access to health insurance coverage. Therefore, under the State Children's Health Insurance Program (SCHIP) provisions of the Budget Reconciliation Act of 1997 (Section 4913), states were required to continue Medicaid eligibility for all children who lost SSI benefits because of the changes in the definition of childhood disability until the child's 18th birthday.

IMPACT OF SCHIP

The intent of Section 4913 was to assure that those children who are terminated from SSI through the reevaluation process continue to be covered under the Medicaid Program. However, although this provision appears to be straightforward, a number of complex issues had to be addressed. Starting in November 1997, the HCFA issued a series of "Letters to State Medicaid Program Directors" related to the implementation of this provision. In response to reports that children were being terminated, in spite of the provisions of Section 4913, the November 13, 1997[19] HCFA directive stated that it was the responsibility of the state Medicaid agency to proactively reinstate any children who had been terminated in error, and that families could not be required to reapply in order to regain lost Medicaid benefits. Further, state Medicaid Programs were required to use "all available means" to identify and locate such children.

Some state programs could not readily identify children who qualified for Medicaid because of SSI because the program information systems did not include data on beneficiaries' SSI status. In response to this problem, HCFA worked with the Social Security Administration, as is described in an October 2, 1998 letter to Medicaid Directors,[20] to provide state Medicaid programs with electronic lists to the states of SSI children who no longer met the new definition of disability and had exhausted SSA's administrative appeal process or never appealed their original decision.

The November 1997 HCFA instructions also specify that those children who are terminated from SSI but continue to receive Medicaid as a result of SCHIP will be required to continue to meet the SSI disability criteria that were in effect prior to the passage of the Personal Responsibility and Work Opportunity Reconciliation Act of 1996. As with financial eligibility, the state Medicaid agency would have responsibility for monitoring and redetermining disability status. The determination of disability, based on SSI criteria and procedures, is a complex and highly specialized task, which is carried out by state Disability Determination Services Units, under contract from SSA.

The Title XXI/SCHIP legislation assures continuing Medicaid benefits to those who lose SSI, but this legislation does not extend Medicaid coverage to the estimated 267,000 children who would have qualified for SSI between 1996 and 2002 if the SSI eligibility criteria had not been changed. There are no provisions within the SCHIP legislation that help to assure that these children are given priority for coverage under Title XXI.

CONCLUSION

The Supplemental Security Income (SSI) program for children has recently undergone significant changes that will reduce the number of children who receive cash benefits through this program. However, the SSI program, along with state Title V CSHCN programs, state Title XVI Medicaid programs, and the new Title XXI Child Health Insurance program (three other programs authorized under the Social Security Act), continues to provide low-income children with special needs supports they need to become self-supporting members of our society.

BIBLIOGRAPHY

Crocker, A.C. Improved Support for Children with Disabilities. *Pediatrics.* 1991;88:1057–1059.

Perrin, J.M. and Stein, R.E.K. Reinterpreting Disability: Changes in Supplementary Social Security Income for Children. *Pediatrics.* 1991;88:1047–1051.

Perrin, J.M., Kulthau, K., McLaughlin, T.J., Ettner, S.L., Gortmaker, S.L. Changing patterns of conditions among children receiving SSI disability benefits. *Arch Pediatr Adolesc Med.* 1999;153:80–84.

Schulzinger, R. *Advocates Guide to SSI for Children.* 3rd ed. Washington, DC. Judge David L. Bazelon Center for Mental Health Law. 1998.

REFERENCES

1. American Academy of Pediatrics, Committee on Children with Disabilities. Continued Importance of Supplemental Security Income (SSI) for Children and Adolescents with Disabilities. *Pediatrics* 2001:107;4:790–793.

2. House Report No. 92-231 (Ways and Means Committee), May 26, 1971, reprinted at 1972 U.S.C.C. & A.N. 4989, 5133–5134.

3. Senate Report No. 94-1265 (Finance Committee), December 16, 1975, reprinted at 1976 U.S.C.C. & A.N. 6019, 5133–5134.

4. In 1973 these programs were known as "Crippled Children Services Programs."

5. For information about supports and services available through state Title V CSHCN programs, see Reiss J & Lamar DL. (2000) "Directory of State Title V CSHCN Programs: Eligibility Criteria and Scope of Services." Gainesville, FL: Institute for Child Health Policy (http://cshcnleaders.ichp.edu/TitleVDirectory/).

6. Sullivan v. Zebley 493 US 521. 1990.

7. Alaska, Idaho, Kansas, Nebraska, Nevada, Oregon, Utah.

8. Connecticut, Hawaii, Illinois, Indiana, Minnesota, Missouri, New Hampshire, North Dakota, Ohio, Oklahoma, Virginia.

9. P.L. 92-603, §209(b), 86 Stat. 1329, 1465 (1973).

10. Prior to 1998, this figure was reported by SSA as 296,298. In 1993 SSA approximately 35,000 cases previously classified as children were reclassified as adults. In 1998, SSA recalculated its estimated for the number of SSI child recipients for years 1974–1997. See *Children Receiving SSI: December, 1995* and *Children Receiving SSI: 1998* (Office of Research, Evaluation and Statistics, Social Security Administration).

11. *Social Security: Rapid Rise in Children on SSI Disability Rolls Follows New Regulations* (GAO/HEHS-94-225, Sept 9, 1994). Washington, DC: US General Accounting Office (www.gao.gov).

12. A *Desktop Guide to SSI Eligibility* is available from SSA. See: http://www.ssa.gov/pubs/11001.pdf

13. Social Security Administration. *Disability Evaluation Under Social Security*. Baltimore, MD: SSA; 2001. Publ No 64-039. (http://www.ssa.gov/disability/professionals/bluebook/).

14. Section 1614(a)(3)(A) of the Social Security Act.

15. See *Supplemental Security Income: Growth and Changes in Recipient Population Call for Reexamining Program* (GAO/HEHS-95-137, July 7, 1995) and *SSA Initiatives to Identify Coaching* (GAO/HEHS-96-96R, May 15, 1996).

16. Interim final rules were published on February 11, 1997, in Volume 62, Number 6408 of the *Federal Register*. Final rules were published on September 11, 2000, in Volume 65, Number 176, Page 54747–54790 of the *Federal Register*.

17. Categories of children afforded special protections are those participating in the following five programs: SSI; Katie Beckett Home and Community-Based Waiver Program; Title V CSHCN Block Grant; Federal foster care or adoption assistance; and foster care or out-of-home placements funded from other sources. See US General Accounting Office. *Medicaid Managed Care. Serving the Disabled Challenges State Program* (GAO/HEHS-96-136, 1996).

18. For a discussion of the impact of these safeguards, see Mitchell JB, Khatutsky G, and Swigonski NL. Impact of the Oregon Health Plan on Children With Special Health Care Needs. *Pediatrics* 2001:107;4, 736–743.

19. For a copy of this letter see http://www.hcfa.gov/medicaid/bbakids.htm

20. For a copy of this letter see http://www.hcfa.gov/medicaid/bba10298.htm

ARTICLE 5

MANAGED CARE AND CHILDREN

Dana Hughes and Sarah Arzaga

INTRODUCTION

Since the early 1980s, the health care system in this country been radically transformed from one dominated by fee-for-service arrangements to one increasingly dominated by managed care. Within this short period of time, the number of Americans enrolled in some form of managed care reached an estimated 67 million by 1997. Twenty-six states have more than 20% of their populations in HMOs, and HMO enrollment now represents more than 25% of the entire U.S. population.[1] Recently released population-based data from the 1996 Medical Expenditure Panel Survey indicate that managed care is becoming the norm for children's health care delivery in the United States. By early 1996, more than half (57%) of privately insured children were enrolled in managed care plans.[2]

The significance of this change is only partially understood today. Managed care, in a variety of forms and names, has been a means of financing and delivering health care for more than 50 years. The number of persons enrolled in managed care plans was, however, relatively low until recently. Thus, the extent to which past experience can help predict future effects is limited. However, research on managed care does suggest that this move is likely to at least partially achieve its intended objectives of helping contain costs and improving access to care for some of those enrolled. It may also have some unintended consequences, such as reducing access to needed care for other populations. Managed care may also improve the quality of care for some people, while making it worse for others.

This article provides an overview of managed care and examines the implications that its widespread adoption has for children. In particular, this article examines managed care for children enrolled in Medicaid because of the extraordinary rate at which state Medicaid programs are converting to managed care. The sheer magnitude and speed of this move demand special analysis and scrutiny if lessons are to be learned from this experience. Moreover, because children who are Medicaid beneficiaries are generally from low-income families or are disabled,

281

they may be more vulnerable to changes in how health care is delivered and financed.

WHAT IS MANAGED CARE?

The term *managed care* refers to a variety of financing and delivery arrangements. The single unifying characteristic of these various approaches is that enrollees are encouraged or required to obtain care through a network of participating providers who are selected by the managed care organization and agree to abide by the rules of that organization.[3] This is in contrast to fee-for-service arrangements, in which patients typically may seek care from any licensed health care professional or organization and providers may perform services based on their individual judgments about what is appropriate or needed.

Within this general approach are a vast number of managed care models, which are derived from three major models:

- *Fee-for-service case management.* Beneficiaries are assigned to a primary care case manager (generally a physician or clinic) that furnishes or arranges primary care services, authorizes use of specialty services, and coordinates such care. Sometimes referred to as *managed indemnity plans* or MIP, these arrangements place providers at no financial risk; instead, they are paid on a fee-for-service basis and receive a monthly case-management fee. This lack of financial risk would lead many not to characterize MIPs as true managed care. However, they are commonly considered as managed care in the context of Medicaid.
- *Partially capitated arrangements.* Plans or providers are placed at risk for only certain services. Each month, the plan or provider is paid a capitated fee covering those specified services for which it is responsible and at financial risk. Other services are reimbursed on a fee-for-service basis as they are rendered.
- *Fully capitated arrangements.* Plans are at full financial risk for all or nearly all services to which the patient is entitled. Plans may provide services within the plan or arrange for them out of plan; they are paid on a capitated basis reflecting the range of covered services and the patient's risk.

MANAGED CARE AND HEALTH CARE DELIVERY FOR CHILDREN

How do these various models influence the delivery of health care for children? Perhaps the easiest way to understand managed care's effect on service delivery is to contrast managed care with fee-for-service. As Table 1 demonstrates, managed care differs from fee-for-service in a number of significant ways. One of the primary distinctions between these two methods of financing and delivering care is the requirement in managed care that patients select providers from a pool prescribed by the plan. Generally, patients select a primary care provider who provides the bulk of care and approves referrals to specialists as he or she deems

TABLE 1 A Taxonomy for Categorizing Health Insurance Plans

	Type of Plan				
	FFS	FFS CM	PPO	POS	HMO
Sponsor assumes financial risk*	-/+	-/+	-/+	-	-
Intermediary assumes financial risk*	+/-	+/-	+/-	+	+
Physicians assume financial risk†	-	-	-	+	+
Restriction on consumer's choice of provider††	-	-/+	-/+	-/+	+
Significant utilization controls placed on provider's practice§	-	+	+	+	+

FFS, traditional fee-for-service indemnity plan; FFS CM, fee-for-service case management; PPO, preferred provider organization; POS, point of service or open-ended health maintenance organization; HMO, health maintenance organization (including independent practice association). - = absent; + = present.

*Sponsor is an employer or government. *Intermediary* is usually a health plan or other entity that serves as an administrative conduit. The left side of the slash reflects a plan in which an employer purchases a full-premium benefit from the insurer. The right side reflects a self-insured (or minimally insured) private plan or government plan in which risk resides with the sponsor.

†Primary care physicians at a minimum, but may also involve other providers.

††In FFS CM, PPOs, and PSOs, consumers' choice is limited through incentives and disincentives rather than mandatory restrictions. They have the option to seek covered care from outside the plan. The right side of the slash reflects care when this "out-of-plan" option is exercised.

§Usually defined as mandated prior authorization for nonemergency hospitalization.

Adapted from Weiner, J.P., and de Lizzovoy, G. Razing a tower of Babel: A taxonomy for managed care and health insurance plans. *Journal of Health Politics, Policy and Law.* 1993;18(1):75–103.

appropriate. This approach limits the patients' choice of primary care providers and eliminates their ability to "self-refer" to care.

In some instances, the list of available providers is quite extensive; in others, it may be more limited. There is, however, an expectation that listed providers are truly available, unless their practice is listed as being closed. This is in contrast to the situation in which all licensed physicians are listed as "available" but, in fact, accept few Medicaid patients. This approach also can serve to ensure linkage to a "medical home" in the form of a primary care provider who is chiefly responsible for a patient's care, which is considered advantageous, if not essential, for children.

Managed care also generally shifts financial risk from the sponsor of coverage—government or employer—to another payer or to providers. For example, under Medicaid managed care, the payer (federal and state governments) shifts its financial risk to participating health plans. Although the payer is still responsible for the premium, financial risk for costs beyond the premium rests with the plan or is passed on in part or in full to providers. From the perspective of the payer, the principal advantage of this approach is that it introduces limits and predictability in expenditures. Although costs may rise from year to year based on renegotiated contracts with plans, the payer knows with some certainty how much will be expended within the time frame of a given contract. This is in stark contrast to fee-for-service arrangements in which the payer is largely unable to either control or predict spending, because retrospective payments are made as services are rendered.

CHALLENGES AND OPPORTUNITIES

Most observers would agree that the transition from fee-for-service arrangements to managed care presents both challenges and opportunities in the provision of services to children, at least in theory. Managed care has the potential to affect access to health care, the quality of care received, and health care costs in countless ways. Proponents of managed care argue that it can result in improvements over fee-for-service through enhanced coordination and convenience of health services, emphasis on prevention, and flexible benefits.[4] Unlike fee-for-service, which merely promises to reimburse patients for the care they obtain, managed care plans have an obligation to provide services to the people enrolled in the plan. This means that the plan has to know who is enrolled and should keep track of the services they receive. A conventional fee-for-service insurer may not even know how many children are covered in a family, let alone whether they have received their immunizations, especially if such services are excluded from the benefit package. A managed care plan should know exactly which children are enrolled and whether their immunizations are up-to-date, thus providing mechanisms to improve access to and coordination of care. Opponents of managed care argue the opposite, citing the potential to create barriers for children through financial disincentives to provide quality care, risk selection, limitations on providers and services, and other system-related obstacles to care, especially specialty and subspecialty care. Which of these perspectives is correct, if either, remains an unresolved question.

Indeed, in the absence of clear empirical evidence, any resolution to this debate is necessarily based on conjecture and speculation. Few data with respect to managed care and children exist to prove one view or the other. Although numerous studies have been conducted on the effect of managed care in general, few studies have been conducted specifically on the impact for children.[5] It is questionable, moreover, whether findings from studies pertaining to adults can be applied to children given how different children's needs for health services are from those of adults.

MANAGED CARE, ACCESS, QUALITY, AND COSTS

As previously stated, few studies have been conducted that examine the impact of managed care on children. What data are available are derived largely from Medicaid demonstration projects conducted in the early and mid-1980s as well as a few more recent studies of Medicaid managed care. Studies examining federally sponsored Medicaid managed care demonstration projects in the 1980s found that use of routine preventive services stays the same or slightly increases under Medicaid managed care compared to fee-for-service.[6-8] However, compliance was below the recommended standards set by the American Academy of Pediatrics and the federal Early Periodic Screening, Diagnosis and Treatment Program.[6,7] A subsequent study found that low-income children who sought care principally in public clinics were more likely to be adequately immunized than those who obtained care through private physicians' offices or health maintenance organizations (HMOs).[9] A more recent study found over 90% of insured children had a usual source of care and over 95% of families generally reported high levels of satisfaction with their children's care. However, the analysis also revealed some problem areas including challenges getting appointments and contacting medical providers by telephone. The study also noted the absence of significant differences in access, satisfaction, and use or quality of care between children enrolled in managed care and traditional health plans.[2] However, a growing body of research suggests that the extent to which managed care improves or impedes children's access to and utilization of quality care depends on the of type of managed care, which children, and the circumstances under which they are enrolled.[10]

Two recent studies examined the experience of children from different payer sources within the same managed care plan. One study, which examined the experiences of children enrolled in a major HMO with Medicaid coverage and commercially insured coverage, found few differences between the two groups in terms of access, utilization, and satisfaction.[2] However, among the differences found were fewer problems finding a personal care provider and fewer problems getting care among the Medicaid beneficiaries. Another study comparing medical care costs of Medicaid and commercially insured children in the same HMO found that income-eligible Medicaid-covered children experienced slightly higher costs than their commercially covered counterparts.[11]

WHY WE DON'T KNOW MORE

Why don't we know more about the impact of managed care on children and how to design optimal programs for them? Although there is a large body of literature based on the Medicaid managed care demonstrations of the 1980s, the applicability of the data from these studies is limited. Indeed, most of the current knowledge available regarding managed care and children is derived from studies of Medicaid recipients.[12] The limitations of this research are based, in part, on the fact that these studies assessed Medicaid managed care programs operating before 1990, when the nature of managed care was dramatically different. Most of the Medicaid managed care demonstration programs were largely voluntary for Medicaid beneficiaries compared with today, when virtually all Medicaid families, especially those on TANF, are required to enroll in managed care plans. This has implications both for the kinds of individuals who are enrolled in managed care (and their health care needs) and for the scope of the transformation to managed care, and hence the ability to make adjustments to address problems that arise. In addition, many of these studies lacked control groups in fee-for-service delivery systems.

Consequently, the findings of studies from the mid-1980s may not be relevant to the current managed care environment. Moreover, virtually no studies have been conducted on nonpoor children in managed care settings. Although conventional Medicaid programs have many of the aspects of fee-for-service from the perspective of the providers, they actually routinely incorporate two important aspects of managed care enrollment and limited co-payments. State Medicaid agencies usually know exactly for whom they are responsible, thus mimicking the responsibility of the managed care plan and the ability to focus on enrolled populations rather than just "users." Reflecting the low-income status of its enrollees, the Medicaid law precludes use of co-payments and deductibles for children and mandates a broad benefit package. Thus, although managed care may offer important "denominator responsibility" and low financial barriers to comprehensive benefits in contrast to coverage for employed populations, this may not be a particular advantage for Medicaid recipients. Similarly, children with special needs covered by targeted programs may find little in the way of additional benefits and coverage under managed care and, in fact, may find that some needed services, particularly specialty care, may be obtained only out-of-plan. For these reasons, as well as the different health care needs of poor and nonpoor children, it is not clear that the results related to children enrolled in Medicaid apply to privately insured children.

The diversity of approaches to managed care further complicates efforts to understand its impact, even among the later studies because different models are likely to have different impact on access and costs. For example, the ability of sponsors, intermediaries, and physicians to absorb risk is so variable that utilization may be more tightly controlled in models in which physicians hold the risk as compared with large employers or large health plans. Care must be taken, therefore, to distinguish between the various approaches when analyzing the impact of managed care on children and designing programs for them.

Lack of strong evidence about the impact of managed care on children is also a function of fundamental problems with the current state of knowledge about measuring the impact of health services in general; these problems with research in health services prohibit a fuller understanding of managed care. There is little agreement about which outcomes to monitor, which measurements of outcomes to use, and which are the appropriate comparison groups, particularly with respect to children. After years of effort, researchers have managed to produce a handful of basic quality-of-care measures. The measures that do exist tend to be applicable to high-prevalence health conditions experienced by large numbers of individuals (such as prenatal care and immunization rates) rather than low-prevalence conditions that affect relatively few individuals with high health needs but that may constitute a better test of quality in the case of a prepaid health care system that has a built-in incentive to underspend on its enrollees.

SUMMARY AND RECOMMENDATIONS

The adoption of managed care in place of fee-for-service health care is rapid and widespread. Between 1975 and 1994, the number of Americans who received care in health maintenance organizations alone rose by more than sevenfold, from 6 million to 51.1 million.[13] Use of managed care is also pervasive in the Medicaid program. From 1991 to 1999, the proportion of all Medicaid beneficiaries enrolled in managed care—either capitated or in primary care case management models—rose from about 10% to 55%. Only two states do not have at least some Medicaid beneficiaries in managed care plans.[14]

This dramatic shift to managed care has significant implications for children. Most observers agree that, if well designed and executed, managed care may have the potential to reproduce for children the cost savings, improved quality, and greater access that it has for middle-class adults. However, the evidence in support of managed care, although convincing for middle-class adult populations, is inconclusive and sometimes contradictory when considering children. As already mentioned, information derived from the managed care experiences undertaken thus far offer limited guidance about what constitutes optimal design and implementation for children, with the exception of Medicaid managed care.

Policymakers and program planners concerned about children currently face a significant dilemma. The movement toward managed care has developed an undeniable momentum. At the same time, there is very little empirical evidence to demonstrate that this is an appropriate direction or to indicate ways to maximize the potential benefits and minimize the potential harm. At a minimum, this lack of conclusive data suggests the need to slow the conversion momentum until information can be gleaned from the current experiences about the impact on children, and modifications made, as needed. In particular, there is a need for research on the impact of managed care on nonpoor children, for whom there is virtually no reliable information available. A commitment to and investment in research and monitoring by the federal and state governments, philanthropic organizations, and health plans are key to this effort.

We do have enough information to suggest the need for explicit steps to ensure that managed care plans address the needs of children and, as appropriate, the needs of poor children. At the very least, this means that plans must have available providers who are trained in pediatrics, particularly for children with special health care needs. In addition, health plans for Medicaid-enrolled populations must adapt their plans to this group's unique needs and circumstances. The principal distinctions between Medicaid-enrolled children and other children can provide guidance as to some of the aspects of plans that should be examined and possibly altered.

REFERENCES

1. Health Insurance Association of America. Source book of health insurance data. 1999-2000. Washington, DC: Health Insurance Association of America, December, 2000.

2. Newacheck, P.W., Hung, Y.Y., Marchi, K.S., Hughes D.C. The Impact of managed care on children's access, satisfaction, use, and quality of care. *Health Services Research.* June, 2001; 36:(2):315–34.

3. Rosenbaum, S., Serrano, R., Mager, M., Stem, G. Civil rights in a changing health care system. *Health Affairs.* 1997;16(l):90–105.

4. Saucier, P. *Public managed care for older persons and persons with disabilities: Major issues and selected initiatives.* Waltham, MA: The Center for Vulnerable Populations, 1995.

5. Miller, R.H., Luft, H.S. Managed care: Past evidence and potential trends. *Frontiers of Health Services Management.* 1993;9(3):3–37.

6. Heinen, L., Fox , P.D., Anderson, M. Findings from the Medicaid competition demonstrations: a guide for states. *Health Care Financing Review.* Summer 1990; 11:55–67.

7. Hurley, R.E., Freund, D.A., Gage, B.J. Gatekeeper effects on patterns of physician use. *Journal of Family Practice.* 1991;32:167–173.

8. Freund, D.A., Lewit, E.M. Managed care for children and pregnant women: Promises and pitfalls. *The Future of Children.* 1993;3(2):92–122.

9. Wood, D., Halfon, N., Shervourne, C., Grabowsky, M. Access to infant immunizations for poor, inner-city families: What is the impact of managed care? *Journal of Health Care of Poor and Uninsured.* 1994;5:1–12.

10. Simpson, L., Fraser, I. Children and managed care: What research can, can't, and should tell us about impact. *Medical Care Research and Review.* 1999;56:(Suppl 2):13–36.

11. Ray, G.T., Lieu, T., Weinick, R.M., Cohen J.W., Firemen B., Newacheck, P.W. Comparing the medical expenses of children with Medicaid and commerical insurance in an HMO. *American Managed Care.* 2000; 6(7):753–60.

12. Health Management and Gini Associates. *Evaluation of the Michigan Medicaid program's physician sponsor plan, 1989–1990, Part I.* Analysis of cost effectiveness issues in the AFCD population. Lansing, MI: Health Management Associates and Gini Associates, 1991.

13. Troy, T.N. Does managed care work? *Managed Healthcare.* July, 1996;6(7):20–41.

14. United States General Accounting Office. *Medicaid stronger efforts needed to ensure children's access to health screening services.* GAO-01-749. July, 2001;1–35.

ARTICLE 6

ADOLESCENT HEALTH

Donald E. Greydanus, Dilip R. Patel,
and Elizabeth K. Greydanus

INTRODUCTION

Adolescence is the critical process in which the individual leaves the dependency of childhood and enters a period in which dramatic changes occur, eventually resulting in what society calls adulthood. It is a complex developmental time that involves sociological, psychological, and physiological issues. It is a unique bridge that accepts the achievements and failures of childhood and sets in motion the changes necessary to establish adulthood. Since the goal of this period is to develop an adult who is autonomous and capable of functioning at intellectual, sexual, and vocational levels that are acceptable to society, anyone interested in children or adults should be interested in the health of our adolescents.

In early adolescence the brain undergoes significant changes under the influence of pubertal hormones, such as estrogen and testosterone. There is considerable growth of the brain, including central nervous system areas that direct impulsivity and social behavior; other parts of the body also undergo profound change. Eventually, an adult-like individual appears who soon takes his or her place in society. Many potential problems, medical and/or psychological, await this youth as s/he heads toward adulthood and independence. This chapter reviews the current health status of American youth (Table 1), outlines some of the problems encountered in helping them, and concludes with some suggestions to improve their health. We all have a stake in our adolescents, for they profoundly affect our present and will continue to affect our future. How we care for our children says much about us as a society, whether for good or for ill. How our children and adolescents are treated will determine much about the future of the United States as the 21st century unfolds.

DEMOGRAPHY OF THE ADOLESCENT POPULATION

There are one billion adolescents (10–19 years of age) in the world, making up over 20% of the world's population; there are one billion humans who are between 15 and 24 years of age and about 50% of the world's population is now under age 25 years.[1] (See http://www.unicef.org/sowc00/map/.htm.) In 1974, the number of American youth aged 12–17 years was 25 million; in 1990 this was about 19.2 million and was 22.1 million in 1999. There are over 50 million adolescents (aged 10–19) in the United States in the beginning of the 21st century.

HEALTH STATUS OF ADOLESCENTS

About 31% of youth have a chronic illness or handicap (including 6% with illness that limits daily activity); the potential behavioral complications of such difficulties on adolescent growth and development should be considered by those interested in health care.[2] Although 70% of this group have one condition, 21% have two conditions, and 9% have three or more conditions. Approximately 84% of children with severe illness now reach age 20.[3] The impact chronic illness has on the lives of our children and adolescents is considerable.[4–6]

Demographic information on specific illnesses include such statistics as: (a) one million teenagers with epilepsy, (b) over one million with asthma, (c) 100,000 with diabetes mellitus, (d) eight million with refractive errors (myopia,

---

TABLE 1 ADOLESCENT HEALTH TOPICS

Obesity
Disorders of the Lower Respiratory Tract
Cardiac Disorders
Diabetes Mellitus
Mental Health
Abuse
Sexual Behavior
    Adolescent Pregnancy
    Sexually Transmitted Diseases
    The Adolescent Sexual Offender
Substance Abuse
Youth Violence
Mortality
    Homicide and Suicide
    Motor Vehicle Accidents
Runaway and Homeless Youth
Incarcerated Youth

---

hyperopia, or astigmatism) including 100,000 with partial or limited vision, and (e) over one million with significant hearing loss. The overall illness prevalence in the 10–17 age group is 315 per 1,000. The following are the prevalence rates (shown in parentheses as the numbers per 1,000 teens) for various illnesses: musculoskeletal disorders (20.9), asthma (46.8), frequent, severe headaches (45.8), heart disease (17.4), deafness and hearing loss (17.0), blindness and vision impairment (16.0), speech defects (18.9), and diabetes (1.5).[3]

Hypertension, recurrent migraine headaches, and severe dysmenorrhea are each experienced by about 10% of youth. Recent studies suggest that 25% of adolescent females have an eating disorder: bulimia nervosa, anorexia nervosa, or exogenous obesity. Approximately 80% or more of youth develop acne vulgaris and the majority have dental problems, particularly dental caries. Estimates are that the average 15-year-old youth has 10 "diseased" teeth (decayed, filled, or missing).

Obesity

Obesity, with a prevalence of 22%, is one of the most important problems affecting the health and well-being of the American population.[7] This is not a new problem, but rather a rapidly increasing one. The reasons for this are multifactorial; each must be appreciated and perhaps addressed before solutions to obesity are practical. Obesity has increased among both pediatric and adult individuals both in the United States and around the world. There has been a significant decrease in the average amount of physical activity. In part, the decline in activity levels can be traced to the advent of video games, computers, cable television, VCRs, public and private transportation systems, and employment opportunities that do not require great amounts of physical exertion. Since increased weight gain is due to the intake of excess calories, it is inevitable that persons who eat similar amounts of food as generations prior, but expend less energy, will gain weight. The 1999 Youth Risk Behavior Surveillance study from the Centers for Disease Control and Prevention notes that 76.1% of American high school students do not eat five or more servings of fruits and vegetables, that 70.9% have no daily physical education classes, and that 16% are at increased risk of becoming overweight.[8]

Obesity has a major impact on the physical and emotional well-being of many people. Adult obesity is an independent risk factor for cardiovascular diseases, diabetes mellitus, stroke, arthritis, and some cancers. Psychological complications have been associated with obesity in adolescents, including depression, poor self-image, and difficulties in both the home and social environment (including school). Obese female teens are at increased risk of becoming adults who did not complete high school, remain unmarried, and remain in poverty. The correction of obesity is associated with an improvement of risk factors, most notable of which are related to cardiovascular- and diabetes-related events. It is important that obesity be addressed early in childhood because it is clear from adult studies that outcomes are better for those adults who are not obese when they are young adults. Further, it is during the adolescent years (if not sooner) that most people develop lifestyle habits that will likely be a foundation of their adult behaviors.

Disorders of the Lower Respiratory Tract

One of the most important factors in the production of bronchitis in youth is nicotine addition.[9] Tobacco use and addiction is a common problem in all parts of the world, due to the heavy global advertisements of the tobacco industry, the social acceptance of tobacco use, the highly addictive nature of this drug, and many other factors. The immediate effects (such as bronchitis and nicotine addiction) and the long-term effects (including lung cancer, emphysema, and heart disease) are staggering. Major efforts must be made by society to reduce or eliminate nicotine addiction so as to reduce (delay) morbidity and mortality in these individuals later in their lives.

Effects of marijuana smoke (with chronic cough and bronchitis) are just now being realized. Since the smoke is often more potent than cigarette smoke, and since it is often held in the lung for longer times, serious pulmonary problems can be expected with chronic marijuana use.

Asthma. Asthma is one of the most common medical conditions in the adolescent throughout the world. Its prevalence in all ages is on the rise in many countries where data is available, including a 46% increase in Australia, 4.6% in Japan, 34% in New Zealand, 5.1% in Taiwan, and 4.3% in the United States.[10] The reasons for this geographic variation are not known, although it is likely tied to a complex interaction of local environmental factors, medical care practices, and, perhaps, genetics. Though the disease is often diagnosed in childhood, adolescence is a time when many previously asthmatic individuals improve or even when the diagnosis may first be made. It is the most common medical reason for teenagers missing school. Despite the availability of better medications and increasing awareness of this disorder as a public health problem, the mortality of asthma has been increasing around the world. Research has noted a 111% increase in asthma mortality from the mid-1970s to the mid-1980s in individuals 5 to 34 years of age in the United States.[10]

In the United States, African American teenagers experience about a three- to fourfold increase risk of dying from asthma as compared to their White peers. The reasons for this are unknown, although higher asthma morbidity and mortality in the United States has been linked to inner city populations with low socioeconomic status. Additional factors in the United States that are associated with this increased morbidity and mortality include mental illness, substance abuse (including alcohol), lack of medical care, and belonging to a dysfunctional family. In America, costs for some 17 million asthmatics exceeds $6.2 billion dollars, including direct medical costs and indirect costs from lost work and school days. Reducing asthma morbidity and mortality in our youth is a major challenge for medicine and society in the 21st century.

Cardiac Disorders

Coronary heart disease is the major cause of death in the adult population, and it may begin in adolescence.[11] Thus, teenagers as well as adults should be screened for the many associated risk factors: obesity, high blood pressure, diabetes, ciga-rette smoking, limited exercise, and hyperlipidemia. Frequently genetically determined, primary abnormalities of lipid metabolism are a major risk factor for the early development of coronary artery disease. Dietary habits formed in ado-lescence influence dietary choices as adults, even in those adolescents without overtly abnormal total cholesterol or serum lipid profiles. Autopsy data suggest that atherosclerotic changes begin long before adulthood—even in those persons without inherited or other disorders of a lipid metabolism.

Diabetes Mellitus

The most common endocrine disorder in youth is diabetes mellitus. Current stud-ies note that the incidence of Type I diabetes is increasing by 2.5% to 3% through-out the world—in both low and high incidence areas.[12] The incidence is project-ed to be 50 per 100,000 a year in Finland and over 30 per 100,000 in many parts of the world—a 40% increase from 1998 to 2010. It will be under 2 per 100,000 in China, under 5 in Japan, 22 in the United States, and 36.7 in West Australia. Type 2 diabetes is increasing globally as well, probably, in part, due to the increasing incidence of obesity around the world.[13]

Mental Health

A major cause of disability (32%) among 10-to-18-year-olds is the result of men-tal (psychosocial, behavioral, developmental, or psychiatric) disorders. Approxi-mately 20% of 9-to-17-year-olds have a behavioral or emotional disorder, and studies note that 9% to 17% of 9-to-17-year-olds have an emotional disorder that limits their life functioning in school, at home, with family members, and/or other arenas.[14,15]

Depression appears to be common in youth. Some research reports that 13% to 28% of youth are mildly depressed, 7% moderately depressed, and 11.3% severely depressed.[16] A National Institute of Mental Health-sponsored epidemio-logical study of 9-to-17-year-olds noted a 6% prevalence of depression (4.9% with major depression).[17] In 1999, 28.3% of high school students (35.7% of females versus 21% of males) felt sad and/or hopeless enough for at least two weeks that they stopped doing some usual activity.[8] In this same 1999 survey, approximately 19% of depressed adolescents report seriously contemplating sui-cide (24.9% females versus 13.7% males) while 14.5% of teens (18.3% of females versus 10.9% of males) have made a specific plan to attempt suicide; 7.8% of these teens actually made an attempt at suicide over the previous 12 months of the survey.[8] In this 1999 study, 2.6% of youth made a suicide attempt over the previous 12 months of the survey, which resulted in injury, poisoning, or an overdose that had to be treated by a doctor or nurse.[8] This survey looked at youth who are in school; the rates are projected to be even higher in those who have left school.

School dysfunction is a major problem for youth as well. Various studies of urban students indicate up to 10% of enrolled youth are always absent from school, up to 30% are absent on any given day, and as many as 20% or more of 14-to-15-year-olds simply drop out of school.[18] School phobia is estimated at 17 per 1,000 school age children.[18] The severe negative effects of such school failure on the future of these unfortunate individuals and society at large is incalculable —especially in this ever increasingly technical world.

In 1982 the Children's Defense Fund reported on 3 million children under age 18 years with serious mental health disorders, noting that *most* were *not* receiving needed mental health care.[19] While mental health disorders of children and youth have increased over the past several decades, services for these individuals with mental health problems (including substance abuse disorders) have been reduced.[20,21] Treatment of these conditions over the past 30 years has been complicated by a managed care cost-containment system that has markedly reduced inpatient psychiatric beds in favor of community-based programs with an emphasis on outpatient management.[22]

Abuse

There are approximately 3 million reported annual cases of abuse in those under age 18 years; in 1994 reported abuse cases were subdivided into *neglect* in 53%, *physical abuse* in 26%, *sexual abuse* in 14%, and *emotional abuse* in 5%.[23] Research notes that 25% of 10-to-16-year-olds report being victims of violence in 1994.[24] Sexual abuse was noted in 13% of females and 7% of males in the eighth and tenth grades.[25] Forced coital behavior is reported in over 70% of sexually active females under age 14 years, 60% for those under age 15.[26] The 1999 Youth Risk Behavior Survey reports that 8.8% of high school students have been sexually assaulted, 12.5% of surveyed females versus 5.2% of the males.[8] Twelve months before this survey, 8.8% of high school students report they were hit, slapped, or physically hurt by their girl- or boyfriend.[8] A study in the United States concluded that 27% of *adult* females and 16% of *adult* males report a history of sexual abuse.[27] The child or adolescent who is subjected to violence and abuse may become an adult with serious sequelae, including diverse mental health disorders.[28,29]

Sexual Behavior

In the United States, millions of sexually active youth produce about one million pregnancies and over 6 million sexually transmitted diseases each year.[29] The 1999 Youth Risk Behavior Survey (YRBS) notes that 49.9% of all high school students are sexually experienced (coitally experienced), with a range of 45.1% for Whites, 54.1% for Hispanics, and 71.2% for African Amerian youth.[8] This report notes that 8% are coitally active before age 13 (12.2% in males and 4.4% in females), and 16% of youth have four or more partners (19.3% of males and 13.1% of females).[8] Youth who have experience with more than one partner usually practice *serial monogamy*—having one partner and then moving on to others, but usually one at any particular time.[30] There is an increased coital rate with increased drug/alcohol use and those engaged in survival sex.

Adolescent Pregnancy. Approximately one million adolescent pregnancies occur each year in the United States.[29,30] There was a decrease in adolescent pregnancies from 1973 (when abortion was legalized in the United States) until 1986; it increased in numbers from 1986 until 1991 and has decreased since then, except for the teen 15 years of age and younger (Table 2). In 1992 there were 12,200 adolescent pregnancies in those under age 15, versus 6,780 in 1960. Currently, approximately 43% of American adolescent females become pregnant at least once before age 20. Adolescent females account for 13% of all U.S. births (4,158,212 in 1992) and 26% of all abortions (about 400,000).[31]

TABLE 2 AMERICAN ADOLESCENT BIRTH RATES

Year	Birth Rate per 1,000 Females 15–19 Years of Age
1950s–1960s	Highest rates
1970	66
1986	50.2
1990	60
1997	53
1998	51
1999	49.6
2000	48.5
2001	45.9

The 1996 birth rate of 54.7 per 1,000 females aged 15 to 19 years (49.6 in 1999) in the United States is the *highest* among all developed nations and is in stark contrast to Japan, for example, where the rate is 4 per 1,000 or the Netherlands, where the rate is 7 per 1,000 in the same age group. Similar rates include 26 in Canada and 31 in the United Kingdom. Also, the abortion rate among American adolescent females is higher than the teen pregnancy rate in many countries (as Sweden, Netherlands, France, others). The abortion rate per 1,000 females ages 15 to 19 years is 36 in the United States versus 6 in Japan. The reason for this discrepancy is thought not to be any lesser sexual activity among youth in other European countries but rather that sexuality and family life education, as well as the provision of contraceptive services, is seriously lacking in the United States by comparison.[31]

In the United States, 1 in 10 adolescent females becomes pregnant each year; 90% or more are unintended. In adolescents, 14% of the pregnancies end in miscarriages, 35% in abortions, and 51% in live births. In 1992, 25% of births to adolescents were not first births, representing a 12.5% increase in *repeat* childbearing during adolescence since 1985. The 1992 data note a birth rate of 112.4 per 1,000 females aged 15–19 in the African American population versus 51.8 for the 15-to-19-year-old White female. In 1992, 10.9% of the White mothers were under age 20 (producing 505,415 live births) versus 22.7% of African Americans who were mothers under age 20 (with 153,248 live births), 20% of Native American mothers who were under age 20 (with 7,877 live births), and 5.6% of Asian or Pacific Islander mothers who were teens (with 8,404 live births). In 1999 the total number of births was 3,957,829 with teens under 20 accounting for 484,794 or 12.3% of all births. There were 172,608 births to mothers at or under 17 years of age or 4.4% of all births.

Risks of Adolescent Pregnancy. In general, the obstetric risks for pregnant adolescents are not greater than with adults, *if* the pregnant teenager receives prenatal services that begin early, remain constant, and are comprehensive.[30,31] However, lack of or failure to seek appropriate prenatal care compromises the outcome all too often. Thus, the risks are not because of age alone (15 to 19 years), but additional factors that compromise health care and that lead to a two- to four-times increase in maternal mortality rates for teens versus adults. There may be an increased risk for maternal preeclampsia due to age, but other problems (as increased premature labor, spontaneous abortion, and stillbirths) are related to such issues as limited health care, educational level, socio-economic status, and parity. For example, primiparous females of all ages have increased risks for eclampsia, preeclampsia, and chronic hypertension compared to non-primiparous individuals. Those under age 15 years may not be fully developed and problems with birth may occur due to small uterine size and the continued growth of the young mother, perhaps compromising her fetus' nutritional support. Some teens may not seek early prenatal care out of shame for the pregnancy.

Risks for Children of Adolescents. Over 4 million newborn babies die each year in the world, most due to poor prenatal care afforded the mother. Over the past 40 years, the American neonatal mortality rate has been reduced to 7.6 per 1,000 live births; however, the rate for African Americans and for all Americans under age 15 is 15 per 1,000 live births. Low birth weight is a major part of this mortality: 14% of first-born infants whose mothers are 14 years of age or less, weigh less than 2,500 grams at birth; this is in contrast to 5.8% noted with mothers who are 25 to 29 years of age. If these young mothers have additional infants during their teen years, the babies tend to be smaller and have a higher risk for death versus babies of older mothers. Also, prematurity is noted in 14% of infants with mothers under 15 years of age, versus 6% in 25-to-29-year-old mothers. Prematurity, low birth rate, and increased neonatal/infant morality rates are increased with limited prenatal care, poverty, poor nutrition, incomplete pubertal growth, reduced family support, limited education, drug abuse (including alcohol and tobacco), and sexually transmitted diseases.

There is also increased illness and death for infants (30% increase in the first year of life) whose mothers are 17 years of age or less (regardless of parity) and for 18-to-19-year-old multiparous mothers. These infants are in the hospital more than infants of adult mothers, and are subject to injuries, including burns and poisonings. The mortality rates are nine times higher due to violence (including accidents) and sudden infant death syndrome (SIDS).

Children whose mothers were teens at birth tend to have more problems in school, due to lower intelligence, reading ability, and communication scores, along with increased developmental delay, hyperactivity, and impulsiveness. Young teen mothers in America do not physically nor sexually abuse their children more than adult mothers, but they do neglect their children more than adult mothers—especially if they have more than one child. A young teen may not be mature enough to be sensitive to her child's needs, may have limited parenting skills, and may provide inappropriate discipline. These children become teenagers at increased risks for teenage pregnancy and sexually transmitted diseases.

Though 38% of American youth live in low-income families, 61% of teens who have an abortion and 83% of teens who deliver come from low-income families. These teen parents are at increased risk for not completing their education and not getting out of poverty during their teen and adult lives. They also are at increased risk of having further pregnancies before they reach 20—this worsens the already noted psychosocial risks of teen pregnancy. The number of unmarried adolescent mothers who are head of their households in the United States and the number of these families living in poverty have increased over the past 30 years.

Are these negative consequences of teen pregnancy inevitable: No! For example, factors that increase the teen mother's chances of finishing school include: being raised in a small family, having both parents with a "good" education, and having a mother who is employed. Attention to underlying complications (such as poverty, limited education, limited work skills, and reduced access to quality health care) can reduce or even remove the increased risks for these negative psychosocial outcomes.[30,31]

Marriage. Only 11% of 15-to-19-year-old American females are married before age 18 years. The percentage of teen births occurring outside of marriage rose from 15% in 1960 to 80% in 1999. Unfortunately, American teen mothers tend to have higher divorce rates (approximately 70%) if they marry and tend to have limited contact (support) from the child's father. The teen mother and her partner are less likely to marry now (versus 20 or more years ago) simply because of the pregnancy.

Sexually Transmitted Diseases. There are many types of sexually transmitted diseases (STDs) that can affect youth. Current studies in the United States identify over 14 million STD cases from all age groups, including 1–2 million new cases of gonorrhea each year, 4 million new cases of chlamydia each year, 12 million existing human papillomavirus (HPV) cases, and 30 million existing herpes simplex virus (HSV) cases.[29,32] Those between 15–29 years of age acquire 86% of these STDs; one in 6–7 sexually active teens acquires an STD each year, resulting in 5–6 million STDs in the 15-to-24 age group each year! There are about 3 million STDs reported in the 10-to-19-year-old age group each year. There are also unknown millions of asymptomatic, unreported STDs in adolescents each year in the United States. The cost in terms of preventable health care spending is staggering, and the complications of STDs are severe, especially for females; these include pelvic inflammatory disease, chronic pelvic pain, ectopic (tubal) pregnancy, and poor pregnancy outcomes, among others.

Studies note that youth (aged 15–19) have the highest rates of chlamydia, gonorrhea, cervicitis (endocervicitis), syphilis, and hospitalizations due to pelvic inflammatory disease. Worldwide, those 15–24 years have the highest STD risk.[29] Inner city, minority youth in the United States are at the highest STD risk—having two to three times the STD rate as compared to American suburban Caucasians.

In the United States, there are an estimated 3,000 youth with overt HIV infection and 23,000 in the 21-to-24-year age group (out of 200,000 cases in the United States), and a growing syphilis incidence that is now complicated by the HIV epidemic.[29,33] There is an estimated one million Americans who are infected with HIV; it is unknown how many are teenagers who will eventually die from HIV in their third or fourth decade of life. Approximately 20% of adults with HIV infection acquired it as a teenager and one in four individuals newly diagnosed with HIV infection is under age 22. African Americans are 14% of the American population, yet bear 28% of the AIDS cases in America.

The Adolescent Sexual Offender. The sexual victimization of children by adolescents has become a serious, yet often ignored problem in our society.[34] Adolescents under the age of 18 years account for 20% of arrests for all sexual offenses (excluding prostitution), 20% to 30% of rape cases, 14% of aggravated sexual assault offenses, and 27% of child sexual homicides.[34] About 0.5% of all adolescents are ever arrested for violent crimes, of which sexual offending represents a small subset. Known offenders represent only a fraction of the number of actual cases of child and adolescent sexual abuse.

Substance Abuse

The socio-medical phenomenon of alcohol and illegal drug use among adolescents in the United States remains one of the most serious health issues facing society in the 21st century.[35] Alcohol use contributes to 25% to 50% of the deaths in adolescents (due to motor vehicle accidents, suicide, others).[35] The most widely used drugs are marijuana, tobacco, and alcohol among youth from all socioeconomic and ethnic backgrounds. Following a slightly reduced prevalence early in the 1990s, the use increased until 1997 with a slight dip after that. Lifetime prevalence of illicit drug use for any drug is 26.8% for those in the eighth grade, 45.6% for 10th graders, and 54% for 12th graders.[36] Lifetime prevalence for alcohol use is 51.7% for 8th graders, 71.4% for 10th graders, and 80.3% for 12th graders.[36] Cigarette use for this group, respectively, is 40.5%, 55.1%, and 62.5%.[36] The 1999 YRBS report notes that 50% of high school students had consumed alcohol over the past 30 days of the survey, 26.7% had used marijuana over the past 30 days, and that 32.8% currently used tobacco (cigarettes, cigars, and/or smokeless tobacco).[8] There is increasing drug use among younger teens, many beginning their first use at 12 to 13 years of age (or even younger). The greatest risk for long-lasting dysfunctional patterns of substance use is the onset of use before age 15 years. One of every three young persons in the United States comes from a home in which alcohol has been an abused substance. Children of alcohol and other drug abusers are at increased risk for abusing drugs themselves.

Youth Violence

Violence remains an important cause of physical and psychosocial morbidity among adolescents in the United States.[37–39] According to the United States Department of Education, in schools there were 188,000 incidents of physical attacks not involving weapons, 11,000 fights involving weapons, and 4,000 incidents of sexual assaults. In an average month, there are 525,000 attacks (including shakedowns and robberies), and 125,000 threats against teachers in United States public secondary schools. Approximately 5,000 teachers suffer actual physical harm in a given month. A 1998 survey of 15,686 American students in grades 6 through 10 noted that 29.9% reported moderate or frequent involvement in bullying behavior: 13% as a bully, 10.6% being bullied, and 6.3% as both.[40] A vast majority of children and adolescents (especially inner city youth [70% to 95%]) have witnessed a violent act such as robbery, stabbing, shooting, murder, or domestic violence. African Americans and other minority ethnic groups experience a disproportionate share of violence. Young African American females are four times more likely and African American males 11 times more likely to be killed than Caucasian teenagers. Violence in school is often highlighted in the media following unfortunate incidents. Fortunately, the estimated odds of dying a violent death in school in the year 1999 were 1 in 2 million.[39] However, the consequences of witnessing or being involved in school violence are incalculable.

The medical costs as a result of violence are enormous.[38,39] In the long run it is less expensive to prevent youth violence than to treat its lifelong consequences. It is estimated that 3% of the total U.S. medical expenditure goes to treat interpersonal violence-related injuries annually. Firearm injuries cost between $1.4 and $4 billion annually for direct treatment. Because of lifelong effects of serious firearm injuries, another $19 billion are lost in indirect costs such as loss of future earnings. The direct costs to treat domestic violence related injuries are estimated to be $44 million annually and for child abuse about $500 million annually. The comparative costs and benefits of prevention and intervention of youth violence are shown in Table 3.[39]

Mortality

Violence accounts for about 75% of deaths in youths 15 to 24 years of age.[37–44] In 1999, nearly three-fourths of deaths among Americans 10 to 24 years of age resulted from only four causes: motor vehicle accidents (30%), other uninten-

TABLE 3 COMPARATIVE COSTS AND BENEFITS OF PREVENTION AND
INTERVENTION OF YOUTH VIOLENCE

Age	Program	Estimated Cost per Participant ($)	Benefits per Dollar Cost ($)	
			Benefits to the Taxpayer (Criminal Justice System Benefits)	Benefits to the Taxpayer and Victims
Early Childhood	Perry Preschool Program	13,938	0.66	1.50
	Syracuse Family Development Research Program	45,092	0.19	0.34
	Prenatal and Infancy Home Visitation by Nurses	7,403	0.83	1.54
Middle Childhood	Seattle Social Development Project	3,017	0.90	1.79
Adolescent Non-Juvenile Offender	The Quantum Opportunities Program	18,292	0.09	0.13
	Big Brothers Big Sisters of America	1,009	1.30	2.12
Adolescent Juvenile Offender	**Community-Based**			
	Multisystemic Therapy	4,540	8.38	13.45
	Functional Family Therapy	2,068	6.85	10.99
	Multidimensional Treatment Foster Care*	1,934	14.07	22.58
	Intensive Supervision (probation)**	1,500	0.90	1.49
	Institutional-Based			
	Boot camps**	−1,964	0.42	0.26

Source: Washington State Institute for Public Policy, 1999.
*Costs calculated relative to costs of treatment in a regular group home.
**Costs calculated relative to costs of regular probation.

tional injuries (10%), homicides (20%), and suicides (13%).[37,41,44] Violence-related deaths have increased over the last quarter of the 20th century, with a 400% increase in motor vehicle accidents, a 400% increase in homicide rates, and a 600% increase in suicide rates.[18] The leading cause of adolescent deaths is accidents, most of which are car accidents; many of these involve the use of drugs, especially alcohol. The second and third leading causes of deaths for males aged 15 to 19 are suicide and homicide; they are the third and fourth causes of death for females aged 15 to 19. Homicide is the third leading cause of death for youth 10 to 14 years of age, and suicide the fourth leading cause of death. The male is more likely to be involved as a victim and as a victimizer, while the female is more likely to be involved in suicide attempts and as a sexually abused victim. Male teenagers die at a two times greater rate than female adolescents.

Homicide and Suicide. Mortality rates have increased for adolescents from the early 1960s to the late 1980s; these rates have stabilized since then, except for an increase in the rate for African American males, due to increased homicide rates.[37] The mortality rate for African American males more than doubled in the 1980s and was three times the rate from natural causes.[44] Firearm homicide rates for Black males are 11 times greater than for White males; White males were more than twice as likely as Black males to commit suicide with firearms.[37] Easy access to guns in the home increased the risk for suicide in these youth in their homes.[45]

In general, homicide is more likely to occur in the inner city than suicide, while suicide is more prevalent in suburban America. Approximately four to five thousand teens commit suicide each year; the suicide rate in 15-to-24-year-olds is over 13 per 100,000 in contrast to 5.2 in 1960.[46] In 1988 the suicide rate for 15-to-19-year-olds was 11.3 (versus 2.7 in 1950) and 15.0 for 20-to-24-year-olds (versus 6.2 in 1950).[46] Suicide is the second leading cause of death for White males 15–24 years of age; chronic illness is a factor in some of these cases.[47] Suicide is increased in certain ethnic groups, such as Alaskan American, Asian American, and Native American youth.[47] Each year, four to five thousand youth are murdered (14 to 15 deaths per 100,000 population aged 15–24 years, versus 5.9 in 1960). The homicide rate for Black male teens is over five times that of White males. The 1997 death rate for the Black male teen was 921 deaths per 100,000, 60% higher than for White males and the highest age-adjusted death rate of any race or sex group.[48]

Motor Vehicle Accidents. Thirty percent of deaths in 15-to-20-year-olds result from motor vehicle crashes (MVAs), the number-one cause of deaths among teens.[41] In 1998, 3,427 drivers between 15 and 20 years of age were killed, and 348,000 were injured in motor vehicle accidents. Fourteen percent (7,975) of all drivers involved in fatal crashes (56,543) were 15 to 20 years old, and 16% (1,801,000) of all drivers involved in police-reported crashes (11,368,000) were young drivers. In 1998, 37% of male drivers aged 15–20 years involved in fatal crashes were speeding at the time of the MVA. Fifty-three percent of teen motor vehicle crashes in 1997 occurred on weekends, with 41% between 9 P.M. and 6 A.M. In 1997, 19.3% of high school students (14.5% female; 23.2% males) rarely or never wore seat belts when riding in a car or truck driven by someone else. The economic toll of 1998 police-reported crashes involving these young drivers in the United States is estimated to exceed $31.8 billion.[41]

A number of factors influence driving-associated morbidity and mortality. For the adolescent driver, psychosocial development and inexperience contribute to increased risk-taking and dangerous driving behavior. Alcohol-related factors are of special significance. Miles driven per week, truancy, drug abuse, and number of evenings out are all positively associated with driving-after-drinking behavior, whereas positive academic performance and religiosity reduce this deadly behavior. The United States National Highway Traffic Safety Administration notes that

30% of Americans will be involved in an alcohol-related crash at some point in their lives.[41] In 1998, 57% of deaths from MVAs were alcohol-related accidents; 21% of drivers 15–20 years of age who were killed in these crashes were legally intoxicated.

According to the 1999 Youth Risk Behavior Survey, 33.1% of high school students had ridden one or more times with a driver who had been drinking alcohol during the preceding 30 days.[8] Thirteen percent of students nationwide (8.7% females; 17.4% males) had driven a vehicle one or more times after drinking alcohol.[8] According to a 1995 Centers for Disease Control and Prevention (CDC) survey, 35.1% of college students (18–24 years) had ridden with a driver who had been drinking; 27.4% of these college students had driven after drinking during the 30 days preceding the survey.[41]

Runaway and Homeless Youth

It is estimated that there are several hundred thousand adolescents who run away from home and are homeless in the United States.[49] The *Runaway and Homeless Youth Act* (Title III of the Juvenile Justice and Delinquency Prevention Act) defines runaways as "juveniles who leave and remain away from home without parental permission."[49] Some are "situational runaways" who leave home for a day or so after an argument with a parent. Others are "throwaways" who have parents who abandon them, ask them to leave, or severely abuse (neglect) them— forcing them to leave home.[50] Some youth have no family contact and have lived in various institutions or foster homes; these "systems youth" eventually leave to live on the street.

The most detailed U.S. government study looked at 40 urban counties and included 430 shelters; this study estimated there were 253,600 homeless children and youth under age 16 years; this included over 9,000 living in cars, abandoned buildings, bus terminals, and other areas.[51] Others estimate there are over 450,000 runaways and 127,000 throwaways.[50] There are also several hundred thousand youth who live with their families, but lack access to a conventional dwelling or residence.[52] Homeless youth are subject to many dangers of the street—as physical/sexual abuse, substance abuse, sexually transmitted diseases, various medical disorders, and others. Their main medical treatment is usually through the emergency room, if they receive any care at all.

Incarcerated Youth

There are over 800,000 youth in jail-like facilities in the United States, whether jails, detention centers, lock-ups, or others.[53-55] They have various health care needs and often are not eligible for health care coverage. Over 75% of these youths have health care problems that need to be addressed.[55] They represent a very vulnerable and high-risk group of youth in America.

BARRIERS TO ADOLESCENT CARE

Confidentiality

American laws have gradually recognized that youth (minors) have some legal rights, allowing them to seek medical evaluation and treatment without parents' knowledge.[18,56,57] The inability of many youth to seek medical services without parents' permission combined with the refusal of various health care professionals to treat adolescents under such circumstances has resulted in many youth refusing to seek health care. Considerable confusion is found in this arena and the laws as well as their interpretation may vary from state to state.

Definitions of laws in the area of confidentiality are developed from a compilation of Supreme Court rulings (federal and state) and their interpretations. During the first century of the founding of the United States, there were minimal rights for youth. This has been called the "era of parental autonomy," in which parents had complete autonomy over their children. Children were expected to obey parents, and punishment resulted from parents or others (police officials, for example) if there was disobedience. The "era of child welfare" emerged at the end of the 19th century when it was recognized that children were different from parents and needed to be protected from them in some instances. The adult was then punished if the child was abused by parents or legal guardians. Juvenile courts were developed and child labor was controlled. Minors, however, were still not allowed to make contracts of their own with health care providers.

Common law tradition has held that to treat a minor without appropriate parental permission is an "unauthorized touching" and legally called "assault and battery." The current "era of the rights of minors" was ushered in in 1967 with a legal case—in re Gault.[18] This case involved a 15-year-old male who was sentenced by a court to several years of institutionalization after a conviction of placing obscene phone calls to a teacher. The parents brought forth a lawsuit based on the concept that the minor was entitled to, but denied, the right of a legal representative, cross examination, and other measures which would help him mount a legal defense.

In 1976 the Danforth case emerged, placing the rights of a minor to obtain an abortion against the parents' rights to stop it. The Court noted that the minor had a right to such a procedure even against the parent's permission, under certain conditions:

The State may not impose a blanket provision requiring the consent of a parent or person in loco parentis as a condition for abortion of an unmarried minor during the first twelve weeks of her pregnancy .... The State does not have the Constitutional authority to give a third party an absolute, and possibly arbitrary, veto over the decision of the physician and his patient to terminate the patient's pregnancy. Minors, as well as adults, are protected by the Constitution and possess Constitutional rights .... Any independent interest the parent may have in the termination of the minor daughter's pregnancy is no more weighty than the right of the competent minor mature enough to become pregnant.[18]

Such issues are quite complex and are far from being resolved, especially for the abortion issue. However, it seems clear that youth can give consent for medical treatment in some situations and do not necessarily have to involve parents in all cases. In general, it is best to involve parents in such matters, but such is not always possible or feasible. A nonofficial legal concept has emerged over the past generation—the *mature minor doctrine*. This implies "emancipated" minors may seek and receive some medical treatment without parental approval or knowledge.[18,56] However, the interpretation of "emancipation" can be vague and vary according to different criteria that have been used in various states. Being familiar with one's own state rules and philosophy is strongly recommended for those who deal with such teenagers. As an example, Table 4 identifies some of these specific concepts as they apply in many states. The avoidance of confidentiality for youth by insurance companies and various clinicians limits the number of adolescents who are willing to seek care for diverse high-risk behaviors—such as sexual activity and drug use.

TABLE 4 VARIOUS CRITERIA FOR EMANCIPATION

---

1. Age (often over 18, but varies from 14–19)

2. Marriage

3. Parenthood

4. Runaway status (financially independent)

5. Individuals away from home with parent's permission

6. Individuals at home who are "essentially independent"

7. Education (as high school graduates)

8. Member of armed forces

9. Certified by physician and others

Reimbursement

Another problem that has persisted and that encourages clinicians not to treat youth is lack of adequate reimbursement for services rendered. Insurance coverage for youth is a combination of public and private insurance payment. Private insurers, in an attempt to save money expenditure on health care, have covered less and less in the way of health care for youth, especially as managed care contracts have become more popular with employers.[58,59]

Since private insurance (employee-based) is not comprehensively covering the health care needs provided for youth, coverage increasingly has relied on

Medicaid and/or State Children's Health Insurance Programs (SCHIP). Medicaid was first enacted in 1965 as Title XIX of the Social Security Act. It became the largest source of health care funding for low-income women, children, and adolescents. As it was developed, the federal government outlined basic rules of coverage and the states developed their own programs to meet these rules. A complex series of ever-changing laws has emerged seeking to define this coverage. In the 1980s and 1990s, complex laws removed cash assistance and developed eligibility criteria based on federal poverty levels. In 1989 a variety of changes were made to the Early and Periodic Screening, Diagnosis and Treatment Program (EPSDT). Though coverage through Medicaid has recognized the need for preventive services and various services for teens with chronic illnesses and disabilities, the reimbursement to clinicians who wish to see these teens, has remained low—discouraging many clinicians from caring for these youth.

Many youth remain uninsured, especially those with chronic health problems who are in poor health, the poor, and those from ethnic minorities; these youth often cannot find confidential care, receive minimal preventive care, and often rely on hospital emergency departments for their health care.[60] The uninsured mainly come from low-income families in which the head of the family works at a low-income job that provides no insurance.[61] They often have minimal understanding of eligibility rules. In 1988, 13.7% of youth (12–17 years) had no health insurance, including 33% of those below the federal poverty line.[59] In 1992, there was no insurance for 14.9% of the 10-to-14-year-olds, 19.9% for 15-to-19-year-olds and 25.2% for 19-to-21-year-olds.[59] In 1995, there were 9.8 million children and youth (under age 18) without insurance; this became 11 million in 1996 and 10.7 million in 1997; approximately 15% of those under age 18 did not have any insurance. In the 1990s, two-thirds of the uninsured were under 35 years of age— 42.1 million persons in 1999 versus 43.9 million in 1998.[62] Ethnic groups often fared poorly; for example, Hispanics who were 13% of the population were 25% of the uninsured.[63]

In 1996, Congress passed the Personal Responsibility and Work Opportunity Reconciliation Act (PRWORA) or Welfare Reform, as it is often known.[64] It sought to reduce welfare dependence and increase the economic independence of poor families in the United States. Welfare reform also sought to extend Medicaid benefits to children who will lose benefits due to PRWORA. The SCHIP was enacted to help children in this regard.

The SCHIP was enacted in 1997 as part of the Balanced Budget Act of 1997 (a new Title XXI of the Social Security Act—42 U.S.C. 1397 et seq. #35). This represents an allocation of $48 billion dollars to the states (50 states and Washington, D.C.) in an attempt to provide further health insurance to low-income children and adolescents (under 19 years of age) who are not covered by Medicaid; this includes $20.3 billion from 1997 to 2002 and a total of $48 billion over 10 years.[65] It is an effort to provide coverage for uninsured children while others were losing coverage ("leaky-bucket coverage") because of welfare reform sending mothers off to low-paying jobs.[62] The states have been given a number of options, including expanding their Medicaid program, developing a state-specific program, or combining their Medicaid and SCHIP. The states have been given much freedom in terms of establishing eligibility levels, outreach activities, benefit packages, and others.[66] Welfare reform has eliminated the Temporary Assistance to Needy Family Program (TANF) in favor of this block-grant program, allowing each state to decide how to assist such families.[67,68]

However, problems in reimbursing for comprehensive care of adolescents still remain. There is considerable state to state variation in coverage and the United States continues to struggle with the rising cost of health coverage.[66,69] Medicaid and SCHIP do not match the recommendations of the American Academy of Pediatrics, the American Medical Association's Guide to Preventive Services or the government's Bright Futures.[70,71] The EPSDT participant rates have lagged below the Health Care Financing Administration's (HCFA) goal of 80%. There is much state to state confusion over what family planning services will be covered, disagreement over whether or not all teenagers are covered for reproductive services, and severe restrictions on abortion services. It is difficult for adolescents to obtain comprehensive mental health services, whether for depression, eating disorders, substance abuse or other conditions. Teens are often left out of coverage.

The need for confidentiality in services to youth is often not recognized by insurance plans. There are a limited number of health care professionals who are trained to work with youth, and the coverage for many services for youth remains poor. When access to primary and comprehensive care is limited, youth often seek care in emergency rooms in the United States. In 1994, adolescents represented nearly 16% of the visits to emergency medicine departments.[72] Youth should be encouraged and allowed to see their regular clinicians for health care and use the emergency medicine departments at hospitals for emergency care only.[72]

RECOMMENDATIONS FOR THE FUTURE

Provide Comprehensive Insurance Coverage for Children and Adolescents

Insurance coverage for our children has been in turmoil for many decades.[19–22,53–55,58–69,73,74] It was recognized in the 1990s and before, that many of those under age 21 were not provided adequate insurance coverage, discouraging needy patients from needed health care and discouraging health care providers from caring for these persons.[74] Though many children and adolescents need health care for immediate and chronic problems, they are denied this care in America, especially for mental health and substance abuse disorders.[4,15,35,36,75,76] There is no acceptable reason for this and no reason to keep our children in the middle of the continuing insurance crisis.[73] All elements of society must come together and provide comprehensive insurance coverage for all our children— they are our future and it remains inexcusable, even in this era of welfare reform, to limit their care as we currently do.

Deal with Confidentiality Issues

The health care professional should learn how to relate to youth. Involving parents as much as possible is usually recommended when health care professionals work with youth. However, some teenagers will seem more eager than others to talk alone to a health care professional. Young adolescents (11–14 years of age) often prefer the assistance of parents, but late adolescents (18 years and older) do not, and middle adolescents (14 to 18 years) typically place the health care provider in a very delicate position because the provider must relate to both parents and youth.[18,59] In general, the very young teenager, the critically ill, and the mentally challenged individual do need active parental involvement.

When possible, confidentiality must be carefully approached and provided.[56,57] Young concrete-thinking teenagers are especially eager for health information but may be unable to provide detailed answers to the health care provider's questions. A questionnaire focusing on health issues and interviews with parents and teens may be helpful in this regard. In general, documentation data from as many sources as possible are extremely helpful in evaluating complex situations that involve diverse family dynamics and individual personality complications. Encouraging youth to talk with their parents openly, and even providing them with examples of how to do so, is an important part of the clinician's role.

Youth must be given some sense of confidentiality and shown that the health care professional is not merely an unfiltered conduit of information from the youth to the parent. These young patients must be given some reassurance that what they say will be held in acceptable confidence. However, the youth must realize that there are some limits to this aspect. Federal and state laws specify what information must be reported to parents and police departments. For example, individuals who are severely depressed and threatening suicide or those presenting with a risk of physical harm to others must not be allowed to go through with these serious issues untreated and unchecked. Sexual or physical abuse of a minor is also an area governed by legal mandates. Clinical judgement is necessary in deciding who to tell and how to handle such problems. Specific documentation of these situations must be kept in the patient's files. In some states, there are legal mandates specifying who must be notified and in what time frame. However, appropriate health care for youth should not be denied by the health care professional or insurance managers because of insensitivity to well-known psychosocial issues of adolescence.

Provide Comprehensive Sexuality Education

Limited sexuality education can be invoked as a partial explanation for the tragic statistics of American adolescent sexuality (i.e., high rates of unwanted pregnancy, STDs, sexual assaults) noted throughout the country.[8,18,23,34] If youth are sexually active, simply discouraging/banning sexuality education on cultural and religious bases does not fully resolve the issues. Limited knowledge of sexuality can be very dangerous for the youth of America and elsewhere.[77,78]

Youth are naturally curious about sexuality and often experiment widely, especially starting in mid-adolescence.[8,18,30,31] The current American society stresses the enjoyment of human sexuality but often, paradoxically, ignores the potentially negative consequences of unwise, unprotected sexual experimentation. Many adolescent males eagerly experiment with their sexuality, often without regard for others. Part of this is the "normal" narcissistic stage of adolescent sexuality, while part of it is concurring with American society's encouragement in which sexual advertisements eagerly expose youth to various high-risk behaviors and in which sex as well as violence without consequences are promoted. The modern media (such as cable, television, videos) have a profound effect on America's and the world's youth. Only limited attempts have been made to modify the media's portrayal of sexual behavior without responsibility.

Approaches to reduce unwanted adolescent pregnancies and sexually transmitted diseases vary. For example, sexuality education has been part of the school curriculum in Finland since 1970 and is also required in Sweden. Low teen pregnancy rates are noted in these and other countries (as the Netherlands) where comprehensive sex education and easy access to contraceptives are provided.

It is very costly to provide limited sexuality education to youth and then deal with the consequences of sexually transmitted diseases and pregnancy.[30-33] For example, in its Aid to Families and Dependent Children (AFDC) program, the U.S. government spent about 5 billion dollars for homes headed by females who are or were teen mothers.[31,79] Research notes that the younger the teen is when pregnancy and birth take place, the more likely it is that she will need government help to provide for herself and her children.[30,31] Public costs from teenage childbearing totaled $120 billion from 1985 to 1990 in the United States, and it has been noted that $48 billion could have been saved if each birth had been postponed until the mother was at least 20 years old.[79] (See http://www.cdc.gov/nccdphp/teen.thm—1999.) Prevention of unwanted adolescent pregnancy and sexually transmitted diseases are important goals of all elements of society.[32,78, 80]

RECOMMENDATIONS FOR PREVENTION OF UNWANTED ADOLESCENT PREGNANCY AND SEXUALLY TRANSMITTED DISEASES

We recommend the following principles in this regard:

1. Adolescents can be taught that abstinence is an important goal while they are preparing to become adults.[80] They can be taught a number of strategies preventing negative consequences of sexual behavior:
   a. How to avoid sexual abuse
   b. How to resist unwanted sexual advances (including "date rape")
   c. How to negotiate peer pressure
   d. How to avoid media messages for sexual behavior without responsibility

2. Teenagers who are mothers and fathers should receive parental, school, and society support to become the best possible parents to reduce potential negative consequences of teenage pregnancy[30,31]

3. The teenage mother must be taught how to avoid repeat pregnancy until she is emotional and financially ready for more children.[80]

4. Pregnancy prevention programs should be tailored to the needs of each region, involving multidimensional solutions.[30,31] Cultural and religious beliefs of each person must be respected.[80]

5. Sexual abuse of children and adolescents throughout the country must be eliminated.[8,23–29,81,82]

6. Adolescents who become sexually active must be taught how to effectively use contraceptives ("safe sex") and receive access to contraception, including emergency contraceptives.[80,83,84]

RECOMMENDATIONS FOR PREVENTION OF YOUTH VIOLENCE

The 2001 Report of the Surgeon General makes the following recommendations:[38]

1. Continue to build the science base, seeking to understand the causes and best management strategies for violence.

2. Accelerate the decline in gun use by youths in violent encounters.

3. Facilitate the entry of youths into effective intervention programs rather than incarcerating them.

4. Disseminate model programs with incentives that will ensure fidelity to original program design when taken to scale.

5. Provide effective training and certification programs for intervention personnel.

6. Improve public awareness of effective interventions.

7. Convene youth and families, researchers, and private as well as public organizations for a periodic youth violence summit.

8. Improve federal, state, and local strategies for reporting crime information and violent deaths.

REFERENCES

1. Population Reference Bureau, *Population Today* 27(8): 2, 1999 (September) (http://www.prb.org).

2. Newacheck PW, McManus MA, Fox HG: Prevalence and impact of chronic illness among adolescents. *Am J Dis Child* 145:1367–1373, 1991.

3. Gortmaker Sl, Perrin JM, Weitzman M et al.: An unexpected success story: Transition to adulthood with chronic physical health conditions. *J Res Adolesc* 3:317–336, 1993.

4. Greydanus DE, Wolraich ML (Eds.). *Behavioral Pediatrics* NY: Springer-Verlag, 1–471, 1992.

5. Patel DR, Rowlett JR, Greydanus DE: Youth with chronic conditions in transition to adult health care. *Adolesc Med* 5:543–554, 1994.

6. Hofmann AD: "Chronic illness and hospitalization" in: *Adolescent Medicine*, Third Edition. AD Hofmann & DE Greydanus (Eds.) Stamford, CT: Appleton & Lange. Ch. 33: 740–754, 1997.

7. Hofmann AD: "Obesity" in: *Adolescent Medicine*, Third Edition. AD Hofmann & DE Greydanus (Eds.). Stamford, CT: Appleton & Lange. Ch. 30: 663–682, 1997.

8. Kann L, Kinchen SA, Williams JG et al.: Youth Risk Behavior Surveillance-United States, 1999. *Morb Mort Week Rep* 49 (No. SS-5): 1–94, 2000.

9. Patel DR & Homnick DN: Pulmonary effects of smoking. *Adolesc Med* 11:567–576, 2000.

10. Grant EN, Wagner R, Weiss KB: Observations on emerging patterns of asthma in our society. *J Allergy Clin Immunology* 104 (2 pt.2): S1–9, 1999.

11. Navas-Nacher EL, Colangelo L, Beam C et al.: Risk factors for coronary heart disease in men 18 to 39 years of age. *Ann Intern Med* 134:433–439, 2001.

12. Onkamo P, Väänänen S, Karvonen M et al.: Worldwide increase in incidence of Type I diabetes—The analysis of the data on published incidence trends. *Diabetologica* 42:1395–1403, 1999.

13. American Diabetes Association. Type 2 diabetes in children and adolescents. *Diabetes Care* 23 (3):381–389, 2000.

14. Kazdin AE: Adolescent mental health: Prevention and treatment programs. *Amer Psychol* 48(2): 127–141, 1993.

15. Manderscheid R, Somenschein MA (Eds.): *Mental Health, United States*. Washington, DC: Center for Mental Health Services, U.S. Government Printing Office, 1996.

16. Kaplan S, Hong G, Weinhold C: Epidemiology of depressive symptoms in adolescents. *J Am Acad Child Psychiatr* 23:91–98, 1984.

17. Shaffer D: Description, acceptability, prevalence rates and performance in the MECA study. J Am Acad Child Adolesc Psychiatr 35(7): 865–77, 1996.

18. Greydanus DE, Pratt HD: *Adolescence: A Continuum From Childhood to Adulthood*. Third Edition. Des Moines, IA: Iowa Department of Public Health 132 pages, 1995.

19. Knitzer J: *Unclaimed Children: The Failure of Public Responsibility to Children and Adolescents in Need of Mental Health Services*. Washington, DC: Children's Defense Fund, 1982.

20. American Academy of Pediatrics. Insurance coverage of mental health and substance abuse services for children and adolescents: A consensus statement. *Pediatrics* 106(4): 1–4, 2000.

21. American Psychiatric Association: *Issues affecting mental health coverage for children.* Washington, DC: American Psychiatric Association, 1999.

22. Stroud B & Friedman R: "The system of care concept and philosophy" in: *Children's Mental Health: Creating a System of Care in a Changing Society.* B. Stroll (Ed.). Baltimore, MD: Paul H. Brooks Pub. Co., 1996.

23. United States Department of Health and Human Services, National Center on Child Abuse and Neglect. *Child Maltreatment, 1994: Report from States to the National Center for Child Abuse and Neglect.* Washington, DC: U.S. Government Printing Office, 1996.

24. Finkelhor V, Dziuba-Leatherman J: Children as victims of violence. *Pediatrics* 94:413–420, 1994.

25. Wilson M, Joffe A: Adolescent Medicine. *JAMA* 273(21): 1657–1659, 1995.

26. Finkelhor V, Hotaling G, Lewis I: Sexual abuse in a national survey of adult men and women: Prevalence, characteristics and risk factors. *Child Abuse Negl* 14:9, 1990.

27. Felitti VJ, Anda RF, Nordenberg D et al.: Relationship of childhood abuse and household dysfunction to many leading causes of death in adults: The Adverse Childhood Experience (ACE) Study. *Am J Prev Med* 14(4): 245–257, 1998.

28. Silverman A, Reinherz H, Giaconia F: The long-term sequela of childhood and adolescent abuse: A longitudinal community study. *Child Abuse & Neglect* 20:709–723, 1996.

29. Alan Guttmacher Institute: *Into a New World: Young Women's Sexual and Reproductive Lives.* pages 1-56, New York: The Alan Guttmacher Institute (120 Wall Street, NY, NY USA 10005), 1998. (www.agi-usa.org).

30. Adolescent pregnancy—Current trends and issues: 1998. American Academy of Pediatrics. Committee on Adolescence. *Pediatrics* 103(2): 516–520, 1999.

31. Greydanus DE: "Adolescent pregnancy and abortion" In: *Adolescent Medicine*, Third Edition. AD Hofmann & DE Greydanus (Eds.). Stamford, CT: Appleton & Lange. Ch. 27: 589–604, 1997.

32. Centers for Disease Control and Prevention. 2001 Guidelines for treatment of sexually transmitted diseases. *MMWR* 47 (RR-1): 1–116, 2001.

33. Centers for Disease Control and Prevention. HIV/AIDS Surveillance Report. *Morb Mort Week Rep* 9:1–43, 1997.

34. Pratt HD, Patel DR, Greydanus DE et al.: Adolescent sexual offenders. *International Pediatrics* 16:73–80, 2001.

35. Greydanus DE: Substance abuse in adolescents. *International Pediatrics* 17:1–3, 2002.

36. Johnston L: *National Survey Results on Drug Use from the Monitoring of the Future Study, 2000.*

37. Pratt HD, Greydanus DE: Adolescent violence: Concepts for a new millennium. *Adolesc Med* 11:103–125, 2000.

38. *Youth Violence: A Report of the Surgeon General.* April 2001. www.surgeongeneral.gov/library/youthviolence (accessed 4/23/01).

39. *Youth and Violence. Report of the Commission for the Prevention of Youth Violence.* December 2000 (www.ama-assn.org/violence[accessed 4/23/01]).

40. Nansel TR, Overpeck M, Pilla RS et al.: Bullying behaviors among U.S. youth: Prevalence and association with psychosocial adjustment. *JAMA* 285:2094–2100, 2001.

41. Patel DR, Greydanus DE, Rowlett JD: Romance with the automobile in the 20th century: Implications for adolescents In a new millennium. *Adolesc Med* 11:127–139, 2000.

42. Reiss D, Richters JE (Eds.): *Children and Violence.* NY: NY: Guildford Press, 1993.

43. Widom CS: The Cycle of Violence. *Science* 244:160–16, 1989.

44. Centers for Disease Control and Prevention. Homicide among 15 to 19 year old males—United States 1963–1991. *Morb Mort Week Rep* 43:725–727, 1994.

45. Resnick MD, Bearman PS, Blum RW et al.: Protecting adolescents from harm. Findings from the National Longitudinal Study on Adolescent Health. *JAMA* 278 (10): 823–32, 1997.

46. Centers for Disease Control. *Youth suicide prevention programs: A resource guide.* Department of Health & Human Services. Public Health Service. National Center for Injury Prevention and Control. Atlanta, GA, p. 2, September, 1992.

47. Jenkins RR: "Suicide" In: *Nelson Textbook of Pediatrics.* Eds: RE Behrman, RM Kliegman & HB Jenson. Philadelphia, PA: WB Saunders Co., ch. 110:559–560, 2000.

48. *Advance Data—Vital Health Statistics.* Atlanta, GA. Centers for Disease Control and Prevention, 1999.

49. Farrow JA, Deisher W, Brown R et al.: Health and health needs of homeless and runaway youth: A position paper of the Society for Adolescent Medicine. *J Adolesc Health* 13:717–726, 1992.

50. Finkelhor D, Hotaling G, Sedlak A: *Missing, Abducted, Runaway and Throwaway Children in America.* First Report: Numbers and Characteristics. Washington, DC: US Department of Justice, Office of Juvenile Justice and Delinquency Prevention, May, 1990.

51. U.S. General Accounting Office: *Homeless Children and Youths.* Washington, DC: US Government Accounting Office, June, 1989.

52. Health needs of homeless children and families. Committee on Community Health Services. American Academy of Pediatrics. *Pediatrics* 98(4): 351–353, 1996.

53. Health care for incarcerated youth: Position paper of the Society for Adolescent Medicine. *J Adolesc Health* 27:73–75, 2000.

54. U.S. Congress, Office of Technology Assessment. *Adolescent Health-Volume II: Background and Effectiveness of Selected Prevention and Treatment Services.* Washington, DC: U.S. Government Printing Office, 1991.

55. American Academy of Pediatrics. Committee on Adolescence. Health care for children and adolescents in the juvenile correctional care system. *Pediatrics* 107(4): 799–803, 2001.

56. Hofmann AD: "Consent and confidentiality" In *Adolescent Medicine*, Third Edition. AD Hofmann, DE Greydanus (Eds.). Stamford, CT: Appleton & Lange. Ch. 6: 61–73, 1997.

57. *Confidential care for minors.* Code of Medical Ethics. Council on Ethical and Judicial Affairs. 5.055. American Medical Association. p. 86–87, Chicago, IL, 1997.

58. Freund DA, Lewit EM: Managed care for children and pregnant women: Promises and pitfalls. *Future of Children* 3(2): 92–122,1993.

59. English AA: Changing health care environment and adolescent health care: Legal and policy changes. *Adolesc Med* 8(3): 375–384, 1997.

60. Andrulis DP, Bauer TA, Hopkins S: Strategies to increase enrollment in children's health insurance programs: A report of the New York Academy of Medicine. *J Urban Health* 76 (2): 247–279, 1999.

61. Sochalski J, Villarruel AM: Improving access to health care for children. *JSPN* 4(4): 147–154, 1999.

62. Schroeder SA: Prospects for expanding health insurance coverage. *N Engl J Med* 344 (1): 847–852, 2001.

63. Shi L: Vulnerable populations and health insurance. *Med Care Research and Rev* 57(1): 110–134, 2000.

64. Smith LA, Wise PH, Chan KW et al.: Implications of welfare reform for child health: Emerging challenges for clinical practice. *Pediatrics* 106(5): 1117–1125, 2000.

65. Weinick RW, Wegers ME, Cohen JW: Children's Health Insurance, access to care and health status: New findings. *Health Affairs* 17:127–136, 1998.

66. Friedman B, Jee J, Steiner C et al.: Tracking the States Children's Health Insurance Program with hospital data: National baselines, state variations and some cautions. *Med Care Res Rev* 56(4): 440–455, 1999.

67. Center for Law and Policy Reform. *A summary of H.R. 3734: The Personal Responsibility and Work Opportunity Reconciliation Act of 1996.* Washington, DC: Center for Law and Social Policy, August, 1996.

68. Greenberg M, Savner S: *A brief summary of key provisions of The Temporary Assistance for Needy Families Block Grant of H.R. 3736: The Personal Responsibility and Work Opportunity Reconciliation Act—1996.* Washington, DC: Center for Law and Social Policy. August 13, 1996.

69. Blumenthal D: Controlling health care expenditures. *N Engl J Med* 344 (10): 766–769, 2001.

70. Fleming M, Elster AB, Klein JD et al.: *Lessons Learned.* National Development to Local Implementation of Guidelines for Adolescent Preventive Services (GAPS). Chicago, IL: American Medical Association, 1–51, 2001.

71. Green M: *Bright Futures: Guidelines for Health Supervision of Infants, Children and Adolescents.* Arlington, VA: National Center for Education and Child Health. 1994.

72. Meggs WJ, Czaplijski T, Benson N: Trends in emergency department utilization, 1988–1997. *Acad Emeg Med* 6:1030–35, 1999.

73. Dudley RA & Luft HS: Managed care in transition. *N Engl J Med* 344 (14): 1087–1092, 2001.

74. English A, Kaplan D and Morreale M: Financing adolescent health care: The role of Medicaid and CHIP. *Adolesc Med* 11:165–182, 2000.

75. Satcher D: Global mental health: Its time has come. *JAMA* 285 (13):1697, 2001.

76. Institute of Medicine. *Psychiatric, Neurological and Developmental Disorders: Meeting the Challenge in the Developing World.* Washington, DC: Institute of Medicine, 2001.

77. Greydanus DE, Senanayake P, Gaines MJ: Reproductive health: An international perspective. *Ind J Pediatr* 66:339–348, 1999.

78. Greydanus DE, Pratt HD, Dannison LL: Sexuality education programs for youth: Current state of affairs and strategies for the future. *J Sex Educ Ther* 21:238–54, 1995.

79. U.S. House of Representatives Ways and Means Committee. *Overview of Entitlement Programs: 1994* Green Book: U.S. Government Printing Office, p. 324, 1994.

80. Greydanus DE, Patel DR & Rimsza ME: Contraception in the adolescent: An update. *Pediatrics* 107(3): 562–573, 2001.

81. Mitchell KJ, Finkelhor D & Wolak J: Risk factors for and impact of online sexual solicitation of youth. *JAMA* 285:3011–14, 2001.

82. Dupe SR, Anda RF, Felitti VJ et al.: Childhood abuse, household dysfunction, and the risk of attempted suicide throughout the life span. Findings from the Adverse Childhood Experiences Study. *JAMA* 286:3089–3096, 2001.

83. Sionean C, DiClemente RJ, Wingood GM et al.: Psychosocial and behavioral correlates of refusing unwanted sex among African-American adolescent females. *J Adolesc Health* 30:55–63, 2002.

84. Greydanus DE, Rimsza ME and Newhouse PN: Sexuality and disability in adolescence. *Adolesc Med* 13:500–514, 2002.

U NIT 4

HEALTH ISSUES

INTRODUCTION

As we begin the 21st century, health issues have become one of the nation's most prominent concerns. This unit offers authoritative insights into several major health areas: women's health, immunizations, oral health, injury prevention, attention deficit hyperactivity disorder, HIV and AIDS, sexually transmitted diseases, child abuse and neglect, homelessness, substance abuse, and infant mortality.

The first area, women's health, involves more than reproduction. Some gender-related conditions are cardiovascular disease (including obesity, diabetes, and smoking), diseases of the bones and joints (osteoarthritis, osteoporosis), autoimmune diseases, and cancers (especially of the breast and reproductive system). Women's health issues permeate discussions of complementary and alternative therapies, as well as the medicalization of natural events such as birth. The Collaborative Initiative of Johns Hopkins University and the Maternal and Child Health Bureau have made important steps toward the goal of a women's and perinatal health policy agenda.

In the area of prevention, the decline in certain serious diseases in the United States over the previous century is due in large part to the development and deployment of vaccines. Immunization campaigns and strategies, especially for pre-school children, are very cost-effective: For every vaccine dollar spent, our nation can save up to thirty dollars in direct and indirect costs. But barriers to complete immunizations remain.

Other prevention-oriented health issues are next considered in this unit—oral health, emergency services, and injury prevention. Oral health in general and the prevalence of dental caries and periodontal disease in particular remain concerns, especially in some segments of our population. Life-saving and preventive emergency services, especially for children, vary widely across the states, in part because regulations, funding mechanisms, and education for prevention and care vary widely. Much progress has been made in understanding injuries and their prevention. In injury prevention, the recognition that injuries are not accidents, that they are not random or unpreventable, has been a major step forward. The concepts of primary, secondary, and tertiary prevention have led to more integrated models of injury prevention and intervention.

The neurodevelopmental problem of attention deficit hyperactivity disorder (ADHD) has individual, familial, and societal implications. The diagnostic criteria

317

remain behavioral, though blood and imaging studies show promise. Although research has led to varying treatments, monitored stimulant medications remain the mainstay of therapy.

There are over 15 million new cases of sexually transmitted diseases in the United States each year. Some are curable (mostly bacterial) and some are incurable (such as genital herpes and human papillomavirus). Prevalence is higher in women, as the infection may be "silent" or asymptomatic. Since 1981, we have grappled with the epidemic of HIV and AIDS. That epidemic extends worldwide and is of horrendous proportions. Modes of transmission are now more clearly understood; new medications have allowed for long-term survival of infected individuals. These medications have been shown to be safe and effective for administration to pregnant women, helping to reduce the disastrous impact upon children.

Child abuse and neglect are problems with which individuals and society must cope long after the abusive event, because suicide, depression, learning problems, and the cycle of violence reverberate for years. Similarly, substance abuse remains a persistent social problem, with important health consequences for individuals and families. Substance abuse presents special problems for adolescents, pregnant women, and unborn babies.

Homelessness, especially for women and their children, is a persistent and growing problem. Many of the homeless are children who are vulnerable to the psychological and intellectual harm associated with homelessness.

A commonly accepted indicator of the health status of a nation is its infant mortality rate. Within the United States, differences in this rate by race and ethnicity are marked. Prematurity, low birth weight, congenital anomalies, and sudden unexpected infant death syndrome (SIDS) all play a role in infant mortality, as recorded by the National Center for Health Statistics. Although great progress has been made, our country has much room for improvement in this health issue and the others presented in this unit.

ARTICLE 1

WOMEN'S HEALTH CARE

Mary Brucker

INTRODUCTION

In China there is a saying that "women hold up half the sky." In the United States, women represent 51 percent of the total population. In groups categorized by increasing age, the percentage climbs. For example, 60% of the U.S. population over the age of 65 are women, 70% of those over 85. Centenarians are among the fastest growing demographic segments in the United States, and these individuals are predominately female. However, despite living for close to a decade longer than their male cohorts, women are more likely to suffer poor health, including more chronic disease and greater disability from health conditions.

For many years, women's health care involved a discussion of pregnancy, birth, and postpartum only. Yet women's health is a field of study that encompasses more than reproductive activity. Although perinatal care is a vital component of women's health care, it has become obvious that other important areas are gender influenced. Reproduction no longer encompasses the majority of a woman's life. At the turn of the last century, a woman's life expectancy was 48.3 years. However, by the beginning of the 21st century, her life expectancy is 78.8 years. Thus, she lives one-third of her life after her body no longer has reproductive capacity. One of the challenges of women's health care today is to move beyond considerations only of reproduction, while seeking balance in care.

A difficulty in seeking balance in health care is that gender differences do exist and, for some diseases, the clinical pictures are different. For others, treatments may differ in terms of efficacy or side effects. Some conditions are more common among women than among men, or vice versa. Other diseases have more significant sequelae for women than for men. Since much of the research on gender differences is relatively new, much remains to be discovered.

Larger questions also have emerged in gender studies relative to health. For example, what is the impact of the environment and the health care infrastructure on the delivery of women's health care services? Socio-economically, women are more likely to be poor than are men, often influencing access to care.

Ecoestrogens from water pollutants appear to affect women's menstrual cycles and may negatively influence fertility and, for those pregnant, fetal well-being. Numerous factors such as culture, spiritual beliefs, and genetics all are involved in women's health. For some women with a specific condition, American health care provides the best care in the world, yet for other women, access to the care is denied or restricted. Disparity of care is not exclusively gender-linked, although gender plays a role. The role of the government in women's health care is an emerging one as many people ask similar questions. These questions are important because women's health care is important.

IMPORTANCE OF WOMEN'S HEALTH

Women are the decision-makers for approximately 75% of all health care decisions in the United States. Approximately 66% of health care expenditures are spent on women's behalf. The majority of health care visits, as well as pharmaceutical purchases, are made by women. The central role of women in the family means that women tend to be the broker or manager for health care for her entire family, not simply herself. Based on her culture, she may define her family to include parents, siblings, nonblood-related "relatives," as well as a partner and children. Thus, the connection of women to health care has impact upon a larger segment of the population than is conveyed by the numbers specific to the gender alone.

Women seek care for a variety of reasons. Between 1997 and 1998, approximately 500 million visits were made by women to health care providers in ambulatory settings. Using an age-adjusted annual rate, these visits represent approximately 4.6 visits per woman per year. The rate of all visits increased in each age category, ranging from an average of 3.8 per woman 15–44 years of age to 7.1 visits per woman 65 years of age or older. The most commonly cited reason for a visit, general medical examination, was reported only for 7% of the ambulatory visits. Six percent of the visits were for regular prenatal care. Therefore, the reasons for visits seem to be wide and varied. Among the other more common reasons were treatment of disorders of the gastrointestinal system, respiratory system, and vision. No reason for care accounted for more than 10%, and the top five categories accounted for less than 20% of all visits. Thus, 80% of health care visits made by women are for specific health issues, aside from pregnancy. As women age, they tend to use different types of health care providers. Women under the age of 45 years are more likely to use primary care providers, outpatient departments, and emergency departments than their older counterparts.[1]

CAUSES OF MORTALITY AMONG WOMEN

The leading causes of death traditionally have been the same for women and men, that is, cardiovascular disease and cancer. Yet gender differences exist between men and women regarding these two types of conditions.

Cardiovascular Disease

Consider the popular press, in which the stereotypical picture of a heart attack is one of a middle-aged businessman clutching his chest. Yet heart disease also is the number one killer of women. Fifty percent of deaths in women can be attributed to heart disease or stroke. Compared to men, women on average develop heart disease approximately a decade later. Often the disease is asymptomatic until a myocardial infarction occurs. The symptoms of this same cardiovascular event tend to be different among men and women, often causing a diagnostic conundrum. A man having a heart attack usually experiences sudden severe crushing chest pain. However, a woman more commonly presents with shortness of breath, fatigue, and jaw pain, which she experiences over hours, rather than minutes.

Health care providers in emergency rooms often have misdiagnosed a woman's heart condition because of the difference in the clinical picture. Failing to diagnose a myocardial infarction has resulted in unnecessarily treating a woman for psychological stress or respiratory viruses and losing valuable time. Moreover, it is likely that the cardiovascular condition is more severe in the symptomatic woman than in her male counterpart. Almost twice as many women as men who have a heart attack die within one year of the event.

In addition to myocardial infarctions, women and men both experience another major cardiovascular disease, hypertension. However, of all the generally accepted subgroups, the one with the highest incidence of hypertension is that composed of African American women.[2] General risk factors for cardiovascular disease include various modifiable conditions such as smoking, obesity, and sedentary lifestyle.

Cardiovascular Risk: Smoking. Historically, women have adopted smoking later in age than men, due to perceived social constraints. In 2001, the U.S. Surgeon General released a report titled, "Women and Smoking." The main theme of the report was that smoking *is* a woman's issue. Although a higher percentage of men smoke than women, the gap has narrowed, and today more than 20% of American women smoke. Most women begin smoking as adolescents. Smoking among adolescents declined in the 1970s, but increased in the 1980s, obliterating most successes. In the 1990s, smoking again demonstrated a decline among adolescents, although it remains a concern.[3]

Unfortunately women smokers not only risk cardiovascular disease, but also lung cancer, emphysema, and cardiovascular disease. Smoking presents a unique problem for women due to reproductive issues. Infants born of smoking mothers have decreased birth weight and a slightly increased risk of intrauterine growth restriction. Although smoking cessation may be more difficult for women than men, women can and do stop smoking. Few gender differences in factors related to successful quitting have been identified. However, only one-third of women who stop smoking during pregnancy are still smoke-free one year after the birth of their child. Tobacco-industry marketing often targets women, and particularly girls, for smoking by making the product appear socially desirable and indicative of independence. Models who are healthy and attractive often are used to promote the unhealthy behavior.[4]

Cardiovascular Risk: Obesity. Obesity has been reported as an epidemic in the United States.[5] Controversy exists about the level at which a person is determined to be overweight and the level at which obesity occurs. Various sources use a body mass index (BMI) from 25 to 30 kg/m[2]; the higher the value, the more over-weight/obese the individual. Figure 1 illustrates the number of Americans who report their weight as a BMI of 30 kg/m[2] or more. Self-reporting often indicates under-representation of a condition, yet approximately 20% to 25% of adults report being obese, with men and women having similar BMI's until the age of 60, when women are more likely to be considered obese. When a relatively liberal value of a BMI of greater than 25 kg/m[2] is employed, 51% of American women are overweight or obese. Even using a conservative value of greater than 27.3 kg/m[2], more than one-third of women are overweight/obese. Sedentary lifestyle most likely contributes to the problem and appears to be increasing, with approximately 30% of women reporting no leisure-time activity in the latest National Health Interview Survey.[6] As illustrated in Figure 2, only 10% to 15% of women reported regular participation in light or moderate leisure-time physical activity.

FIGURE 1

Self-reported prevalence of obesity among adults aged 20 years and older, by age group and gender: United States, 2000

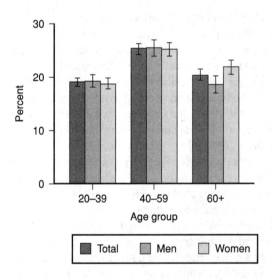

Data Source: Sample Adult Core component of the 2000 National Health Interview Survey.

FIGURE 2

Percentage of adults aged 18 and older who regularly participated in light or moderate leisure-time physical activity, by age group and gender: United States, 2000

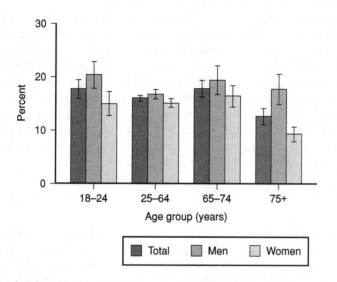

Data Source: Sample Adult Core component of the 2000 National Health Interview Survey.

Cardiovascular Risk: Diabetes. Women with type II diabetes have a significantly increased risk of cardiovascular disease. As the incidence of obesity increases, so does the incidence of diabetes. The two conditions are often intertwined, as obesity is associated with insulin-resistance or type II diabetes. Type II diabetes is likely responsible for approximately 90% to 95% of all diagnosed cases of diabetes. In addition to obesity, risk factors for type II diabetes include older age, family history of diabetes, prior history of gestational diabetes, impaired glucose tolerance, physical inactivity, and race/ethnicity. African Americans, Hispanic/ Latino Americans, American Indians, and some Asian Americans and Pacific Islanders are at particularly high risk for type II diabetes. Recent studies have indicated that the development of type II diabetes may be delayed by the adoption of better health habits. A longitudinal cohort study of more than 84,000 women over 16 years found that overweight or obesity is the single most important predictor of diabetes, followed by lack of exercise, poor nutrition, smoking, and abstinence from alcohol (consumption of a limited amount of alcohol has a *protective* effect against diabetes). Modifying these behaviors may result in a significant delay in developing type II diabetes.[7]

Although the incidence of type II diabetes is approximately the same for men and women at slightly more than 8%, only women experience gestational diabetes, a condition exclusive to pregnancy. Gestational diabetes becomes a challenge for management in pregnancy and later: Some studies have indicated that the risk of later developing type 2 diabetes is 40% higher for those with gestational diabetes than it is for women who did not have gestational diabetes. Type I diabetes is the least common type, usually occurring among children and young adults, and it most frequently requires exogenous insulin.

Diabetes is a chronic disease with major health consequences. For example, the leading cause of blindness is diabetic retinopathy, usually among people with type I diabetes. Retinopathy also may be a complication experienced by individuals with type II diabetes, but the most common severe complication for them is the elevated risk of coronary heart disease (CHD). Traditionally, women have been regarded as having a lesser risk of coronary heart disease than men, at least for essentially a decade after menopause. All diabetics have a significantly increased risk of CHD, but the diabetic woman has approximately twice the risk of a diabetic man, of the same age, for unknown reasons. Diabetics also are at higher risk for stroke, hypertension, and depression.[8]

Cancer

When mortality is categorized according to age, the most common cause of death in women younger than age 75 is cancer. Like men, the leading cause of cancer death in women in the United States is cancer of the lung and bronchus.[8] Screening is difficult for this condition, as numerous studies of chest X rays and sputum analysis have failed to demonstrate any impact on mortality. Recent research suggests that low-dose CT scan may be valuable in identifying early disease with subsequent early treatment and better outcome. However, the most effective management for lung cancer is prevention. Pulmonary malignancies are well associated with modifiable lifestyle and workplace issues of smoking and asbestos exposure. As aforementioned, smoking remains a major issue for women and most likely will continue to be a problem, especially as young girls and women adopt smoking behaviors.

Regarding other cancers, both men and women are approximately as likely to die of colorectal and pancreatic cancers. However, for women, certain cancers are unique because they are associated with the female reproductive system.

Reproductive Cancers: Breast Cancer. Second to cancer of the lung or bronchus, the most common cancer for male mortality is that of prostate cancer. For women, the second highest cancer mortality is associated with breast cancer. Breast cancer has the highest incidence of all cancers experienced by women, but progress in detection and treatment over the second half of the last century means it is no longer an automatic death sentence. It is estimated in 2001 that while 239,900 new cases of breast cancer were diagnosed, 40,600 women died of the disease. Breast cancer can be diagnosed and treated early. Current recommendations include self breast examinations regularly, starting at the age of 20; clinical breast examinations by a health care professional at least every three years during ages 20–39, and annually thereafter; and annual mammograms, starting at age 40. The latter recommendation remains a controversial area, as many credible scientists continue to debate the usefulness of mammograms before the age of 50.

Mammograms have been well accepted by most women. Women of color are less likely to receive regular mammograms than white women, and lack of access to screening and diagnostic methods has been postulated as one of the major reasons for a higher death rate among black women. Today, certain organizations such as the Susan B. Komen Foundation and the American Cancer Society recognize the disparity and assist in arranging community access for women without commercial insurance. Mammograms are able to locate masses too small for palpable detection. They also can identify tissue that is atypical, suggesting a higher than usual risk of cancer development. However, mammograms are not universally acknowledged as ideal screening devices. Although many scientists debate the efficacy for women younger than 50, Gotzche and Olsen caused some debate in the literature when they reported that the two rigorous, well-designed, long-term population-based studies (in Sweden and Canada) failed to find any association between breast cancer survival and the routine use of mammograms, even after the age of 50.[9] These researchers questioned the advisability of mammograms as a screening device, particularly citing the use of resource dollars. Their findings are not in concert with other research, and it may be anticipated that the federally funded Women's Health Initiative may provide more insight into this debate when its preliminary data become available, approximately in 2005. Furthermore, breast cancer screening has benefited from emerging technological advances, and it is likely that advanced mammogram and ultrasound techniques may revolutionize the manner of screening and diagnosis of breast cancer in the future.

Risks for breast cancer, unlike lung cancer with clear and modifiable risks, remain enigmatic. Some breast cancers clearly have a genetic component. Discovery of the genes BRCA1 and BRCA2 initially was met with great enthusiasm and hope for breast cancer cure, until it was recognized that these genes were associated with a minority of cases of breast cancer, probably 5% or less. In the quest to identify factors that increase the risk of breast cancer, studies have linked fat intake, alcohol ingestion, sedentary lifestyle, late childbearing, nulliparity, lack of breastfeeding, high body mass index, and other factors to development of breast cancer. However, with the exception of one risk factor, all others have failed to have clear, consistent associations. The one undisputed, nonmodifiable risk factor is that of gender. Although men can develop breast cancer, it is uncommon; breast cancer essentially is a disease of women.

Forms of treatment of breast cancer include pharmaceutical agents such as the selective estrogen receptor modulators (abbreviated as SERM) that are antagonistic to the estrogen receptors in such areas as breast, but not in other areas such as bone. A large federally funded study has revealed that prophylactic treatment of women at high risk for breast cancer can reduce their risk by more than 45%. However, treatment is not without cost, since increased rates of endometrial cancer and thromboembolic disease were associated with the drug. Moreover, the women were studied for 5 years, and data now suggest that the protection tends to decrease after that point, leading providers to question when such drugs should be given, particularly since breast cancer is directly related to age.[10]

Reproductive Cancers: Ovarian Cancer. Although of lesser incidence than breast cancer or even endometrial cancer, ovarian cancer is more lethal. Ovarian cancer has a genetic link, and also is associated with BRCA1 and BRCA2. However, unlike breast cancer where a clinical breast exam by a health care professional may be useful, a bimanual pelvic exam often may fail to find subtle changes, especially if the woman has any central fat deposits, and even if she is of normal weight. Blood tests like the CA125 have high specificity but low sensitivity, indicating a good use for diagnosis, but not for screening. Ovarian cancer has a predilection for seeding the peritoneum with cells, causing metastasis to occur, often before the disease has become symptomatic.

Other Reproductive Cancers. Endometrial cancer, or cancer of the uterine corpus, is diagnosed in more than 35,000 women annually, and more than 6,000 die from it every year. Women at risk are those who are overweight and nulliparous. Certain drugs, such as estrogen without progesterone and some of the SERMs, encourage a constant proliferative environment that often leads to endometrial hyperplasia, which is itself a precursor to endometrial cancer. There is no routine screening for the disease. However, perimenopausal and postmenopausal women with irregular bleeding should be assessed by an endometrial biopsy. Cervical cancer, most likely related to sexually transmitted infections, has been routinely screened by Pap smears since the 1950s. Early detection and treatment of abnormalities has resulted in a decrease of 75% of cervical cancers.[8]

Maternal Mortality

Approximately one woman dies every day in the United States due to a condition related to pregnancy, childbirth, or postpartum. Although this is a dramatic drop from the pre-antibiotic early years of the 20th century, the current rate of approximately 7.5 maternal deaths per 100,000 births essentially has remained static for the last two decades.

The United States ranks 20th among all countries in maternal death, primarily because of the disparity between black and white women. The risk of maternal death is 18 to 22 per 100,000 births for black women, while it is only 5 to 6 per 100,000 births for white women. In 1996, if maternal mortality for black women were equal to that of white women, the U.S. rate would have dropped almost a third, from 7.6 per 100,000 to 5.1 per 100,000 births.[11] The major causes of maternal mortality continue to be hemorrhage, pregnancy-induced hypertension, infection, and ectopic pregnancy. Not all of these conditions are preventable, but early recognition and treatment can provide a positive impact. The phrase "Safe Motherhood" was coined to discuss advocacy for changes to decrease maternal mortality. Although less frequent than in underdeveloped countries, maternal mortality continues in the United States at a rate that can be decreased. Reduction of maternal mortality, and the racial disparity associated with it, is a goal of the Healthy People 2010 program.

MORBIDITY AMONG WOMEN

The paradox concerning women's health is that women live longer than men, but often suffer greater disability from disease. Some of the diseases are conditions that demonstrate significant differences between men and women. Diseases associated with mortality, such as cardiac disease, diabetes, and cancer clearly affect the quality of life among those afflicted with them. But so do other conditions that are not major causes of death. Women report this gender disparity as illustrated in Figure 3 where, when compared to men, fewer women assess their health as excellent (38.9% to 35.6%). The following illustrate some of the more common gender-biased conditions.

FIGURE 3

Percent distribution of respondent-assessed health status, by gender, all ages: United States, 2000

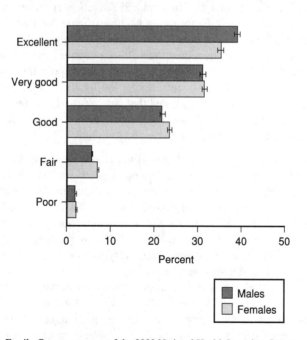

Data Source: Family Core component of the 2000 National Health Interview Survey.

Sexually Transmitted Diseases

Women and newborns are disproportionately likely to bear the burden of long-term consequences of sexually transmitted diseases. This topic is discussed in depth elsewhere in this book, but it is appropriate to note here the women are more likely to be infected by a male partner than vice versa. Because of the reproductive ramifications, STDs among women can result in significant perinatal and neonatal disease. Of particular note are perinatal transmission to the newborn infant from a mother with acquired immunodeficiency virus, herpes, and hepatitis. Even a health-promoting activity such as breastfeeding is potentially harmful if the woman is HIV positive. Sexually transmitted diseases may render a woman infertile due to pelvic inflammatory disease (PID) caused by chlamydia or gonorrhea, or tubal scarring associated with PID may result in a life-threatening ectopic pregnancy. Occasionally severe infections can result in need for hysterectomies or other major surgeries.[8]

Musculoskeletal Conditions

Osteoarthritis. As they age, women are far more likely than men to experience osteoarthritis, especially of the knee and hip.[12] The cartilage, ligaments, and other structures wear away, causing chronic pain and limitation of movement, particularly among mature women. Even young healthy women are more likely than men to injure the ligaments of their knees. Female basketball players are more likely to suffer cruciate tears than their male athletic counterparts. It has been theorized that a woman's pelvis and wider hips may predispose these injuries by placing greater strain on the ligaments, and/or the ligaments may be weaker in women in general. It also has been noted that certain injuries are more likely to occur during different phases of a woman's menstrual cycle, suggesting that the hormonal milieu also has a role in muscle and joint health.[13]

Osteoporosis. Bone loss is not a disease limited to women; however, women experience the loss to a greater degree than do men. In large part this decrease is associated with the decrease in estrogen potency found in the postmenopausal woman's body. Estrogen is a major component in the continuing cycle of a woman's normal bone mineralization and demineralization process. During the perimenopausal period, the types of estrogen shift from predominantly estradiol, a potent ovarian estrogen, to estrone, a relatively weak estrogen derived from a nonovarian, peripheral conversion process.

Contrary to what may be reported in the popular press, not all women have a similar risk for osteoporosis. Women with a family history of the disease; those that are underweight or who smoke; and women on a number of drugs such as steroids are more likely to develop the disease. Obese women, those who are African American, and women leading active lives rather than sedentary ones are among those who are less likely to develop the condition.

Much research exists on the subject of osteoporosis, especially using bone mineral density (BMD) measurements. However, the methods to obtain bone mineral densities are heavily dependent on a multitude of factors including technological process, site of measurement, ethnicity, and even altitude. Although the search for the optimal BMD method continues, other studies explore the risk of fracture in longitudinal research, recognizing that perhaps the important consideration is that of spinal and hip fractures. For example, following a hip fracture, 20% die in the first year after the event, only 50% are able to walk without assistance, and 28% will require long-term care. While awaiting definitive studies, many commercial insurance companies cover the costs of BMD testing. Since 1998, Medicare also will cover the screening tests.

Psychiatric Disorders

Both women and men may suffer from psychiatric disorders. However, depression is almost twice as likely among women as men. It has been estimated that 25% of women in the United States have stated that they have been significantly depressed at some time in their lives. Treatment of depression and anxiety is different for women than for men. There is an increasing body of research suggesting that male and female brains react differently to hormones and chemicals. Women produce less serotonin (mood regulating agent), and the serotonin produced largely is modulated by estrogen. Thus women respond better to drugs affecting the serotonin system (e.g., Prozac) while men tend to respond better to drugs that also affect norepinephrine, a neurotransmitter secreted by the adrenal glands and by nerve endings during stress.[8]

Drug Usage

According to the National Household Survey on Drug Abuse, in 2000, men are more likely to be users of illicit drugs than women (7.7% compared to 5.0%). However, the nonmedical use of psychotherapeutic agents (e.g., analgesics, tranquilizers, sedatives) was similar for both women and men.[14]

According to findings from the Sloane Survey, women use more pharmaceutical therapeutic agents than men in all age groups, with the exception of people 65 years of age or over, at which point no significant gender difference exists. The agents in the survey included over-the-counter and prescription drugs. The overusage of pharmaceuticals may in part be explained by the use of female hormonal contraceptive agents, since no similar drugs exist for men. For both men and women, the most commonly used agents are over-the-counter analgesics. But hormones, either for contraceptive use or perimenopausal/postmenopausal treatment, comprised the next most commonly used drugs for women.[15] This finding is consistent with the observation that even in the 21st century, contraception remains predominantly a woman's responsibility.

Autoimmune Diseases

A woman's immune system appears to have a control mechanism that is lacking in man's. For example, it seems that women may be able to have more aggressive responses to bacteria. Yet, during pregnancy the response is markedly decreased, in order to accommodate the intrauterine conceptus. In spite of the fact that this system is highly sophisticated, or perhaps due to it, women are more likely to develop autoimmune diseases like lupus, rheumatoid arthritis, and multiple sclerosis. All of these diseases are conditions in which the immune system attacks healthy tissue.[8]

Gastrointestinal Conditions

Assuming that a man and a woman are eating the same food, both type and amount, digestion differs between them. Even masticating food is different. Women's saliva seems to be chemically different, causing digestion to require a longer period of time. Slower transport throughout the alimentary canal results in women being the more likely of the two genders to experience chronic constipation and other gastrointestinal conditions. Women also metabolize chemicals differently. This variation of metabolism is most apparent with common drugs. For example, beta-blockers take longer to metabolize and dosages may need to be different for men and women. Clearance of aspirin is slower for women than men. A woman's liver metabolizes alcohol more slowly than a man, resulting in more alcohol remaining in the blood stream and affecting a woman more profoundly even when compared to a man who may be of similar size and who drank an equivalent amount.[8]

Genitourinary System

The rate of urinary incontinence (UI) among women is at least twice that of men. Incontinence is of particular note since it tends to be both embarrassing as well as potentially socially limiting for women. Among risk factors for UI are multiple vaginal births and obesity. Although long ignored, UI is an area of current active research, especially as the American population ages.[8]

Other Systems

Numerous other examples of differences between genders exist. There is data from drug studies that suggest pain receptors may be different for women and men. Women appear to respond more favorably to kappa opioids and less favorably to nonsteroidal anti-inflammatory drugs like over-the-counter analgesics. Estrogen receptors have been found in tissue throughout the body and newer research has identified at least two types of receptors, alpha and beta, found in varying degrees among men and women. Further studies may elucidate information about these receptors and most likely help explain at least some of the differences between the genders.[8]

Social Issues and Morbidity

The National Violence Against Women Survey discovered that physical assault is common among American women. More than 50% of women said they were assaulted as a child by an adult, and almost 2% were assaulted within the previous year. Far more than men, women were likely to have been raped and/or physically assaulted by a current or former partner, with 25% reporting such behavior sometime during their lives and 1.5% during the last 12 months. One million women reported being stalked by an adult. In each case, women are more vulnerable than men. They are more likely to be seriously physically injured during a violent incident and are most likely to be injured by a partner.[8]

Disability

In summary, for all categories of age, women are more likely than men to suffer disability. Women also are more likely to have difficulty with activities of daily living, yet are less likely than men to have assistance.

SUCCESSFUL AGING

Most discussion on aging concentrates on morbidity and mortality. Yet many mature women have a high level of functioning in their older years. Studies often have focused on individuals in institutions, leading to a biased picture. Much of geriatric research concentrates on women, although the situation (e.g., visual loss, hearing impairment) may not be different between the genders. However, more women are in the older age category to be studied.

Successful aging is best accomplished by employing health promotion behaviors. These practices such as maintenance of normal weight, avoidance of smoking and illicit drug use, regular exercise, and healthy diet can prevent several diseases or conditions linked to mortality and morbidity.

MEDICALIZATION OF NATURAL EVENTS

Birth is a quintessential female experience. For millennia, birth remained a woman-centered event, reflecting the local culture in its trappings, but essentially unchanged. Within the last century, birth in first-world countries has moved from the home to the hospital. Technology has become a major component of even a low-risk birth. Many of the technological changes have been unqualified advances such as antimicrobial therapy. Yet other changes commonly assumed to be advances fail to have scientific evidence to that effect. For example, in 1999 84% of women giving birth in the United States had their fetuses monitored electronically.[16] Although it is commonly accepted as a routine today, numerous studies have indicated that monitoring low-risk women lacks evidence as to decreased perinatal morbidity/mortality and is linked to higher rates of cesarean section births. Tocolytic agents, or pharmaceutical intervention to quell preterm labor, are frequently employed, yet data generally suggest that they prolong preterm labor by 48 hours or less. Use of technology may result in increased untoward effects, such as exhausting economic resources at least or beginning a cascade of interventions that most likely were unnecessary. Thus, many providers and consumers advocate an adoption of technology that is scientifically based on effectiveness.

Birth is not the only area of medicalization. Hormonal contraception has enabled women in the second half of the 20th century to control if and when they desire to be pregnant. As with any technology, some risk is involved. Hormonal contraception has been linked to complications such as thromboembolic disease. However, within the last decade various noncontraceptive benefits have emerged. For example, women who have used combination oral contraception are less likely to have a lifetime risk of endometrial cancer. Today, there is a discussion of manipulation of hormonal contraception so that not only is birth control obtained, but a woman can avoid the inconvenience of menses. New drugs are soon to be marketed as agents that will allow a woman to choose when and if she wishes to have her period. Some women already experience this phenomenon by continuously using combination oral contraceptives.[17]

Menopause is yet another example of a natural female event. Yet use of hormones allows women to ameliorate or even avoid some of the common discomforts, even though research has found that they are no more than minor nuisances to the majority of women.[18] Perimenopausal and postmenopausal estrogen has been found to increase bone mineral density and positively impact lipid levels, although cardiovascular protection is controversial. Again, the technology is not risk-neutral since the hormonal therapy is associated with thromboembolic disease and potentially increased risks of cardiac events in women with a preexisting history.[19]

Female sexual response also is a natural female event. Today, hormones such as testosterone are being prescribed to increase female libido and sildenafil citrate (Viagra) is being used by some providers for women. In each case the evidence is less than clear about which women might benefit from the treatment, if any.

COMPLEMENTARY AND ALTERNATIVE THERAPIES: BACK TO NATURE

Although certain aspects of care have used increased technology, there appears to be a growth in attempting to naturalize therapy, or return to low technology. One example of this is the explosion of alternative therapies. The National Center for Complementary and Alternative Medicine, a branch of the National Institutes of Health, has found that the percentage of Americans who use alternative therapies rose from approximately 33% in 1990 to more than 42% in 1997. The most commonly used therapies were herbal medicine, massage, megavitamins, self-help groups, folk remedies, energy healing, and homeopathy. In 1997, Americans spent more than $27 billion on these therapies, which is more than out-of-pocket spending for all U.S. hospitalizations.[20] Not only have many Americans used alternative therapies, the Sloane Survey revealed that they do so regularly, with 14% of the U.S. population reporting using at least one herbal agent in the week preceding the survey.[15] It has been found that the use of alternatives could be found in all ethnic groups and social strata.[21] These methods often were employed as adjuncts or complemental therapy to treatments in the medical mainstream. Use of alternative therapies often implies use of alternative providers. Over the past decade there has been a growth in nonphysician providers, including those generally considered outside the medical mainstream such as homeopathic practitioners, acupuncturists, and herbologists as well as physician assistants, nurse practitioners, nurse anesthetists, and nurse-midwives. The last mentioned is a provider whose scope of practice focuses on women. The final U.S. natality statistics released for 1999 revealed that in 1975 98.4% of women delivered their babies in a hospital attended by a physician. Only 1% of births were attended by a midwife. In 1999, 91.7% of women delivered their babies in a hospital attended by a physician, and 7% were cared for by midwives. Approximately 95% of the midwifery births in 1999 were by Certified Nurse-Midwives, with the vast majority in a hospital. Of the approximate 1% of births out of the hospital, approximately two-thirds were in homes, followed by those taking place in freestanding birthing centers.[16]

SUMMARY

In conclusion, women's health is a field unto itself. Women have unique needs and risks, and they are not necessarily related to childbearing. Much remains to be studied. Research about women's health has been limited by lack of funding and interest. The creation of the United States Office of Women's Health in 1990 has increased research in the area. Yet issues regarding recruitment of women of color, poor women, and hard-to-find populations continue to present challenges and limit generalizability of research findings.

Women hold up half the sky. More investigation into gender differences and commonalities whether they be biological, psychological, or social can impact the public health for the entire country.

REFERENCES

1. CDC (Centers for Disease Control and Prevention) and NCHS (National Center for Health Statistics). *Utilization of Ambulatory Medical Care by Women: United States 1997–1998.* 2000.

2. Tsang T.S., Barnes M.E., Gersh B.J., and Hayes S.N. Risks of coronary heart disease in women: Current understanding and evolving concepts. *Mayo Clinic Proceedings.* 2001;75(12):1289–303.

3. CDC (Centers for Disease Control and Prevention). *Women and Smoking: A Report of the Surgeon General,* 2001.

4. Kelly A., Blair N., and Penchacek T. Women and smoking: Issues and opportunities. *Journal of Women's Health & Gender Based Medicine.* 2001;10:515–8.

5. Jeffrey R. W. Public health strategies for obesity treatment and prevention. *American Journal of Health Behavior.* 2001;25(3):252–9.

6. CDC (Centers for Disease Control and Prevention). *National Health Interview Survey:2000.* 2001.

7. Hu F.B., Manson J.E., Stampfer M.J., Colditz G., Liu S., Solomon C.G. and Willett W.C. Diet, lifestyle and the risk of type 2 diabetes mellitus in women. *New England Journal of Medicine* 2001;345(11):790–7.

8. Goldman M. and Hatch M. *Women and Health.* San Diego: Academic Press, 2000.

9. Gotzche P.C. and Olsen O. Is screening for breast cancer with mammography justifiable? *Lancet.* 2000;355:129–134

10. Gail M. H., Costantino J. P., Bryant J., Croyle R., Freedman L., Helzlsouer K. and Vogel V. Weighing the risks and benefits of tamoxifen treatment for preventing breast cancer. *Journal of the National Cancer Institute,* 1999;91(21): 1829–1846

11. CDC (Centers for Disease Control and Prevention). Maternal Mortality— United States, 1982–1996. *MMWR.* 1998;47:705–7.

12. Cheng Y., Macera C. A., Davis D. R., Ainsworth B. E., Troped P. J. and Blair S. N. Physical activity and self-reported, physician-diagnosed osteoarthritis: Is physical activity a risk factor? *Journal of Clinical Epidemiology.* 2000;53(3):315–22.

13. Wojtys E. Association between the menstrual cycle and anterior cruciate ligament injuries in female athletes. *American Journal of Sports Medicine.* 1998;26(5):614–9.

14. DHHS (Department of Health and Human Services). *National Household Survey on Drug Abuse: 2000.* 2001.

15. Kaufman D.W., Kelly J.P., Rosenberg L., Anderson T.E. and Mitchell A.M. Recent patterns of medication use in the ambulatory adult population of the United States: The Sloane Survey. *Journal of the American Medical Association.* 2002;287,337–44.

16. Ventura S. J., Martin J. A., Curtin S. C., Menacker F. and Hamilton B. E. Births: Final data for 1991. *National Vital Statistics Report.* 2001;49(1):1–99.

17. Shakespeare J., Neve E. and Hodder K. Is norethisterone a lifestyle drug? *British Medical Journal.* 2000;320(7230):291.

18. Porter M., Penney G.C., Russell D., Russell E. and Templeton A. A population based survey of women's experience of the menopause. *British Journal of Obstetrics and Gynaecology,* 1996;103:1025–8.

19. Hulley S., Grady D., Bush T., Furberg C., Herrington D., Riggs B. and Vittinhoff, E. The Heart and Estrogen/Progestin Replacement Study (HERS) Research Group Randomized trial of estrogen plus progestin for secondary prevention of coronary heart disease in postmenopausal women. *Journal of the American Medical Association.* 1998;280:605–11.

20. Eisenberg D.M., Davis R.B., Ettner S.L., Appel S., Wilkey S., Van Rompay M. and Kessler R.C. Trends in alternative medicine use in the United States, 1990–1997: Results of a follow-up national survey. *Journal of the American Medical Association.* 1998. 280(18):1569–75.

21. Borkan J., Neher J.O., Anson O. and Smoker B. Referrals for alternative therapies. *Journal of Family Practice.* 1994. 39(7):545–50.

ARTICLE 2

WOMEN'S HEALTH CARE: ISSUES AND CHALLENGES

Mary Brucker

INTRODUCTION

In 1999, the U.S. Department of Health and Human Services Public Health Service published the results of a collaborative initiative with the Johns Hopkins University School of Public Health and the Maternal and Child Health Bureau, Health Resources and Services Administration. The objectives of the collaboration were to uncover new viewpoints and to stimulate new partnerships toward a goal of a women's and perinatal health policy agenda. The group identified a number of reasons for the appropriateness of timing of the collaboration. Among these reasons were rapidly changing health care delivery systems, social welfare policy reforms, and a resurgence of women's activism. Among the initial health care problems that the group identified was the historical approach to perinatal care as a distinct specialty, often totally apart from the larger context of women's health care. Loss of the connection between perinatal care and overall women's health care caused each area to suffer. Other problems that the group identified included the multiple societal roles that women play today; the issues of a problem-based focus, rather than a wellness focus; and the variety of health-related challenges that women find throughout their life. Based on these discussions, the group pointed out four main perspectives:

Holistic perspective, with a wellness approach that encompasses the multiple influences of biological, psychological, and social factors

Lifespan perspective, to recognize that transitions across a woman's life give rise to different health and psychological needs

Social role perspective, in order to acknowledge the multiple societal roles of a woman

Woman-centered perspective, in order to view women's gender-specific experiences as normal rather than abnormal when compared to men's

Using these four perspectives, the collaborative group explored past and current practices. The group conducted a massive literature review and employed a panel of experts to develop recommendations. These recommendations were organized according to six major domains: social policy; surveillance and quality assurance; service availability, coordination, and organization; financing of health programs and services; health communication and education services; and development of workforce competency and capacity.

SOCIAL POLICY

No policy develops in a vacuum. Health care policies for women evolve within a society and therefore reflect how the society views women. For example, historically women have suffered from social inequities in terms of education, work, and politics. Such inequities generally prevented women from assuming policy decision-making positions until more recent generations. Women of color and socioeconomically challenged women continue to be disadvantaged and may be underrepresented when policies are made. Current social policies also may be inconsistent for women, based on whether they were developed within the context of perinatal care, women's health care, or society in general. The collaboration identified policies regarding the incarceration of pregnant women who are addicted to drugs as an example of this tension.

Among the basic recommendations of the group was to promote a coherent policy agenda for women, pregnant or not, and to encourage policies that improve women's access to resources. These resources are not limited to health care, but include safe community environments, higher education, jobs, housing, pay equity, economic development, child care, domestic violence laws, and gun control. One policy goal was to support processes that aid women in developing skill and confidence in articulating their goals and making their own decisions.

Five large areas summarize the strategies to facilitate the development of a coherent social policy. These five areas included promoting coordination and collaboration among the large number of groups involved in perinatal and women's care advocacy. For example, in the legislative arena, policy and program coordinating committees should be developed to eliminate redundancies as well as gaps. A second strategy would be to require federal agencies to address women's health and/or access to care for any proposed social policies. Promotion of informed decision-making and legal protection for women to improve access to health services is another strategy. This approach encourages women to develop and to use their autonomy in making decisions for themselves. Establishment and maintenance of privacy in health care through establishing safeguards is yet another strategy to help women through development of social policies. A final strategy would address health concerns of women with respect to changes in ethnic, cultural, and racial composition of the American population.

The research implications for social policies are clear. According to the collaborative group, social policies, including those recently adopted, should be analyzed with respect to their impact on women's health care. In summary, the domain of social policymaking is one that is complex and will require long-term, sustained focus. At the same time, as women develop more skill and status in politics, the area of women's health needs becomes clearer and more apparent.

SURVEILLANCE AND QUALITY ASSURANCE

Quality assurance is more than a nominal patient chart review in a hospital. Quality assurance is a process that includes measurement as compared to a standard, and surveillance is the necessary process during which information is gathered. Several challenges exist for women's health care surveillance and quality assurance. For example, standards may be multiple and possibly overlapping, such as in Healthy People 2010; standards may be perceived as contradictory if they are established by a variety of groups involved in care of women, each with a slightly different approach, or perceived as simply lacking for certain subgroups. More data are available with current technology, but multiple providers and potential fragmentation of the systems may result in dissemination of less useful data to persons or groups to whom they may be of most importance. The evidence-based approach to clinical practice has revealed that many generally accepted standards lack evidence to underpin their significance. The collaborative group advocated three major strategies: to develop and promote standards of care for women and providers; to create a process to identify needed data, collect them, and distribute them; and to acknowledge the importance of quality assurance functions and leadership.

The federally sponsored development and publication of *Bright Futures for Children* is a national guidelines initiative in the area of pediatrics. A similar publication for women could develop health status goals for women as a result of collaboration of the major health care groups, such as the American College of Obstetricians and Gynecologists and the American Academy of Pediatrics. Moreover, the document could incorporate components of health care provider education in women's health care, emphasize coordination of care, and provide a set of standards of care based on evidence-based clinical practice findings. From this activity, a single, integrated, standardized health record could be derived. A single health record is common in other countries, but the fragmentation of services in the United States requires that time be spent in obtaining a health history every time a woman receives care in a new site. Development of a universal record could save untold dollars and hours in the delivery of health care.

Quality assurance is based upon a set of measurable indicators. Once health status goals for women are developed and a set of standards is derived from the goals, measurable indicators can be devised. These indicators also should be based on conceptual or theoretical frameworks that recognize the pathways linking women to health outcomes. Perinatal care should be included. The indicators should not simply be at the provider level, but should include information about the women and the system itself. The measurements must be encompassing, so that preconceptional through postpartum care is included, and the measurements should reflect age, race, ethnicity, and other health-related determinants. Community-level needs should be recognized through development of a set of measures that document resources to support the lives and health of women. In addition to the above, the group recommended that performance measures should specifically assess and monitor linkages and coordination between/among providers, and include biological and psychosocial services and outcomes.

The collaborative group further suggested that information flow systems be improved and that there be a commitment to develop a confidential record with assurance for privacy. Additional activities to promote quality assurance and surveillance for women's health care included an emphasis on quality improvement mechanisms. Simple assurance that quality is present does not reflect the dynamic process of quality improvement. Among the suggestions for quality improvement are development of a monitoring system on topics related to women's and perinatal health care; creation of an annual national report; establishment of incentives for states and communities to demonstrate improvement; assessment of unmet health needs and establishment of a priority methodology to guide resource allocation; creation of ongoing data collection mechanisms; and assurance that the routinely collected data are used appropriately and distributed widely. In order to promote these activities, the group also advocated that accountability be clearly established; that guidelines for processes be specific regarding operations and administration; and that local, state, and federal public health agencies be promoted and facilitated, especially given that many public health functions are being privatized and some activities such as collection of population-based data are being threatened.

The challenge to the recommendations in the domain of surveillance and quality assurance may be strongest among the groups most concerned for the health care of women. The diversity of these groups provides both the advantage of a wide scope of knowledge and the disadvantage of investment by each group in their own specific approach or interest area. Development of a consensus document such as *Bright Futures for Women* may prove to be a challenge.

SERVICE AVAILABILITY, COORDINATION, AND ORGANIZATION

Most men have a single point of entry into the health care system, often a family practice or general internist physician. Yet women often enter the system through care by an obstetrical or gynecological provider, then use multiple providers for different health issues, especially preventive care. Continuity of care for women is often nonexistent, or at best, threatened in many current systems. Health care of women, including perinatal care, should be integrated.

The goals that were proposed by the coalition included the development of holistic service models; promotion of community accessibility to quality, culturally competent, coordinated care; integration of women's and perinatal health issues in federal and local agencies; and promotion of integrated models of care that are culturally based and reflective of different times in a woman's life. The strategies recommended by the group included supporting and funding the development and assessment of holistic models that are women-centered; deploying health care providers into positions and activities that support holistic, integrated models (e.g., community workers into schools to discuss ways to prevent obesity); and supporting demonstration models that combine health screening and treatment. Other strategies focused on identification of collaborative strategies to ensure public health accountability in an era of managed care; recognition of gender-relevant issues that are often overlooked, like domestic violence; preservation of safety net services for women; and protecting their access to sensitive reproductive services. Additional strategies include increasing accessibility to health care and community outreach, especially for the underserved. Models and methods of coordination of women's health services should be established and tested, while screening services should be implemented to the fullest extent. Complexities in governmental programs should be decreased. Oversight processes based on infant mortality reviews should be implemented as a strategy to improve the coordination of services at various levels for such issues as perinatal substance abuse, chronic illness, and breast cancer.

In regard to research, it was recommended that studies be conducted to document the health benefits and costs of coordination, as well as costs of lack of coordination of care. Research studies also were recommended to address women's health care utilization and service quality based on provider and organization, since there is a paucity of evidence in this area. Among the identified potential constraints are the start-up costs, both in dollars and time, to establish meaningful collaborations. Information-sharing mechanisms are another concern. Furthermore, issues remain regarding provider education for quality, coordinated health care of women.

FINANCING OF HEALTH PROGRAMS AND SERVICES

For many women, health care presents problems due to costs. Some women have no health care insurance. Other women have some insurance, but limited coverage. For many, preventive care remains poorly funded in spite of potential long-term benefits. Private administration of Medicaid managed care has resulted in the attenuation of public health departments in many local areas, thus decreasing the safety net of care for poor women. National categorical funding of care has discouraged, rather than promoted, coordination of care. The goals identified by the collaborative initiative were to support affordable universal health insurance for all, increase population-based health services, and maintain core public health functions.

The recommended strategies included encouraging all health plans to provide a comprehensive benefits package; ensuring that women have health care insurance that continues regardless of changes in jobs, marital status, pregnancy, loss of Medicaid eligibility, or documentation status; promoting parity in coverage for mental health and substance abuse services as outlined in federal statutes; promoting increases in funding for public health population services; promoting regionalization of perinatal care through cost sharing and risk-adjusted reimbursement; and mandating a specific communication and education set-aside within all federally funded women's and perinatal health services, to include health promotion as integral to women's health. Funding remains an issue entrenched in politics. The potential constraints are based on the political environment of the times. Recession generally indicates that more women are financially challenged, while the government has less fiscal means to provide support. However, studies demonstrating cost-effectiveness of integrated, community-based care may be more potent during times of cost constraint, providing an opportunity for changes in financial processes.

HEALTH COMMUNICATION AND EDUCATION SERVICES

More women than men experience chronic disease, yet many chronic diseases could be ameliorated or even prevented by early implementation of healthy habits. Early smoking, drinking, poor nutrition, and sedentary lifestyles may result in profound ill effects later in life. Education about healthy behaviors, coupled with encouraging a woman to make her own decisions, can facilitate a woman's autonomous health decisions with positive lifelong effects. The collaborative group suggested that the policy goal in this domain was to design and to implement health education strategies that improve the woman's ability to make personal healthy choices and navigate the health care system appropriately.

Specific areas of health communication and education strategies such as healthy body images, age-appropriate screening, and critical thinking skills were recommended. Another strategy included designing health communication and education programs that reflect the multiple demands that are placed upon women by individuals and society. Yet another strategy is implementing community partnerships and collaboration in health communication and education. The most effective of these communication and education practices for women's and perinatal care should be identified by rigorous research. These practices may be mass-media endeavors at the population level, or on the individual level. Research into communication patterns between a woman and her providers, or into barriers to adherence to prescribed treatment patterns, should be pursued.

Many studies have been conducted regarding changing consumer behaviors linked to mass-media messages for advertising purposes. However, the effectiveness of health education, either mass-media or individual, remains largely unproven. As research results emerge, the effective methods should be widely shared. Areas of consensus provide opportunities for action. For example, many of the Healthy People 2010 objectives could provide a common ground for stakeholders to develop and study health education messages.

DEVELOPMENT OF WORKFORCE COMPETENCY AND CAPACITY

As the body of knowledge about the health care of women grows, so does the challenge of dissemination of information into clinical practice. Not only should providers be knowledgeable, but they should be sensitive to the needs of women, especially in the context of racial, ethnic, age, and cultural diversity of the population and of women. Just as women are diverse, so are providers. Health care providers for women include professional and lay providers. The goal identified by the group in this area was to encourage girls and young women to consider health careers, and to promote resources to support these individuals.

Strategies that were identified to facilitate reaching the goal included understanding and promoting diversity by promoting education of women to care for women; providing means to make education within reach of those interested in health care, especially among the low-income groups and people of color; reconsidering affirmative action; and enhancing science and math education for girls, especially in the early years of school. Other strategies included promoting women as leaders within all health professions; using national guidelines, such as the proposed *Bright Futures for Women*, to promote education that emphasizes appreciation of gender issues; comprehensive care of women; multidisciplinary education; and additional provider skills in population-based health sciences, evidence-based practice, and collaborative practices. Cultural competency and sensitivity should be hallmarks of all providers of women's care, and providers should have more facility in coordination of women's and perinatal services across the life span, including specific gender issues. Additional strategies included improving providers' communication skills and the development of new funding methods of women's health care.

Among the research needed in the workforce domain are studies in forecasting health professional demand and supply. This forecasting should be focused on the needs of women, as well as the workforce mix needed (e.g., number and types of physicians, nurse practitioners, nurse-midwives, dieticians, social workers, and physician assistants). The lack of documentation of numbers and types of providers needed today results in potential confusion and implementing the above strategies. However, the sheer volume of information on women's health care may spur changes in education of providers. Moreover, new educational technologies such as asynchronous distance education provide new methods of teaching/learning.

SUMMARY

The collaborative initiative, which included Johns Hopkins University and the Maternal and Child Health Bureau, Health Resources and Services Administration, undertook a large task when they sought to uncover new viewpoints and to stimulate new partnerships toward a goal of a woman's and perinatal health policy agenda. Their recommendations (organized according to six major domains: social policy; surveillance and quality assurance; service availability, coordination, and organization; financing of health programs and services; health communication and education services; and development of workforce competency and capacity) provide a general framework as well as specific actions to be undertaken in the area of women's health care.

REFERENCES

Grason, H., Hutchins, J. and Silver, G. *Charting a Course for the Future of Women's and Perinatal Health*. HRSA: Washington. 1999.

ARTICLE 3

CHILDHOOD IMMUNIZATIONS

Lance E. Rodewald and Jeanne M. Santoli

INTRODUCTION—THE IMPORTANCE OF CHILDHOOD IMMUNIZATION

Routine immunization is a health intervention that saves both lives and dollars. The decline in vaccine-preventable disease incidence in the past several decades has been dramatic, saving the lives and improving the health status of millions of children. In the United States, compared with no vaccination program, vaccination saves from $2 (for hepatitis B vaccination) to $30 (for DTP vaccination) for every dollar spent, and compared with prevaccination-era disease levels, the current U.S. disease levels are from 97% to 100% lower.

Failure to vaccinate not only places children at risk of vaccine-preventable disease, but also is associated with failure to receive other important aspects of primary care. For example, compared with completely immunized children, under-immunized children make fewer health supervision visits, are one-sixth as likely to be screened for anemia, and half as likely to be screened for lead exposure.

From 1989 to 1991, there was a resurgence in measles in the United States that was caused by low immunization coverage levels in preschool children. The resurgence demonstrated that high immunization coverage levels in school-age children were insufficient to prevent epidemics, and that coverage in preschool children must also be high in order to prevent disease transmission. Major efforts were undertaken to understand barriers to preschool immunization, to develop interventions that raise coverage levels, and to add capacity to the immunization delivery system.

In 1994, the Childhood Immunization Initiative (CII) was launched. The three goals of the CII to be achieved by 1996 were to (1) reduce most vaccine-preventable disease to zero, (2) increase vaccination levels for 2-year-old children to at least 90% for the initial and most critical doses in the vaccine series, and 70% for a more recent vaccine, hepatitis B, and (3) build a vaccine delivery system to maintain these achievements in the United States. A fourth goal was that by the year 2000, a comprehensive infrastructure would be in place to provide the full series of vaccines for at least 90% of all children.

As a result of programmatic interventions, vaccination coverage levels rose. Currently, for preschool children, coverage levels are at or near record highs, and incidences of vaccine-preventable disease are at record lows. By 1996, the disease reduction goals of the CII were met or nearly met, and the immunization coverage goals were met or exceeded, including coverage among the five major race/ethnicity groups in the United States.[1] Table 1 presents the CII coverage goals as well as national coverage levels from 1992 and 2000.

Despite these successes, much work remains. Even though the gap in coverage among preschool children by race/ethnicity has been substantially narrowed, there remains a persistent gap by poverty. Nationally, there was a 13.6 percentage point difference in coverage levels across the poverty line in 1996 and a 10.0 percentage point difference in 1999.[2] Moreover, we have not developed a comprehensive infrastructure that can maintain coverage of 90% or greater for all children. The Institute of Medicine recently reviewed the roles of the states and the federal government in supporting immunization programs and services. A key finding of this review was that new challenges and reduced resources have led to "an instability in the public health infrastructure that supports the U.S. immunization system."[3]

WHAT PREVENTS TIMELY VACCINATION OF PRESCHOOL CHILDREN?

During the 1990s, a number of investigators studied the barriers that prevent timely immunization of preschool children.[4] Barriers to childhood vaccination are predominantly confined to preschool children because all states have school vaccination requirements that effectively ensure that greater than 95% of all school enterers have completed their recommended series. Thus, the problem is failure to receive timely vaccination, not failure to eventually be vaccinated.

There are several potential barriers that turn out *not* to be significant barriers when examined closely. First, many have speculated that parental attitudes toward vaccination can explain underimmunization; however, the evidence shows otherwise[5]—parents are very supportive of protecting their children through vaccination. Second, attitudes of providers have remained very positive toward routine vaccination and have not been found to correlate with immunization coverage levels.[6,7] And third, the vast majority of preschool children have access to an immunization provider. For example, according to the 1993 National Health Interview Survey, 93% of undervaccinated children 19 to 35 months of age had a usual source of primary care. Having access to a primary care provider and using services are not the same, however.

Findings in the recent literature about significant barriers to vaccination are several. First, poverty and its associated factors—such as residence in a single parent family, transportation difficulties, and large family size—have consistently been identified as a barrier to timely immunization.

Second, cost of vaccination is a barrier that is mediated through referral to health department clinics. Parents prefer to have their children receive their immunizations by the same provider that delivers other components of primary

TABLE 1 VACCINATION COVERAGE LEVELS AMONG CHILDREN AGED 19–35 MONTHS, BY SELECTED VACCINES, UNITED STATES, 1992[1] AND 2000[2]

Vaccine/Dose	Childhood Immunization Initiative 1996 Goals	NHIS[1] January– December 1992[1]	NIS[2] January– December 2000[2]
		% (95% CI)[3]	% (95% CI)[3]
DTP/DT[4]			
>3 Doses	90%	83 ± 2.2	94.1 ± 0.5
>4 Doses	—	59 ± 2.9	81.7 ± 0.8
Poliovirus			
>3 Doses	90%	72.4 ± 2.3	89.5 ± 0.6
Haemophilus influenzae type b (Hib)			
>3 Doses	90%	28.2 ± 2.6	93.4 ± 0.5
Measles-Containing Vaccine (MCV)[5]			
>1 Doses	90%	82.5 ± 2.3	90.5 ± 0.6
Hepatitis B			
>3 Doses	70%	—	90.3 ± 0.6
Combined Series			
4DTP/3Polio/1MMR[6]	—	55.3 ± 2.8	77.6 ± 0.9
4DTP/3Polio/1MMR/3Hib[7]	—	—	76.2 ± 0.9

[1]National Health Interview Survey (NHIS), household data only; children in this survey year were born between February 1989 and May 1991.

[2]National Immunization Survey (NIS), household and provider data collected during 2000; children in this survey year were born between February 1997 and May 1999.

[3]Confidence interval.

[4]Diphtheria and tetanus toxoids and pertussis vaccine/Diphtheria and tetanus toxoids (DTP/DT).

[5]Goals are for MMR (i.e., measles-mumps-rubella vaccine); estimates are for MCV.

[6]Four or more doses of DTP/DT, three or more doses of poliovirus vaccine, and one or more doses of MCV.

[7]Four or more doses of DTP/DT, three or more doses of poliovirus vaccine, one or more doses of MCV, and three or more doses of Hib.

Sources: CDC. Status report on the Childhood Immunization Initiative: national, state, and urban area vaccination coverage levels among children aged 19–35 months—United States, 1996. *MMWR* 1997; 46(29):657–664.

CDC. National, State, and Urban Area Vaccination Coverage Levels Among Children Aged 19–35 Months—United States, 2000. *MMWR* 2001; 50(30):637-641.

care. For example, Lieu and colleagues[8] showed that 62% of parents of families at health department clinics had a source of preventive care other than the immunization clinic, and that most would have preferred to receive their vaccines at these sources. Cost was named by these parents as the main barrier to immunizations at primary care sources. The RAND Health Insurance Experiment showed that less health insurance coverage for vaccination resulted in lower vaccination rates.[9] More recent data have shown that immunization delay is greatest for children lacking insurance coverage,[10] and that once previously uninsured children receive full insurance coverage for vaccination services, their use of health department clinics drops dramatically, their use of primary care providers increases significantly, and their immunization coverage levels improve.[11]

A third barrier is the role that provider practices play in underimmunization. Few providers assess their performance on immunizations; few operate recall/reminder systems; and many opportunities to immunize children are missed in primary care offices.

A fourth barrier is an information gap in the knowledge of children's vaccination status. Providers generally overestimate the immunization coverage levels of their patients, and parents tend to believe that their children are up-to-date on their immunizations. For example, in the 1994 National Health Interview Survey, 78% of parents of underimmunized children thought that their child was completely immunized. A prerequisite for vaccination is to know who is in need of vaccination. Thus, the role of individual-specific information is critical.

STRATEGIES TO ADDRESS VACCINATION BARRIERS

In 2000, the Task Force for Community Preventive Services made recommendations for evidence-based strategies to raise vaccination coverage levels among children, adolescents, and adults.[12] These recommendations were based upon a systematic review of published literature from 1980 to 1997.[13] Table 2 summarizes the recommendations relevant to children and adolescents. The sections that follow provide details about several of the strategies recommended by the Task Force and currently being implemented in the United States.

System-Based Interventions

To address vaccine cost and referral to health department clinics, the Vaccines for Children Program (VFC) was created in 1994. The Vaccines for Children program is an entitlement program that provides free vaccine to public and private providers for use in children without health insurance, those receiving Medicaid, and those who are American Indians or Alaska Natives. Children with commercial health insurance that does not cover vaccination can receive VFC vaccine as well, but only when vaccinated in federally qualified health centers. Providers enrolled in the VFC program benefit by not having to pay for vaccine and by the ability to charge a state-determined fee for the administration of the vaccines. The VFC program has been shown to reduce the rate of referral from private providers to health department clinics for immunizations.[14]

Measurement systems have been established to improve monitoring of vaccination coverage levels. Beginning in 1991 an immunization supplement to the

TABLE 2 RECOMMENDATIONS FROM THE TASK FORCE FOR COMMUNITY
         PREVENTIVE SERVICES ON RAISING IMMUNIZATION COVERAGE LEVELS
         AMONG CHILDREN AND ADOLESCENTS[1]

Increasing Community Demand for Vaccinations

Client reminder/recall	Strongly recommended (C)
Multicomponent interventions that include education	Strongly recommended (C)
Vaccination requirements for childcare, school, and college	Recommended (C, A)

Enhancing Access to Vaccination Services

Reducing out of pocket costs	Strongly recommended (C)
Expanding access in health care settings (when part of multicomponent intervention)	Strongly recommended (C)
Vaccination programs in Women, Infants, and Children (WIC) settings	Recommended (C)
Home visits	Recommended (C)

Provider-based Interventions

Provider-based reminder/recall	Strongly recommended (C, A)
Assessment and feedback of vaccination providers	Strongly recommended (C)

[1]Recommendations followed by a "C" apply to children; those followed by an "A" apply to adolescents.

Source: Task Force on Community Preventive Services. Recommendations regarding interventions to improve vaccination coverage in children, adolescents, and adults. *Am J Prev Med.* 2000;18(1S):92–96.

National Health Interview Survey was initiated to measure the immunization status of children less than seven years of age at the national level. In 1994, the National Immunization Survey (NIS) was initiated. This ongoing survey, conducted on a quarterly basis by the CDC, measures the immunization coverage of preschool children using provider-verified vaccination histories. The NIS measures state and urban area coverage, and the aggregated results have been used to monitor progress toward the Healthy People 2010 goals. For clinic level management, CDC developed the Clinic Assessment Software Application (CASA) to measure clinic-based immunization coverage levels and to help clinics diagnose problems with their immunization practices. This assessment tool, a multifunctional public domain software application, is available at http://www.cdc.gov/nip. As these examples illustrate, pairing goals with a system to measure progress is a powerful strategy to improve preschool immunization coverage levels.

Provider-Based Interventions

In 1993, the Standards of Pediatric Immunization Practices were developed and endorsed by the major provider organizations in the United States. The Standards were updated in 2001 and renamed the Standards for Child and Adolescent Immunization Practices to reflect a growing recognition of the importance of adolescent immunization. The revised Standards, listed in Table 3, address 17 important aspects of pediatric vaccinations, including methods to improve practice-based coverage levels. These standards have been shown to be effective at raising coverage,[15] and they have proven to be a powerful set of guidelines for immunization programs to use to enhance their service delivery and that of local area providers.

In particular, three provider-based strategies have been shown to substantially raise vaccination coverage levels: (1) recall/reminder systems to bring underimmunized children back to the provider for vaccination, (2) assessment of provider practice coverage levels with ranked feedback to the providers, and (3) linkage between the U.S. Department of Agriculture's Women, Infants, and Children (WIC) Program. Recall and reminder systems have been known to be effective prevention interventions for decades (there are over 50 randomized controlled trials just for immunizations), so the discussion to follow will concentrate on coverage assessments and WIC linkages.

Conducting practice-based assessments of immunization coverage levels and feeding this information back to the providers in a format that allows them to see how they rank against their peers has been shown to raise coverage levels in health department clinics. For example, in the Georgia health department clinics, median clinic coverage increased from 53% to 89% over a period of six years,[16] and the coverage gains have been sustained since that time.

Although clinic assessments are routinely conducted at all health department clinics in the United States, there is less experience with private practice assessment to date. Some localities, however, do assess private provider practices, and they have found these programs to be effective. Examples include Boston, where median coverage among two groups of private providers increased from 60% to 80% and from 52% to 77% over a four-year period,[17] and Maine, where a one-year, statewide intervention among all private providers (pediatricians and family physicians) resulted in an increase in coverage of 9% points, from 78% at baseline to 87% one year later.[18]

Linkage between the WIC Program and immunizations has also been shown to be a highly effective method to raise immunization coverage levels rapidly. WIC currently enrolls approximately 44% of the nation's infant birth cohort, and because it is a "means-tested" program, it captures a large proportion of the nation's poor children. At a minimum, vaccination-promoting activities in WIC involve: (1) assessment of each child using a documented immunization history and (2) referral of underimmunized children to their immunization provider for needed vaccinations. Monthly voucher pick-up (MVP) for underimmunization requires more frequent visits (monthly) to the WIC clinic for underimmunized children until they become completely immunized. Assessment and referral,

TABLE 3 STANDARDS FOR CHILD AND ADOLESCENT IMMUNIZATION PRACTICES

Standard 1	Vaccination services are readily available.
Standard 2	Vaccinations are coordinated with other health care services and provided in a medical home when possible.
Standard 3	Barriers to vaccination are identified and minimized.
Standard 4	Patient costs are minimized.
Standard 5	Health care professionals review the vaccination and health status of patients at every encounter to determine which vaccines are indicated.
Standard 6	Health care professionals assess for and follow only medically accepted contraindications.
Standard 7	Parents/guardians and patients are educated about the risks and benefits of vaccination in a culturally appropriate manner and in easy-to-understand language.
Standard 8	Health care professionals follow appropriate procedures for vaccine storage and handling.
Standard 9	Up-to-date, written vaccination protocols are accessible at all locations where vaccines are administered.
Standard 10	Persons who administer vaccines and staff who manage or support vaccine administration are knowledgeable and receive ongoing education.
Standard 11	Health care professionals simultaneously administer as many indicated vaccine doses as possible.
Standard 12	Vaccination records for patients are accurate, complete, and easily accessible.
Standard 13	Health care professionals report adverse events following vaccination promptly and accurately to the Vaccine Adverse Event Reporting System (VAERS) and are aware of a distinct program, the National Vaccine Injury Compensation Program (VICP).
Standard 14	All personnel who have contact with patients are appropriately vaccinated.
Standard 15	Systems are used to remind parents/guardians, patients, and health care professionals when vaccinations are due and to recall those who are overdue.
Standard 16	Office- or clinic-based patient record reviews and vaccination coverage assessments are performed annually.
Standard 17	Health care professionals practice community-based approaches.

Source: www.cdc.gov/nip.

coupled with MVP, has been studied most extensively and has produced dramatic improvements in coverage both in a research setting and during large-scale city-wide implementations of the strategy. Other WIC-based interventions are currently being tested, including the use of outreach, recall, and reminder programs to identify WIC clients in need of vaccination.

CHALLENGES FOR THE IMMUNIZATION DELIVERY SYSTEM

There are a number of challenges that will require substantial effort to address, including changes in the public/private split in service delivery, adolescent vaccination, disease surveillance needs, concerns about vaccine safety, and the introduction of new vaccines.

Changes in Public/Private Split in Service Delivery

Delivery of vaccinations to preschool children is being privatized through a set of convergent policy and financial reforms—the Vaccines for Children Program, state-based health insurance reform, the rise of Medicaid managed care, and the creation of the Children's Health Insurance Program. All four of these initiatives have incentives for children to receive their immunizations within a medical home for primary care. The VFC program has an explicit goal of enabling children to receive free vaccine at a private provider office, thus "recoupling" immunizations and primary care for children previously referred to health department clinics for vaccination. State-based insurance reform includes a requirement that health insurance benefits cover the entire cost of vaccination. Managed Medicaid programs are privatizing immunization delivery by requiring vaccination at the child's assigned primary care provider. The Children's Health Insurance Program, created in 1997, provides health insurance to previously uninsured children of the working poor.

Given that this privatization is consonant with programmatic goals, the challenge for the public health community will be to assess and assure the adequacy of vaccination services delivered by others. This is a major challenge because there are over 125,000 private providers. Through collaboration between CDC and state immunization programs, efforts are currently under way to incorporate clinic assessments into routine VFC provider site visits. This collaboration illustrates the assurance role that is becoming an increasingly important function of public health.

Vaccinating Adolescents

There is a large cohort of adolescents in the United States born prior to the recommendation of a number of vaccines for infants. The Advisory Committee on Immunization Practices (ACIP) developed recommendations regarding adolescent vaccination in 1996 to address this issue, and although progress has been made, adolescents remain one of the most undervaccinated age groups in the United States. Time is critical. Certain members of this cohort are already susceptible to several vaccine-preventable diseases, while others may soon begin behavior patterns that place them at risk. Each day, approximately 11,000 adolescents transition through the recommended vaccination age, and as this cohort ages, it becomes more difficult to access them with the health care system.

Important decisions regarding optimal strategies for reaching all adolescents revolve around *who* should provide and pay for the vaccinations. In general, health plans and private providers have responsibility for vaccinating their patients. But parents, other caregivers, or adolescents themselves must assure that provider visits take place. One important strategy to address this problem is the adoption of middle-school entrance requirements, such as a second dose of measles vaccine or completion of the hepatitis B vaccine series. In certain localities, publicly funded clinics and school-based vaccination programs serve as alternative delivery sites.

Improving Disease Surveillance

As disease incidence falls, collecting and reporting complete and accurate information on the remaining cases become increasingly important to improve our understanding of the factors that allow disease transmission to continue, in spite of high vaccination coverage. The occurrence of vaccine-preventable diseases in a community may be a sentinel event that signals the presence of an underimmunized population within the community. Such populations may be small, access health care infrequently, or otherwise be difficult to identify.

Similarly, when the incidence of disease is low, the *quality* of surveillance data begins to limit the precision with which progress toward disease elimination can be monitored. Surveillance indicators that allow monitoring of diagnostic effort are needed to ensure that the absence of reported cases reflects the true absence of disease, rather than the absence of effort to detect disease. In addition, adequate laboratory evaluation of suspected cases is essential. For example, complete serotyping of *H. influenzae* isolates from cases of invasive disease in children is essential to define the factors that allow these cases to continue to occur.

Vaccine Safety

Concerns about vaccine safety from parents and other members of the public have become increasingly common in the past several years. Two factors that play a role in this increasing level of concern are (1) a diminishing level of experience—on the part of patients, parents, and health care professionals—with the diseases that vaccines prevent, and (2) the ready availability of vaccine-related information that may be inaccurate or misleading via the popular press, television, and the Internet.

Although regulatory authorities who license drugs and vaccines do perform post-market monitoring of products, the importance of this task related to vaccines is magnified by the increasing public concern. In order to address the need for enhanced monitoring of vaccine safety, the CDC currently sponsors several ongoing efforts. The Vaccine Adverse Event Reporting System, a passive monitoring system that collects and evaluates case reports of adverse events from providers and the public, is the cornerstone of safety surveillance efforts. All serious adverse events are followed up, and any concerns raised are investigated through more extensive means. Another effort is the Vaccine Safety Datalink (VSD) project, a collaboration with seven large health maintenance organizations. Through standardized databases that capture both vaccines administered within the study population and any medical visits, adverse events that may have followed an immunization can be assessed. A third effort involves an ongoing contract with the Institute of Medicine, whose Immunization Safety Review Committee conducts at least three detailed reviews each year, to assess the scientific evidence around potential adverse events that may result from vaccination, with an emphasis on those of greatest current and potential public health impact. Finally, a network of Clinical Immunization Safety Assessment Centers (CISA) has been established. The primary purposes of this network are: (1) to undertake and improve the clinical evaluation, under standardized protocols, of selected adverse events reported to VAERS; (2) to serve as referral centers for clinical-immunization safety questions from health care providers in the field; and (3) to determine the causes and risk factors for certain adverse events when possible.

New Vaccines

Until the late 1980s, routine childhood vaccination had been a field marked by slow but steady progress. Since that time (and into the foreseeable future) routine vaccination has been anything but routine (see http://www.cdc.gov/nip for an always up-to-date vaccination schedule). Advances in biotechnology are bringing new combination vaccines, vaccines against additional diseases, improvements in existing vaccines, and changes in the vaccination schedule.

A critical issue involves paying for vaccines that are likely to become increasingly more expensive due to advances in biotechnology. To keep up with the expanding immunization schedule, federal and state dollars, which currently finance approximately 60% of all vaccine purchased in the United States, will need to increase. Insurers and health plans will need to routinely revise their benefit packages to incorporate new vaccines. In addition, those insurers and health plans that do not include routinely recommended vaccinations as a covered benefit should be encouraged to do so. Providers will also have to bear some upfront costs for new vaccines, particularly just after they are recommended, but before managed-care contracts have been revised or renegotiated. Finally, the parents of children underinsured with respect to vaccination will likely face increased out-of-pocket expenses when seeking to obtain vaccination for their children.

VISION FOR THE NATIONAL IMMUNIZATION DELIVERY SYSTEM

Essential Roles of Immunization Programs

Vaccinating children requires a strong partnership between public health and private medicine. Population-level responsibility for immunization rests with federal, state, and local public health agencies, even when others perform direct-service delivery. Because the public health role is important to the success of the entire system, the Institute of Medicine (IOM) recently described the essential roles of federal and state immunization programs in their report "Calling the Shots; Immunization Finance Policies and Practices."

The IOM description of the public health role in assuring immunization is in the form of a solved puzzle, in which each piece and its interaction with the other pieces is essential for the whole system to be effective. At the center of this system is the primary reason for immunization programs—the control and prevention of infectious diseases. Directly surrounding this fundamental goal are four key pieces: (1) assuring the purchase of recommended vaccines for the total population of U.S. children and adults—in particular, vulnerable or higher risk populations; (2) assuring access to vaccines within the public sector when private health care services are not adequate to meet local needs; (3) conducting population-wide surveillance of immunization coverage levels and vaccine safety to identify significant disparities in coverage, gaps in delivery of immunization services, and vaccine safety concerns; and (4) sustaining and improving immunization coverage levels within child and adult populations. Finally, the sixth piece of the puzzle, which provides the foundation for the five other pieces, is the efficient use of adequate and stable resources to achieve the national immunization goals.

The IOM recognized that vaccine purchase alone is not sufficient to assure the administration of vaccine and protection of the population from vaccine-preventable diseases. Rather, an infrastructure capable of conducting all six roles of immunization programs is necessary to achieve fully the benefits offered by vaccination.

Partnerships

Partnerships with private, nongovernmental organizations are one key component in assuring protection against vaccine-preventable diseases throughout the population. CDC's National Immunization Program has developed strong partnerships that promote and support international and national programs.

Through a competitive process, the National Immunization Program provides funding for collaborative programs with partners such as (1) national provider organizations (the American Academy of Pediatrics, the American Academy of Family Physicians, the National Medical Association, the Ambulatory Pediatric Association, the Society for Adolescent Medicine, the American Nurses Association, the National Association of School Nurses, the American Pharmaceutical Association, and the National Association of Community Health Centers), (2) national minority organizations (the Congress of Black Churches, the National Alliance for Hispanic Health, and the National Asian Women's Health Organization), and (3) national coalition groups (the Immunization Action Coalition and the National Partnership for Immunization). In addition, the National Immunization Program works closely with the Association of State and Territorial Health Officials and the National Association of City and County Health Officials. Each of these organizations works at the national level and with local affiliates to promote immunization through education, communication, and targeted interventions.

Finally, partnerships with other federal agencies are important. Currently, the immunization program is partnering with the Center for Medicare and Medicaid Services (CMS, formerly known as HCFA) to promote the Vaccines for Children Program and with the U. S. Department of Agriculture to promote WIC linkages.

REFERENCES

1. CDC. Vaccination coverage by race/ethnicity and poverty level among children aged 19–35 months—United States, 1996. *MMWR* 1997; 46(41):963–969.

2. Klevens RM, Luman ET. U.S. children living in and near poverty: Risk of vaccine-preventable diseases. *Am J Prev Med* 2001;20(4S):41–46.

3. Institute of Medicine, Division of Health Care Services and Division of Health Promotion and Disease Prevention. *Calling the Shots.* National Academy Press: Washington, DC, 2000.

4. The National Vaccine Advisory Committee. The Measles Epidemic: The Problems, Barriers, and Recommendations. *JAMA* 1991;266:1547–1549.

5. Strobino D, Keane V, Holt E, Hughart N, Guyer B. Parental Attitudes Do Not Explain Underimmunization. *Pediatrics* 1996;98:1076–1083.

6. Szilagyi PG, Roghman KJ, Campbell JR, Humiston SG, Winter NL, Flauberts RF, Rodewald, LE. Immunization practices of primary care practitioners and their relation to immunization levels. *Archives of Pediatrics and Adolescent Medicine* 1994;148:158–166.

7. Zimmerman RK, Schlesselman JJ, Mieczkowski TA, Medsger AR, Raymund M. Physician concerns about vaccine adverse events and potential litigation. *Archives of Pediatrics and Adolescent Medicine* 1998;152:12–19.

8. Lieu TA, Smith M, Newacheck P, Langthorn D, Venkatesh P, Herradora R. Health Insurance and Preventitive Care Sources of Children at Public Immunization Clinics. *Pediatrics* 1994;373–378.

9. Lurie N, Manning WG, Peterson C, Goldberg GA, Phelps CA, Lillard L. Preventive care: Do we practice what we preach? *Am J Pub Health* 1987; 77:801–804.

10. Zimmerman R, Janosky J. Immunization Barriers in Minnesota Private Practices: The Influence of Economics and Training on Vaccine Timing. *Family Practice Research Journal* 1993;13:213–224.

11. Rodewald L, Szilagyi P, Holl J, Shone L, Zwanziger J, Raubertas E. Health Insurance for Low-Income Working Families. *Arch Pediatr Adolesc Med* 1997;151:798–803.

12. Task Force on Community Preventive Services. Recommendations regarding interventions to improve vaccination coverage in children, adolescents, and adults. *Amn J Prev Med* 2000;18(1S):92–96.

13. Shefer A, Briss P, Rodewald L, Bernier R, Strikas R, Yusuf H, Ndiaye S, Williams S, Pappaioanou M, Hinman AR. Improving Immunization Coverage Rates: An Evidence-based Review of the Literature. *Epidemiological Reviews.* 1999; 21:96–142.

14. Zimmerman R, Medsgar A, Ricci E. Impact of Free Vaccine and Insurance Status on Physician Referral of Children to Public Vaccine Clinics. *JAMA* 1997;278:996–1000.

15. Pierce C, Goldstein M, Suozzi K, Gallaher M, Dietz V, Stevenson J. The Impact of the Standards for Pediatric Immunization Practices on Vaccination Coverage Levels. *JAMA* 1996; 276:626–630.

16. LeBaron C, Chaney M, Baughman A, et al. Impact of Measurement and Feedback on Vaccination Coverage in Public Clinics, 1988–1994. *JAMA* 1997;277:631–635.

17. Link D. Sharpen Your Aim: Increasing Immunization Rates in the Preschool Population, in *Improving Childhood Immunization: A Public Health and Private Provider Partnership*, Report of the Thirtieth Ross Roundtable on Critical Approaches to Common Pediatric Problems. Columbus, OH: Ross Products Division, Abbott Laboratories Inc., 1999, pp. 79–84.

18. Massoudi MS, Walsh J, Stokley S, Rosenthal J, Stevenson J, Miljanovic B, Mann J, Dini E. Assessing immunization performance of private practitioners in Maine: Impact of the assessment, feedback, incentives, and exchange strategy. *Pediatrics* 1999 103(6 Pt 1):1218–1223.

ARTICLE 4

EMERGENCY MEDICAL SERVICES AND CHILDREN: A GROWING CONCERN

David Heppel

INTRODUCTION

One wintery Sunday in Utah a family was leaving church. Some of the family had crossed the highway to get to their car. Without warning five-year-old Kacey raced to join his brothers . . . and into the path of an oncoming 16-wheeled tractor trailer. The truck severed one leg and mangled the other. Kacey's hold on life was tenuous. Within minutes paramedics arrived and took him to the nearest hospital. There he was stabilized and flown by helicopter to Salt Lake City and the regional Level I trauma center. The flight nurse on the transport had pediatric training, which served her well in maintaining Kacey's blood pressure during the flight. Her paramedic partner also had received pediatric training. This training, along with pediatric protocols instituted by the EMS system, allowed them to deliver Kacey in the best condition possible. At Primary Children's Hospital, the trauma team was waiting. Because of advanced communication, the hospital team knew the type and extent of injury and had assembled all of the appropriate specialists to deal with Kacey's injuries. A combination of medical skill, a very effective EMS system, and the remarkable spirit of a five-year-old resulted in a positive outcome to this very difficult situation. Unfortunately, Kacey's other leg could not be saved. However, after two months of hospital recovery and rehabilitation and two years of physical therapy as an outpatient, he is able to walk home from school, ski, and enjoy numerous other activities on his two prosthetic legs. According to his father, Kacey does whatever he wants to do.[1]

355

This is a true story. No one wishes a child to become ill or injured, but if such an event occurs, everyone wishes to have available the skills and resources that assisted Kacey's recovery. As citizens, we take as an article of faith that an ambulance, helicopter, or some other sort of emergency vehicle will be available promptly when we need it, that the people who emerge from that vehicle will have the knowledge and tools to assist appropriately, and that the vehicle will transport us to a care center that either will be able to provide definitive care or will further stabilize and then transport us to the definitive facility. We assume these resources are available for ourselves and for our children. In some places, they are; in others, they are not.

EMERGENCY MEDICAL SERVICES FOR CHILDREN

The Emergency Medical Services (EMS) system is an intersection of the public health, public safety, social services, and the personal health care systems. The care provided is almost exclusively individual, while the logistics of care delivery are basically population focused. An excellent Emergency Medical Services for Children (EMSC) system cannot exist in the absence of an excellent EMS system. Children comprise only about 10% of EMS transport runs and between 20% and 30% of emergency room visits.[2] Necessarily, the primary population focus of the EMS system is on adults, particularly adult trauma and cardiac victims. The adult EMS system forms the foundation of pediatric care. Without a functional adult EMS component, there is little hope of having a functional pediatric component. Likewise, without a functional adult trauma care capacity, the probability of effective pediatric trauma care is highly unlikely.

Historical View

Historically, the development of an EMS systems approach has been associated with those human endeavors which have created the greatest trauma—primarily wars. Historians generally credit Napoleon's chief physician with creating the first prehospital system designed to transport and triage injured from the battlefield.[3] In the United States, the Civil War provided the "opportunity" to develop first aid and transport systems. Civilian services began shortly thereafter. Emergency Medical Services operated with a range of human resources from hospital physicians to fire fighters to lay volunteers and with a range of transportation resources, including funeral home hearses. In the early 1960s, advances in rescue breathing and cardiac resuscitation provided the impetus for expansion of emergency services, especially in urban areas. The Vietnam War provided another environment in which the value of an EMS system was demonstrated.

Federal Support

In 1966, *Accidental Death and Disability: The Neglected Disease of Modern Society* was released by the National Academy of Sciences.[4] This document identified injury as the leading cause of death of young Americans while also recognizing the relatively poor resources of the nation's health care system to address this problem. The recommendations from this study were a major stimulus for improving the EMS. In the same year, Congress passed the Highway Safety Act, which gave the Department of Transportation the responsibility to assist states in developing regional EMS systems and also provided resources for provider training. This began the leadership efforts of National Highway Traffic Safety Administration in the development of EMS systems. The first nationally recognized emergency medical technician training curriculum was developed in 1969, beginning an effort to implement national training standards that continues to the present.

In 1973 additional federal support appeared in the form of the Emergency Medical Services Systems Act.[5] The Act provided resources, through the Department of Health and Human Services, to support a program of planning, operations, expansion, improvement, and research. During the 1970s the EMS Act was a major financial resource for many states to develop EMS systems. Resources of the EMS Act were combined with other health programs into the Preventive Health and Health Services Block Grant created by the Omnibus Budget Reconciliation Act of 1981. Block granting allowed states to shift resources to areas of greatest need. The impact on EMS programs has varied significantly across states, but the prevailing view is that support for EMS diminished. In 1990 the Trauma Care Systems and Development Act began support for development of state trauma systems. Funding for the program was modest but did provide some important catalytic support for states. The program ended in 1995 and has recently been revived. It is too early to assess the impact of its second life.

ELEMENTS OF AN EMERGENCY MEDICAL SERVICES SYSTEM

What are the necessary elements of an Emergency Medical Services system? The EMS Systems Act of 1973 identified 15 components: Manpower, Training, Communications, Transportation, Facilities, Critical care units, Public safety agencies, Consumer participation, Access to care, Patient transfer, Coordinated patient record keeping, Public information and education, Review and evaluation, Disaster plan, and Mutual aid. The National Highway Traffic Safety Administration's statewide EMS systems technical-assessment program[6] has 10 essential components: Regulation and policy, Resource management, Human resources and training, Transportation, Facilities, Communications, Public information and education, Medical direction, Trauma systems, and Evaluation. More recently, as part of the EMS Agenda for the Future effort, the following attributes have been identified as necessary for excellence in EMS.[7]

Integration of Health Services

EMS focuses on meeting the immediate needs of acutely ill or injured individuals. Traditionally this is done in relative isolation from other components of the personal health care delivery system and the public health system. Such an arrangement limits the opportunity of EMS to address community prevention efforts and to assist in appropriate follow-up of patients, particularly those who are not transported to hospital. In an enlightened system, EMS will achieve its potential to be an integral piece of the personal and public health system. It will become involved in collecting community data and sharing such information with other community providers.

EMS Research

Emergency Medical Services is a relatively new academic specialty. The first medical residency program in EMS was established in 1972. Certification in pediatric emergency medicine began in 1992. The research base in EMS is relatively modest, with most efforts addressing single interventions or topic issues and not the overall system. EMS clearly lags behind other health specialties in developing an evidence base for practice. There are limited financial resources available for EMS research and a rather small cadre of researchers involved. The many components of EMS (prehospital, emergency department, critical care unit, acute care hospital, transfers between hospitals) substantially increase the complexity of studying the EMS system.

Legislation and Regulation

There is significant variation among states' enabling legislation. Although all states have statutes, the degree of comprehensiveness and flexibility is wide. If EMS is going to be a functional public health resource, there needs to be a state mechanism to ensure overall system accountability, adaptability to specific local geographic and socio-economic conditions, and availability of resources for technical assistance and training support for local EMS systems.

System Finance

Presently EMS is supported through a variety of funding mechanisms. There are variations in mechanisms of financial support just as there are variations in legislation and regulation among states. In the governmental arena, EMS may be supported through general revenue funds or specific revenue sources such as surcharges on motor vehicle registrations, taxes on telephone bills, or dedicated funds from motor vehicle moving violations. Government as buyer of health care also may contribute to EMS through insurance programs such as Medicaid. In the private arena, selling of subscriptions for EMS services, reimbursement through third-party payers, and various charitable activities account for additional financial support. Stability of funding is a not inconsequential issue. In recent years, concern about appropriate utilization of health care services has had significant impact on EMS. Whether to transport and to where have financial repercussions.

Human Resources

EMS is provided by a wide variety of individuals with a wide variety of skills and knowledge: dispatchers, firefighters, police, emergency medical technicians (EMTs), nurses, physicians. EMTs and paramedics are responsible for the greatest amount of prehospital care. It is estimated that there are close to 600,000 EMTs in this country with 70,000 of them achieving paramedic status.[8] Many of the EMTs are volunteers, particularly in rural areas. Keeping up skills and knowledge has time requirements that may not be possible for volunteers to meet. For whatever reasons, the percentage of volunteers is diminishing. Being an EMS provider, both prehospital and hospital, is tough work. Physical injury, psychological stress, and exposure to infectious agents are all part of the job. Career advancement and mobility are variable, due in part to varying licensing requirements between states and, in some instances, within a state. All of these factors contribute to challenges to the system to recruit and retain sufficient personnel.

Medical Direction

Medical direction is responsible for assuring that appropriate standards of EMS care are achieved. It includes assuring appropriate education of EMS personnel, assuring that appropriate treatment protocols and standing orders are part of the EMS system, developing and implementing communications protocols, assuring appropriate equipment for the system, and maintaining a quality improvement program. In a number of programs it also means direct, real-time supervision of EMS providers in the field. Medical direction is provided by physicians, hopefully but not necessarily with special competency in EMS. Additional support is frequently provided by nurses, EMTs and paramedics, administrators, and other physicians. Most, but not all, EMS programs have some degree of medical direction.[9] To have an excellent system, medical direction must be provided by trained individuals with sufficient resources to assure that the tasks of the system can be discharged appropriately. They must assure appropriate and uniform practice parameters within the system and must assure active collaboration with other members of the health care community. Medical direction should exist at the state level and in all local EMS systems.

Education Systems

The education and training needs in EMS expand as the field becomes more sophisticated. In hospital, continuing education requirements are a part of medical and nursing professions. The primary concerns in this arena are the amount, content, and quality of continuing education activities. Basic training and education also are addressed through the professions. (For example, residency and fellowship training in emergency medicine.) Prehospital training is not so clearly defined. Although national guidelines describe training for four levels of prehospital providers (First Responders, EMT-Basic, EMT-Intermediate, and Paramedic), across the country there exists a wide variety of emergency medical technician certifications with different associated educational requirements. Continuing education requirements likewise are variable. In a changing medical environment lifelong learning is essential. The EMS system requires adequate national core curricula that are renewed on a regular basis. Particularly for the prehospital provider, training aids that can be accessed conveniently both geographically and over time are essential. The Internet provides a means of access that can open new avenues for learning. Particularly for the prehospital volunteer, the Internet may be the best method for keeping competent.

Public Education

The EMS system has the potential to be a significant resource for educating the public, although this potential is inconsistently realized. Programs to promote injury and illness prevention and appropriate and effective use of the EMS system are two areas of immediate focus for the EMS system. Given EMS's position in the community, it also is well situated to distribute information about health insurance and health care access in general, health care services, and consumer educational materials on health care quality. This public health education role provides an opportunity for collaboration with other components of the public health system; this role promotes health services integration.

Prevention

Emergency Medical Services is focused on guaranteeing rapid, competent, appropriate response and treatment of injury and illness. It is an important responsibility. However, no matter how quick the first responder, no matter how skilled the EMT, no matter how quick the transport, no matter how talented the emergency room staff, no matter how facile the surgeon, no matter how effective the rehabilitation, emergency medical services can never be as successful as a successful injury prevention program. Prevention is the responsibility of all of the health care system, but it is a particular responsibility for EMS. EMS systems have important monitoring and surveillance roles to play in addition to clinical responsibilities. As with public education, prevention efforts provide opportunities for EMS to partner with other public health and safety organizations.

Public Access

Arguably, the most important step in seeking emergency care is the initial contact with the system. Most people expect that the system can be accessed by telephone and, more specifically, by using telephone number 911. The advantage of using 911 is clear. Eighty-five percent of the public knows it, a figure that drops to approximately 35% to 45% when a seven-digit number is used.[10] The majority of the U.S. population does indeed have 911 access. Approximately 64 of the more than 3,000 counties do not. Within the majority which does have 911, many but by no means all of the call centers have enhanced capability to identify the geographic location of the call, an important piece of information in an emergency. Cell phones, from which upwards of 30% of 911 calls are made, currently are not able to be located geographically. The Federal Communications Commission has asked cellular providers that this capacity, which is costly, be added. It will take a while to do so, and some groups have raised privacy issues.

Communication Systems

Communication is a critical component of an EMS system. It is the first opportunity of the EMS system to intervene in an emergency situation. It is the means by which emergency services are dispatched to the scene. It is a means of coordinating activities of EMS and other public safety agencies. It is the means by which medical direction can be received by EMS personnel in the field. It is the means by which information on the patient can be shared with a receiving emergency room and hospital. The first contact with the EMS system is through the dispatcher at the public safety answering point (911). These individuals, responding to fire and public safety as well as medical calls, have varying skills and knowledge bases and thus varying abilities to provide information to callers in the "pre-arrival" phase of EMS. Although there is a national standard curriculum for emergency medical dispatchers, the curriculum and associated standards are not employed everywhere.[7] The communications equipment used by the system needs to be capable of handling the load of transmission of the system, and the equipment used by the various components of the system (prehospital transport, emergency room, hospital, public safety) must be compatible. The degree of sophistication of telemetry (e.g., transmission of EKGs, global positioning tracking of emergency vehicles) must be agreed to by system providers. These needs present a variety of challenges to the EMS system and require a variety of knowledge and understanding to address.

Clinical Care

The EMS system is intended to provide immediate medical attention to individuals with medical or traumatic emergencies and to transport those individuals to the closest appropriate source of definitive medical care. Initially, the overwhelming purpose of EMS was transport. Even though this is still the primary purpose, and the purpose upon which most third-party reimbursement is based, immediate medical attention is increasingly important. Care in the field and during transport has become increasingly sophisticated and complex. Even "basic" EMS providers are performing procedures that no EMS provider did thirty years ago. Increased clinical care holds the promise of improving the patient's condition, bringing some of the resources of the emergency department to the patient sooner. Presently, standards of prehospital care, at any level of sophistication, differ across the country. Therefore, the care received may very well differ. This is due to differences in credentialing and practice laws between states and standards of practice within states. For any given condition, what is done and who does it are not necessarily done based on national norms. Research has been done and is currently being performed to identify best practices and most appropriate resources, but much remains to be addressed.

Information Systems

In order to improve EMS it is critical that the system know what it is doing now. To achieve this end, components of the EMS system must collect information using the same definitions and in a similar fashion to assure data can be aggregated in order to have sufficient power to draw conclusions. It is also important that the data from EMS can be linked with information from other components of the health system so that overall outcomes can be studied. A significant amount of progress has been made during the past decade to achieve these ends, but these systems are not yet in place.

Evaluation

As with all care, EMS needs to ascertain the quality of its activities and the impact of its efforts and use this information to plan and implement system improvements.

Suffice it to say that EMS is a multifaceted, complex system in which a large number of factors must function well in order for the system to be successful.

TRAUMA CARE

A major component of emergency medical services and considered a system in its own right is trauma care. The American College of Surgeons Committee on Trauma (ACSCOT) historically has been the major influence on development of trauma services and systems. Starting in 1976, ACSCOT has published information on the components and organization of trauma centers from the most sophisticated to those having basic competence in handling trauma situations (Levels I, II, and III). In the ACSCOT vision, these centers are linked in regional networks so that complex patients can be stabilized in the more basic centers and transported within the system to those centers with greater capacity. Alternatively, the system is also designed so that critical patients may be transported directly to the primary (Level I) center if medically indicated. In its most recent guideline, *Resources for Optimal Care of the Injured Patient* (1999),[11] ACSCOT has expanded its categorization of trauma centers to include a designation for initial trauma care in rural/remote areas (Level IV). This alteration allows for a more inclusive system of care that takes into account the variation in health care resources across the country. There are eight key criteria necessary for trauma system development identified by ACSCOT: authority to designate, certify, identify, or categorize trauma centers; a formal process for such designation; use of ACS standards to designate centers; use of on-site verification of services by outside experts; authority to limit the number of trauma centers based on need; existence of prehospital triage protocols; existence of a monitoring process; and statewide coverage. In 1999, five states met all 8 criteria, 14 states met 7 of the criteria, 14 states met 6, 10 reported meeting between 1 and 5 criteria, and 8 states had no trauma system in place.[12] The most difficult criterion to achieve was the ability to limit the number of trauma centers (10 states); the next most common deficiency was statewide coverage.

In the view of ACSCOT, a trauma system must be directed by an organization with the authority to designate components included in the system (or, more importantly, to not designate some components that wish to be in the system) and to have sufficient resources to administer and monitor the system. This organization ultimately is responsible for the overall outcome of the system.

Rapid Access, Appropriate Care

A trauma system must assure rapid access to appropriate care. Prehospital services, mentioned earlier, are crucial components of the trauma system. Beyond the initial field triage decisions, the system requires rapid and accurate interhospital transfer decisions based on defined protocols. Hospitals designed to care for trauma must work together, not only during the acute event but also in triaging back through the system during rehabilitation and ultimately back to the patient's medical home. Coordination among acute care providers and among rehabilitation providers is equally important for the system to function with maximum efficiency.

Assessment and Prevention

A trauma system recognizes that system success is measured not only by survival rates but also by the quality of that survival. Measurement of system function and patient outcomes, both by the system itself and by outside evaluators, is an ongoing responsibility of a trauma system. And, related to this is the responsibility to conduct research to improve the system's effectiveness and the clinical care provided. Finally, a trauma system has a responsibility to attempt to prevent the occurrence of traumatic events in the first place. Thus, injury prevention programming also is an important role.

Economic Challenges

The economic circumstances of health care have impacted EMS and trauma care. In the 1990s health care reimbursement for trauma centers declined. Providers financially have been caught between their responsibility to treat all presenting patients regardless of reimbursement considerations (EMTALA[13]) and a decreasing ability to provide those services in a constricted economic environment. Addressing these economic challenges in a changing health care system has been and continues to be a major concern of the EMS/Trauma community.

A SPECIAL EMS FOCUS FOR CHILDREN

Although the EMS system must respond to each patient's individual needs, there are certain populations which require special consideration—for example, children. The EMS system is designed primarily for adults. Children have different illnesses from adults; sustain different types of injury; have different anatomy; have different physiology, both normal and pathologic, from adults; are different developmentally both emotionally and cognitively from adults. And, children are different from each other. An infant is different from a toddler, who is different from a preschooler, who is different from a school-aged child, and who is different from an adolescent.

Children's Anatomy

Children are different from adults in that they are physically smaller. They are not, however, simply miniature adults. Children have a greater surface area relative to body volume than adults. This characteristic is important in that, all things being equal, children are at much greater risk of heat and fluid loss than adults. The airway of a child is smaller than that of an adult. Obstructions, either foreign bodies or inflammation or swelling, which would only minimally impair respiration in adults can be catastrophic in children. Additionally, the anatomic relationship of the larynx in the posterior pharynx makes endotracheal intubation technically more difficult than in adults. Smaller blood vessels make delivery of intravenous fluids and medications technically more challenging. Body proportions are different depending on the child's age, with, for example, the head being relatively larger and heavier in the younger age groups which makes it more vulnerable to injury. (Children are significantly more likely to have sustained an unintentional injury to the head than are adults.) Bones are "softer" and less likely to fracture while the body still sustains significant injury.

Children's Physiology

Children's physiology is different from adults'. Children have normal heart rates and respiratory rates that are considerably higher than an adult's. The younger the child, the higher the normal rates. If not careful, an emergency provider can conclude that a child with normal vital signs is in trouble or may miss a child who is crashing because the respiration and heart rates are normal for adults. Normal blood pressure for a child, on the other hand, is lower than adult levels and changes as the child ages. A child's response to stress is different from an adult's. A child's cardiovascular system may be able to sustain blood pressure in the face of a volume of blood loss that would cause an adult to exhibit vital sign changes. Thus, there is a risk that emergency personnel may underestimate the significance of a child's situation.

Children's Communication

Children are by definition developing both cognitively and emotionally. Infants have a very limited repertoire of ways to communicate discomfort and pain. Toddlers are able to express feelings but to a relatively simple degree. As children age, their ability to communicate and therefore their ability to inform health care providers of their distress improves. A child is a developing organism: The young child has a better developed motor capacity than an ability to comprehend danger. The adolescent may comprehend danger but may have a sense of mastery of situations that is overly optimistic. Emotionally, children evolve in interaction with their surrounding society and that social experience may influence their abilities to be active, reliable participants in their emergency care.

Children's Diagnoses

These differences between children and adults, and among children of different ages, can make identification and treatment of serious conditions especially challenging. If chest pain rarely means cardiac problems in a child, what does it mean? How to identify the child with meningitis from among the many with illnesses manifesting as fever, irritability, and lethargy; how to recognize that a child's blood pressure is about to drop; how to recognize impending respiratory arrest all take awareness and experience. It is difficult for EMS providers to gain such experience.

A CONTINUUM OF CARE FOR CHILDREN

To assist the EMS system to better address the care of children is the mission of the Emergency Medical Services for Children (EMSC) program of the federal government. The program addresses a continuum of care from prevention to prehospital, to emergency department, to acute hospital and critical care, to rehabilitation.

A Medical Home

EMSC views the care of children as beginning and ending with a "medical home." As described by the American Academy of Pediatrics, a medical home is an approach to providing care that is "accessible, continuous, comprehensive, family centered, coordinated and compassionate...delivered or directed by physicians who are able to manage or facilitate essentially all aspects of pediatric care."[14] (The AAP Policy Statement identifies six characteristics of a medical home.) The medical home is an important source of information for the EMS system concerning the child and family and is the location to which the child and family will return after moving through the EMSC system. A good system will have integrated a means of identifying a child's medical home as soon as possible and a mechanism to communicate with the medical home. In addition to providing injury-prevention counseling for the family, the medical-home provider should prepare the family to access the EMS system, maintain communication with the family and the EMS system during an acute emergency, working with rehabilitation service providers, and be prepared to act as the child and family's advocate as the child reintegrates into the community. The involvement of the medical home and EMS is an important component of integration of health services concept as described in *EMS Agenda for the Future.*[7]

Prevention

Prevention of illness and injury is the ideal outcome of the efforts of the health care system. No emergency medical services system can match a successful injury-prevention program. After the first birthday, injury kills more children than all other causes combined, and the number of children sustaining nonfatal injuries is overwhelming. EMS providers are particularly well-situated to promote injury prevention efforts, are able to access information on injury patterns in the community, have credibility in the community, and are painfully aware of the consequences of unsuccessful injury-prevention efforts. Illness also can respond to prevention efforts, immunization being the most obvious example. Although at first EMS may not appear to have a role to play in this arena, particularly in rural/remote areas EMS providers have acted to administer immunizations quite successfully.

Prehospital Care

Prehospital care of children requires special knowledge, skills, and equipment. As noted previously, children have different responses than adults to the insults of illness and injury. Even though prehospital providers, either those providing bystander care or EMS personnel themselves, will more than likely encounter an adult patient, they must be prepared to deal with a child. Because they do so relatively infrequently, their knowledge is at greater risk of decay than with adults. They, therefore, may be more anxious when dealing with a child, which, in turn, may make it even more difficult to act clearly and appropriately.

The EMSC program has attempted to reduce this stress and to increase a sense of competence among prehospital providers by assisting states in instituting special educational and training programs that address children's special needs. These programs address both the cognitive information necessary to treat children and the technical skills necessary to successfully intervene. Starting an intravenous line in a child requires a degree of precision beyond that needed for most adults. The needles, for example, are not only smaller but are usually of different type than the catheters for adults. The vein into which the needle is placed is obviously smaller. Assuming that the provider successfully places the IV line, how much fluid should be given? There is a much greater margin for error in adults than children. Should drugs be administered? What kind? What is an appropriate dose? Most emergency meds for adults are designed to be unit doses; that is, the provider gives the entire amount in the container. Unit doses are rarely available for children, especially in EMS vehicles. If a unit dose is not appropriate, how can the proper amount be determined? Most pediatric dosing is done based on the child's weight. How does a prehospital provider determine weight? If a child needs assistance in breathing, what is the proper respiratory rate? If a child requires intubation in order to breathe, what are the differences in technique for placing that tube? A child's anatomy is such that it is relatively easy to insert the tube in the esophagus rather than the trachea. How far should the tube be inserted? In small children and infants it is, unfortunately, relatively easy to insert the breathing tube too far and ventilate only a portion of the child's lungs. These and other issues are addressed in training courses specifically designed for children's needs.

Equipment

Training is useful only to the extent that the trained prehospital provider has access to appropriate equipment to employ that training. Presently, there is a gap between what experts in EMSC believe should be available to prehospital providers and what actually is available in most circumstances. In 1996, only two states required all essential EMSC-recommended pediatric equipment and supplies on basic life-support ambulances and five states required all essential EMSC-recommended equipment and supplies on advanced life-support units.[15] The *2000 Equipment List* published by the Commission on Accreditation of Ambulance Services did not include all essential EMSC-recommended equipment and supplies.[16] Additional work is necessary to assure that the promise of improved services for children becomes a reality.

Emergency Departments

Hospital emergency departments (ED) are generally reasonably equipped and staffed to respond to pediatric emergencies. As with the prehospital provider, the emergency staff is much more likely to see adult patients and thus has more experience with them. However, pediatric patients make up a significant minority (between 20% and 30%) of ED visits, resulting in a greater degree of provider familiarity than in the prehospital situation. Within the general category of competence there exists a range of skills and resources. At one end of the spectrum is a small, frontier facility that may function as an ED and may be staffed only on an as-needed basis. This facility treats relatively few patients and therefore treats relatively few children. The staff is likely to have relatively little particular pediatric experience and also not likely to have specific pediatric training and continuing education. The purpose of these emergency facilities primarily is to stabilize and transfer on to a hospital with greater capacity. Although somewhat limited in their ability to deliver definitive care, these facilities play an important role in assuring access to emergency services in all areas of the country. At the other end of the spectrum are the emergency departments associated with pediatric trauma centers or general trauma centers with a pediatric capacity. These EDs are likely to be staffed with personnel who are either pediatric specialists or who have a substantial amount of pediatric experience. As important, the ED is supported by a pediatric inpatient service, possibly a pediatric intensive care unit, and all of the components of a trauma center. Most emergency departments, of course, fall between these two extremes with inpatient support that also varies.

Rehabilitation

The circle of EMSC care, beginning with prevention, is closed by rehabilitation. As the EMS system is better able to cope with the specific therapeutic challenges presented by children, more children are surviving critical injury and illness. For some, with survival comes the possibility of temporary or permanent disability. The goal of rehabilitation is to return the patient to as high a level of functioning as possible, ideally to pre-incident functioning. For children, the concern not only is a return to function but also the capacity to continue the developmental processes of childhood. Quality of life is a major concern of the EMSC program. Early initiation of treatment, from the moment of the incident through the entire therapeutic process, diminishes the child's morbidity and time away from normal life activities. Communication between the acute care EMS providers and the more chronically focused rehabilitation community has not always been strong. The EMSC program, as part of its system approach, has supported integration of acute and rehabilitative services through its state programs and through grants that target specific rehabilitation issues in the EMS world.

FEDERAL EMERGENCY MANAGEMENT SYSTEM FOR CHILDREN

The Federal EMSC program started in the mid-1980s with a simple but encompassing charge: "to support a program of demonstration projects for the expansion and improvement of emergency medical services for children who need treatment for trauma or critical care."[17] Originally intended to support only states, the legislation was amended to identify medical schools as potential grantees as well. In the early years, the modestly funded EMSC program supported demonstration grants in a few states. The law limited grants to four per year. To expand the impact of the program, existing state grantees would "adopt-a-State" to provide specific help to states not receiving direct support. In the Northwest, for example, Oregon assisted Washington. They then both helped Idaho, and all three subsequently assisted Nevada.

As the EMSC appropriation increased and the experience of the grantees expanded, categories beyond the original state demonstration grants came into being. Since it was clear that different states were at different levels of sophistication in providing EMS to children, the program evolved different grant programs to address initial planning needs (planning grants), to implement new approaches to EMSC service delivery (implementation grants), and to maintain an ongoing concern about children's issues within the basic EMS program (partnership grants). All states and most territories now have received support, with most states having progressed to the partnership program. Additionally, a "targeted issues" grant category was created to address common needs of all states such as training curricula for prehospital providers, types of pediatric equipment needed for ambulances and emergency departments, and development of treatment protocols for use in the field. These efforts, and collaboration with agencies focused on professional education and research, have allowed the EMSC program to provide a support base for pediatric aspects of EMS.

CHALLENGES FOR THE FUTURE

What challenges lie ahead? Reliable financial support for EMS in general and EMSC in particular is a critical concern. The variation in funding mechanisms, as noted earlier, is substantial. In uncertain economic times, it is not at all clear that the present patchwork quilt will hold together. Moreover, EMS and EMSC will necessarily be influenced by the evolution of our efforts to contain costs in the larger health care system. The ascendancy of managed care in the 1990s certainly had a significant impact on the delivery of EMS. As costs again increase, there is no reason to believe that new cost-containment efforts will not equally significantly impact the system.

Quality-of-care issues will continue to be of great importance. Medical mistakes have received a great deal of attention in 2001. The high-stress environment of EMS is an unfortunately fertile ground for misadventures. Efforts to standardize and simplify clinical interventions, such as unit dosages of pharmaceuticals and standardized equipment, will free the clinician to focus on the condition of the patient. Clinical practice guidelines will support care providers who infrequently treat children while not restricting the skills and experience of more seasoned pediatric emergency providers.

Cultural competence is an important characteristic of a good health care system. In emergency situations, it is even more critical. The stress of an emergency taxes the best of communicators. Not knowing or appreciating a patient and family's beliefs and view of the world compounds communications problems. Although it is vitally important to have the technical knowledge and skill to address critical illness and injury, it is equally important to have the knowledge and skill to communicate clearly. With a greater and greater degree of cultural diversity in this country, such knowledge and skill are more and more difficult to fully obtain.

Integration of emergency medical services for children into the general emergency medical services system and integrating both into the public health system remain a challenge. Some achievements take a long time. This goal has been part of the EMSC program since its inception in 1984. That we are into the 21st century and continue to need to make progress in this area demonstrates: (1) the challenge that children face in receiving their due from the health care system in general; (2) the challenge of collaboration among intersecting but differing cultures of emergency care providers; and (3) the continuing challenge of integrating the medical perspective and the public health perspective, a challenge that has dogged us for almost a century. On a positive note, much progress has been made. In the clinical arena, pediatric specialists and emergency medicine generalists are collaborating on standards of care and on designation of facilities for pediatric care. Most EMS programs are taking population-based approaches to care and are intimately involved in public health efforts, especially in the area of injury prevention. As we move further into the 21st century we can look forward to a more coherent approach to addressing emergency medical needs. Hopefully, we also can look forward to a more coherent approach to addressing overall health needs; in other words, a public health approach.

REFERENCES

1. Feely HB, Athey JL. 1995. *Emergency Medical Services for Children: 10 Year Report*. Arlington, VA: National Center for Education in Maternal and Child Health.

2. Yamamoto LG, Wiebe RA, Maiava DM, Merry CJ. A One-Year Survey of Pediatric Prehospital Care. *Pediatric Emergency Care* 1991, 7: 206–214.

3. Brewer LA. Baron Larrey 1766–1862. *Journal of Thoracic and Cardiovascular Surgery* 1986, 92: 1096–1098.

4. National Academy of Sciences, National Research Council. *Accidental Death and Disability: The Neglected Disease of Modern Society*. Washington D.C.: National Academy Press, 1966.

5. *Emergency Medical Services Systems Act of 1973*: Public Law 93–154, Title XII of the Public Health Service Act. Washington D.C.: 1973.

6. National Highway Traffic Safety Administration. *EMS System Development: Results of the Statewide EMS Assessment Program*. Washington D.C.: U.S. Department of Transportation (DOT HS 808 084), 1994.

7. National Highway Traffic Safety Administration. *Emergency Medical Services: Agenda for the Future*. Washington D.C.: U.S. Department of Transportation (DOT HS 808 441), August 1996.

8. Keller RA. 1992 EMS Salary Survey. *Journal of Emergency Medical Services* 1992, 17(11): 62–73.

9. Snyder JA, et al. Emergency Medical Services System Development: Results of the Statewide Emergency Medical Service technical assessment program. *Annals of Emergency Medicine* 1995, 26: 146–152.

10. Eisenberg M, Hallstrom A, Becker L. Community Awareness of Emergency Phone Numbers. *American Journal of Public Health* 1981, 71: 1058–1060.

11. American College of Surgeons. 1999. Resources for Optimal Care of the Injured Patient. Chicago: ACS.

12. Bass RR, Gainer PS, Carlini AR. Update on Trauma System Development in the United States. *The Journal of Trauma: Injury, Infection and Critical Care* 1999, 47(3): S15–20.

13. Emergency Medical Treatment and Active Labor Act of 1985.

14. Ad Hoc Task Force on Definition of Medical Home. The Medical Home (RE9262). *Pediatrics* 1992, 90: 90(5): 774.

15. Committee on Ambulance Equipment and Supplies, National Emergency Medical Services for Children Resource Alliance. Guidelines for Pediatric Equipment and Supplices for Basic and Advanced Life Support Ambulances. *Annals of Emergency Medicine* 1996, 28(6): 699–701.

16. Commission on Accreditation of Ambulance Services. Commission on Accreditation of Ambulance Services Equipment List 2000. Glenview IL: Commission on Accreditation of Ambulance Services, 2000.

17. *Emergency Medical Services for Children, Public Health Service Act, Section 1910.*

ARTICLE 5

ORAL HEALTH IN MATERNAL
AND CHILD HEALTH

Paul S. Casamassimo

INTRODUCTION

Major gains have been made in the oral health of Americans in the last half of the 20th century. Women and children have been beneficiaries of many improvements in oral health, including a dramatic decrease in dental caries and increased availability of fluoridated water supplies. Despite better oral health for many, others within the maternal and child health (MCH) community continue to experience significant disease and limited access to care. Minority groups, the poor, recent immigrants, the uneducated, and those living in nonfluoridated communities constitute segments of society that have not benefited equally from advances in oral health science and practice and whose access to care remains limited. For those people in these groups, oral disease constitutes a silent epidemic, according to the 2000 report of the Surgeon General, *Oral Health in America, A Report of the Surgeon General.*[1] This chapter reviews the advances in oral health status of the MCH population and briefly discusses issues that have affected and will likely continue to affect that status into the next century. Table 1 orients the reader to several segments of the MCH populations and their oral health issues.

The major oral health issues facing the MCH population can be summarized, using a variety of sources,[1-7] as the following:

1. The need to reduce preventable infectious diseases of dental caries and periodontal disease, with particular emphasis on the distribution of disease in certain MCH populations
2. Problems with access to oral health care, particularly for poor and minority MCH populations
3. Limited availability of public health measures such as early dental screenings, dental sealants, water fluoridation, and referral of special needs populations to established care pathways

4. Inadequate systemic infrastructure that is needed to deliver consistent services nationally, establish standards and policies, and advocate for MCH oral health issues
5. Weak integration of oral health services into general health at all levels

TABLE 1 SELECTED MATERNAL AND CHILD HEALTH POPULATIONS AND RELATED ORAL HEALTH ISSUES

MCH Population Cohort	Oral Health Issues
Pregnant women	Poor periodontal health is linked to prematurity of offspring; lifestyle can influence oral health of child; periodontal inflammation is exacerbated by hormonal change; and pregnant women do not access care during pregnancy. It is not clear how maternal nutrition affects offspring's oral health.
Perinatal/Infancy	Maternal transmission of virulent microflora is possible, influencing offspring caries susceptibility. Fluoride benefits begin at six months of age. First dental visit is encouraged.
Preschool/Head Start	One in five children have dental caries at this age. Access to care is limited because of socio-economic status and limited cooperation.
Homeless	Lack of access to care and increased caries rate are common.
HIV patients	Increased caries rate, periodontal diseases, and oral pathology due to immunocompromised status characterize this population. Stigma makes access to care limited.
Special health care needs	Access to care is limited and a major health issue. Craniofacial and other condition-related problems are common and complicate care.

REDUCTION OF ORAL DISEASES

Dental caries and periodontal disease are the major conditions affecting MCH populations. Both are preventable infectious diseases that affect all age groups.

Dental Caries

Dental caries is an infectious disease of teeth causing acid breakdown of enamel and dentin, abscess formation, and eventual loss of teeth. Treatment and prevention of dental caries account for most dental expenditures in this country. Over the last three decades, dental caries in permanent teeth has declined dramatically in children so, on average, about 50 percent of children do not have dental caries in their permanent teeth.[8] This statistic belies the fact that dental caries remains the most common infectious disease and is now clustered in selected populations in high severity.

Caries is primarily a disease of childhood, but its effects reach into adulthood. By age 17, over 80% of children have dental caries of their permanent teeth. Employed women, 18–19 years of age, have almost 13 decayed or filled tooth surfaces (DFS, a measure of mean caries experience). This climbs to a DFS of 25 by ages 35 to 39.[2] Black women in this age group have a lower caries rate, but also a lower rate of filled surfaces, suggesting less access to care.

Overall, minorities tend to have more untreated disease, and the historical trend to having less dental caries than whites appears to be reversing.

Several other trends in dental caries appear to be developing in MCH populations and these have implications for the future. First, recent studies have noted a clustering of dental caries into a smaller group of children, so that roughly 25% of children experience 75% of dental caries.[4] Many of these children are from at-risk populations including the poor and minorities. Clustering represents an opportunity to identify risk factors and apply risk profiling to those with varying susceptibility, so resources can be used more efficiently. Unfortunately, the care system's approaches to management of dental caries lag well behind the clustering phenomenon. For example, many public health measures remain global rather than targeted at high-risk groups. Insurance and entitlement programs are not designed to offer risk-based benefits to those most severely affected.

A second trend concerns caries in primary teeth. Early childhood caries, or ECC, is a new term that refers to dental caries in primary teeth. Data from this country and from other industrialized nations suggest that ECC is no longer declining.[9] The explanation for this remains elusive, but may relate to increasing use of inappropriate bottle feeding, inability of some segments of the population to gain access to preventive measures like fluoride or professional visits, and increasing numbers of immigrants. A major factor may also be the prevailing standard of care that delays the first dental visit until three years of age.[10] Those most severely affected are poor and minority children. Native American children, for example, routinely experience dramatically high rates of primary caries, often double that of white children of similar age. Poor black children also often have higher rates of primary caries as well.[11]

The third trend notable for children is the continued presence of baby bottle tooth decay (BBTD) as a subcomponent of ECC. BBTD occurs when very young children are pacified with a bottle containing a liquid with fermentable carbohydrate, most often sugar. This is usually done at night, but also occurs during waking hours when parents or caretakers use the bottle for behavior modification. Studies place the prevalence of BBTD at well over 50% of Native American children and at 20% of other at-risk groups such as Head Start children. BBTD creates immediate and long-term consequences for oral health. The caries pattern created is rapid and severe in many cases, requiring extensive restorative treatment. The age of the affected child often mandates that treatment be done using sedation or general anesthesia to manage behavior, adding expense and risk. A 1996 study of Iowa Medicaid reported that the average additional (nondental) cost of treatment was $1,812 in 1994 for 317 children 5 years of age and under, adding over a half-million dollars to overall treatment charges.[12]

Just as troubling for future caries management in this youngest segment of the MCH population afflicted with BBTD is the well-documented phenomenon of increased susceptibility of these children to future caries throughout childhood[13] even when intensive caries preventive strategies are used. Current preventive strategies stress education, but it should be noted that recent research suggests that BBTD has deep cultural linkages and a strong relationship to societal stresses on parents and thus may be resistant to preventive education.[14]

Periodontal Disease

Periodontal disease is the other major infectious disease of concern in the MCH population. Periodontal disease is an umbrella term to describe infections and deteriorating conditions of the gingival tissues and bone supporting teeth. Gingivitis is a minor form affecting the gums and is reversible in most cases with good oral hygiene. Periodontitis involves irreversible destruction of bony support of teeth as the result of infection by oral microorganisms. In adults, periodontal disease accounts for more tooth loss in later decades as opposed to dental caries.

For the majority of young children, gingival problems are minor. However, periodontal conditions affect one out of two adolescents[1] and the first signs of bone loss (as measured in millimeters of loss of gingival attachment to the tooth) appear during this period. Early onset periodontitis (EOP), defined as attachment loss greater than 3 millimeters, is not common, but most recent national data suggest that 10% of African Americans, 5% of Hispanics, and 1.3% of whites are affected in the 15–17 year age group. EOP is also associated with increased caries.[15]

Women of childbearing age experience periodontal problems that increase with age, although women overall fare better than men of comparable age.[1] National data available from the 1985–86 Oral Health Survey of Adults and Seniors show gingival bleeding in 37% to 46% of employed women 18–39 years of age. In this same group, up to 15.7% had periodontal pockets suggestive of attachment loss.[2] Periodontitis is a finding in diabetes, a systemic condition that occurs in higher rates in minorities. Very recent research suggests that there may be an association between periodontal disease in mothers and prematurity in their offspring.[16] In addition, there may be an association between periodontal disease and heart disease.[17]

The implications of these most recent associations could be significant and make prevention of periodontal disease a major oral health priority in the next decade and beyond. At present, periodontitis prevalence in adults seems stable as compared to 1986 levels.[6] The concern that periodontal disease, like dental caries, is higher in the poor and minority populations may also direct future policy and programmatic decisions. Recent emphasis placed on research into this disease and its prevention may be more a factor of the baby-boom generation's aging than the disease's impact on oral health.

In summary, oral health has improved, but many within the MCH population have seen only minor gains and others have experienced none. Clearly some children and many women have benefited from the decline in permanent tooth dental caries. Racial and income differences continue to exist for dental caries and periodontal disease, particularly for untreated disease.

ACCESS TO CARE

In 1996–97, 63% of women had a dental visit within a year, with a slightly lower percentage for those 25–34 years of age. Higher percentages were noted for those with higher education and income levels. Whites tend to seek dental care more often than nonwhites[18] and tend to seek it more frequently with shorter intervals between visits.[5]

The cost of care is a major factor in access. In 1992, dental care accounted for a little over 5% of health care expenses.[5] Data from the 1995 Behavior Risk Factor Surveillance System indicate that about 44% of adults do not have dental insurance,[19] yet all but 3% of total expenditures for oral health services are private dollars. Only 38% to 48% of women, 18–44 years of age, have dental insurance. About 50% of 5–17-year-olds have some form of dental insurance, primarily through an employed parent. Reaching the age of majority causes a dip in insurance coverage, which takes about a half-dozen years to reverse.

Table 2 provides a snapshot of age, race, insurance, and oral health care utilization for U.S. children and adults.

MEDICAID

Any discussion of access to oral health care for MCH populations must include consideration of Medicaid. The establishment of Medicaid in 1965 intended to ensure the poor access to health care. The Early and Periodic Screening Diagnosis and Treatment Program of Medicaid requires states to pay for oral health services for children and to ensure that they are delivered. States may or may not offer dental services for adults and have the discretion to limit services. Dental per capita expenditures under Medicaid actually decreased between 1975 and today, in contrast to all other medical benefits of the program.[5] Edelstein[20] reports summary statistics for the program period 1993–95 that are reflective of the limited success of the Medicaid dental program:

- Only 18 percent of all Medicaid eligible recipients (children, adults, handicapped, and elderly) received any dental treatment.
- Combined state and federal spending for dental services was $1 billion annually.
- Dental expenditures accounted for 1% of total Medicaid expenditures.

- Annual per enrolled beneficiary expenditures were $43 and for each beneficiary who had at least one dental visit were $241.

TABLE 2 ORAL HEALTH STATUS AND UTILIZATION OF DENTAL SERVICES FOR U.S. CHILDREN (CH) AND ADULTS (AD)

Condition or Variable	Poor*		African American		Hispanic		U.S. Mean	
	Ch	Ad	Ch	Ad	Ch	Ad	Ch	Ad
Percentage of untreated coronal dental caries	—	—	27.2	22.1	—	23.0	15.3	8.12
Percentage with private dental insurance	7.8	13.3	31.9	35.6	28.7	31.2	44.3	43.9
Percentage with dental sealants	4.3	n/a	4.2	n/a	5.1	n/a	10.9	n/a
Percentage with at least one visit in preceding year	48.8	42.7	49.9	43.9	47.9	45.2	61.7	57.7
Average number of dental visits per year	1.1	1.4	1.0	1.3	1.6	1.5	2.1	2.1

* Income less than $10,000.

Some states have converted dental programs to managed care/HMO style programs. None of these has operated long enough to make conclusions about their effect on oral health of recipients. Success of HMO-driven systems, capitation, carve-outs, gate-keeping, and other aspects of managed care remains to be seen. The additional layer of administration provided by such arrangements can hinder participation by both recipient and provider.

Numerous state and government reviews of Medicaid dental services have noted consistent problems with the program.[21,22] Providers cite low fees, extensive paperwork, rigorous regulation, poor patient compliance, and limitation of allowable services that creates a dual standard of care and ethical dilemmas for dentists. More recently, participating dentists have left the system because of concerns about Medicaid agency personnel who question treatment decisions and employ extrapolation techniques that project billing errors across an entire population. Recipients complain of limited access due to lack of providers and transportation costs to reach providers who will accept Medicaid.

If Medicaid is to work, the above problems need to be addressed. Creative approaches to attract providers such as stipending training programs to develop sensitive providers are needed. Fees need to approach usual and customary private fee structures to be competitive. Quality standards that eliminate the dual standard of care need to be developed and disseminated as guidance. Formative rather than punitive auditing practices need to be developed and applied. Acuity needs to be factored into populations and appropriate steps taken to account for the higher disease rates in the covered population. On a national and state level, regular evaluation of program success needs to be instituted. A consistent and comparable database must be developed for this purpose.

Medicaid reform is occurring in isolated states with both fee increases for providers and administrative improvements. Progress is slow because of legislative and budgetary controls and competition by nursing homes, medical professionals, and hospitals for similar improvements. Both legislative and executive branches note the failures of Medicaid, and in an impending change, they may fashion a block-grant format with greater state flexibility, a direction supported by state governors.

STATE CHILD HEALTH INSURANCE PROGRAM

In 1997, Congress enacted the State Child Health Insurance Program (Title XXI), also called SCHIP or CHIP, entitling states to federal monies for child health assistance. States can expand Medicaid or create new programs to cover children up to 200% of poverty. Children from "working poor" families, unable to purchase health insurance, will benefit from CHIP. When Medicaid is the vehicle chosen by a state for CHIP, dental benefits including EPSDT, must be provided. However, states choosing alternatives to Medicaid need not offer dental benefits. At the writing of this chapter, only one state plan does not include dental benefits of some type, which on face value, suggests better access to care.

Oral health advocates have expressed concerns over any of three options of SCHIP—Medicaid, no dental coverage, or new programs that include dentistry. If Medicaid is expanded, the program brings with it problems noted earlier in this chapter. It is possible that access will not be improved, even though more children are eligible, since the forces keeping away providers remain. In addition, the sudden addition of eligible recipients, many of whom have significant treatment needs, may overwhelm and drive away existing providers. A state opting for no dental coverage ignores the significant treatment needs of the very populations the legislation intends to serve. States choosing new programs, such as "benchmarks" equivalent to those dental plans offered their state employees, may inadvertently impose restrictions or limit services because of co-payment provisions, gate-keeping, and other subtle benefit limitations.

In summary, improvement of access to oral health for MCH populations is a complex problem whose detailed discussion is well beyond the scope of this chapter. When one considers that about 35% to 40% of the MCH population lives below or within 175% of the poverty level, improved access will revolve around improvement in public programs. The following significant issues stand in the way of meeting access goals; they include but are not limited to:

1. Decreased funding for public health clinical programs
2. Competing programs within states for limited dollars, such as within-state MCH block grants
3. Inadequate provider pool, particularly pediatric dentists and dentists willing to be Medicaid providers
4. Complex and conflicting eligibility requirements affecting women and dependent children
5. Dependency of a disproportionate percent of the MCH population on publicly funded clinical care programs

PUBLIC HEALTH MEASURES

Fluoride

Fluoride is the public health measure that can be credited with reducing the dental caries rate in this century. About 144 million Americans (56%) have access to fluoridated water, with most of these served by public water systems. This includes over 60 million children. In addition, recent estimates are that 93% of children 2 to 16 years of age use a fluoridated dentifrice. Almost all toothpaste sold in the United States contains fluoride.[23]

Fluoride consumed during tooth development strengthens enamel against carious attack by food acids after eruption. Fluoride consumed daily acts on teeth already erupted to remineralize, thus arresting or reversing early caries. Some antibacterial effect has been attributed to fluoride as well. Its negative effects in this country are limited to fluorosis or tooth mottling and toxicity when consumed in concentrated form. The MCH population thus benefits from fluoride passively in drinking water and foodstuffs produced within fluoridated communities. Dentifrice swallowed also contributes to the fluoride load of young children. Topical effects of fluoride are also gained from foodstuffs and water consumed as well as from home application in dentifrice and professionally applied fluoride treatments.

The major fluoride issues for the MCH population relate to (1) increasing the percentage of the population receiving optimal fluoride in communal water systems and (2) addressing increasing fluorosis in the population due to a halo effect caused by ubiquitous sources in the food chain and dentifrices. Although clearly a public health issue, fluoride has been pushed into the political spotlight by various groups across the political spectrum, including those concerned with government's intrusion into privacy and environmentalists. It is unlikely that major changes will occur in the availability of fluoride in water supplies. A more likely scenario is a relatively stable percentage of Americans exposed to fluoridated water and more exposed to topical and systemic fluoride via existing and new personal and professionally applied vehicles, such as fluoride varnishes. Today, three states—Washington, Iowa, and North Carolina—are piloting nondentist application of fluoride varnish by primary care medical providers who tend to see very young children more regularly, but data on outcomes is yet to be released.

Dental Sealants

The other major anti-caries preventive measure is dental sealants. These are plastic coatings applied to teeth by dentists or other trained professionals before dental caries begins. Since most dental caries of posterior teeth occurs in their pits and grooves, sealants offer a potential major anti-caries effect.

Sealants can be placed in private offices as well as in public health settings such as mobile clinics or school-based programs. A Year 2000 goal is to have 50% of children with sealants on at least one tooth,[24] but goals for 2010 are less ambitious and simply seek to increase the prevalence of sealants over baseline measures. Currently, only about one in five 5- to 17-year-old children has dental sealants on the permanent teeth. The number of children with sealants has risen from 1986–87 when about 7 to 8% of children had sealants. Access to care plays an important role in obtaining sealants; racial gradients in who has sealants tend to disappear when access to care is equaled.[25]

Public funding provides sealants to those in low-income groups who are also the ones who experience most dental caries. Thus, policies and programs providing sealants are important. Similarly, sealants represent a sound, low-cost preventive measure that needs to be a part of all private and public dental coverage programs. When combined with fluorides, which protect enamel surfaces between teeth, a major caries reduction can be anticipated.

INFRASTRUCTURE FOR ORAL HEALTH

Dental disease can be debilitating. In 1989, over 164 million hours of work were missed because of dental problems. In addition, 117 hours of school were lost per 100 students.[5] Despite the morbidity associated with oral problems, the lack of life-threatening consequences makes it a low priority when compared to other social and health issues. This second-class status may contribute to the lack of emphasis given dental health in many arenas and, to some degree, to the infrastructural problems[2,6] at local, state, and national levels.

Dental health is administered by dozens of federal agencies. At the state level, resource allocation varies greatly, as does the oversight of oral health issues. Even though diversification and decentralization have some benefit, oral health is put at risk when there is no critical mass to advocate for effective programming, to advocate for funding, and for other important functions. An additional theme in dealing with infrastructural weakness in MCH oral health is the lack of a cohesive family focus for oral health. This has resulted in fragmentation of effort, failure to formulate standards, and failure to generate minimal and consistent guidance for clinical care programs.

An important consideration for the future is to consolidate efforts to develop a strong infrastructure for policy, clinical programming, research, development of standards, advocacy, and health care promotion. The recent creation of the National Oral Health Resource Center[26] is a beginning in consolidating information within a single database. Congressional efforts to produce an omnibus oral health bill to embrace current disparate federal programs under one banner is still a possibility, in spite of the tendency of the executive branch to the contrary.

INTEGRATION OF ORAL HEALTH INTO GENERAL HEALTH

In recent years, some effort has been made to integrate oral health into general health considerations. On the one hand, such an effort establishes competition for interest and resources; on the other, it consolidates oral health as an important health component. One notable example is the Bright Futures project, created to establish preventive health supervision guidelines for children.[27] This joint project of HCFA and MCHB of DHHS melded oral health into overall health considerations. Another example is the participation of oral health in state block grants. Seventy-five percent of federal funding for state dental programs comes from MCHB Block Grants to States, or about $12–15 million in a recent budget cycle.[26]

Additional integration is occurring slowly through networking with groups sharing MCH focus. Oral health is integrated in WIC programming and Head Start. Professional and child advocacy groups advocating for children have established coalitions and oral health related organizations have become a part of these efforts. In the private sector, professional groups like the American Academy of Pediatric Dentistry and the American Academy of Pediatrics have co-developed guidelines on sedation, child abuse, and other aspects of MCH that are shared.[28]

Recent research points to oral health and access to care as pivotal issues for special needs populations.[29] Team management, where oral and systemic health are integrated, is a successful approach to care for these groups. Management of children with craniofacial deformities, most commonly cleft lip and palate, provides one of the most successful models of integration of oral health into a health pathway. In most states, multidisciplinary teams manage the care of children with these deformities. Physicians, psychologists, speech and language therapists, and other health providers join with orthodontists, pediatric dentists, oral surgeons, and prosthodontists to render care to these children, beginning as early as in the first year of life. In response to a 1987 Surgeon General's report on children with special health care needs,[30] national standards were developed to guide the care of these children.[31] Even though strict protocols vary from team to team, these standards describe the appropriate interventions of surgery, audiology, dentistry, genetics, nursing, otolaryngology, pediatrics, psychology/social work, and speech and language, as well as credentialing and quality assurance. Some states utilize a handicapped children's service or bureau to ensure access and payment for services as well as to coordinate services in areas where team access is limited or non-existent.

Future improvement of oral health will require that integration continue and expand, and that the role of oral health in such MCH areas as systemic health, school readiness, behavior, and early development be clarified and better understood.

SUMMARY

Maternal and child oral health has improved over the last generation because of better preventive education, availability of dental care, and increased recognition of the role of preventive therapies including fluoride. The impact of oral health on systemic health has become clearer and presents opportunities to improve the health of mothers and children. Challenges remain as (1) the predominant dental diseases of dental caries and periodontal disease concentrate within the poor and minority populations and (2) access to dental care remains a significant problem for these groups. Public programs to finance oral health care must be revamped to give equal access to care to all, and research must be done to address lingering disease prevalence in the poor and minorities. Provider education must begin to account for social components of health care seeking behavior and cultural competency of those who serve the public in order to reduce oral health care disparities.

REFERENCES

1. USDHHS. *Oral Health in America: A Report of the Surgeon General.* Rockville, MD: USDHHS, NIDCR, 2000.

2. Steffensen JEM, Brown JP. Public Health Service Workshop on Oral Health of Mothers and Children: Background Issues Papers, September 10–12, 1989. *J Public Health Dent* 50: 355–472, 1990, Special Issue.

3. USDHHS. *Equity and Access for Mothers and Children, Strategies from the Public Health Workshop on Oral Health of Mothers and Children, September 9–12, 1989.* NCEMCH: Washington, DC, DHHS Publication No. HRS-MCH-90-4, 1990.

4. Association of Maternal and Child Health Programs. *Position Statement on Oral Health in Children and Youth.* 1993.

5. USPHS Oral Health Coordinating Committee. *Toward Improving the Oral Health of Americans: An Overview of Oral Health Status, Resources, and Care Delivery* (Final Draft), March, 1993.

6. Gift HC, Drury TF, Nowjack-Raymer RE, et al. The state of the nation's oral health: Mid-decade assessment of healthy people 2000. *J Public Health Dent* 56:84–91, 1996.

7. Nowak AJ, Johnsen D, Waldman HB, et al. *Pediatric Oral Health,* Center for Health Policy Research, George Washington University: Washington, DC, 1992.

8. Brunelle JA. *Oral Health of U.S. Schoolchildren. National and Regional Findings.* DHHS Publication No. (NIH) 89-2247. U.S. Government Printing Office, Washington, DC, 1989.

9. Brown LJ, Kingman A, Brunelle JA. Most U.S. schoolchildren are caries free: This is no myth. *Public Health Rep* 110:531–533, 1995.

10. American Academy of Pediatrics, Committee on Psychosocial Aspects of Child and Family Health. *Guidelines for Health Supervision.* AAP: Elk Grove, IL, 1988.

11. Edelstein BL, Douglass CW. Dispelling the myth that 50 percent of U.S. schoolchildren have never had a cavity. *Public Health Rep* 110:522–530, 1995.

12. Damiano PC, Kanellis MJ, Willard JC, et al. *A Report on the Iowa Title XIX Dental Program.* Public Policy Center and College of Dentistry, University of Iowa, Iowa City, April, 1996, pp. 21–22.

13. Nowak AJ. Rationale for the timing of the first oral evaluation. *Pediatri Dent* 19:8–11, 1998.

14. Benitez C, O'Sullivan D, Tinanoff N. Effect of a preventive approach for the treatment of nursing bottle caries. *ASDC J Dent Child* 61:46–49, 1994.

15. Albandar JM, Brown LJ, Loe H. Clinical features of early-onset periodontitis. *JADA* 128:1393–99, 1997.

16. Offenbacher S, Katz V, Fertig G, et al. Periodontal infection as a possible risk factor for preterm low birthweight. *J Periodontol* 67:1103–13, 1996.

17. Loesche WJ, Schork A, Terpenning MS. Assessing the relationship between dental disease and coronary heart disease in elderly U.S. veterans. *JADA* 129:301–311, 1998.

18. Bloom B, Gift HC, Jack SS. Dental Services and Oral Health; United States, 1989. National Center for Health Statistics. *Vital Health Stat* 10(183), 1992.

19. Centers for Disease Control and Prevention. Preview: *MMWR* 46:(50), December 19, 1997.

20. Edelstein BL. *Public Funding of Dental Coverage for Children: Medicaid, Medicaid Managed Care and State Programs.* Children's Dental Health Project: Washington, DC, 1998, p. 11.

21. U.S. Congress, Office of Technology Assessment: *Children's Health Services Under the Medicaid Program – Background Paper.* OTA-BP-H-78, US Government Printing Office: Washington, DC, October, 1990.

22. Department of Health and Human Services, Office of the Inspector General. *Children's Dental Services Under Medicaid, Access and Utilization.* US Government Printing Office: Washington, DC, OEI-09-93-00240, April, 1996.

23. Pendrys DG. Risk of fluorosis in a fluoridated population. *JADA* 126:1617–24, 1995.

24. PHS, Office of the Assistant Secretary for Health, Office of Disease Prevention and Health Promotion. *Healthy People 2000: National Health Promotion and Disease Prevention Objectives.* DHHS Publication No. (PHS) 91-50212. US Government Printing Office: Washington, DC, 1990.

25. Brown LJ, Kaste LM, Selwitz RH, et al. Dental caries and sealant usage in U.S. children 1988-91: Selected findings from the third national health and nutrition examination survey. *JADA* 127:335–43, 1996.

26. Rosetti J. Maternal and Child Health Bureau: *Oral Health Activities and Projects.* Unpublished report, 1998.

27. Green M. *Bright Futures: Guidelines for Health Supervision of Infants, Children and Adolescents.* National Center for Education in Maternal and Child Health: Arlington, VA, 1994.

28. American Academy of Pediatric Dentistry. Reference Manual 1994–95. *Pediatr Dent* 16:1–96, 1994.

29. Newacheck P, McManus M, Fox HB et al. Access to health care for children with special health care needs. *Pediatrics* 105: 760–66, 2000.

30. Office of Maternal and Child Health. *Surgeon General's Report: Children with Special Health Care Needs.* USDHHS, PHS: Washington, DC, June 1987.

31. American Cleft Palate-Craniofacial Association. *Parameters for Evaluation and Treatment of Patients with Cleft Lip/Palate or Other Craniofacial Anomalies,* March 1993.

ARTICLE 6

THE PROGRESS AND POTENTIAL
OF INJURY PREVENTION

Allen Bolton, Martha Stowe,
Paul Boumbulian, and Mary McCoy

INTRODUCTION

"I never thought it would happen to us." This is a refrain often heard in emergency rooms of children's hospitals throughout the nation. Injuries happen suddenly and seemingly unexpectedly, but the impact may be long lasting. The welfare of a family can change in an instant as a result of a car wreck, a fall, a drowning, or a blast of gunshot. In fact, injuries are the leading cause of death for persons aged 1 to 44.

The costs of injuries can be staggering financially and emotionally. The cost of injury in the United States in 1996 was $260 billion.[1] Viewed another way, each year in our country injuries cost the equivalent of $960 per man, woman, and child. The emotional cost of learning to live without a limb, eyesight, or a loved one cannot be measured.

The good news is that injuries are preventable. Great strides are being made in developing interventions that reduce injuries.

INJURIES IN PERSPECTIVE

Definitions

An injury is physical damage to the body caused by acute exposure to mechanical, chemical, thermal, or electrical energy, or by the absence of essentials such as heat or oxygen. Without a transfer of energy, injury does not occur.[2,3]

Injuries are not accidents. "Accident" implies randomness or unpredictability, traits which are uncharacteristic of injuries.[3-6] Robertson writes that "accident is also intertwined with the notion that some human error or behavior is responsible for most injuries." That focus detracts from examinations and interventions that

385

would include the multitude of other factors that contribute to injuries and their severity.[7] These other factors are often more amenable to change than is human behavior, thereby breaking the causal chain of events that would otherwise lead to injury. The causal chain or epidemiological triangle will be explained later in this article.

Injuries in a Public Health Perspective

Injuries are a public health problem. In a landmark publication, public health leader Dr. William Foege stated, "Injury is the principal public health problem in America today (1985)." His statement was based on the impact of injuries on the health of the population. He and the Committee on Trauma Research explained that, historically, injury and infectious diseases have been the major causes of premature death throughout the world.[3,6] Since the beginning of the 20th century, public health measures have significantly reduced infectious disease mortality. However, public health has devoted relatively little attention and few resources to the prevention of injury. Figure 1 illustrates significant downturns in death rates from four infectious diseases between 1910 and 1999, while relatively little

FIGURE 1

Death rates from injuries and infectious diseases by year, 1910–1999

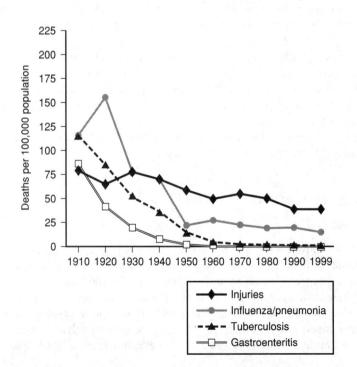

progress was made in the reduction of injury deaths.[4] Public health interventions were key to each dramatic decrease in these infectious disease categories. For example, enactment of the nation's first Water Quality Standards Act and the widespread adoption of pasteurization of milk in the early 20th century are public health interventions that contributed to large reductions in the death rate from gastroenteritis.[8] Public health, as you will read in this chapter, did not become significantly involved in injury prevention until the 1980s.[6,9,10]

Magnitude of the Injury Problem

In 1998, there were 146,941 injury deaths in the United States resulting in an age-adjusted death rate of 48.3 per 100,000 population. This represents 6% of all deaths in the United States.[11] Additionally, 8% of all hospital discharges and 37% of all emergency room visits were due to injury in 1998.[12,13] There were 13.8 emergency department visits for injury per 100 U.S. residents.[13] Office-based physicians treated another 89.8 million trauma patients during the same year. This is equal to 33.3 visits per 100 persons and represents 10.8% of all physician office visits.[14] Overall, injuries are responsible for 12% of medical spending in the United States or about $44 billion in direct health care costs per year.[9,15,16] Medical care for trauma represents the second largest category of medical expenditures in the United States.[1,17] Figure 2 depicts the volume of injuries that our health care system encountered in 1998.

FIGURE 2

Burden of injury: United States, 1998

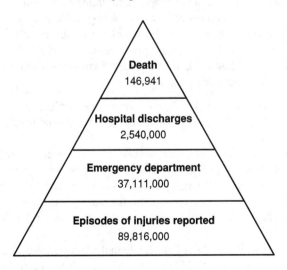

Injury is the fourth leading cause of death for the entire human life span but has a disproportionate impact on children and youth. Between the ages of 1 and 44, it is the leading cause of death in our country.[1,11] In fact, injuries are the leading cause of life-years lost.[4,18] More than 4 million years of potential life are lost prematurely due to injuries.[19] For children aged 1–4, injuries account for 45% of all deaths. For older children aged 5–14, they are responsible for 52% of all deaths. Seventeen percent of childhood hospitalizations are related to injury.[1]

The largest numbers of injury deaths were for age groups 15–24, 25–34, and 35–44. By ages 45–54 and 55–64, deaths from diseases of the heart and malignant neoplasms are three and four times the total number of injury deaths in those respective age groups. For the population over age 65, the incidence of injury is lower than in any other age group, but elderly patients are more likely to die from their injuries. Injury is the seventh leading cause of death among this age group.[11]

Intentional and Unintentional Injuries. Injuries are categorized as intentional or unintentional. Intentional injuries are inflicted with the purpose of causing harm or death. Intentional injuries include homicide, suicide, physical, sexual, emotional abuse, and assault. Unintentional injuries do not result from an intention to do harm or be harmed. Unintentional injuries may include falls, car wrecks, drowning, poisoning, and burns.[3]

Unintentional injuries were responsible for 67% of injury-related deaths in 1998. The leading cause of fatal unintentional injuries was motor vehicles followed by falls, poisonings, suffocation, burns, and drownings. In each of these categories there were also fatalities classified as intentional. Among intentional injury deaths, 63% are classified as suicides. Firearms are the leading mechanism of fatal injury for homicides and suicides, representing nearly two-thirds and over one-half of the deaths in these categories, respectively.[11]

In 1998, motor vehicle injuries represented 28.8% of all injury deaths (78% of which were to motor vehicle occupants, 13% to pedestrians, and 6% to motorcyclists).[11,20] Firearms were responsible for 20.9% of the fatalities. Poisonings were third with 12.5% of the total, and falls accounted for 9.1%. Suffocation represented 7.5% of the fatalities. Drownings and burns were responsible for 3.5% and 2.3% of the deaths in each category.[11]

Fatal and Nonfatal Injuries. Leading causes or mechanisms of injury vary by age categories. Table 1 details the leading causes of fatal and nonfatal injury for different age groups.

Risk of injury and death also varies greatly by sex, race, and income level. Unintentional and intentional injury death rates are higher for males than for females in each age group. The rate of nonfatal injury is also higher for males in all age categories up to age 65. At that point, the rate for females begins to exceed males.[21] The death rate for injuries for the least-educated was three times the rate for the most-educated adults.[22]

In 1998, the age-adjusted injury death rate in the United States was 22% lower than in 1981.[23] The majority of this decrease occurred in the early 1980s and can be largely attributed to improvements in transportation safety. In Table 2, the age-adjusted death rates for unintentional injuries show impressive reductions for all

TABLE 1 LEADING FATAL AND NONFATAL INJURIES BY AGE

Ranking of Mechanism of Injury

Age	Fatal	Nonfatal
0–1	Suffocation Motor vehicle	Falls Motor vehicle
1–4	Drowning Motor vehicle	Falls Struck by person/object
5–14	Motor vehicle Firearms	Falls Struck by person/object
15–24	Motor vehicle Firearms	Motor vehicle Struck by person/object
25–64	Motor vehicle Firearms	Falls Motor vehicle
65+	Falls Motor vehicle	Falls Motor vehicle

Source: Table compiled from sources 11 and 21.

TABLE 2 AGE-ADJUSTED DEATH RATES FOR INJURY BY ETHNICITY

	All Races	White	Black	Hispanic
Unintentional Injuries				
1950	57.5	55.7	70.9	NA
1998	29.2	28.7	35.4	27.4
Homicide				
1950	5.4	2.6	30.5	NA
1998	7.2	3.2	25.9	9.8
Suicide				
1950	11.0	11.6	4.2	NA
1998	10.4	11.8	6.1	6.0

Source: Compiled from data in source 21, updated with web-based Injury Statistic Query and Reporting System, CDC http://www.cdc.goc/nicpc/wisquars.html.

ethnic categories during the past half-century. Data on Hispanic residents were not reported for 1950. In 1998, the homicide rate was the lowest in three decades. Despite the overall decline in homicide mortality, it is still the leading cause of death for young black males 15–24 years of age.[22] Suicide rates have remained relatively stable during this period.

Risk Factor for Injuries. Unintentional injuries and homicide occur more often in low-income populations. In fact, studies reveal that socio-economic status is more closely associated with injury rates, excluding suicide, than is ethnicity.[1,4,24] In a recent study of injuries and deaths in house fires in Dallas, Texas, low-income populations were shown to be at significantly higher risk of injury than those with high median income (relative risk of 8.1).[25] See Figure 3.

A significant risk factor for unintentional and intentional injuries is alcohol. For motor vehicle-related incidents, approximately 20% of serious injuries and 50% of fatalities are related to alcohol use. Likewise, studies indicate alcohol may be involved in as many as half of all residential injury deaths. For intentional injuries, alcohol is also a major contributor. Various studies of violence have found alcohol involved in 33% to 60% of homicides and in a high proportion of

FIGURE 3

Annual rate of injuries related to house fires and prevalence of functioning smoke detectors in houses that have had a fire, according to the median income of the census tract, in Dallas from 1991 to 1997

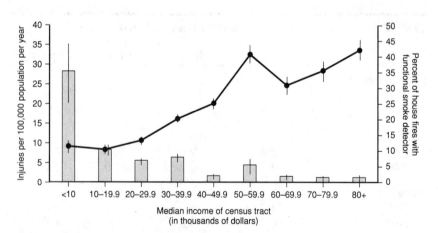

Columns represent the annual rates of injury (injuries per 100,000 population per year). The curve represents the prevalence of functioning smoke detectors (percentage of house fires in houses with functioning smoke detectors). Vertical bars represent standard errors

Source: New England Journal of Medicine, 2001; Vol. 344, No. 25: 1911–1919. Reprinted with permission.

nonfatal injuries. The contributory effect of the use of other drugs on the incidence of injury has also been documented; however, the role of alcohol is better understood and is a more prevalent drug.[3]

HISTORY OF INJURY PREVENTION

Tracing the Roots

In the early part of the 20th century injury prevention efforts focused largely on the "fault" or behavior of the victims with little consideration or understanding of other variables that helped produce injury. It was the work of Hugh De Haven in 1942 that first looked at methods of preventing injury other than changing human behavior. As a World War I pilot who survived a crash, he studied how vehicle and restraint system designs could minimize the damage done by crash forces. He demonstrated that humans can be "crash packaged" in automobiles so that in the event of a crash, the human body can be protected.[3]

A few years later in 1949, John E. Gordon was the first to characterize injuries like classic infectious diseases. He identified epidemic episodes, seasonal variation, geographical, socio-economic, and rural–urban distributions for trauma. Gordon recognized that injuries are not caused by a single cause but by the interaction of forces between an agent and host in a permissive environment. Although this line of thinking was correct and significantly advanced the understanding of injury epidemiology, Gordon's description of agents was not accepted.

In 1961 James Gibson, an experimental psychologist at Cornell University, was the first to actually delineate the agents of injuries as physical energy, "either mechanical, thermal, radiant, chemical or electrical."[2] Shortly after Gibson's paper was published, Dr. William Haddon, Jr. modified the description of energy transfer to include negative agents, that is, the absence of heat or oxygen.[3] Dr. Haddon, a physician-epidemiologist, developed his analysis into preventive approaches. He is widely regarded as the founding father of injury prevention. In 1966, Dr. Haddon became the first administrator of what is known today as the National Highway Traffic Safety Administration. For many years after that government appointment he was the president of the Insurance Institute for Highway Safety. In both roles, he made significant contributions to the safety of transportation in the United States.

By 1983, a handful of professionals across the country were conducting research on the causes and prevention of trauma. In that year Congress commissioned a study of injury research, and the role of government in injury prevention and treatment. In response, the Institute of Medicine (IOM) convened a Committee on Trauma that published its findings and recommendations in the landmark publication *Injury in America*.[3,6] Congress responded to the Committee's recommendations by appropriating funds for the establishment of a federal lead agency for injury prevention at the CDC. The Division of Injury Epidemiology and Control (DIEC) was established at CDC in 1985.

In 1989, a Committee was reconvened to review the progress of DIEC. The result was a recommendation to Congress that the issue warranted Center rather than Division status at CDC. In 1992, the National Center for Injury Prevention and Control (NCIPC) was created from the DIEC. It is the primary federal agency responsible for injury prevention research outside of transportation safety. In 1997, another Committee on Trauma was convened by the IOM for the purpose of reviewing progress within the field since 1985 and making recommendations about the future of injury prevention. Their report, Reducing the Burden of Injury, was released in 1999.[1]

Basic Concepts/Underlying Principles—The Epidemiological Approach

Haddon, Baker, Robertson, and others have explained the epidemiological triangle that has been applied to the study of diseases is also applicable to injuries.[2,4,7,26,27] The epidemiological triangle has at its three points: (1) agent, (2) host, and (3) environment. All three factors must interact to cause disease or injury. Every injury is produced when an *agent* transfers energy to a *host* or human body in an *environment* that permits and even facilitates injury. For example, a speeding, unhelmeted, teenage motorcyclist (host) driving a bike that is capable of speeds over 150 mph (agent) on a dark, rain-slick rural road (environment) is a scenario in which injury is probable. Thus, interventions to prevent diseases or injuries alter or eliminate one or more of these factors.

Haddon further refined our understanding of injury causation when he conceptualized the Haddon Matrix. See Figure 4. The matrix examines agent, host, and environmental factors over three time periods relevant to injury production and severity: pre-event, event, post-event. The matrix clearly shows the preventive value of the epidemiologic view in traumatic events.

FIGURE 4

The Haddon Matrix

Factors*

Phases	Agent/Energy	Host/Human	Environment
Pre-event	Exceeding speed limit	Drinking alcohol	Poor visibility
Event	No airbag	Unrestrained occupant	No divided road
Post-event	Gas tank wall	Frail elderly occupant	Rapid EMS time

*Example uses a motor vehicle collision.

The pre-event phase covers factors that determine whether a potentially injury-producing event will occur. The event phase includes factors that determine whether injuries are produced by the event. And the post-event phase includes factors that determine if injury severity can be reduced.[3,28]

Prevention Stages

Applying epidemiology to injuries underscores their preventable nature. Injuries are not random events. They are caused by the alignment of factors that can be both anticipated and altered. In other words, injuries are predictable and controllable.

There are three possible prevention stages, sometimes called *injury control*. The first stage, *primary prevention*, is the prevention of the incident that might have caused the injury. Avoiding a car wreck by utilizing a designated (sober) driver exemplifies primary prevention. The second stage, *secondary prevention*, involves preventing or reducing the severity of injury once a traumatic incident (i.e., a car wreck, a fight, etc.) occurs. The use of safety belts and the deployment of airbags in a collision are two examples of secondary prevention techniques. The third stage, *tertiary prevention*, consists of efforts to reduce morbidity after injury and restore injury victims to maximum functional potential. Proper nursing care using special cushions, beds, and weight-relief techniques are tertiary prevention methods aimed at preventing pressure sores in patients with spinal cord and traumatic brain injuries.[29-31]

Prevention Strategies

Injury prevention or control strategies can be categorized as active or passive. Generally, *passive strategies*, or those that work automatically and do not require any action on the part of the individual(s) being protected, have been most successful. Engineering changes that have made roadways less hazardous are passive strategies that have saved thousands of lives during the past three decades. *Active strategies* require that people alter their behavior and repeat the new, safer behavior every time they are exposed to a certain risk. Wearing a helmet when riding a motorcycle is an active injury prevention strategy that requires considerable effort and some expense on the part of the motorcyclist. Those at risk must believe the justification for this safe behavior, select and buy the safety device, and wear the helmet each time they ride. Most injury prevention strategies combine both active and passive elements, but those that emphasize a passive approach have resulted in greater sustained reductions in injury.[2,27,29,32]

In addition to the active/passive categorization, injury prevention countermeasures have traditionally fallen into one of three strategies: (1) engineering or technology, (2) enforcement of policies/regulations, and (3) education.[3,6,18] The work of groups such as the Injury Prevention Center of Greater Dallas suggests that a fourth strategy of "community change" can be added.

Engineering is a passive injury prevention strategy that has led to significant reduction in injuries throughout the 20th century. Safer roads, safer automobiles, safer toys, safer residential and commercial construction, and safer drug packaging are all examples of engineering or technological interventions that have reduced injury.

Safety policies or regulations and their enforcement are important for the reduction of certain types of trauma. In 1978, Tennessee became the first state to pass a law requiring small children to be transported in child safety seats. Passage of the law resulted in a modest increase in child-safety seat usage. However, the greatest impact came after law enforcement agencies in the state began enforcing the law. Regulatory interventions are effective but somewhat less so than technological interventions. One reason is that with regulations some action is required by the individual being protected, which means that individuals cannot assume an entirely passive role. Additionally, the effectiveness of policies may be highly dependent upon the manner and consistency of enforcement efforts, or upon the public's perception of their enforcement.[9]

Educational interventions can be effective, especially in combination with other strategies, but alone they are the least effective of the three single strategies. Education is an active strategy. After safety information is communicated to at-risk individuals, it is necessary for those receiving the message to change personal behavior each time they are at risk. Some well-designed, well-executed educational interventions have been shown to be effective at reducing trauma. The Willy Whistle pedestrian safety curriculum and The Injury Prevention Project (TIPP) of the American Academy of Pediatrics are two such examples.[3,33] However, education is most effectively used as a complementary effort to other types of injury countermeasures.

Haddon's 10 Strategies. Between 1962 and 1970 Haddon developed and refined a list of 10 strategies to interfere with the transfer of energy that produces injury. These strategies are inclusive of the active/passive categorization and address primary, secondary, and tertiary prevention. They are:

1. Prevent the creation of the hazard
2. Reduce the amount/quantity of the hazard
3. Prevent the release of a hazard that already exists
4. Modify the rate or spatial distribution of the hazard
5. Separate, in time or space, the hazard from that which is to be protected
6. Separate the hazard from that which is to be protected by a material barrier
7. Modify relevant basic qualities of the hazard
8. Make what is to be protected more resistant to damage from the hazard
9. Begin to counter the damage already done by the hazard
10. Stabilize, repair, and rehabilitate the object of the damage[2,3]

Changing the social norms and expectations of a community about safety is also a strategy to prevent injuries. Two decades of success in child-restraint device usage and in alcohol-impaired driving have been largely due to a shift in societal norms related to these two injury prevention issues.[1] If the community mores include the view that drinking and driving is unacceptable, there will be a decrease in drinking and driving. If the community is appalled by children riding unrestrained, more children will be restrained. The values of a community dictate the behavior of the community. The task becomes to work with the community to change or develop the values of the community in ways that encourage safe behavior. Social norms can be influenced by legislation, enforcement, and grassroots movements such as Mothers Against Drunk Driving (MADD) on a national scale or the Lidköping example of the world's first Safe Community.[34]

FUTURE OF INJURY PREVENTION

Population Demographics

Between 2000 and 2050, the population of the United States is expected to increase 47% from 275 million to 404 million. With this increase the population will become more racially diverse and the number of those over age 65 is expected to grow 196%. Among ethnic groups, the projected growth of the Hispanic population is expected to rise from 12% of the population in 2000 to 24% of the population in 2050, a particularly impressive growth (see Figure 5).

FIGURE 5

U.S. population projections by race/ethnicity

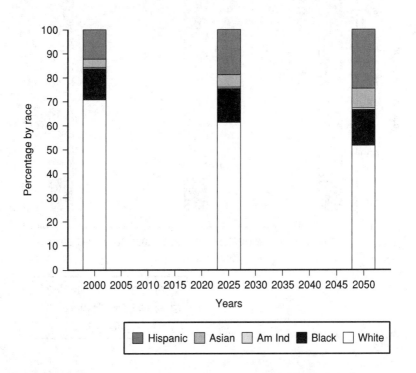

These population projections will affect the future of trauma care and injury prevention because injury patterns vary across ethnic populations. The growth in the proportion and number of Hispanic residents will thus be challenging from an injury perspective. Hispanics are at disproportionate risk for transportation-related injuries, injuries resulting from violence, and injuries involving alcohol.[21]

In fact, the increasing diversity of the U.S. population is expected to amplify existing cultural and attitudinal differences among racial and ethnic groups in regard to injury prevention. A new "breed" of injury prevention professionals that are competent to deal with these differences will be needed.

During the second decade of the 21st century, the proportion of elderly residents will rise dramatically.[35] By 2050, one in four Americans will be over age 64.[36,37] Every age group will grow during the next 50 years, but the increase in the number of residents over age 64 will be particularly challenging from an injury-prevention standpoint. The elderly have the highest rates of hospitalization for injury and the highest fatality rates for injury over any other age groups[4] (see Figure 6).

FIGURE 6

U.S. population projections by age

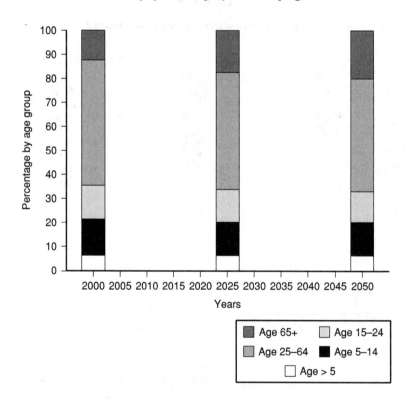

Intervening at the Clinical Level–The Medical Model

The Ongoing Provision of Trauma Care. States and health care providers have established trauma care systems that are regional or statewide networks of acute care facilities for the treatment of trauma patients. Fully developed trauma care systems provide injury prevention strategies through policy and education; prompt recognition of injurious events with rapid response by emergency medical services; advanced communication and medical control for EMS; on-scene triage and transportation to appropriate medical facilities; designated trauma care facilities; interfacility transfer agreements; rehabilitation facilities; and standardized trauma care data systems.[38] Studies have shown that preventable injury deaths decrease after implementation of trauma care systems. Nevertheless, less than one-quarter of the U.S. population is served by these systems.[39,40]

Trauma centers, particularly Level I trauma centers, are the hub of trauma systems. One of the main reasons for fledgling efforts to develop trauma care systems is the economic instability of designated trauma centers. A study of trauma center closures identified the level of uncompensated care, high operating costs, and inadequate reimbursement from government medical assistance programs as the three primary reasons hospitals discontinue trauma services.[17] Particularly vulnerable from an economic standpoint are trauma centers located in large urban areas. Their vulnerability is due to the large volume of poor and uninsured injured patients they treat.[41,42]

The survival of trauma centers and the expansion of trauma systems in the United States is desirable and will be dependent upon the ability to manage the demand for trauma care services. Demand management limits the number of people who need the service and provides only the appropriate level of care for those who are in need of it. The key strategy for managing the demand for trauma care services is to prevent injuries.[17,42–44]

The Incorporation of Prevention into Clinical Practice. By providing routine medical care to injured patients, medical personnel are involved in tertiary prevention. However, studies and expert opinion indicate an increasing need for and efficacy of physician involvement in primary prevention of injuries.[18,30,33,45–48] There are at least three roles for physicians in injury prevention:

1. *Screening and counseling.* The physician's role in screening and counseling patients to modify high-risk behaviors is a proven strategy to reduce injuries and is a role that should be expanded. Particularly impressive is the involvement of pediatricians in this role over the past decade. Evaluation of The Injury Prevention Program (TIPP), an office-based counseling schedule developed by the American Academy of Pediatrics, has shown a 13:1 benefit-cost ratio.[33]

2. *Advocacy.* Physicians can influence public policy regarding trauma prevention. Dr. Abraham Bergman, a Seattle pediatrician, was instrumental in the adoption of national standards for fire-retardant material in children's sleepwear, and Dr. Robert Sanders lobbied the Tennessee legislature (and subsequently many other state legislatures) to achieve passage of the nation's first mandatory child safety seat law.[3]

3. *Collaborative research.* Scientists in other areas, such as epidemiology, economics, and sociology can contribute to injury prevention research, but the physicians who treat injured patients have perspectives and insights that are invaluable to collaborative research.

Each of these three roles will require significant modification in the manner in which physicians are trained.[18,38] Institutions will also need to re-examine physicians' performance and perhaps alter how physician compensation is determined.

Intervening at the Community Level–The Public Health Model

At this point in the evolution of the field of injury prevention and control, many "easy gains" have come through passive strategies such as technology and the semi-passive strategy of legislation/enforcement. Although there is still work that can be done to advance these types of strategies, the very active strategy of enlisting community participation is a primary new direction.

Community participation is "the involvement of people in designing and implementing research and interventions intended to benefit them."[49] There are varying degrees of participation from shared decision making at one end of the spectrum through passive compliance to tokenism. Green emphasizes that the more engaged community members are, the more successful the project is likely to be.[50] Although the concept has been around health care since at least the 1960s, the power of community participation was first recognized in the 1980s North Karelia Project. This program sought to reduce cardiovascular disease risk factors such as smoking, cholesterol, obesity, and others in a community in Finland. Residents became alarmed to learn of their community's excessive mortality rates and initiated the project's media efforts, counseling, and education programs; food labeling efforts; and other activities with the aid of health professionals. After 15 years of experience, the North Karelia Project not only reduced risk factors, but it actually produced a decrease in heart disease mortality.[50] Other examples of injury prevention programs that have incorporated community participation to change risky behavior and reduce the incidence of trauma are slowly emerging.[51–56]

Dr. David Satcher, the assistant Secretary of Health, stated in the mid 1990s, "If public health doesn't work at the level of the community, it doesn't work." He was referring to a new initiative at CDC, Safe America, which was aimed at translating knowledge about injury prevention into action within communities. Even though the program at CDC was new, the idea was not. The World Health Organization (WHO) began testing and promoting such community-level strategies in Sweden in 1978.[53] The WHO model for community-based injury prevention has now been embraced and refined by the U.S. government's two lead agencies on injury prevention, the National Center for Injury Prevention and Control and the National Highway Traffic Safety Administration.

Safe Communities. The Safe Community model includes several steps. Data are collected to identify where, how, when, and to whom injuries are occurring. Stakeholders in a community are gathered to consider the data and choose the issue to address. Proven interventions are chosen by the community with the help of injury professionals. The interventions are implemented with the community. Throughout the process evaluation is conducted to assure that in fact a reduction in injuries has occurred as a result of the interventions.[29,34] In the United States, work from groups such as the Injury Prevention Center of Greater Dallas has been able to demonstrate that the Safe Communities model works to enhance safety. Working with an extremely impoverished, young, first-generation Hispanic population near downtown Dallas, the Center and community were able to increase child safety-seat usage from 18% to over 80% over five years. This usage rate has been sustained in this densely populated neighborhood for over two years.

Challenges in Injury Prevention

The primary challenges facing injury-prevention professionals as we begin an era of working with communities to reduce injury are: (1) evaluation, (2) health systems bias, (3) a breakdown in society's traditional sense of community, and (4) a lack of understanding by the community of the need and efficacy of injury prevention.

Challenge: Evaluation. Evaluation methods for community-level interventions are difficult because they do not conform to traditional notions of evaluation. They are not performed in a controlled environment, they may be extremely long term, or they may rely upon indicators or surrogate measures rather than true outcomes. Research needs for the future are outlined later in this chapter, but they will be important for their impact on appropriate evaluation strategies for community-level interventions. Especially appropriate for evaluation of community-participation programs are the recommendations made for more prevention research and analytic epidemiologic studies. Schwab and Syme claim the information we gather from participatory interventions is not "normal science." It is not normal because it is not driven by scientists but by the community. It does not seek universal truths but local or situational truths. Nevertheless, practitioners must embrace the "experience and partnership of those we are normally content simply to measure."[49]

Challenge: Health Systems Bias. A second major obstacle is something we term *health systems bias.* Injury-prevention professionals typically receive little or no training in community development, and few seem to appreciate the skills necessary to be successful in such an uncontrolled environment. The majority of injury prevention professionals are affiliated with health systems, such as hospitals, academic medical centers, and health departments. This affiliation is likely to set up working barriers because there is a stark contrast between the values of such a system and the values of communities. Systems value hierarchical top-down order while communities value active consent of the people. Systems depend upon clients or consumers while communities depend upon citizens. In Greek, the root word for *client* means "one who is controlled." *Citizen* means "one who holds the power."[57]

Another difference is that health systems define people and communities by disease or injury problems. This perspective is that communities are a collection of deficiencies while communities define themselves according to their capacities or assets. Finally, systems produce standardized outcomes while communities require creativity to produce unique outcomes.[57]

Challenge: Interconnectedness of Community. The third obstacle we identify is a growing loss of society's traditional "sense of community." Communities have traditionally been a group of individuals with a high degree of interconnectedness provided by geographic proximity and shared economic, religious, cultural, ethnic, or political values.[48] This interconnectedness is what we define as a *sense of community.* The continuing breakdown of extended family networks and the increasing mobility of individuals are factors that negatively affect this sense of interconnectedness among citizens. Today, *community* is often defined by a workplace, a club, a church, or other more institutional setting rather than by the location where one lives. Any such community units may be engaged in injury control. Injury prevention specialists must be able to identify appropriate community units in which to anchor intervention strategies.

Challenge: Engaging the Population. Although most of the population understands the threat of HIV or cancer, few would name injuries as a dire health issue. The fourth challenge to injury prevention professionals is to help the population understand that injuries are a threatening health issue and that injuries can be prevented. Earlier in this chapter, we spoke of the need to address and change some social norms in order to effect change in injury-related behaviors of the population. Techniques to raise the priority communities place on injury risks must be appreciated and learned by injury-prevention specialists.

Needs Within the Field of Injury Prevention

Research. Ultimately, injury-prevention efforts have one or more of the following goals: to reduce the incidence of injury, the severity of injury, or the costs associated with injuries. To accomplish any of these ideals, research to determine the effectiveness of injury prevention efforts must be increased.[6,10,45,58] This type of prevention research should be conducted with community-level practitioners in mind. Prevention studies should consider the feasibility of replicating, within communities, prevention initiatives that have fared well under "study conditions." Injury-prevention programs must be subjected to evaluation; the results must be reported in the professional literature and disseminated widely to practitioners at the community level.

Although descriptive epidemiological studies have dominated injury prevention research to date and continue to have some value, Rivara and Wolf advocate a larger commitment to analytic epidemiology. Analytic epidemiology uses case-control or cohort designs to discern causal factors that influence the risk of injury. By identifying causal factors, these types of studies are more likely to yield information that will result in the development of effective intervention strategies.[58] These types of studies require more resources, planning, and analytic capabilities than descriptive studies but yield superior information for prevention.

Descriptive epidemiological studies continue to be warranted if they address significant injury issues within the population. Much of the previous research of this type has focused on injury issues that are of academic interest yet of little interest or value to communities. Research that examines injuries that are "frequent but of low severity, infrequent and severe, or both infrequent and not severe" is common, costly, and has relatively little value in the actual prevention of trauma.[58] However, injuries that are frequent, severe, and for which there are not definitive descriptive studies are important to investigate.[33,34,58] The involvement of trauma care personnel, including EMS, emergency physicians, trauma surgeons, emergency nurses, or medical examiners/coroners, in the selection of injury-prevention research issues may help investigators avoid conducting irrelevant descriptive studies.

The primary question to be asked of any injury-prevention researcher, whether conducting a prevention, analytic epidemiologic, or descriptive epidemiologic study, is "does the study provide *new* information that will lead to the better understanding of and prevention of injury within the population?" With extremely limited research resources in this area, if the answer to this question is no, the study should be abandoned in favor of more practical research applications.[4,58]

Data. Implicit in the discussion so far in this chapter is the need for data on which to base injury-prevention priorities and judge the effectiveness of injury-prevention efforts. There are currently significant gaps in our understanding of the incidence, causes, and costs of injuries. To improve the quality of the information available to injury-prevention practitioners, the following actions are necessary.

The International Classification of Disease Codes (ICD-9 and ICD-10 codes), which is a worldwide classification system for diagnoses used by health care facilities, includes a Supplemental Classification of External Causes of Injury and Poisoning (E-codes). ICD-9 is the ninth revision of the classification system that has been in use since 1980. ICD-10 is the tenth revision released in 1993 and implemented in the United States in 1999. ICD codes are widely used by health care facilities largely because they are directly tied to reimbursement. The supplemental E-codes provide information on the mechanism of injury (e.g., automobile crash, bicycle crash, and fall). Increasing the reporting of E-codes on emergency department and hospital admission/discharge databases is a priority for the next century.[3,6,38,47,59]

Linking various injury databases would also provide information that would enhance the prevention of injuries. The first category for which this linking capacity is being developed is motor vehicle crashes.[60,61] Traffic crash records from law enforcement are being successfully linked to medical records from EMS, hospitals, and, in some cases, coroners. Other categories of injury such as fires and violence are also appropriate targets for linkage efforts.[25,47,48,59,61] Even though efforts to link such information raise concerns about issues such as confidentiality and propriety, advances in computer technology and in society's increasing ability to manage information are expected to make the linkage of such injury databases commonplace. Some communities are organizing each of the response groups to use common identifiers that will greatly enhance the ability to link data.

Another pressing data need is the development and implementation of uniform data sets for trauma care and rehabilitation. Currently, we do not know the extent to which acute care and rehabilitation systems are utilized. Nor do we know the overall efficacy, including the cost-effectiveness, of such systems. To realistically look at the continuum of injury prevention from primary through tertiary phases, such a uniform system is necessary.[38,59] In each of the enhanced injury surveillance systems described in this section, there is needed a uniform method for assessing and coding injury severity and data from which injury costs can be calculated.[45,47]

Understanding and Expertise in Community-Based Interventions

Injury-prevention efforts must be based in agencies or institutions that lend themselves to community-based interventions. Injury-prevention professionals must understand both injury prevention and community development. Successful health system/community interactions appear to depend on at least four practices of professionals with the systems: (1) professionals should not take a lead role in community programs, and they must demonstrate that they respect the wisdom of the community; (2) professionals have useful health information for citizens that should be shared in understandable forms; (3) professionals should use their resources to expand the power of citizens and the community instead of bringing attention or resources to the system; and (4) professionals should not look at the injury (or deficit) as what is important but should look at the community's capacities (or assets) to deal with such issues.[57]

Human and Financial Resources. Finally, no chapter on the future of injury prevention would be complete without the admonition that more resources are needed in order for the field to meet its life- and cost-savings potential. Resources are needed in two areas: personnel and funding. The need for additional training of medical personnel has already been cited. There is also a need for increasing the number of other scientists whose primary research focus is injury prevention and for increasing the number of community-level injury prevention practitioners. Without a properly trained "workforce" in this area, the field cannot advance. Injury-prevention experts need to come from a variety of fields including social work, media relations, public health, community development, and education. Training will come from a combination of the increasing number of colleges and universities that offer courses in injury prevention, from health departments and other agencies that offer workshops and seminars, and from an explosion of injury-prevention information available through professional publications and electronic media such as the Internet.

Financial resources are also necessary. It was estimated in the early 1990s that approximately 3% of health care funding was spent on prevention of any kind. The proportion spent on injury prevention was a fraction of 1%.[6,18] In perspective, in the 1980s injuries were the leading cause of premature life-years lost followed by cardiovascular diseases and cancers. Yet, federal funding for injury prevention was one-tenth that for cancer and one-sixth that for cardiovascular diseases.[6,10,45]

Since the 1980s HIV/AIDS has become a leading cause of premature death while funding for AIDS research has grown commensurate with its increasing threat to society. Injury prevention should receive funding in proportion to its impact on the health of the nation. It is recommended that governments not be the only sources to increase their spending on injury prevention. The corporate and non-profit sectors also have a lot to gain from investing in injury-prevention research and programs. However, potential funding agencies need to understand that a long-term investment is needed because change at the community level takes time. It may take five or more years to see a change in targeted injury rates.

REFERENCES

1. Bonnie RJ, Fulco CE, Liverman CT (Eds). *Reducing the burden of injury: Advancing prevention and treatment.* Washington, DC: National Academy Press; 1999.

2. Haddon W. Advances in the epidemiology of injuries as a basis for public policy. *Pub Health Reports* 1980;95:411–421.

3. National Committee for Injury Prevention and Control. *Injury prevention, meeting the challenge.* New York City, New York: Oxford University Press; 1989.

4. Baker SP, O'Neill B, Ginsburg MJ, Li G. The injury fact book, second edition. New York City, New York: Oxford University Press; 1992.

5. Christoffel T, Teret SP. *Protecting the public, legal issues in injury prevention.* New York City, New York: Oxford University Press; 1993.

6. National Research Council and the Institute of Medicine. *Injury in America, a continuing public health problem.* Washington, DC: National Academy Press; 1985.

7. Robertson L. *Injury epidemiology.* New York City, New York: Oxford University Press, 1992.

8. Hanlon JJ, Pickett GE. *Public health administration and practice, eighth edition.* St. Louis, MO: Times Mirror/Mosby College Publishing; 1984.

9. Bolton A, Boumbulian P, Anderson A. Public health enemy number one: Injury in America. *Metropolitan Universities* 1995;6:23–34.

10. Committee to Review the Status and Progress of the Injury Control Program at the Centers for Disease Control. *Injury control.* Washington, DC: National Academy Press; 1988.

11. Murphy SL. *Deaths: Final data for 1998. National vital statistics reports, 48(11).* Hyattsville, MD: National Center for Health Statistics; 2000.

12. Popovic JR, Hall MJ. *1998 National hospital discharge survey, advance data from vital and health statistics, (316).* Hyattsville, MD: National Center for Health Statistics; 2000.

13. McCaig LF, Burt CW. *National hospital ambulatory medical care survey: 1999 emergency department summary, (313).* Hyattsville, MD: National Center for Health Statistics; 2000.

14. Woodwell DA. *National hospital ambulatory medical care survey: 1998 summary, (315).* Hyattsville, MD: National Center for Health Statistics; 2000.

15. Rivara FP, Grossman DC, Cummings P. Injury prevention, first of two parts. *NEJM* 1997;337:543–548.

16. Miller TR, Lestina DC, Galbraith MS, Viano DC. Medical care spending—United States. *MMWR* 1994;43:581–586.

17. Elliott DC, Rodriguez A. Cost effectiveness in trauma care. *Surg Clinics N Am* 1996;76:47–62.

18. Martinez R. Injury prevention, a new perspective (editorial). *JAMA* 1994;272:1541–1542.

19. Christoffel T, Gallagher SS. *Injury prevention and public health: Practical skills and strategies*. Gaithersburg, MD: Aspen Publications; 1999.

20. National Highway Traffic Safety Administration. *Traffic Safety Facts 1998: Complication of Motor Vehicle Crash Data from the Fatality Analysis Reporting System.* Washington, DC; 1999.

21. National Center for Health Statistics. *Health, United States, 1996–1997 and injury chartbook.* Hyattsville, MD; 1997.

22. National Center for Health Statistics. *Health United States, 2000 with adolescent health chartbook.* Hyattsville, MD; 2000.

23. National Center for Health Statistics. *Vital statistics system for number of deaths.* Hyattsville, MD.

24. Singh GK, Yu SM. U.S. childhood mortality, 1950-1993: Trends and socioeconomic differentials. *AJPH* 1996;86(4):505–512.

25. Istre GR, McCoy MA, Osborn L, Barnard JJ, Bolton A. Deaths and injuries from house fires. *NEJM* 2001;334(25):1911–1916.

26. Robertson LS. *Injuries: Causes, control strategies, and public policy.* Lexington, MA: Lexington Books, 1983.

27. Waller JA. *Injury control: A guide to the causes and prevention of trauma.* Lexington, MA: Lexington Books, 1985.

28. Runyan CW. Using the Haddon matrix: Introducing the third dimension. *Injury Prevention* 1998;4:302–307.

29. Stanford GG, Bolton A. Injury prevention—The ultimate solution for reducing death and disability for traumatic injury in Dallas. *Dallas Med J* 1994;80:454–457.

30. Institute of Medicine. *Disability in America, toward a national agenda for prevention.* Washington, D.C.: National Academy Press, 1991.

31. Teutsch SM. A framework for assessing the effectiveness of disease and injury prevention. *MMWR* 1992;41:1–12.

32. Rivara FP, Grossman DC, Cummings P. Injury prevention, second of two parts. *NEJM* 1997;337:613–618.

33. Miller TR, Galbraith M. Injury prevention counseling by pediatricians: A benefit-cost comparison. *Pediatrics* 1995;96:1–4.

34. Andersson R. Community safety promotion at local, regional, and national levels. *IJ Consumer Safety* 1995;2(2):61–70.

35. Day JC. *Population projections of the United States by age, sex, race, and Hispanic origin: 1995 to 2050.* Washington, DC: US Government Printing Office; 1996.

36. Population projections of the United States by age, sex, race, Hispanic origin and nativity: 1999 to 2100. Population Estimate Program, Population Division, U.S. Census Bureau, Washington DC. 2000 (http://www.census.gov/population/www/projections/natsum-t3.html).

37. Hackler C, ed. *Health care for an aging population*. Albany, NY: State University of New York Press; 1994.

38. Waxweiler RJ, Rosenberg ML, Fenley MA, eds. *Injury control in the 1990s, a national plan for action: a report to the second world conference on injury control*. Association for the Advancement of Automotive Medicine; 1993.

39. Eastman AB. Blood in our streets: The status and evolution of trauma care systems. *Arch Surg* 1992;127:677–681.

40. Goldfarb MG, Bazzoli GJ, Coffey RM. Trauma systems and the costs of trauma care. *Health Services Research* 1996;31:71–95.

41. Bazzoli GJ, Meersman PJ, Chan C. Factors that enhance continued trauma center participation in trauma systems. *J Trauma* 1996;41:876–885.

42. Cornwell EE, Berne TV, Belzberg H, Asensio J, Velmahos G, Murray J, Demetriades D. Health care crisis from a trauma center perspective, the LA story. *JAMA* 1996;276:940–944.

43. Skolnick AA. Injury prevention must be part of nation's plan to reduce health care costs, say control experts (commentary). *JAMA* 1993;270:19–24.

44. Fries JF, Koop E, Beadle CE, Cooper PP, England MJ, Greaves RF, Sokolov JJ, Wright D. Reducing health care costs by reducing the need and demand for medical services. *NEJM* 1993;329:321–325.

45. Rice DP, Mackenzie EJ. *Cost of injury in the United States, a report to Congress, 1989*. San Francisco, CA: Institute for Health & Aging, University of California and Injury Prevention Center, The Johns Hopkins University; 1989.

46. Tengs TO, Adams ME, Pliskin JS, Safran DG, Siegel JE, Weinstein MC, Graham JD. Five hundred life-saving interventions and their cost-effectiveness. *Risk Analysis* 1995;15:369–390.

47. Berger LR, Mohan D. *Injury control, a global view*. New Delhi, India: Oxford University Press, 1996.

48. Bolton A, Stanford G, Elston R. *Summary of an international congress: safe communities, the application to large urban environments, KI Red Report 358*. Sundbyberg, Sweden: Karolinska Institute, 1997.

49. Schwab M, Syme SL. On paradigms, community participation, and the future of public health (commentary). *AJPH* 1997;87:2049–2051.

50. Green LW, Kreuter MW, eds. *Health promotion planning: an educational and environmental approach, 2nd ed.* Mountain View, CA: Mayfield, 1991.

51. Gielen AC, Collins B. Community-based interventions for injury prevention. *Fam Community Health* 1993;15:1–11.

52. Baker EL, Melton RJ, Stange PV, Fields ML, Koplan JP, Guerra FA, Satcher D. Health reform and the health of the public, forging community health partnerships. *JAMA* 1994;272:1276–1282.

53. Svanstrom L, Schlep L, Ekman R, Lindstrom A. Falkoping, Sweden, ten years after: Still a safe community? *Int J Consumer Safety* 1996;3:1–7.

54. DiGuiseppi CG, Rivara FP, Koepsell TD, Polissar L. Bicycle helmet use by children: Evaluation of a community-wide helmet campaign. *JAMA* 1989;262: 2256–2261.

55. Plautz B, Beck DE, Selmar C, Radetsky M. Modifying the environment: A community-based injury reduction program for elderly residents. *Am J Prev Med* 1996;12:33–38.

56. Bablouzian L, Freedman ES, Wolski KE, Fried LE. Evaluation of a community based childhood injury prevention program. *Injury Prevention* 1997;3:14–16.

57. McKnight JL. Two tools for well-being: health systems and communities. *Am J Prev Med* 1994;10:23–25.

58. Rivara FP, Wolf ME. Injury research: Where should we go from here (commentary)? *Pediatrics* 1989;84:180–181.

59. US Department of Health and Human Services. *Healthy people 2000, national health promotion and disease prevention objectives.* Washington, DC: US Government Printing Office; 1991.

60. Johnson SW, Walker J. *The crash outcome data evaluation system (CODES).* National Highway Traffic Safety Administration, DOT HS 808 338; 1996.

61. National Highway Traffic Safety Administration. *Getting started: A guide to developing safe communities.* DOT HS 808 404; 1996.

ARTICLE 7

ATTENTION-DEFICIT HYPERACTIVITY DISORDER

Laurel K. Leslie and Martin T. Stein

INTRODUCTION

Attention-deficit hyperactivity disorder (ADHD) is one of the most common and persistent disorders of childhood and adolescence. Research regarding the prevalence, etiology, diagnosis, and treatment of ADHD has burgeoned over the last decade. Recent research combined with clinical expertise was summarized in a National Institutes of Health Consensus Conference in 1998 (National Institutes of Health, 1998) as well as published guidelines for identification and treatment of ADHD by the American Academy of Child and Adolescent Psychiatry (American Academy of Child and Adolescent Psychiatry [AACAP], 1997) and American Academy of Pediatrics (American Academy of Pediatrics, 2000. In press).

The Centers for Disease Control have also targeted ADHD as one of several childhood disorders with pressing public health implications. ADHD qualifies as a disorder of public health import for several reasons, including its estimated prevalence as well as its prominence among childhood and adolescent disorders. With respect to its prevalence, the Centers for Disease Control estimate that more than two million children and adolescents in the United States may have ADHD (Centers for Disease Control & Division of Birth Defects, 1999). A recent evidence-based report further addressed the issue of prevalence (Agency for Health Care Policy and Research, 1999). Previous reports on the prevalence of ADHD examined samples of children from referral populations in tertiary care centers and may reflect unknown sampling biases. The recent report reviewed studies conducted in communities, schools, and primary care settings. The report estimated that prevalence rates for ADHD ranged from 4% to 12% in the general population, compared with the published rate of 3% to 5% in the psychiatric (referred) literature (Agency for Health Care Policy and Research, 1999). Not only is ADHD common in children and adolescents, it is also one of the few chronic conditions identified frequently in childhood. According to the American Academy of Pediatrics, ADHD is one of the three most common chronic disorders seen in primary care settings, the other two

407

being asthma and chronic otitis media with effusion (Leslie LK, Rappo P, Abelson H, Jenkins RR, & Sewall SR, 2000).

ADHD is also important from a public health perspective in that it has significant individual, familial, and societal implications. The symptoms associated with ADHD interfere with attainment of many of the normal developmental milestones of childhood and adolescence, such as academic, fine motor, and social and adaptive skills. Children with ADHD often experience school failure, poor family and peer relations, as well as other emotional, behavioral, and learning problems. Studies that have followed youth identified with ADHD have demonstrated poor academic attainment, impaired functioning in their families, lower self-esteem, and an increase in driving-related accidents (Robin, 1998). Marital stress and/or poor sibling relationships are also common. The social and economic burden of ADHD through the lifespan has not been investigated, but is anticipated to be substantial.

This article briefly reviews available evidence regarding the symptoms, etiology, and diagnosis of ADHD, drawing heavily on recently published reports (National Institutes of Health, 1998; Agency for Health Care Policy and Research, 1999; American Academy of Pediatrics, 2000). Implications regarding diagnosis are then reviewed. The article follows with current recommendations regarding treatment, with a particular focus on treatment strategies in the school setting. It is the authors' perspective that ADHD should be targeted for secondary prevention measures, specifically, the identification of school-age children in early stages of ADHD's natural history, and the implementation of treatment techniques that hold the potential to decrease the individual, familial, and societal toll of this disorder.

ADHD: ITS SYMPTOMS, ETIOLOGY, AND DIAGNOSIS

ADHD is characterized by varying degrees of inattention and/or hyperactivity/impulsivity beyond what would be expected for a child's developmental level. Criteria for the disorder have been carefully researched and published recently in the *Diagnostic and Statistical Manual of Mental Disorders*, fourth edition (DSM-IV) (American Psychiatric Association, 1994). The DSM-IV identifies 18 specific symptoms children with ADHD are found to have more frequently than their peers (see Table 1). Many school-age children have some of these symptoms, either transiently or in a mild form, and it is important to establish the high frequency of symptoms in order to make the diagnosis of ADHD. The combination of symptoms displayed allows for the identification of three different subtypes of ADHD: a hyperactive/impulsive subtype (ADHD-HI), in which a child has at least 6 of 9 hyperactive/impulsive symptoms; an inattentive subtype (ADHD-IA), in which a child has at least 6 of 9 inattentive symptoms; and a combined subtype (ADHD-CT), where a child shows at least 6 symptoms in both categories. The DSM-IV also states that children and adolescents with this disorder must be distinguished from children with other disorders by determining that symptoms: (1) began prior to the age of 7 years, (2) occur across multiple settings (e.g., in school, home, other

TABLE 1 DSM-IV CRITERIA

A. Either 1 or 2

1. Six (or more) of the following symptoms of *inattention* have persisted for at least 6 months to a degree that is maladaptive and inconsistent with developmental level:
   Inattention
   a) Often fails to give close attention to details or makes careless mistakes in schoolwork, work, or other activities
   b) Often has difficulty sustaining attention in tasks or play activities
   c) Often does not seem to listen when spoken to directly
   d) Often does not follow through on instructions and fails to finish schoolwork, chores, or duties in the workplace (not due to oppositional behavior or failure to understand instructions)
   e) Often has difficulty organizing tasks and activities
   f) Often avoids, dislikes, or is reluctant to engage in tasks that require sustained mental effort (such as schoolwork or homework)
   g) Often loses things necessary for tasks or activities (e.g., toys, school assignments, pencils, books, or tools)
   h) Is often easily distracted by extraneous stimuli
   i) Is often forgetful in daily activities

2. Six (or more) of the following symptoms of *hyperactivity-impulsivity* have persisted for at least 6 months to a degree that is maladaptive and inconsistent with developmental level:
   Hyperactivity
   a) Often fidgets with hands or feet or squirms in seat
   b) Often leaves seat in classroom or in other situations in which remaining seated is appropriate
   c) Often runs about or climbs excessively in situations in which it is inappropriate (in adolescents or adults, may be limited to subjective feelings of restlessness)
   d) Often has difficulty playing or engaging in leisure activities quietly
   e) Is often "on the go" or often acts as if "driven by a motor"
   f) Often talks excessively
   Impulsivity
   g) Often blurts out answers before questions have been completed
   h) Often has difficulty awaiting turn
   i) Often interrupts or intrudes on others (e.g., butts into conversations or games)

B. Some hyperactive-impulsive or inattentive symptoms that caused impairment were present before 7 years of age

C. Some impairment from the symptoms is present in 2 or more settings (e.g., at school [or work] or at home)

D. There must be clear evidence of clinically significant impairment in social, academic, or occupational functioning

E. The symptoms do not occur exclusively during the course of a pervasive developmental disorder, schizophrenia, or other psychotic disorder and are not better accounted for by another mental disorder (e.g., mood disorder, anxiety disorder, dissociative disorder, or personality disorder).

Code based on type:

314.01 Attention-Deficit/Hyperactivity Disorder, Combined Type: If both criteria A1 and A2 are met for past 6 months

314.00 Attention-Deficit/Hyperactivity Disorder, Predominantly Inattentive Type: If criterion A1 is met but criterion A2 is not met for past 6 months

314.01 Attention-Deficit/Hyperactivity Disorder, Predominantly Hyperactive, Impulsive Type: If criterion A2 is met but criterion A1 is not met for past 6 months

314.9 Attention-Deficit/Hyperactivity Disorder Not Otherwise Specified

Reprinted with permission from the *Diagnostic and Statistical Manual of Mental Disorders*, 4th Ed. (DSM-IV). Copyright 1994. American Psychiatric Association.

activities, and with peers), and (3) are associated with clinically significant functional impairment (American Psychiatric Association, 1994).

The DSM-IV also stresses the importance of identifying other medical, psychosocial, behavioral, or neurological conditions that may either mimic the symptoms of ADHD or co-occur in the same child. These conditions may cause the behavioral and attentional difficulties a child is experiencing or compound a child's level of impairment. Common medical conditions can include side effects of prescribed medications or abused substances, and/or hearing or vision problems. Psychosocial problems include environmental or familial stressors that lead a child to display symptoms of hyperactivity/impulsivity or inattention. Common psychiatric conditions to investigate include both externalizing (oppositional and disruptive disorders) and internalizing (anxiety and depression) disorders. Neurological conditions to investigate include learning disabilities, neurodevelopmental syndromes, tic disorders, mental retardation, cerebral palsy, seizure disorders, and developmental delays.

Children with ADHD often have associated conditions; almost 30% of children with ADHD have at least one co-existing mental health condition or learning problem (Agency for Health Care Policy and Research, 1999). These co-existing conditions can affect a child's needs, treatment options, and disease outcome (Costello et al., 1996; Foley, Carlton, & Howell, 1996). Calculated mean prevalence rates of co-occurrence are 35% for Oppositional Defiant Disorder, 26% for Conduct Disorder, 26% for Anxiety, and 18% for Depression (Agency for Health Care Policy and Research, 1999). It has also been estimated that 11% to 22% of children with ADHD may also have Bipolar Disorder (Biederman, Russell, Soriano, Wozniak, & Faraone, 1998). Learning disabilities have also been noted in 12% to 25% of children with ADHD; the prevalence of learning disabilities in different studies reflects different definitions of learning disabilities (Agency for Health Care Policy and Research, 1999; Smith & Strick, 1997; Arnold et al., 2000).

Limitations of the DSM-IV Criteria

The diagnostic criteria should be recognized as a description of a set of behaviors; the diagnosis of ADHD has several limitations. First, the DSM-IV diagnostic criteria do not provide insight into the etiology of ADHD. Many etiologies have been proposed for ADHD such as functional brain impairment, genetic conditions, biochemical alterations, dietary habits, parenting styles, and environmental stressors such as large, overly stimulating classrooms and excessive television viewing. Recent studies utilizing brain imaging, molecular genetics, and neurochemical analyses strongly suggest that ADHD is the final common pathway of several potential disorders of neurodevelopmental origin (Brown et al., 2001; Agency for Health Care Policy and Research, 1999). However, currently, blood tests, electroencephalograms, brain imaging studies, and computerized tests of sustained attention and impulsivity are neither sufficiently sensitive nor specific to determine the diagnosis of ADHD. The diagnosis rests on collecting information from multiple settings to determine if a child meets the DSM-IV criteria for ADHD. The DSM-IV criteria thus require collaboration between families, schools, and primary care clinicians.

Second, limitations of the DSM-IV criteria can result from its dichotomous approach to a diagnostic decision: either a child has ADHD or does not. However, clinically, the symptoms associated with ADHD often present along a continuum with hyperactive/impulsive and inattentive behaviors spanning the occasional occurrence to the behavioral extremes associated with a child with ADHD and severe functional impairment. The American Academy of Pediatrics' recent publication of the *Diagnostic and Statistical Manual for Primary Care Providers* (DSM-PC) attempts to reframe symptoms associated with ADHD in a more dimensional nature spanning normal developmental variations, problem behaviors, and behavioral disorders (American Academy of Pediatrics, 1996). The DSM-PC provides an important conceptual model for ADHD-like behaviors but provides little diagnostic help for families, teachers, and clinicians trying to determine the nature and degree of a child's problems.

The DSM-PC also introduces a third limitation of the DSM-IV criteria: the lack of a developmental perspective in terms of symptom presentation across the lifespan. The 18 criteria in the DSM-IV are very specific for school-aged children and activities they often engage in. The diagnosis as it is currently framed leaves families, schools, and primary care clinicians less certain about the diagnosis and management of ADHD in preschool children, adolescents, and adults. The DSM-IV also does not comment on common developmental "stumbling blocks" for school-aged children presenting with ADHD-like symptoms. Clinicians and teachers with experience have noted that certain behaviors may present as problematic in certain grades because of the increased academic and social demands required. For example, children with the hyperactive and combined subtypes of ADHD often present with behavior problems in kindergarten or first grade; in contrast, children with the inattentive form of ADHD may not experience significant problems until 4th, 6th, or 9th grade—these are grades in which the academic and organizational skills demanded escalate substantially.

In addition, while the DSM-IV provides for a diagnosis for children who demonstrate several of the symptoms associated with ADHD with an insufficient number of symptoms to meet the DSM-IV diagnostic criteria, specifically ADHD-Not Otherwise Specified (ADHD-NOS), there is no clarity on how to determine if a child meets criteria for this diagnosis. Children out of the school-age range or with insufficient symptoms remain a diagnostic and treatment dilemma and require careful review by a professional with specific expertise in ADHD and related disorders.

Public Health Perspectives

The current state of our knowledge regarding ADHD, its prevalence, etiology, and diagnosis, has several important public health implications. First, given the high prevalence rates of ADHD, school personnel, families, and primary care clinicians should be alert to the possibility of this disorder in children who have behavioral or attentional difficulties in school and/or at home. Second, because the diagnosis of ADHD rests on the documentation of symptoms that are associated with functional impairment from multiple informants, school personnel, families, and primary care clinicians need to work collaboratively to document specific symptoms and their effect on a child's current functioning. School personnel and families also need to be cognizant of the fact that there currently are not any biological markers or computerized tests that allow for diagnostic specificity. The role of the primary care clinician is as an unbiased observer who acts to synthesize and interpret information regarding a child's behavior, identify other medical or psychosocial problems that might be causing and/or exacerbating the child's symptoms, refer for further evaluation where needed, and provide appropriate medical treatment.

The third public health perspective on ADHD is that, in the absence of accurate blood tests or imaging studies for making the diagnosis of ADHD, families, school personnel, and clinicians must share their expertise to develop better symptom descriptions for behavioral and attentional difficulties and improve diagnostic specificity. Both health and education professionals should recognize, however, the significant expertise from clinicians, educators, and developmental psychologists that has gone into the development of the DSM-IV criteria for ADHD. The diagnostic process for ADHD is similar to other neurodevelopmental and mental health conditions such as depression, anxiety disorders, and autistic-spectrum disorders. Similar to ADHD, these conditions are diagnosed based on the demonstration of behavior symptoms that cause functional impairment in children, adolescents, and/or adults.

A fourth public health implication is less obvious but of sufficient importance to merit discussion. Many clinicians and school personnel limit the help they can provide to children and families by an overemphasis on the dichotomous nature of the DSM-IV criteria, focusing primarily on ruling in or out the diagnosis of ADHD. Those children whose behaviors meet criteria for ADHD are targeted for a course of treatment; however, children who show some symptoms with mild to moderate impairment, but whose behaviors do not meet criteria, may garner little help with respect to their functional needs. These children legitimately deserve as careful an assessment of their symptoms and functioning with targeted strategies for addressing identified areas of compromise.

ADHD: TREATMENT

Treatment strategies for ADHD over the last several decades have been based on both clinical expertise and research. Four primary modalities have been recommended, usually in combination: medications, primarily stimulants; psychosocial interventions directed at the child, home, and school; classroom accommodations; and parental education. Other treatments are usually related to the co-existing conditions and learning disabilities that an individual child demonstrates. Of the four primary modalities, stimulant medications (methylphenidate [Ritalin] and dextroamphetamine) and psychosocial interventions have been subjected to a number of research studies addressing the effectiveness of these interventions, both individually and in combination. Although other psychotropic medications have been used to treat ADHD, few have been subjected to rigorous research trials (Hoagwood, 1998). Classroom accommodations and parental education have also not been subjected to any rigorous research testing, although experienced teachers and clinicians as well as parents will attest to more smoothly functioning classrooms, ease of homework completion, and self-efficacy for a child with ADHD who has received these interventions.

Research Studies

The most rigorous and long-term study to date is the Multimodal Treatment Study of Children with Attention Deficit Disorder (MTA). The MTA study enrolled 579 children carefully diagnosed with the combined subtype of ADHD at 6 sites across North America (Arnold, Abikoff, Cantwell, Conners et al., 1997; Arnold et al., 1997; Arnold et al., 2000). On enrollment, the children ranged from 7 to 9 years of age, including a number of children from different racial/ethnic backgrounds, family structures, and income brackets. Children were randomized to one of four conditions: (1) stimulant medication only, in which the type of stimulant medication, its dose, and time interval were carefully titrated, monitored, and adjusted for the needs of each individual child; (2) behavioral treatment only (including intensive individual and group programs of behavioral management targeted at ADHD symptoms for children, teachers, and parents, and a summer-camp experience for children focused on principles of behavior management); (3) combined treatment (both medication and behavioral); and (4) community care (parents were given a list of providers in the community to choose source of care).

Statistical and clinical gains for core ADHD symptoms were noted for the titrated stimulant medication only group and the combined treatment group compared to the behavioral treatment only and community care groups; results indicated there was not a significant augmentation in outcomes with the use of intensive behavioral management over medication use alone. Of particular importance was the fact that children in the medication group, in which 67% of the children were on medication, showed significant improvement in symptoms compared with those receiving community care. This suggests that medication use without careful attention to type of stimulant, dose, and interval as was used in the MTA study will *undertreat* children's symptoms. Recently published results continue to demonstrate significant gains for the children receiving titrated medication alone or in combination with behavioral approaches in three major domains of outcome: core ADHD symptoms, symptoms of oppositional-defiant or conduct disorder, and the need for parental discipline (Arnold et al., 2000).

Results of the MTA study suggest that carefully monitored stimulant medication use is the single most efficacious treatment for ADHD and thus a critical component of treatment for ADHD. An initial trial of stimulants has been shown to be effective for about 70% of children diagnosed with ADHD (Swanson et al.,

1998; Wolraich et al., 1990). The percentage increases to over 90% if an alternative stimulant is tried following failure of an initial stimulant (Jensen & Payne, 1998). Stimulant medication choice, dosage, and time interval must be carefully titrated to meet the needs of each individual child (Abikoff, 1998); several trials may be necessary before the most effective medication type and dosage is identified. What is the role of psychosocial interventions? Psychosocial interventions such as parent education and behavior modification are appropriate and have been shown to be beneficial in reducing ADHD symptoms (Pelham, Wheeler, & Chronis, 1998). However, individual psychotherapy, play therapy, and cognitive therapy have not been shown to reduce core ADHD symptoms; these nonbehavioral therapies may benefit some children with ADHD who have associated mental health conditions responsive to these therapies.

Psychosocial interventions have several theoretical advantages that deserve further exploration in research studies: (1) use in combination with medication may allow for a reduced dose, (2) the therapeutic benefits of stimulant medication usually occur during the day, whereas behavioral interventions may be used in the late afternoon or evening in place of an additional dose of medication, (3) disruptive disorders have been shown to respond to behavioral modification, and (4) psychosocial treatment may help to enhance a parent's positive perception of his/her child and of his/her own parenting abilities. Recent results from the MTA study also suggest that medication in combination with behavioral approaches may be particularly effective for children with ADHD and associated anxiety disorders or children in single-parent households (Arnold et al., 2000). In addition, not all children and families accept the use of medication treatment for ADHD or respond to stimulants (Spencer, Biederman, Wilens, Harding et al., 1996). It should be noted, however, that those psychosocial interventions with demonstrated effectiveness in the literature are usually quite intensive including the behavioral intervention in the MTA study, Pelham's nine-week summer day camp for children with ADHD (Pelham & Hoza, 1996), and Frankel's social skills training sessions for parents and children (Frankel, Myatt, Cantwell, & Feinberg, 1997). Because they are not available through schools or health insurance plans, these types of intensive interventions are often difficult to access for the majority of children.

Several other treatment strategies deserve further mention. Although the prevalence rate of learning disabilities in children with ADHD in community settings is unclear, the documentation of 17% learning disabilities in children with ADHD in the MTA study suggests that learning disabilities are not uncommon (MTA Cooperative Group, 1999a,b). Families, teachers, and clinicians need to make sure that the behavioral problems associated with ADHD are not masking co-existing learning disabilities. These will require formal testing for learning problems, identification of areas of disability, and specific learning interventions under an Individualized Education Program (IEP) as stipulated under the Individuals with Disabilities Education Act (Public Law 94-142, amended in 1997 under Public Law 105-17) (U.S. Department of Education, 2001). These learning disabilities will usually fall into the category of language-based disorders of learning or impaired mathematics performance. Children with ADHD may also demonstrate dysgraphia, related to poor visuomotor ability or fine motor control, and pragmatic language disorders related to language use in social contexts. Children with ADHD also show other learning problems, including inconsistent performance, delayed acquisition of core reading and math skills, and poor meta-cognitive abilities (organization, time management, and breaking tasks down into smaller components). These problems can often be inappropriately attributed to laziness or lack of motivation. Direct remediation of learning problems, bypass strategies, and meta-cognitive skills training are all-important academic tools to utilize in planning curricula for children with ADHD (Smith & Strick, 1997).

Similarly, the MTA study documented that 54% of children had co-existing disruptive disorders and 34% had anxiety or depression (Arnold et al., 2000). Referral to a mental health professional may be indicated for pharmacological or clinical treatment of a co-existing mental health disorder. Mental health professionals may also play an important role if there is significant familial stress related to a child's ADHD or psychopathology in the family, including domestic violence, substance abuse, and other conditions. Children with severe emotional impairment secondary to any mental health disorder, including ADHD, are also eligible for development of an intensive behavioral management plan under the IEP mechanism described above.

Intervention Outcomes

The question is often asked as to whether or not treatment of ADHD changes a child's outcomes in the long run. Recognizing the chronicity and functional impairment resulting from ADHD, even with treatment, suggests the need to reframe this question (e.g., Can interventions be implemented to act as secondary preventive measures to protect against more severe outcomes?). Unfortunately, long-term prospective studies on children with optimal ADHD treatment are lacking. A meta-analysis by Swanson and colleagues (Swanson, McBurnett et al., 1993) concluded that the impact of stimulant medications on academic achievement was significantly less than the impact on behavior and cognition. In addition, many children with ADHD continue to show symptoms as they enter adult life, including troublesome interpersonal relationships with family members and peers, career underachievement, and poor self-esteem (Frankel, Cantwell, Myatt, & Feinberg, 1999; Goldman, Genel, Bezman, & Slanetz, 1998). However, these earlier studies have not adjusted for the onset of treatment and the intensity of intervention offered. More recent retrospective studies demonstrate that treatment may be protective against poor outcomes. For example, children treated for ADHD with stimulant medication are less likely to experiment with substances during adolescence compared to their untreated peers with ADHD (Biederman, Wilens, Mick, Spencer, & Faraone, 1999). Families, school personnel, and clinicians often observe that children whose symptoms are recognized, assessed, and managed at an early age will show improved self-esteem and success in the classroom, both essential for normal psychosocial and educational development.

TREATMENT GUIDELINES: MEETING THE OBJECTIVES

The American Academy of Pediatrics treatment guidelines (American Academy of Pediatrics, In press) were developed based on the available evidence to date and have several important public health considerations. These guidelines recommend that families, school personnel, and clinicians first recognize that ADHD is a chronic neurodevelopmental condition that will require ongoing, collaborative care. Second, clinicians, parents, and the child, in collaboration with school personnel, should specify appropriate target outcomes for the ADHD symptoms as well as any co-existing conditions that will guide management decisions. Third, treatment strategies should be systematically monitored to determine impact and adverse side effects through the acquisition of information from parents, teachers, and children. If the selected management for a child has not met targeted outcomes, clinicians, parents, and school personnel should collaboratively evaluate the original diagnosis, use of all appropriate treatments, adherence to the treatment plan, and the presence of previously unidentified co-existing conditions. Mechanisms for communication may include phone, facsimiles, e-mail, or face-to-face conferences; tools may include narratives notes, behavioral checklists, daily report cards regarding behavior, and routine school reports.

Table 2 summarizes treatment modalities as a function of their objective. The American Academy of Pediatrics treatment guidelines (American Academy of Pediatrics, In press) state that the strength of evidence regarding the effect of stimulant medication use is strong; children appropriately diagnosed with ADHD deserve discussion of possible stimulant medication use. Medication is an effective strategy for several treatment objectives including the core ADHD symptoms, classroom performance, relationships with others, and improved self-esteem and self-efficacy. If medication is given, it should be carefully titrated and monitored for effects on ADHD symptoms and side effects. Titration requires collaboration between child, family, school personnel, and clinician. School personnel are particularly critical for determining if a dose is impacting on a child's behavior and attention and if the dosing interval is sufficient for smooth functioning during the day. Families are important for determining symptom reduction in the afternoon and early evening as well as for tracking any potential side effects of the medications. Advocacy work must continue for research to develop medications that can be taken once daily and for insurance companies to cover these medications as they do not require nursing or administrative staff time and decrease stigma for children.

Second, psychosocial interventions to address areas of impairment related to ADHD as well as co-existing mental health conditions must be available, affordable, and with sufficient intensity to improve outcomes. Families, school personnel, and clinicians will need to advocate for the passage of mental health parity legislation that permits more open access to behavioral health for children and families, no matter what their insurance type. Mental health parity legislation should include mechanisms to improve communication between families, school personnel, and clinicians so that disorders of childhood, like ADHD, can be more collaboratively managed. Utilization review mechanisms should also not provide

TABLE 2 TREATMENT OBJECTIVES AND MODALITIES

Treatment Objective	Treatment Modalities
Decrease ADHD symptoms	Medication and/or behavioral management
Address co-existing medical and neurological disorders	Medical management
Address co-existing mental health disorders	Mental health treatments (psychopharmacology and behavioral/psychological therapies)
Address co-existing learning disabilities	IEP process and services necessary to address IEP goals
Address co-existing environmental and familial stressors	Stressor-specific interventions

Address difficulties in academic performance	Medication
	Behavioral modification
	Classroom accommodations through
	   IEP mechanism:
	      Direct remediation
	      Bypass strategies
	      Meta-cognitive skill development
	      Behavioral management plan

Address difficulties in peer relationships	Medication Social skills training Behavioral and psychological therapies
Address difficulties in familial relationships	Medication Behavioral modification Family counseling

Foster developmental trajectory:
   Developmental skills acquisition
     (*cognitive, fine and gross motor, and*
     adaptive)
   Self-esteem
   Self-efficacy
   Decision-making capabilities
	Above measures as secondary prevention
	Supportive relationships with adults in home and in other settings

Foster child and familial competency:
   Improve knowledge regarding ADHD in general and in child specifically
   Improve sense of self-efficacy
   Increased decision-making capacity regarding care for child with ADHD
	Educational resources
	Respect for family as consumers of medical, behavioral, and school-related services
	Self-assessment skills regarding ADHD symptoms and level of functioning
	Family therapy

barriers to care for children with ADHD and their families but guarantee quality of care.

Third, school systems need to examine their approach to ADHD in light of recent research findings. ADHD must be seen as a neurodevelopmental disorder; characteristic features of ADHD like inconsistent performance should not be interpreted as lack of motivation but as symptomatic of ADHD. Systematic strategies need to be developed to address the behavioral and academic needs of children with ADHD. Specifically, training in social skills and in metacognitive skills must be incorporated at the school setting. School personnel working with children with ADHD will need cross-training in both behavioral management strategies as well as different learning styles. Lastly, parents, school personnel and clinicians must be alert to possible anxiety and depression or learning disabilities that may co-exist with ADHD and impact on a child's academic and personal development.

Fourth, while there is no research documenting effectiveness, the authors of this paper recognize that poor child and parental self-esteem and self-efficacy are common in families with a child with ADHD. School personnel and clinicians must be sympathetic to parental and child self-concepts and work to instill self-confidence in both the parent and child. This may be particularly important if a child's parent also demonstrates symptoms of ADHD and/or learning disabilities, a possibility that is not uncommon given the likelihood of a strong genetic component to ADHD. Considering the chronic nature of ADHD, parents and children must be encouraged to take ownership of the condition, working as equal partners with clinicians and school personnel, to manage the difficulties of ADHD and build on their individual strengths.

Lastly, ongoing research on the identification and treatment of ADHD must continue. Although the MTA study has improved our understanding of children with the combined subtype of ADHD, questions still remain about the treatment of the inattentive form of ADHD. Prospective studies are also needed to investigate the question: If strategies are put in place at an earlier age, can symptoms be controlled, impairment minimalized, and projected outcomes improved?

REFERENCES

Abikoff H. (1998). Matching patients to treatments. *NIH Consensus Conference on Diagnosis and Treatment of ADHD.*

Agency for Health Care Policy and Research. (1999). *Diagnosis of Attention-Deficit/Hyperactivity Disorder (Technical Review No. 3).* Rockville, MD: Author.

American Academy of Child and Adolescent Psychiatry (AACAP). (1997). Practice parameters for the assessment and treatment of children, adolescents, and adults with attention-deficit/hyperactivity disorder. *Journal of the American Academy of Child & Adolescent Psychiatry, 30*(10 Suppl), S85–121.

American Academy of Pediatrics. (1996). *The Classification of Child and Adolescent Mental Diseases in Primary Care.* Washington, DC: American Academy of Pediatrics.

American Academy of Pediatrics. (2000). Clinical practice guidelines: Diagnosis and evaluation of children with attention-deficit/hyperactivity disorder. *Pediatrics,* 105, 1158–70.

American Academy of Pediatrics. (In press). *Clinical practice guideline: Treatment of school-aged children with Attention-Deficit/Hyperactivity Disorder.*

American Psychiatric Association. (1994). *Diagnostic and statistical manual of mental disorders.* 4th ed. Washington, DC: American Psychiatric Association.

Arnold L. E., Jensen, P. S., Hechtman, L., Hoagwood, K., Greenhill, L., and MTA Cooperative Group. (2000). *Do MTA treatment effects persist? New follow-up at 2 years.* Paper presented at the American Academy of Child and Adolescent Psychiatry, New York.

Arnold L. E., Abikoff H. B., Cantwell D. P., Conners C. K. et al. (1997). NIMH collaborative multimodal treatment study of children with ADHD (MTA): design challenges and choices. *Archives of General Psychiatry,* 54(9), 865–870.

Arnold L. E., Abikoff H. B., Cantwell D. P., Conners C. K., Elliott G. R., Greenhill L. L., Hechtman L., Hinshaw, S. P., Hoza B., Jensen P. S., Kraemer H. C., March J. S., Newcorn J. H., Pelham W. E., Richters J. E., Schiller E., Severe J. B., Swanson J. M., Vereen D., and Wells K. C. (1997). NIMH collaborative multimodal treatment study of children with ADHD (MTA): design, methodology, and protocol evolution. *Journal of Attention Disorders,* 2(3), 141–158.

Biederman J., Russell R., Soriano J., Wozniak J., & Faraone S. V. (1998). Clinical features of children with both ADHD and mania: does ascertainment source make a difference? *Journal of Affective Disorders, 51*(2), 101–12.

Biederman J., Wilens T., Mick E., Spencer T., and Faraone S. V. (1999). Pharmacotherapy of attention-deficit/hyperactivity disorder reduces risk for substance use disorder. *Pediatrics, 104*(2), e20.

Brown R. T., Freeman W. S., Perrin J. M., Stein M. T., Amler R. W., Feldman H. M., Pierce K., and Wolraich M. L. (2001). Prevalence and assessment of attention-deficit/hyperactivity disorder in primary care settings. *Pediatrics, 107*(3), E43.

Centers for Disease Control (1999) *Attention-Deficit/Hyperactivity Disorder: A Public Health Perspective* [Web Page]. URL http://www.CDC.gov/ncbddd/fact/adhd.htm [2001, April 25].

Costello E. J., Angold A., Burns B. J., Stangl D. K., Tweed D. L., Erkanli A., and Worthman C. M. (1996). The Great Smoky Mountains study of youth: Goals, design, methods, and the prevalence of DSM-III-R disorders. *Archives of General Psychiatry,* 53, 1129–1136.

Foley H. A., Carlton C. O., and Howell R. J. (1996). The relationship of attention deficit hyperactivity disorder and conduct disorder to juvenile delinquency: legal implications. *Bull Am Acad Psychiatry Law,* 24(3), 333–45.

Frankel F., Cantwell D. P., Myatt R., & Feinberg D. T. (1999). Do stimulants improve self-esteem in children with ADHD and peer problems? *J Child Adolesc Psychopharmacol,* 9(3), 185–94.

Frankel F., Myatt R., Cantwell D. P., & Feinberg D. T. (1997). Parent-assisted transfer of children's social skills training: effects on children with and without attention-deficit hyperactivity disorder. *Journal of the American Academy of Child & Adolescent Psychiatry, 36*(8), 1056–1064.

Goldman L. S., Genel M., Bezman R. J., and Slanetz P. J. (1998). Diagnosis and treatment of attention-deficit/hyperactivity disorder in children and adolescents. Council on Scientific Affairs, American Medical Association. *JAMA, 279*(14), 1100–7.

Hoagwood K. (1998). A national perspective on treatments and services for children with Attention Deficit Hyperactivity Disorder. *NIH Consensus Conference on Diagnosis and Treatment of ADHD.* Bethesda, MD: National Institutes of Health.

Jensen P. S., and Payne J. D. (1998). Behavioral and medication treatments for Attention Deficit Hyperactivity Disorder: Comparisons and Combinations. *NIH Consensus Conference on Diagnosis and Treatment of ADHD.* Bethesda, MD: National Institutes of Health.

Leslie L. K., Rappo P., Abelson H., Jenkins R. R., and Sewall S. R. (2000). Final report of the FOPE II pediatric generalists of the future workgroup. *Pediatrics, 106*, 1199–1223.

MTA Cooperative Group. (1999a). A 14-month randomized clinical trial of treatment strategies for attention-deficit/hyperactivity disorder. *Archives of General Psychiatry, 56*, 1073–1086.

MTA Cooperative Group. (1999b). Moderators and mediators of treatment response for children with attention-deficit/hyperactivity disorder: The Multimodal Treatment Study of children with Attention-deficit/hyperactivity disorder. *Arch Gen Psychiatry, 56*(12), 1088–96.

National Institutes of Health. (1998). Diagnosis and Treatment of Attention Deficit Hyperactivity Disorder (ADHD). *NIH Consensus Statement, 16*(2), 1–37.

Pelham W. E., and Hoza B. (1996). Intensive treatment: A summer treatment program for children with ADHD. In Hibbs ED, & Jensen PS (Eds), *Psychosocial Treatments for Child and Adolescent disorders* (pp. 311–340). Washington, DC: American Psychological Association.

Pelham W. E., Wheeler T., and Chronis A. (1998). Empirically supported psychosocial treatments for attention-deficit hyperactivity disorder. *Journal of Clinical Child Psychology, 27*, 190–205.

Robin A. L. (1998). *ADHD in adolescents: Diagnosis and Treatment.* New York, NY: Guilford Press.

Smith C., and Strick L. (1997). *Learning Disabilities: A to Z.* New York: Free Press.

Spencer T., Biederman J., Wilens T., Harding M. et al. (1996). Pharmacotherapy of attention-deficit hyperactivity disorder across the life cycle. *Journal of the American Academy of Child & Adolescent Psychiatry, 35*(4), 409–432.

Swanson J. M., Sergeant J. A., Taylor E., Sonuga-Barke E. J. S., Jensen P. S., and Cantwell D. P. (1998). Attention-deficit hyperactivity disorder and hyperkinetic disorder. *The Lancet, 351*, 429–433.

Swanson J. M., McBurnett K. et al. (1993). Effect of stimulant medication on children with attention deficit disorder: A "review of reviews." *Exceptional Children, 60*(2), 154–163.

U.S. Department of Education. (2001) *IDEA '97: The Individuals with Disabilities Education Act Amendments of 1997* [Web Page]. URL http://www.ed.gov/offices/OSERS/IDEA/ [2001, April 26].

Wolraich M. L., Lindgren S., Stromquist A., Milich R., Davis C., and Watson D. (1990). Stimulant medication use by primary care physicians in the treatment of attention deficit hyperactivity disorder. *Pediatrics, 86*(1), 95–101.

ARTICLE 8

THE EPIDEMIOLOGY OF HIV AND AIDS IN THE UNITED STATES

Laurie D. Elam-Evans, Norma S. Harris, and Hazel D. Dean

INTRODUCTION

The first cases of acquired immunodeficiency syndrome (AIDS) were reported in 1981 among five previously healthy young men in Los Angeles.[1] The unusual occurrence of *Pneumocystis carinii* pneumonia (PCP) and Kaposi's sarcoma among a population of gay and bisexual men in California and New York City stimulated an investigation of the unexplained clinical phenomena.[1,2] The Centers for Disease Control and Prevention (CDC) in collaboration with state and local health departments set up a surveillance system in 1981 to track what would become known as AIDS. During the 1980s, surveillance and epidemiologic research revealed that a new agent was being transmitted sexually and through contaminated blood. In 1984, a retrovirus was identified as the etiologic agent of AIDS. This retrovirus was later identified as the human immunodeficiency virus (HIV). Serologic (blood) tests to detect antibody to HIV were subsequently developed and became available in March 1985.[3,4]

Our knowledge of the epidemiology of HIV and AIDS has greatly increased over the past decade. New treatments and therapies are now available, making the interpretation of trends in AIDS incidence increasingly more difficult. This chapter reviews the epidemiology of HIV and AIDS in the United States. We describe HIV/AIDS surveillance, the current state of the epidemic, and provide future directions in conquering the most challenging disease of the 21st century.

HIV/AIDS SURVEILLANCE

Public health surveillance is defined as "the ongoing, systematic collection, analysis, interpretation, and dissemination of outcome-specific data for use in the planning, implementation, and evaluation of public health practice."[5] Figure 1 illustrates how HIV/AIDS surveillance is conducted. Briefly, all states require

FIGURE 1

How HIV/AIDS surveillance works

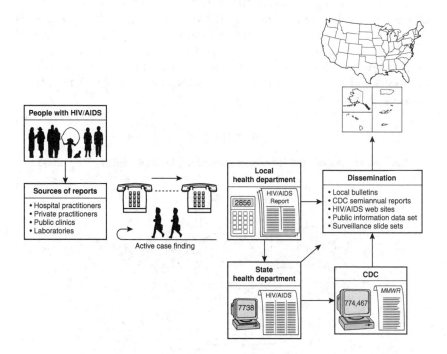

People with HIV/AIDS

Sources of reports
• Hospital practitioners
• Private practitioners
• Public clinics
• Laboratories

Active case finding

Local
health department
HIV/AIDS
Report
2856

Dissemination
• Local bulletins
• CDC semiannual reports
• HIV/AIDS web sites
• Public information data set
• Surveillance slide sets

State
health department
HIV/AIDS
7738

CDC
MMWR
774,467

their laboratories, hospital administrators, physicians, or other health care providers to confidentially report AIDS cases to designated health department officials. Case reports include demographic information; risk factors for HIV exposure; and other variables relevant to the design, implementation, evaluation of prevention and care programs, and monitoring of HIV-related conditions and death. Most states conduct *active* surveillance for AIDS case reporting, in which surveillance case workers at the health department solicit case reports through routine visits to health care providers and laboratory personnel. However, other states conduct *passive* surveillance, in which surveillance case workers wait for the providers to submit case reports to the health department. Regardless of the type of surveillance conducted, each surveillance program is required to evaluate the activities being conducted to ensure accuracy, completeness, representativeness, and timeliness of HIV and AIDS data. State health departments analyze, interpret, and disseminate their own local data. Additionally, these data are stripped of personal identifiers, such as name and address, and are forwarded to CDC where analysis, interpretation, and dissemination are conducted on a national level.

All U.S. states and territories require the reporting of AIDS cases to state or local health departments. As of May 2001, confidential reporting of HIV was implemented in 34 states and the Virgin Islands (Figure 2). Six states and Puerto Rico have implemented a mechanism to use alphanumeric codes instead of names (code-based reporting) to report HIV cases. Three states use a combination approach in which names are initially used to collect data, and then the name is replaced by alphanumeric codes (name-to-code reporting) for reporting HIV cases after epidemiologic follow-up occurs. These latter systems are being evaluated to determine how well they meet standards for completeness, timeliness, and accuracy consistent with historical standards set by confidential name-based reporting of infectious diseases.

FIGURE 2

Current status of HIV infection reporting, United States, May, 2001

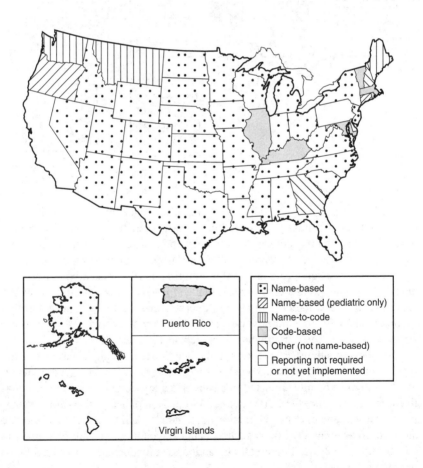

The AIDS data that will be used throughout this chapter are statistically adjusted to correct for differential delays in obtaining reported case data for certain groups or geographic areas and for cases reported with no identified or reported exposure risk. The risk distribution adjustment to estimate reporting delays takes into account differences by exposure risk, geographic area of report, racial/ethnic background, age, sex, and vital status categories, but assumes that delays within these groups have not changed over time.[6] These adjusted data provide a more appropriate presentation of trends in the epidemic and risk characteristics of the affected populations. This chapter will present data on persons in whom AIDS was diagnosed through December 31, 1999.

In this article, the epidemiology of HIV will be provided separately from the epidemiology of AIDS because the data reflect different populations. HIV data are only available and presented for the 33 states and the Virgin Islands that required confidential HIV infection case reporting in 1999.[6] These states represent 44% (320,566) of the cumulative number of U.S. AIDS cases. Additionally, because some persons with HIV have not been tested or were tested anonymously, the reported HIV case data may not be representative of all persons who are infected with or tested for HIV. Furthermore, many factors may influence testing patterns, including the extent to which populations are routinely offered testing or the availability and accessibility to medical care and testing services. However, these HIV data do provide a minimum estimate of the number of persons known to be HIV-infected and reported through December 31, 1999, in the 33 states and the Virgin Islands that required HIV case reporting in 1999.[6] When interpreting the HIV data, it is important to understand that persons with AIDS are counted separately from persons with HIV (not AIDS). This estimate of HIV (not AIDS) cases should be added to the estimate of persons with AIDS to obtain a more accurate assessment of persons affected by the HIV/AIDS epidemic.

AIDS IN MEN

Of the 751,965 adults/adolescents ($\geq$ 13 years old) diagnosed with AIDS through December 31, 1999, 83% were men. The median age at diagnosis for men was 38. The distribution of exposure among men by race/ethnicity is shown in Table 1. Over half (60%) of the cumulative AIDS cases in men were among men who have sex with men (MSM). The distribution of risk categories varies among men within each racial/ethnic group. The AIDS epidemic among African American and Hispanic men consists nearly equally of MSM and injection drug users (IDUs). In contrast, among White men, the AIDS epidemic consists primarily of MSM. In 1999, the rate of newly reported AIDS cases among men was 125 per 100,000 for African American men compared with 16 per 100,000 for White, 54 per 100,000 for Hispanic, 8 per 100,000 for Asian/Pacific Islander, and 18 per 100,000 for American Indian/Alaska Native men.

Since the beginning of the epidemic, a large proportion of AIDS cases occurred in men. Although the incidence of AIDS among men has decreased since 1992, the prevalence of AIDS among men has increased dramatically, from

TABLE 1 ESTIMATED MALE ADULT/ADOLESCENT AIDS INCIDENCE, BY EXPOSURE CATEGORY AND RACE/ETHNICITY, DIAGNOSED THROUGH DECEMBER, 1999, UNITED STATES *

Exposure Category	White (No.)	(%)	Black (No.)	(%)	Hispanic (No.)	(%)	Asian/ Pacific Islander (No.)	(%)	American Indian/ Alaskan Native (No.)	(%)	Total** (No.)	(%)
MSM+	229,218	77	86,583	42	51,401	46	3,729	76	1,085	59	372,473	60
IDU#	29,420	10	78,921	38	43,059	38	441	9	312	17	152,413	24
MSM and IDU	25,104	8	16,817	8	7,983	7	203	4	312	17	50,446	8
Hemophilia or coagulation disorder	3,871	1	724	<1	507	<1	75	2	30	2	5,217	1
Heterosexual contact§	6,505	2	21,265	10	8,302	7	286	6	68	4	36,502	6
Receipt of blood transfusion, blood components, or tissue	3,367	1	1,261	1	666	1	117	2	11	1	5,431	1
Risk not reported or identified	532	<1	2,218	1	314	<1	31	1	6	<1	3,106	<1
Total**	298,017		207,789		112,231		4,883		1,822		625,587	

* These numbers do not represent actual cases of men with AIDS. Rather, these numbers are point estimates adjusted for the delays in reporting of AIDS cases and for redistribution of cases initially reported with no identified risk, but not adjusted for incomplete reporting of cases.

** Total includes 845 men for whom race/ethnicity is unknown.

+ MSM, men who have sex with men; includes men who report sexual contact with other men and men who report sexual contact with both men and women.

IDU, injection drug user.

§ Includes persons who report specific heterosexual contact with a person with, or at increased risk for, HIV infection (e.g., an injection drug user).

Source: Centers for Disease Control and Prevention.[6]

approximately 144,536 cases in 1993 to approximately 252,494 in 1999.[6] Among MSM and MSM/IDU, the estimated incidence of AIDS and the number of deaths among men with AIDS has declined substantially. This decline is temporally associated with the use of highly active antiretroviral therapy (HAART), which became widely available in 1996. The incidence of AIDS cases among MSM appeared to level out in 1998 and 1999. The slowing of the decline in AIDS incidence may reflect that the benefits of treatment in delaying progression to AIDS are limited, that treatment-resistant strains have emerged, or that persons who are not tested and treated until they have AIDS now account for an increasing proportion of new AIDS diagnoses.

HIV IN MEN

As of December 1999, 122,607 cumulative HIV (not AIDS) cases among adults, adolescents, and children (< 13 years old) were reported to the CDC from 33 states and the Virgin Islands, which have confidential HIV reporting. Of these, 120,581 (98%) were among adults or adolescents. Most (72%) of the adults or adolescents with HIV were male; 62% were 25–39 years of age and 45% were MSM. There is concern about recent reports of increased incidence of HIV among a sample of young MSM,[7] in conjunction with other recently reported increases in sexually transmitted diseases and risk behaviors,[8] suggesting a potential resurgence of HIV infection among young MSM. Cumulatively, 47% of the men with HIV were African American, 43% were White, 8% were Hispanic, and nearly 1% were Asian/Pacific Islander and American Indian/Alaska Native.[9]

AIDS IN WOMEN

AIDS was first reported in women in 1981[10] and AIDS incidence rapidly increased through the mid 1990s. The proportion of AIDS cases in women continues to increase, and women accounted for 23% of AIDS cases diagnosed in 1999. Women accounted for 126,378 (17%) of the 751,965 cumulative AIDS cases diagnosed through December 1999.[6] In 1985, more than half (55%) of the AIDS cases in women were acquired through injection drug use. Over time, however, the proportion of AIDS cases acquired through injection drug use has declined and by 1999 accounted for only 35% of cases in women (Figure 3). In contrast, heterosexually acquired infections in women have increased from 27% of AIDS cases in 1985 to 62% in 1999 (Figure 3). In 1994, the proportion of women with AIDS who acquired their HIV infection through heterosexual transmission surpassed the proportion of women infected through injection drug use. Cumulatively, cases acquired through transfusion account for approximately 3% of the AIDS cases in women, with the remaining modes of exposure (hemophilia and cases with no identified risk) accounting for less than 1% of the cumulative cases in women.

FIGURE 3

**AIDS cases diagnosed* in adult and adolescent women,
by mode of exposure, United States, 1985–1999**

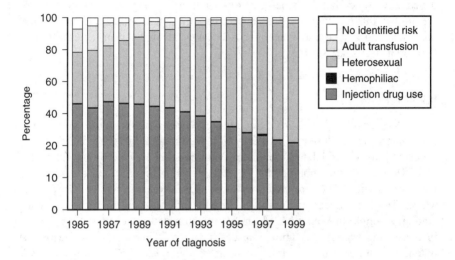

* Adjusted for reporting delays and redistribution of cases with no identified risk.

African American women are disproportionately affected by the AIDS epidemic. In 1999, rates of newly reported AIDS cases in women were 49 per 100,000 for African Americans compared with 2 per 100,000 for Whites, 15 per 100,000 for Hispanics, 1 per 100,000 for Asian/Pacific Islanders, and 5 per 100,000 for American Indian/Alaska Natives.[9] Cumulatively, among women with AIDS, African Americans accounted for 57% of the cases, Hispanics for 20%, Whites for 22%, and Asian/Pacific Islanders and American Indian/Alaska Natives each less than 1%.[6] Cumulatively, 45% of the women with AIDS were 30–39 years of age at diagnosis.

HIV IN WOMEN

The AIDS epidemic in women underestimates the total burden attributed to HIV infection. In addition to the 126,378 cumulative AIDS cases diagnosed in women through 1999, cumulatively, 33,179 women have been reported with HIV infection (not AIDS) by the 33 states and the Virgin Islands, which have confidential HIV reporting.[9] Of the 120,581 cumulative adult or adolescent HIV cases, 28% occurred in women. Of these women, 40% were 25–34 years of age; most (40%)

had heterosexually acquired infections. Sixty-eight percent were African American, 24% were White, 7% were Hispanic, and less than 1% were either Asian/Pacific Islander or American Indian/Alaska Native.[9]

HIV AND AIDS IN WOMEN OF CHILDBEARING AGE

At the end of 1999, 16,318 women 15–34 years of age were reported to be living with AIDS (Figure 4). An additional 15,190 women in this age group who were from the areas that conduct name-based confidential HIV infection surveillance

FIGURE 4

Women 15–34 years of age living with HIV infection* and AIDS, 1999

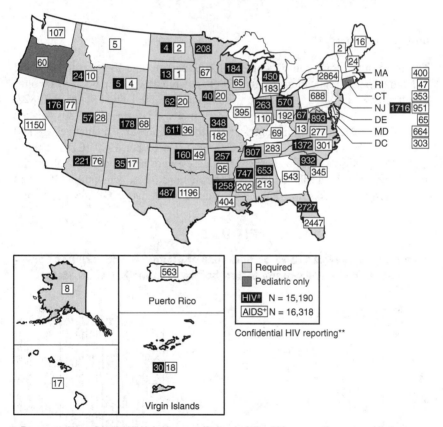

* For areas with confidential HIV infection surveillance. Includes 180 women who were residents of areas without HIV infection surveillance but who were reported by areas with HIV infection surveillance.
** HIV cases reported by patient name.
† Confidential HIV infection surveillance initiated in 1999.
# HIV total includes 5 women who were initiallly reported as pediatric HIV cases who are now 15 years of age with HIV in a non-HIV reporting state.
+ AIDS total includes 2 cases from the U.S. territories and 21 cases with missing state of residence at AIDS diagnosis.

in adults and adolescents were reported to be living with HIV infection (not AIDS) (Figure 4). These numbers are important because these women are of childbearing age and in the years of highest fertility. States with HIV case surveillance data are better able to direct programs and services to these women to enhance efforts to further reduce transmission to newborns. The HIV numbers are underestimates of the true HIV-infected population because (1) they include only women who have been tested for HIV and were reported to the state or local health departments that collect HIV infection case data, (2) a large number of HIV-infected women reside in states that do not have HIV surveillance, and (3) many infected women have not been tested. In most states with HIV surveillance, the number of HIV-infected women in whom AIDS has not developed exceeds the number of women with AIDS. These numbers indicate the burden of HIV morbidity with respect to the medical and social services that are necessary for these women, currently and in the future.

AIDS IN CHILDREN

The increasing proportion of women of childbearing age living with HIV and AIDS has major implications for the AIDS epidemic in children (< 13 years old). The first cases of AIDS in children were reported in the United States in 1982.[11] Since that time, AIDS incidence in children increased during the 1980s, peaked in 1992, and declined significantly after 1994 (Figure 5). Cumulatively, 8,860 pediatric AIDS cases were diagnosed through December 1999 (CDC, unpublished data). Most (93%) pediatric AIDS cases were acquired perinatally, with smaller percentages attributed to blood transfusions (4%), hemophilia (3%), and other unreported risks (<1%) (CDC, unpublished data). Of the perinatally

FIGURE 5

Perinatally acquired AIDS by half-year of diagnosis and receipt of any ZDV among HIV+ women tested before or at birth, United States

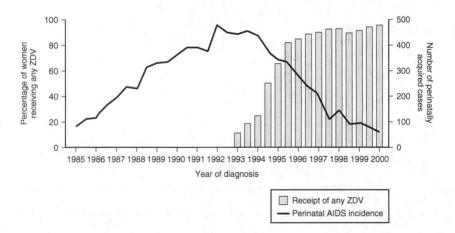

acquired cases, 53% were drug-related; either the mother was an IDU (36%) or the mother acquired her infection heterosexually from an IDU (17%) (CDC, unpublished data). These findings emphasize the importance of addressing substance abuse for HIV-infected women and women at risk for HIV infection. Cumulatively, 59% of the children with AIDS were African American, 23% were Hispanic, 17% were White, and less than 1% were either Asian/Pacific Islander or American Indian/Alaska Native (CDC, unpublished data). The racial/ethnic gap in pediatric AIDS cases has narrowed in the past 5 years but has not been eliminated. In 1999, the rate of AIDS among African American children (2.3 per 100,000) was 23 times higher than among White children (0.1 per 100,000) and 4 times higher than among Hispanic children (0.6 per 100,000).[9] Rates of AIDS were 0.1 per 100,000 for Asian/Pacific Islander children and 0.4 per 100,000 for American Indian/Alaska Native children.[9] This disparity demonstrates the need for outreach to address access to testing and treatment and care services for women in order to achieve further declines in the incidence of perinatally acquired HIV/AIDS.

HIV IN CHILDREN

Cumulatively, 2,026 pediatric HIV infection cases were reported to CDC through December 1999 from the 34 areas with confidential HIV infection reporting.[9] Of these, 87% of the infections were acquired perinatally. Of the cumulative total of children reported with HIV infection, 64% were African American, 23% were White, 12% were Hispanic, and less than 1% were Asian/Pacific Islander or American Indian/Alaska Natives.[9]

PERINATAL HIV/AIDS PREVENTION

Several prevention interventions have successfully reduced the HIV/AIDS epidemic in children. In 1994, the results of the Pediatric AIDS Clinical Trials protocol 076 (PACT protocol 076) showed that giving zidovudine (ZDV) therapy to selected HIV-infected pregnant women and their newborn infants would reduce perinatal HIV transmission from 25% to 8%.[12,13] Also in 1994, the U.S. Public Health Service (PHS) published guidelines for the use of ZDV to reduce perinatal HIV transmission.[14] The use of ZDV has increased significantly since the publication of these guidelines, from 11% of HIV-infected women tested before (prenatal) or at delivery (intrapartum) in 1993 to 94% of those tested in 2000 (Figure 5). In 1995, the PHS published guidelines for universal, routine HIV counseling and voluntary HIV testing of pregnant women.[15] These guidelines were quickly accepted and implemented by health providers and have resulted in a dramatic reduction in perinatal HIV transmission.

Because a substantial number of HIV-infected women do not receive any prenatal care,[16] their infants will not benefit from the advances made through prenatal, intrapartum, and neonatal administration of ZDV. For these women, the development of rapid tests that can be administered during labor together with alternative regimens that include a shorter course of therapy administered during labor and delivery or to the newborn can reduce perinatal transmission rates in the United States. This would also be advantageous internationally in settings where the PACT protocol 076 course is infeasible. A single dose of nevirapine to the mother and to the infant has been shown in Africa to significantly reduce perinatal transmission.[17] Additionally, in the United States, scheduled cesarean delivery before onset of labor and before rupture of membranes reduces the likelihood of vertical transmission of HIV.[18] Although significant progress has been made to prevent HIV/AIDS in children, challenges still remain to totally eliminate perinatal HIV transmission.

GEOGRAPHIC DISTRIBUTION OF AIDS

Although the estimated incidence of AIDS appeared to be leveling in the late 1990s, every state reported AIDS cases in 1999. The AIDS rates per 100,000 population in 1999 are shown for each state, the District of Columbia, Puerto Rico,

FIGURE 6

Reported AIDS rates per 100,000 population, United States, 1999

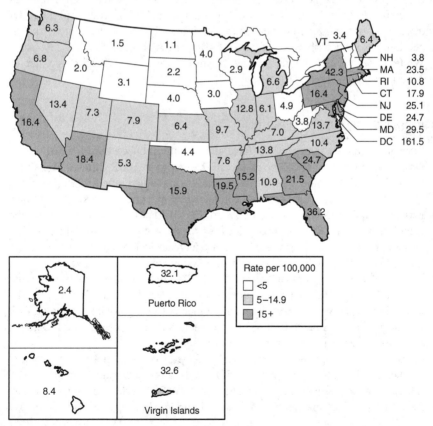

and the Virgin Islands (Figure 6). Areas with the highest rates were District of Columbia (161.5 per 100,000), New York (42.3 per 100,000), Florida (36.2 per 100,000), the Virgin Islands (32.6 per 100,000), Puerto Rico (32.1 per 100,000), and Maryland (29.5 per 100,000). Over 40% of the adult/adolescent AIDS cases reported in 1999 occurred in the South, and 31% occurred in the Northeast. More than three-fourths (82%) of these cases were reported from metropolitan areas of greater than 500,000 population, 10% from metropolitan areas of 50,000 to 500,000, and 8% reported from nonmetropolitan areas of less than 50,000 population. MSM accounted for the majority of cases in three out of four regions— North Central, South, and West—however, in the Northeast, IDUs accounted for the largest proportion of the AIDS cases reported.[19]

GEOGRAPHIC DISTRIBUTION OF HIV

In 1999, 21,419 cases of HIV infection (not AIDS) were reported from 34 areas that conducted confidential HIV case surveillance. Oregon and Connecticut required HIV infection reporting for pediatric cases only. Florida, Texas, New Jersey, and North Carolina reported the greatest number of persons with HIV infection in 1999 (Figure 7).[9] States implemented HIV infection reporting at different times after the HIV antibody test became available in 1985. Additionally, some states are not required by law to report HIV cases that were diagnosed prior to the implementation of HIV reporting in their respective areas.

TRENDS IN HIV/AIDS AMONG RACIAL AND ETHNIC MINORITY POPULATIONS

The United States comprises a diverse population, with 31% of Americans being a member of a racial/ethnic minority group.[20] The proportional distribution of AIDS cases by race and ethnic group has shifted from most cases being reported among White Americans in 1985 to larger numbers being reported among racial and ethnic minorities in 1999. In 1985, more than 60% of the persons reported with AIDS were White.[21] In 1995, for the first time, the number of AIDS cases among African Americans was approximately equal to the number of cases among Whites.[22] In 1996, African Americans represented the greatest proportion of persons reported with AIDS.[23] In 1999, 31,467 (68%) persons reported with AIDS were racial and ethnic minorities.[9] Among racial/ethnic groups, 32% of the persons reported with AIDS were White, 47% were African American, 19% were Hispanic, 1% were Asian/Pacific Islander, and less than 1% were American Indian/Alaska Native.

AIDS Incidence

The annual number of AIDS cases increased through the 1980s, peaked in the early 1990s, and then declined.[24] From 1998 through 1999, AIDS incidence appears to have leveled among all racial and ethnic groups. The same pattern of

FIGURE 7

Reported HIV infections (not AIDS), United States, 1999

N = 21,419*

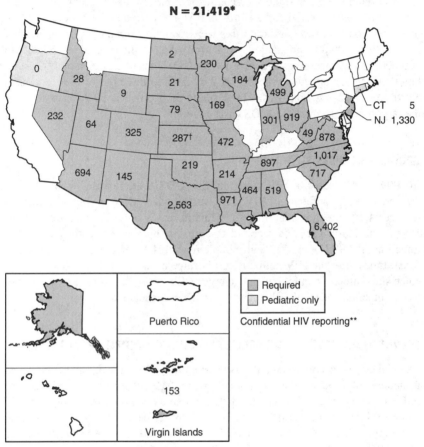

* Includes 361 persons who were residents of areas without HIV infection surveillance
  but who were reported by areas with HIV infection surveillance.
** HIV cases reported by patient name.
† HIV surveillance initiated in July 1999.

decline occurred among all racial and ethnic groups (Figure 8). However, proportionate declines were greater among Whites than among other racial and ethnic groups.

AIDS Prevalence

At the end of 1998, CDC estimated that 800,000 to 900,000 Americans were living with HIV infection (including persons with AIDS).[25] The number of Americans living with AIDS continues to rise, with approximately 320,000 living

FIGURE 8

Estimated incidence of AIDS* for adults/adolescents, by race/ethnicity, United States, 1985–1999

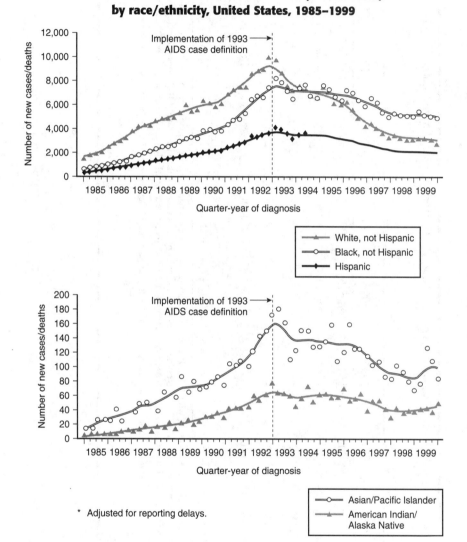

* Adjusted for reporting delays.

with AIDS at the end of 1999. Among Americans living with AIDS, 38% were White, 41% were African American, 20% were Hispanic, 0.8% were Asian/Pacific Islander, and 0.3% were American Indian/Alaska Natives. From 1993 through 1999, there was an 84% increase in the number of persons living with AIDS. The largest proportionate increases in AIDS prevalence have been among African Americans (114%), Hispanics (102%), Asian/Pacific Islanders (101%), and American Indians/Alaska Natives (91%) (Table 2).

TABLE 2 ESTIMATED PERSONS LIVING WITH AIDS, BY RACE/ETHNICITY AND YEAR, 1993 THROUGH 1999, UNITED STATES*

Race/Ethnicity	Year							% Change 1993 to 1999
	1993	1994	1995	1996	1997	1998	1999	
White	80,480	86,703	91,756	98,615	107,273	114,895	122,880	53
African American	60,678	71,863	81,287	92,274	105,306	117,426	129,943	114
Hispanic	31,245	36,524	41,072	46,194	52,121	57,443	62,995	102
Asian/Pacific Islander	1,295	1,460	1,617	1,859	2,094	2,318	2,609	101
American Indian/ Alaska Native	569	662	718	803	888	969	1,085	91
Total**	174,475	197,471	216,796	240,184	268,242	293,702	320,282	84

*These numbers do not represent actual cases of persons living with AIDS. Rather, these numbers are point estimates of persons living with AIDS derived by subtracting the estimated cumulative number of deaths in persons with AIDS from the estimated cumulative number of persons with AIDS. Estimated AIDS cases and estimated deaths are adjusted for reporting delays, but not for incomplete reporting. Annual estimates are through the most recent year for which reliable estimates are available.

**Totals include estimates of persons whose race/ethnicity is unknown. Because column totals were calculated independently of the values for the subpopulations, the values in each column may not sum to the column total.

Source: Centers for Disease Control and Prevention.[6]

New HIV Infections

Approximately 40,000 new HIV infections have occurred each year since 1992.[24] Racial and ethnic minority persons account for a disproportionately high number of new infections. In 1999, CDC estimated that 54% of new infections occurred among African Americans, 26% among Whites, 19% among Hispanics, and 1% among persons of other races. Among newly infected women, approximately 64% were African American, 18% were Hispanic, and 18% were White. Among newly infected men, 50% were African American, 20% were Hispanic, and 30% were White (CDC, unpublished data).

AIDS-RELATED MORBIDITY

AIDS-related morbidity has been defined using a list of clinical manifestations that are a part of the AIDS surveillance case definition. This case definition has expanded over the evolution of the epidemic. Initially, in 1981, *Pneumocystis carinii* pneumonia (PCP) and Kaposi's sarcoma were the opportunistic infections indicative of defective cell-mediated immunity in persons without underlying causes of immunodeficiency.[26] Later, in 1985, this list was expanded to include additional conditions less closely associated with immune suppression.[27] A major revision in 1985 was adding HIV-positive antibody test results. In 1987, presumptive diagnoses of PCP and Kaposi's sarcoma were included, as were conditions such as HIV wasting syndrome and HIV encephalopathy.[28] In 1993, the AIDS surveillance case definition for adults/adolescents ($\geq$ 13 years of age) expanded to include all HIV-infected persons with less than 200 CD4+ lymphocytes/ml or a CD4+ percentage of total lymphocytes less than 14. Additionally, pulmonary tuberculosis, recurrent bacterial pneumonia, and cervical cancer in HIV-infected women were included. As of 2001, the list of AIDS-related illnesses for adults/adolescents includes 26 different AIDS-defining opportunistic infections.[29] The leading illnesses for adults and adolescents are PCP (incidence = 4.7 cases/100 person-years), esophageal candidiasis (incidence = 4.3 cases/100 person-years), and disseminated *Mycobacterial avium* complex infections (incidence = 3.4 cases/100 person-years).[30] Data from the Adult and Adolescent Spectrum of HIV Disease study indicate that incidence of opportunistic infections differs by gender and by mode of exposure.[30] Incidence rates were found to be significantly higher among women for esophageal candidiasis, tuberculosis, cryptosporidiosis, and chronic mucocutaneous herpes simplex virus disease.[30] The incidence rate of Kaposi's sarcoma was significantly higher among men. Also, among men, the incidence rate of Kaposi's sarcoma was significantly higher among MSM whereas the incidence rates of esophageal candidiasis, recurrent pneumonia, tuberculosis, and toxoplasmosis were significantly higher among male IDUs.[30] Among children, PCP is the most common (33%) AIDS-defining condition, followed by lymphoid interstitial pneumonitis (24%), bacterial infection (20%), and HIV wasting syndrome (18%).[31]

AIDS-RELATED MORTALITY

The number of deaths among persons diagnosed with AIDS increased steadily from 1987 through 1994 and stabilized in 1995. However, the number of deaths declined by 24% in 1996, and the decline continued through 1997 (Figure 9). The sudden change in AIDS deaths and incidence of AIDS opportunistic infections suggests that factors such as HAART may be affecting these trends in end-stage HIV disease and death.[32] These trends are consistent with reports of increased survival after AIDS diagnosis with each subsequent year of diagnosis[33] and reports of declines in incidence of AIDS opportunistic infections.[34,35] Between 1998 and 1999, the number of deaths apparently leveled out.[36]

FIGURE 9

Estimated incidence of AIDS, deaths, and prevalence by quarter-year of diagnosis/death, United States, 1985–1999*

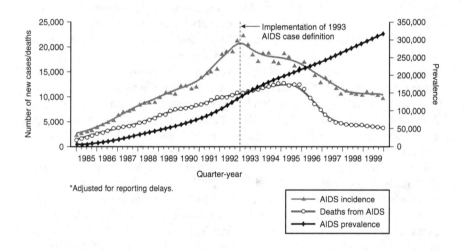

*Adjusted for reporting delays.

The CDC's National Center for Health Statistics compiles death certificate data from 50 states and the District of Columbia on underlying causes of deaths. HIV was first included among the leading causes of death in 1987,[37] at which time, HIV was ranked as the 15th leading cause of death.[37] The rate of death from HIV was 5.5 per 100,000 population, and HIV was responsible for 0.6% of the total deaths in 1987.[37] The ranking moved to 11th in 1989 (the rate of death from HIV was 8.9 per 100,000 population)[38] and gradually climbed to 8th by 1992 (the rate of death from HIV was 13.2 per 100,000 population).[39] HIV remained the 8th leading cause of death until 1997, when it plummeted to 14th (the rate of death from HIV was 6.2 per 100,000 population).[40] In 1998 and 1999, HIV was no longer among the 15 leading causes of death.[41,42] However, in 1999, among persons 25–44 years old, HIV infection was still the 5th leading cause of death for men and women of all races combined.[43] Additionally, HIV was the leading cause of death for Black men, the 3rd leading cause of death for Black women, and the 5th leading cause of death for White men in this age group.[43]

Between 1987 and 1994, deaths due to HIV infection increased an average of 16% annually per year.[40] The age-adjusted death rate due to HIV infection did not significantly differ from 1994 to 1995.[40] However, the death rate decreased 29% from 1995 to 1996, 48% from 1996 to 1997, 21% from 1997 to 1998, and 4% from 1998 to 1999.[42]

FUTURE DIRECTIONS

June 2001 marked the twentieth anniversary of the first reported case of AIDS in the United States. Much has been learned about the epidemic since that time, including the distribution of the populations greatly affected, identification of the virus that causes AIDS, recognition of the need to screen the national blood supply, implementation of clinical trials that identified new therapies, and understanding of the effect of therapy on AIDS incidence, prevalence, and death. Effective HIV therapy was widely available in 1996, and subsequent trends in AIDS incidence and deaths have declined substantially. Because of these treatment-associated declines, AIDS data no longer accurately reflect HIV incidence.

In 1999, CDC published recommendations for expanding the national AIDS surveillance system to include the reporting of HIV infection.[25] Knowledge of the scope of the epidemic at the national, state, and local levels will be greatly enhanced by nationwide HIV reporting and will provide a better estimate of the number of persons infected with HIV disease. Forty-five states have implemented some capacity for HIV infection surveillance although the systems are not uniform or standardized. The remaining states will implement HIV reporting by the end of 2003.

Over the past two decades, the HIV epidemic has expanded increasingly to communities of color, women, heterosexuals, and minority MSM. The challenge for this decade is to develop new and effective prevention strategies that include behavioral and structural interventions that address education and risk reduction (e.g., condom use and needle exchange) in these communities. Additionally, the need for partnerships between public health agencies and communities is even more critical for reducing the number of infections.

The ability to identify recent infections is also critical for developing HIV prevention programs for HIV-infected persons. Recently, a new serologic testing method has been developed to estimate HIV incidence.[44] This technique has been used in limited settings, such as anonymous counseling and testing sites, sexually transmitted disease clinics, and community-recruited survey sites.[7,45,46] The increased use of this testing method will provide additional information to identify on which populations and behaviors to focus additional prevention activities.

In January 2001, the Centers for Disease Control and Prevention published the HIV Prevention Strategic Plan Through 2005.[47] The overall goal of this plan is "to reduce the number of new infections in the U.S. from an estimated 40,000 to 20,000 per year, focusing particularly on eliminating racial and ethnic disparities in new HIV infections."[47] Specific goals are to "(1) decrease by at least 50% the number of persons in the United States at high risk for acquiring or transmitting HIV infection, (2) increase from the current estimated 70% to 95% the proportion of HIV-infected persons in the U.S. who know they are infected, (3) increase from the current estimated 50% to 80% the proportion of HIV-infected persons who are linked to appropriate prevention, care, and treatment services, and (4) strengthen the capacity nationwide to monitor the epidemic, develop and implement effective HIV prevention interventions, and evaluate prevention programs."[47] This strategic plan lays out the blueprint for HIV/AIDS prevention efforts by which CDC will collaborate with numerous partners in other federal agencies, state and local health departments, universities, and community-based and faith-based organizations.

Many initiatives will be implemented in an effort to reach these goals. The Serostatus Approach to Fighting the HIV Epidemic (SAFE) initiative was recently introduced and focuses on expanding voluntary counseling and testing programs to reach all persons living with HIV infection.[48] Through directed awareness and testing programs, SAFE will focus on significantly increasing the number of infected persons who learn their HIV status through voluntary testing, with a goal of 30,000 per year.[48] High-risk persons with negative test results, particularly persons whose partners are living with HIV, will be referred to prevention programs to help them stay uninfected.[48]

Although declines in AIDS incidence and deaths have occurred, prevention, treatment, and care services continue to be needed because approximately 40,000 persons are still becoming infected each year. Achieving declines in HIV incidence will require innovative approaches to increase HIV prevention efforts. The assurance that persons with HIV have access to care and treatment services will optimize their survival and quality of life.

ACKNOWLEDGMENTS

The authors gratefully acknowledge the statistical programming assistance of Jianmin Li.

REFERENCES

1. CDC (Centers for Disease Control). *Pneumocystis* pneumonia—Los Angeles. *MMWR*. 1981;30:250–252.

2. CDC. Kaposi's sarcoma and *pneumocystis* pneumonia among homosexual men—New York City and California. *MMWR*. 1981;30:305–308.

3. CDC. Antibodies to a retrovirus etiologically associated with acquired immunodeficiency syndrome (AIDS) in populations with increased incidences of the syndrome. *MMWR*. 1984;33:377–379.

4. Gallo, R.C., Salahuddin, S.Z., Popovic, M., Shearer, G.M., Kaplan, M., Haynes, B.F., Palker, T.J. Frequent detection and isolation of cytopathic retroviruses (HTLV-III) from patients with AIDS and at risk for AIDS. *Science.* 1984;224:500–503.

5. Thacker, S.B. Historical Development. In: Teutsch, S.M. and Churchill, R.E., eds. *Principles and Practice of Public Health Surveillance.* New York: Oxford University Press, 2001:3–17.

6. CDC. *HIV/AIDS Surveillance Report*, 2000;12 (No. 1):1–43.

7. CDC. HIV Incidence among young men who have sex with men—Seven U.S. Cities, 1994–2000. *MMWR.* 2001;50:440–444.

8. CDC. Resurgent bacterial sexually transmitted disease among men who have sex with men—King County, Washington, 1997–1999. *MMWR.* 1999;48:773–777.

9. CDC. *HIV/AIDS Surveillance Report*, 1999;11(No.2):1–47.

10. CDC. Follow-up on Kaposi's sarcoma and pneumocystic pneumonia. *MMWR.* 1981;30:409–410.

11. CDC. Unexplained immunodeficiency and opportunistic infections in infants—New York, New Jersey, California. *MMWR.* 1982;31:665–667.

12. Connor, E.M., Sperling, R.S., Gelber, R., Kiseley, P., Scott, G., O'Sullivan, M.J., VanDyke, R., Bey, M. Reduction of maternal-infant transmission of human immunodeficiency virus type 1 with zidovudine treatment. *New England Journal of Medicine.* 1994;331:1173–1180.

13. Sperling, R.S., Shapiro, D.E., Coombs, R.W., Todd, J.A., Herman, S.A., McSherry, G.D., O'Sullivan, M.J., VanDyke, R.B., Jimenez, E., Rouzioux, C., Flynn, P.M., Sullivan, J.L. Maternal viral load, zidovudine treatment, and the risk of transmission of human immunodeficiency virus type 1 from mother to infant. *New England Journal of Medicine.* 1996;335:1621–1629.

14. CDC. Recommendations of the US Public Health Service Task Force on the use of zidovudine to reduce perinatal transmission of human immunodeficiency virus. *MMWR.* 1994;43(RR-11):1–20.

15. CDC. US Public Health Service recommendations for human immunodeficiency virus counseling and voluntary testing for pregnant women. *MMWR.* 1995;44(RR-7):1–15.

16. CDC. Success in implementing PHS guidelines to reduce perinatal transmission of HIV. *MMWR.* 1998;47:688–91. [Published errata appear in *MMWR.* 1998;47:718.]

17. Guay, L., Musoke, P., Fleming, T., Bagenda, D., Allen, M., Nakabiito, C., Sherman, J., Bakaki, P. Intrapartum and neonatal single-dose nevirapine compared to zidovudine for prevention of mother-to-child transmission in Kampala, Uganda: HIVNET 012 randomised trial. *Lancet.* 1999;354:795–802.

18. The International Perinatal HIV Group. The mode of delivery and the risk of vertical transmission of Human Immunodeficiency Virus Type 1—A meta-analysis of 15 prospective cohort studies. *New England Journal of Medicine.* 1999.340:977–987.

19. CDC. HIV/AIDS in urban and nonurban areas of the United States. *HIV/AIDS Surveillance Supplemental Report.* 2001;6:1–16.

20. United States Bureau of Census. Census 2000 Brief, CENBR/01-1. *Overview of Race and Hispanic Origin.* Washington, DC: U.S. Government Printing Office. 2001.

21. CDC. *AIDS Surveillance Report.* 1985; 7(No.1):1–34.

22. CDC. *HIV/AIDS Surveillance Report.* 1995;7(No.2):1–38.

23. CDC. *HIV/AIDS Surveillance Report.* 1996;8(No.2):1–39.

24. CDC. HIV and AIDS—United States. *MMWR.* 2001;50:430–434.

25. CDC. Guidelines for national human immunodeficiency virus case surveillance, including monitoring for human immunodeficiency virus infection and acquired immunodeficiency syndrome. *MMWR.* 1999;48(RR-13):1–28.

26. CDC. Update on acquired immune deficiency syndrome (AIDS)—United States. *MMWR.* 1982;31:507–514.

27. CDC. Revision of the case definition of acquired immunodeficiency syndrome for national reporting—United States. *MMWR.* 1985:34:373–375.

28. CDC. Revision of the CDC surveillance case definition for acquired immunodeficiency syndrome. *MMWR.* 1987;36(suppl):1S–15S.

29. CDC. 1993 Revised classification system for HIV infection and expanded surveillance case definition for AIDS among adolescents and adults. *MMWR.* 1992:41(No. RR-17):1–19.

30. Kaplan, J.E., Hanson, D., Dworkin, M.S., Frederick, R., Bertoli, J., Lindegren, M.L., et al. Epidemiology of human immunodeficiency virus-associated opportunistic infections in the United States in the era of highly active antiretroviral therapy. *Clinical Infectious Diseases.* 2000;30:S5–15.

31. Lindegren, M.L., Steinberg, S., Byers, R.H. Epidemiology of HIV/AIDS in children. *Pediatric Clinics of North America.* 2000;47:1–20.

32. Fleming, P.L., Ward, J.W., Karon, J.M., Hanson, D.L., DeCock, K.M. Declines in AIDS incidence and deaths in the USA: A signal change in the epidemic. *AIDS.* 2001;12[suppl A], S55–S61.

33. Lee, L.M., Karon, J.M., Selik, R., Neal, J.J., Fleming, P.L. Survival after AIDS diagnosis in adolescents and adults during the treatment era, United States, 1984–1997. *Journal of the American Medical Association.* 2001;285[10], 1308–1315.

34. McNaghten, A.D., Hanson, D.L., Jones, J.L., Dworkin, M.S. *The effects of antiretroviral therapy and opportunistic illness primary chemoprophylaxis on survival after AIDS.* 5th Conference on Retroviruses and Opportunistic Infections, Chicago, Illinois, February 1998. Abstract #10.

35. Palella, F., Moorman, A., Delaney, K., Loveless, M., Fuhrer, J., Aschman, D., Holmberg, S. *Dramatically declining morbidity and mortality in an ambulatory HIV infected population.* 5th Conference on Retroviruses and Opportunistic Infections, Chicago, Illinois, February 1998. Abstract #198.

36. Fleming, P.L., Wortley, P.M., Karon, J.M., DeCock, K.M., Janssen, R.S. Tracking the HIV epidemic: Current issues, future challenges. *American Journal of Public Health.* 2000;90:1037–1041.

37. National Center for Health Statistics. *Vital Statistics of the United States, 1987.* Vol. II, Mortality, Part A. Washington, D.C.: Public Health Service. 1990. DHHS Pub. No. (PHS) 90–1101.

38. National Center for Health Statistics. *Vital Statistics of the United States,* 1989. Vol. II, Mortality, Part A. Washington, D.C.: Public Health Service. 1993. DHHS Pub. No. (PHS) 93–1101.

39. Kochanek, K.D., Hudson, B.L. Advance report of final mortality statistics, 1992. *Monthly Vital Statistics Reports*; Vol. 43, No. 6, Suppl. Hyattsville, Maryland: National Center for Health Statistics. 1994.

40. Hoyert, D.L., Kochanek, K.D., Murphy, S.L. Deaths: Final Data for 1997. *National Vital Statistics Reports*; Vol. 47, No. 19. Hyattsville, Maryland: National Center for Health Statistics. 1999.

41. Murphy, S.L. Deaths: Final Data for 1998. *National Vital Statistics Reports.* Vol. 48, No. 11. Hyattsville, Maryland: National Center for Health Statistics. 2000.

42. Hoyert, D.L., Arias, E., Smith, B.L., Murphy, S.L., Kochanek, K.D. Deaths: Final Data for 1999. *National Vital Statistics Reports.* Vol. 49, No. 8. Hyattsville, Maryland: National Center for Health Statistics. 2001.

43. Kochanek, K.D., Smith, B.L., Anderson, R.N. Deaths: Preliminary Data for 1999. *National Vital Statistics Reports.* Vol. 49, No. 3. Hyattsville, Maryland: National Center for Health Statistics. 2001.

44. Janssen, R.S., Satten, G.A., Stramer, S.L., Rawal, B.D., O'Brien, T.R., Weiblen, B.J., Hecht, F.M., Jack, N. New testing strategy to detect early HIV-1 infection for use in incidence estimates and for clinical and prevention purposes. *Journal of the American Medical Association.* 1998;280:42–48.

45. McFarland, W., Busch, M.P., Kellog, T.A. Rawal, B.D., Satten, G.A., Katz, M.H., Dilley, J., Janssen, R.S. Detection of early HIV infection and estimation of incidence using a sensitive/less sensitive enzyme immunoassay testing strategy at anonymous counseling and testing sites in San Francisco. *Journal of Acquired Immune Deficiency Syndromes.* 1999;22:484–489.

46. Schwartz, S., Kellogg, T., McFarland, W., Louie, B., Kohn, R., Busch, M., Katz, M., Bolan, G. Differences in temporal trends of HIV seroincidence and seroprevalence among sexually transmitted disease clinic patients, 1989–1998: Application of the serologic testing algorithm for recent seroconversion (STARHS). *American Journal of Epidemiology.* 2001;153:925–934.

47. Centers for Disease Control and Prevention. *HIV Prevention Strategic Plan Through 2005.* Atlanta, Ga: Centers for Disease Control and Prevention; 2001. Available at http://www.cdc.gov/nchstp/od/news/prevention.pdf.

48. Janssen, R.S., Holtgrave, D.R., Valdeserri, R.O., Shephard, M., Gayle, H.D., DeCock, K.M. The serostatus approach to fighting the HIV epidemic: Prevention strategies for infected individuals. *American Journal of Public Health.* 2001;91:1019–1024.

ARTICLE 9

SEXUALLY TRANSMITTED DISEASES
IN THE UNITED STATES

Kimberley Fox

INTRODUCTION

Sexually transmitted diseases (STDs) constitute a substantial public health burden in the United States. Not only are STDs among the most common infections affecting Americans, but they also have sequelae with significant impacts on health at the individual and societal levels. STDs disproportionately impact women and adolescents, particularly those of lower socio-economic status and those of minority race or ethnicity. Advances in diagnostic technologies, expanded modes of service delivery, and new behavioral interventions have improved STD prevention and control programs. Nonetheless, STDs remain a significant public health problem and continue to adversely affect the health of Americans.

MAGNITUDE AND SIGNIFICANCE OF THE STD PROBLEM

Recent estimates suggest that there are over 15 million new cases of STDs in the United States every year.[1] These include over 6 million cases of incurable viral STDs including genital herpes and human papillomavirus infections, and over 8 million cases of curable STDs including gonorrhea, chlamydia, syphilis, and trichomoniasis. Persons of all ages, races, and socio-economic background are affected by STDs. However, adolescents carry a disproportionately high burden: Twenty-five percent of new STD cases occur among these young people.[1] The severity of symptoms associated with STDs range from mild to debilitating; sequelae of untreated infection are frequently serious, including infertility, cancer, and facilitation of HIV transmission (Table 1).

TABLE 1 IMPORTANT SEQUELAE OF SEXUALLY TRANSMITTED DISEASES

Syphilis	• Tertiary disease affecting the cardiovascular system, central nervous system, or other organs • Congenital syphilis • Facilitation of HIV transmission*
Gonorrhea	• Pelvic inflammatory disease and subsequent infertility, ectopic pregnancy, and chronic pelvic pain • Ophthalmia neonatorum • Facilitation of HIV transmission*
Chlamydial infection	• Pelvic inflammatory disease and subsequent infertility, ectopic pregnancy, and chronic pelvic pain • Ophthalmia neonatorum • Facilitation of HIV transmission*
Trichomoniasis	• Probably low birth weight and preterm delivery • Facilitation of HIV transmission*
Genital herpes	• Neonatal herpes • Facilitation of HIV transmission*
Human papillomavirus	• Cervical cancer and other anogenital cancers
Hepatitis B	• Hepatic cirrhosis • Liver cancer

*The preponderance of epidemiologic and biologic evidence suggests that STDs causing genital tract manifestations such as ulcers or mucosal inflammation increase the risk of HIV transmission.[30]

Syphilis

Syphilis is caused by infection with *Treponema pallidum* and can present with a variety of manifestations, including genital ulceration, rash, and neurologic symptoms. Without treatment, infection becomes latent although the initial symptoms of syphilis resolve. Years later, more serious symptoms may appear in up to one-third of infected persons as the disease affects the cardiovascular system, central nervous system, or other organs.[2] Untreated syphilis in the pregnant woman results in congenital syphilis in the fetus in a high proportion of cases, particularly during the first four years of maternal infection. Congenital syphilis may be manifest by fetal death, stillbirth, or a variety of manifestations including rash, hepatosplenomegaly, bony abnormalities, anemia, and central nervous system lesions.[3] Since congenital syphilis is preventable with early and adequate treatment of the mother, screening for syphilis during pregnancy is critical. By 2001, rates of syphilis declined by almost 80% since the peak in 1990;[4,5] to capitalize on this decrease, a national campaign to eliminate endemic transmission of syphilis in the United States was initiated in 1998.[6] An estimated 70,000 total cases of syphilis were diagnosed in 1996;[1] the number of total reported cases has declined from 53,218 in 1996 to 32,221 in 2001; 14,804 of these latter cases represented recently acquired (primary, secondary, and early latent) syphilis.[4] A new challenge will be to address recent increases in syphilis—along with gonorrhea—among men who have sex with men, a group which experienced large declines in STDs in the 1980s.[7,8,9]

Gonorrhea

Neisseria gonorrhoeae infects the urethra, cervix, rectum, and pharynx, with transmission almost exclusively through sexual contact. Symptoms of uncomplicated infection may include dysuria, urethral discharge, vaginal discharge, and rectal pain and discharge, although a minority of cases in men and most cases in women are asymptomatic. Vertical transmission from mother to infant can occur, causing ophthalmia neonatorum, a serious eye infection that can result in blindness if untreated. The major complication of gonorrhea is pelvic inflammatory disease (PID), which occurs in 10% to 20% of women with gonococcal cervicitis and is manifest primarily by lower abdominal pain.[10] Among women with PID, roughly 20% will develop infertility, 18% will have chronic pelvic pain, and 9% will have ectopic pregnancies.[11] Despite a fairly steady rate of decline since 1975,[4,12] an estimated 650,000 cases of gonorrhea occur annually in the United States.[1] Rates of gonorrhea in 2001 are higher than in 1997; although the reasons for this are unclear, increases have been notable in some geographic areas and specific populations such as men who have sex with men, as noted above.[13]

Chlamydial Infections

Chlamydia trachomatis causes syndromes similar to those caused by *N. gonorrhoeae*, with a higher proportion of infections being asymptomatic. At least one-third of urethral infections in men[14] and most infections in women are asymptomatic. Maternal infection can lead to a form of ophthalmia neonatorum less severe than that caused by gonorrhea, and to neonatal pneumonia. Chlamydial infection also is an important cause of PID, with generally mild symptoms yet producing sequelae as severe as those due to gonococcal PID. Expansion of testing for chlamydial infection and improvements in surveillance systems have led to increasing numbers of cases reported and identified.[14] However, rates of chlamydial infection have decreased in some areas with established screening programs.[15,16] Currently, an estimated 3 million cases of chlamydial infection occur annually in the United States.[17]

Trichomoniasis

Vaginal infection with *Trichomonas vaginalis* is among the most common conditions found among women. Symptoms are primarily vaginal discharge and odor, although infection may frequently be asymptomatic. Complications may include low birth weight and preterm delivery in pregnant women.[18] An estimated 5 million cases of trichomoniasis occur annually in the United States.[1]

Genital Herpes

The painful ulcerations known as genital herpes are caused by herpes simplex virus-2 (HSV-2) and, to a lesser extent, HSV-1. However, in the great majority of individuals, these infections are asymptomatic or subclinical. More than 45 million Americans are infected with HSV-2, yet less than 10% of them have been diagnosed with genital herpes.[19] Neonatal herpes results when virus is transmitted from an infected mother to her newborn, usually during delivery. Neonatal herpes frequently causes devastating neurologic consequences or death, even when appropriate therapy is provided.[20] Despite the high prevalence of genital herpes in the general U.S. population, neonatal herpes is rare, with an estimated 2,500 to 5,000 cases annually. The risk of vertical transmission is highest when maternal HSV infection is acquired during pregnancy.[21] An estimated 1 million new cases of HSV-2 infection occur annually in the United States,[1] and the proportion of Americans infected with HSV-2 increased from 16% in the late 1970s to 21% in the late 1980s to early 1990s.

Human Papillomavirus

Infection with human papillomavirus (HPV) is believed to be the most common STD in the United States, with an estimated 5.5 million new cases annually.[1] However, a high proportion of these infections are transient, with a median duration of 8 months.[22] Nonetheless, an estimated 20 million persons in the United States are currently infected with HPV.[23] There are over 30 HPV types that infect genital areas, with "low-risk" types such as HPV-6 and HPV-11 causing genital warts, and "high-risk" types such as HPV-16 and HPV-18 causing the cellular changes that lead to cervical cancer.[24] Recurrent respiratory papillomatosis is a rare, but serious, condition in which HPV (usually HPV-6 or HPV-11) appears to be transmitted from mother to infant during delivery and causes growths on the larynx or pharynx, leading to hoarseness and airway obstruction.[25] Trends in HPV infection are not well documented.

Hepatitis B

Hepatitis B virus causes serious systemic illness, with infection persisting in up to 5% of newly infected adults. Approximately two-thirds of hepatitis B cases are acquired sexually, leading to an estimate of 120,000 sexually transmitted cases annually in the United States.[1] Vertical transmission from a mother with chronic infection is highly efficient; furthermore, 80% to 90% of infants who acquire hepatitis B perinatally develop chronic infection.[26] Screening for chronic infection during pregnancy allows for prevention of vertical transmission. Because transmission occurs primarily during delivery, treatment with specific immune globulin and vaccine within 12 hours of delivery can prevent up to 90% of cases.[27] As many as 5,000 persons in the United States die each year from hepatitis B-related cirrhosis, and another 800 or more die from hepatitis B-related liver cancer.[1] Rates of new infections with hepatitis B appear to be declining, likely due to increased use of the preventive vaccine.[28]

Sexually Transmitted Diseases and HIV Transmission

STDs facilitate HIV transmission through several mechanisms including: disruption of the mucocutaneous barrier, which augments susceptibility; increases in HIV shedding, augmenting infectiousness; and increases in the local concentration of infected or susceptible white blood cells, augmenting both susceptibility and infectiousness.[29] Ulcerative STDs such as herpes and syphilis and nonulcerative inflammatory STDs such as gonorrhea, chlamydia, and trichomoniasis increase the likelihood of HIV transmission by two- to five-fold.[30] Due to these interactions, HIV may spread more quickly through populations with high prevalences of STDs than in populations with low prevalences of STDs, even if sexual behaviors in the populations are similar. Provision of improved STD services led to a 42% reduction in HIV incidence in a multicommunity trial in Africa.[31]

STDS AMONG ADOLESCENTS, WOMEN, AND MINORITIES

For most STDs, rates are highest among adolescents and young adults. Adolescents are uniquely susceptible to STDs for both physiologic and sociobehavioral reasons.[32] For example, in adolescence, the cervix has substantial exposed columnar epithelium, termed cervical ectopy, increasing the susceptibility to *N. gonorrhoeae* and *C. trachomatis*, which infect this cell type specifically. In addition, given infection with either *N. gonorrhoeae* or *C. trachomatis*, adolescents appear to be at greater risk than older women for PID. Rates of STDs among adolescents are also high in part because a high proportion of teenagers engage in sexual intercourse;[33] have concurrent sexual partners;[34] use condoms inconsistently; have inadequate knowledge about STD prevention;[32] delay seeking treatment for STDs due to fear of parental notification;[35] and because of the perception of barriers to care or lack of sufficient self-efficacy to respond to STD symptoms.[36] However, recent data suggest some promising trends, with a decrease in the percentage of youth engaging in sexual intercourse and an increase in the prevalence of condom use among sexually active youth.[33]

Prevalence studies frequently find higher rates of STDs among women, whereas reported incidence rates—for those STDs that are reportable to health authorities—are often higher among men. The asymptomatic nature of most

STDs in women, allowing infections to remain undetected for long periods of time, provides partial explanation for this apparent paradox; additionally, men are more likely to attend STD clinics,[37] where reporting of STDs is more complete than in private settings.[38] Several factors disadvantage women in controlling personal risk for STDs and their sequelae: social contexts that create a gender power differential and therefore limit self-determination of sexual behavior,[39] higher efficiency for many STDs of male-to-female transmission than female-to-male transmission,[40,41] and absence of symptoms in women. Women also more often delay care-seeking and attempt self-treatment.[42]

Racial disparities in STD rates are also notable. For most STDs, rates among African Americans exceed—and for some STDs, greatly exceed—rates among white Americans.[4] Rates among other race and ethnic groups vary. Differential reporting from public and private sources likely contributes to these disparities; however, studies among a nationally representative sample of Americans have also found racial disparities in prevalences of syphilis, chlamydial infection, and HSV-2 infection.[43,44,19] Racial disparities in STD rates likely reflect a complex combination of influencing factors, including poverty, social status, access to medical care, neighborhood of residence, sexual partner choices, and prevalence of practices such as douching.[45–48] In addition, there are population level factors that may increase the incidence of certain STDs among blacks and other minorities compared with whites, namely youthful age composition and a higher number of women than men in the population.[49] This gender imbalance among blacks is important because it contributes to disassortative mixing patterns, whereby individuals at low risk for STDs choose sexual partners at high risk for STDs. Such mixing patterns occur more often when gender imbalance exists, and are responsible for an estimated 30% increase in STD risk among blacks compared to whites in the United States.[50]

RISK FACTORS FOR STDS

The primary risk factor for acquiring an STD is having sex with an infected person. Given that information on the infection status of partners is difficult to ascertain, a number of surrogate markers for STD risk have been identified. For most STDs, young age is a strong risk factor, being both a physiologic factor and a marker for risky behaviors described above. An exception to this is syphilis, which occurs more commonly in adults aged 20 to 40 years. Young age has been closely associated with chlamydial infection, and has been shown to be a risk factor for repeat chlamydial infection and for PID-related sequelae as well.[51,52] Behavioral risk factors for STDs include initiation of sexual exposure at a young age, having multiple sexual partners, and having high-risk partners.[53,54] Specific sexual practices also affect STD risk. Anal intercourse carries an increased risk of transmitting some STDs, while oral sex appears to be less likely to transmit some STDs than other types of sexual contact; however, most STD pathogens can be transmitted through oral sex so this practice should not be considered risk-free.[55,56]

The likelihood that a particular partner is infected is determined in part by the local prevalences of STDs and the partner's sexual behaviors.[54] The social and contextual environment may influence STD prevalence through factors such as discrimination, limited employment opportunity, and economic and social inequities that may promote risky sexual behaviors.[57] The specific contexts of partner recruitment and sexual encounters can be used to identify high-risk acts.[47] For example, partners recruited in drug use settings or sexual acts occurring in anonymous venues carry high risks for STD acquisition. However, STDs that are widely prevalent such as chlamydial infection, genital herpes, or HPV are readily encountered in settings perceived as low risk because these pathogens infect large proportions of the U.S. population.

Biologic factors in addition to age-related cervical ectopy modify the risk for acquiring STDs. Use of hormonal contraceptives also induces cervical ectopy and may increase susceptibility to gonococcal and chlamydial infection.[58] Use of intrauterine devices carries a small increased risk of PID for women with cervical infection.[59] Vaginal douching may increase the susceptibility to STDs by disturbing the natural vaginal flora, and it is clearly associated with higher rates of PID.[60]

CHALLENGES AND OPPORTUNITIES FOR STD PREVENTION

The Hidden Epidemic

In a recent report, "The Hidden Epidemic: Confronting Sexually Transmitted Diseases," the Institute of Medicine (IOM) described biological and social factors that contribute to the spread and hidden nature of STDs.[61] Biologic factors include the asymptomatic nature of many STDs, with the result that most people with STDs are unaware that they are infected. Similarly, the lengthy delay between acquisition of STDs and the appearance of serious complications such as ectopic pregnancy or liver cancer obscures the link between STDs and their complications. Social factors facilitating spread of STDs include inadequate access to care, poverty, and substance abuse. These factors are common among the disenfranchised populations, including sex workers, homeless persons, adolescents and adults in detention, and migrant workers, which have particularly high rates of STDs. These groups are frequently occupied by issues of daily survival, leaving little time and energy for attention to STD medical care or prevention.[62] The Institute of Medicine report also highlights secrecy as a contributing factor to the hidden epidemic. Although sexuality is a normal part of human existence and pervades all aspects of our culture, rarely is there frank discussion of sexuality and related matters such as STDs between sexual partners, peers, parents and children, or health care professionals and patients. The IOM report recommended efforts to overcome barriers to adoption of healthy sexual behaviors; to develop strong leadership, strengthen investment in, and improve information systems for STD prevention; to design and implement essential STD-related services in innovative ways for adolescents and underserved populations; and to ensure access to and quality of clinical services.[61]

A Framework for Prevention

For the spread of an STD to be maintained in a community, each infected person must, on average, transmit infection to at least one uninfected individual.[63] In mathematical terms, this means the reproductive rate of the infection must be greater than or equal to 1. If the reproductive rate stays below 1, the infection will eventually die out in that community. The factors affecting the reproductive rate for STDs have been described with the formula: $R_0 = \beta c D$, where R_0 is the reproductive rate, β is the average probability of transmission per partner sexual contact (transmission efficiency), c represents the rate of partner change, and D is the average duration of infectiousness of an infected person.[63,64] Activities that decrease any or all of these factors will tend to diminish the spread of STDs. Approaches to STD prevention can be classified as impacting the efficiency of transmission, sexual behaviors, or the duration of infection (Table 2).

TABLE 2 FRAMEWORK FOR SEXUALLY TRANSMITTED DISEASE PREVENTION

Prevention approaches aimed at decreasing β, the efficiency of transmission
• Increasing condom use
• Vaginal microbicides (under development)

Prevention approaches aimed at decreasing c, the measure of sexual partner change
• Risk-reduction counseling
• Opinion leaders change behavioral norms

Prevention approaches aimed at decreasing D, the duration of infection
• Screening for curable STDs
• Treatment of sexual partners
• Single-dose therapy
• Improving compliance with therapy
• Improving accessibility of STD services
• Improving healthcare seeking behaviors

Prevention approaches based on the equation describing the reproductive rate of infection, $R_0 = \beta c D$.[62,63]

*In addition, vaccines (e.g., hepatitis B vaccine) decrease the pool of susceptible persons and thereby decrease the opportunities for transmission.

Treatment as Prevention

STD treatment reduces the duration of infection, thus interrupting the spread of disease. Treatment for many STDs, including gonorrhea, chlamydia, syphilis, and trichomoniasis, can be accomplished with single-dose therapy, allowing for directly observed therapy at the time of diagnosis and enhancing the likelihood of therapy completion. A recent advance in STD treatment has been the availability of single-dose therapy, azithromycin, for chlamydial infection.[65] Curative therapy is not available for viral STDs, but advances in treatment for genital herpes have decreased the duration of symptoms and the frequency of outbreaks for many patients. In addition, suppressive therapy for genital herpes—symptomatic or asymptomatic—decreases viral shedding and may prove to decrease the likelihood of transmission.[66]

Screening for STDs

Screening is necessary to detect asymptomatic STDs so that treatment, if appropriate, can be provided. Routine screening for gonorrhea, chlamydia, and syphilis is recommended for pregnant women due to the potential for adverse impact on the neonate.[67] Screening for chlamydial infection is also recommended for all sexually active women aged 25 years or younger and for other women at increased risk of chlamydial infection since this infection is particularly widespread and readily cured with appropriate therapy.[68] Screening for chlamydial infection, which can reduce the risk of PID by as much as 60%,[69] and for gonorrhea, has been advanced by new diagnostic technologies. Nucleic acid amplification tests such as polymerase chain reaction (PCR) and ligase chain reaction (LCR) have substantially improved the sensitivity of testing for *C. trachomatis* and have improved the accessibility of screening for gonorrhea and chlamydial infection because these tests can be performed on urine specimens or self-collected vaginal swabs; a pelvic exam or urethral swab are no longer necessary for chlamydia testing. The use of urine-based testing has increased the feasibility of screening asymptomatic men and has allowed screening to be implemented in nonclinical venues such as schools, jails, and other settings and via street outreach.[70] Self-collected vaginal swabs have had high acceptability rates among adolescents.[71]

Syphilis screening has recently been extended into many additional venues with implementation of the National Plan to Eliminate Syphilis from the United States.[6] Consistent with this approach, screening has increased in settings, such as jails and some emergency rooms, frequented by high-risk populations. Jail testing has proved to be particularly productive, especially among women;[72] jurisdictions with jail screening have found that high proportions of their infectious syphilis cases are identified through this process.[73] With the recognition of the close link between HIV infection and those STDs which cause genital ulcers, syphilis testing has become a routinely available service in many HIV testing venues.

The issues concerning screening for the viral STDs are more complex. New serologic tests for HSV can distinguish between antibodies for HSV-1 and

HSV-2, and have made screening for HSV infection feasible. Issues remain as to the contexts and populations appropriate for HSV screening, the need for confirmatory testing, the specific counseling messages to be provided for those testing positive, and whether suppressive therapy reduces the infectivity of those with asymptomatic infection. Tests that detect HPV DNA in cervical samples have been developed and serologic tests for HPV are under development. Again, issues remain as to the appropriate use of these tests given that HPV infection is highly prevalent, usually asymptomatic, and typically resolves without complication; furthermore, no available therapy is known to cure infection or reduce the risk of transmission. Most promising is the use of tests to detect high-risk HPV subtypes among women with Papanicolau smears showing atypical squamous cells of undetermined significance (ASCUS) to identify those who should undergo colposcopy.[74]

STD Services Access and Utilization

Screening or diagnostic testing and treatment can only take place once the individual encounters STD services. STD services are provided by private physicians or clinics and through public STD or reproductive health clinics.[37] Barriers to utilization include limited hours of service, cost, appointment systems, lack of transportation, cultural differences between providers and patients, and—perhaps most important—the necessity that the patient recognize the need for obtaining services. Given limited public knowledge about STDs, lack of perception of risk, the stigma of STDs, and the asymptomatic nature of many STDs, many infected patients do not actively seek care. Even if care is sought, the failure of many health care providers to address STD issues creates a barrier to the provision of appropriate and complete services.

Improvements in access to STD services are critical to reducing the duration of infection and in preventing complications such as PID and interrupting sexual and vertical transmission. The notification of partners exposed to STDs and associated efforts to bring such persons to clinical settings for assessment and treatment are traditional STD prevention activities. The success of partner notification is limited when patients are unwilling to provide partner information, partners are anonymous, or the affected populations are not amenable to such interventions for physical, social, or cultural reasons. Such population groups include adolescents, for whom traditional partner-notification services are not very effective.[75] The partner notification approach can be expanded to incorporate social network concepts, which may facilitate provision of services to difficult-to-reach groups.[76]

Recent efforts to improve awareness of STDs and access to STD services have led to alliances between public health authorities and organizations serving persons at risk for STDs, including community-based organizations, hospitals, jails, managed-care organizations, and groups of private physicians. Although screening for chlamydial infection has been shown to reduce the incidence of PID[69] and may be cost-saving in some populations,[77] STD screening for asymptomatic persons is not generally covered by traditional health insurance and is not widely available in managed-care organizations. Availability of urine-based testing technologies has allowed the expansion of STD screening into nonclinical and other nontraditional settings.[78] Screening in jails and emergency rooms has identified high prevalences of gonorrhea, chlamydial infection, and syphilis and has the potential for having substantial impact on disease control.[79,80] However, screening programs in these settings have been challenging to sustain. Continued improvements in STD service delivery will require ongoing collaboration with private sector medical providers and other organizations.[81]

Barriers to STD Transmission

Condoms form a physical barrier to particles even smaller than STD pathogens[82] and thus affect β, the efficiency of STD transmission. Male latex condoms, when used consistently and correctly, are highly effective in preventing the transmission of HIV and have varying degrees of effectiveness against other STDs.[83] Condoms do not cover all exposed skin surfaces and so may be more effective in preventing STDs transmitted through mucosal fluids, such as gonorrhea and chlamydia, than those transmitted through skin-to-skin contact, such as herpes, HPV, and syphilis. However, a recent prospective study indicates that condoms provide women a high level of protection against genital herpes.[84] Female condoms have not been well-studied for the prevention of STDs. Chemical barriers such as vaginal microbicides will likely also prove useful in STD prevention. However, the one microbicide that has been commercially available, nonoxynol-9 (also a spermicide), did not prevent STD acquisition and may increase the risk of HIV infection when used in very high doses;[85] it is not recommended for HIV prevention. Other microbicides are undergoing clinical development, and significant work remains to determine the optimal characteristics for product acceptability and usefulness. Implementation of microbicides for STD prevention among adolescents will require special considerations, including post-coital effectiveness.[86]

Behavioral Change

Interventions that effectively alter sexual risk behaviors include both individual-level and community-level interventions. Gender and cultural diversity necessitate the development of interventions appropriate to the attitudes, knowledge, and behaviors of specific groups.[87] The use of enhanced risk-reduction counseling for individuals or small groups has not only altered behaviors, but also decreased cases of STDs among high-risk individuals.[88,89] Interventions that change community norms for sexual behaviors, including condom use, have utilized peer opinion leaders to effectively promote behavior change among gay men.[90] Social marketing of condoms through media campaigns and broadened distribution has been associated with increases in rates of condom use.[91] For adolescents, some school-based sex and STD education programs have been shown to have positive effects such as delaying the initiation of intercourse, reducing the number of sexual partners and frequency of intercourse, and increasing condom use.[92] Self-efficacy is an important component in effecting behavioral change, particularly for adolescents and for women in relationships of unequal power. Prevention programs which focus on empowerment, negotiation, and refusal can provide the underlying skills necessary to effect positive behavioral change.[93]

Vaccination

Currently, the only STD for which there is an available and highly effective preventive vaccine is hepatitis B. Although hepatitis B vaccine is now recommended as a part of standard early childhood immunizations, as of 2001 most adolescents and young adults have not been vaccinated.[94] Despite years of effort, vaccines for other STDs are not yet available.[95] Several companies are actively developing vaccines against HPV and HSV, although early trials have failed to identify candidate vaccines with high levels of protection for both men and women.[96,97] Given the difficulties encountered in implementing hepatitis B vaccination, preparation for other STD vaccines should begin now, with research addressing vaccine acceptability and behavioral changes associated with STD vaccination.[95,96]

Further Information on STD Prevention

Further information may be obtained on the worldwide web at sites for CDC (http://www.cdc.gov), the National Network of Prevention Training Centers (http://depts.washington.edu/nnptc), and the American Social Health Organization (http://www.ashastd.org).

REFERENCES

1. Cates Jr, W. American Social Health Association Panel. Estimates of the incidence and prevalence of sexually transmitted diseases in the United States. *Sex Transm Dis* 1999;26:S2–S7.

2. Gjestland T. The Oslo study of untreated syphilis: An epidemiologic investigation of the natural course of syphilitic infection based on a restudy of the Boeck-Bruusgaard material. *Acta Derm Venereol* 1955;35(Suppl[Stockh]34): I.

3. Ingraham NR. The value of penicillin alone in the prevention and treatment of congenital syphilis. *Acta Derm Venereol* 1951;31:60.

4. Division of STD Prevention. *Sexually transmitted disease surveillance, 2001.* Atlanta, Georgia: Centers for Disease Control and Prevention, 2002.

5. Centers for Disease Control and Prevention. Primary and secondary syphilis—United States, 1999. *MMWR* 2001;50:113–117.

6. Division of STD Prevention. *The national plan to eliminate syphilis from the United States:* Centers for Disease Control and Prevention. 1999.

7. Fox KK, del Rio C, Holmes KK, Hook EW, Judson FN, Knapp JS, Procop GW, Wang SA, Whittington WLH, Levine WC. Gonorrhea in the HIV Era: A reversal in trends among men who have sex with men. *Am J Pub Health* 2001; 91:959–964.

8. Centers for Disease Control and Prevention. Resurgent bacterial sexually transmitted disease among men who have sex with men—King County, Washington, 1997–1999. *MMWR* 1999;48:773–777.

9. Centers for Disease Control and Prevention. Increases in unsafe sex and rectal gonorrhea among men who have sex with men—San Francisco, California, 1994–1997. *MMWR* 1999;48:45–48.

10. Holmes KK, Eschenbach DA, Knapp JS. Salpingitis: Overview of etiology and epidemiology. *Am J Obstet Gynecol* 1980;138:893–900.

11. Westrom L, Joesoef R, Reynolds G, Hadgu A, Thompson SE. Pelvic inflammatory disease and fertility: A cohort of 1844 women with laparoscopically verified disease and 657 control women with normal laparoscopy. *Sex Transm Dis* 1992;19:185–192.

12. Fox KK, Whittington WL, Levine WC, Moran JS, Zaidi AA, Nakashima AK. Gonorrhea in the United States, 1981–1996: Demographic and geographic trends. *Sex Transm Dis* 1998;25: 386–93.

13. Centers for Disease Control and Prevention. Gonorrhea—United States, 1998. *MMWR* 2000;49:538–542.

14. Stamm WE, Koutsky LA, Benedetti JK, Jourden JL, Brunham RC, Holmes KK. *Chlamydia trachomatis* urethral infections in men: Prevalence, risk factors, and clinical manifestations. *Ann Intern Med* 1984;100:47–51.

15. Mertz KJ, Levine WC, Mosure DJ, Berman SM, Dorian KJ. Trends in the prevalence of chlamydial infections. The impact of community-wide testing. *Sex Transm Dis* 1997;24:169–175.

16. Hillis SD, Nakashima A, Amsterdam L, Pfister J, Vaughn M, Addiss D, Marchbanks PA, Owens LM, Davis JP. The impact of a comprehensive chlamydia prevention program in Wisconsin. *Family Plan Perspect* 1995;27:108–111.

17. Groseclose SL, Zaidi AA, DeLisle SJ, Levine WC, St. Louis ME. Estimated incidence and prevalence of genital *Chlamydia trachomatis* infections in the United States, 1996. *Sex Transm Dis* 1999;26:339–344.

18. Cotch MF, Pastorek JG, Nugent RG, et al. *Trichomonas vaginalis* associated with low birth weight and preterm delivery. *Sex Transm Dis* 1997;24:353–360.

19. Fleming DT, McQuillan GM, Johnson RE, et al. Herpes simplex virus type 2 in the United States, 1976 to 1994. *N Eng J Med* 1997;337:1105–11.

20. Whitley RJ, Kimberlin DW, Roizman B. Herpes simplex viruses. *Clin Infect Dis* 1998;26:541–555.

21. Brown ZA, Benedetti J, Ashley R, et al. Neonatal herpes simplex virus infection in relation to asymptomatic maternal infection at the time of labor. *N Engl J Med* 1991;324:1247–1252.

22. Ho GYF, Bierman R, Beardsley L, Chang CJ, Burk RD. Natural history of cervicovaginal papilloma virus infection in young women. *N Engl J Med* 1998;338:423–8.

23. Koutsky L. Epidemiology of genital human papilloma virus infection. *Am J Med* 1997;102(suppl 5A):3–8.

24. Nobbenhuis MAE, Walboomers JMM, Helmerhorst TJM, Rozendaal L, Remmink AJ, Risse EKJ, van der Linden HC, Voorhorst FJ, Kenemans P, Meijer CJLM. Relation of human papillomavirus status to cervical lesions and consequences for cervical-cancer screening: A prospective study. *Lancet* 1999;354:20–25.

25. Quick CA, Watts SL, Krzyzek RA, Faras AJ. Relationship between condylomata and laryngeal papillomata: Clinical and molecular virological evidence. *Ann Otol Rhinol Laryngol* 1980;89:467–471.

26. Hyams KC. Risks of chronicity following acute hepatitis B virus infection: A review. *Clin Infect Dis* 1995;20:992–1000.

27. Xu ZY, Duan SC, Margolis HS, et al. Long-term efficacy of active postexposure immunization of infants for prevention of hepatitis B virus infection. *J Infect Dis* 1995;171:54–60.

28. Mast EE, Mahoney FJ, Alter MJ, Margolis HS. Progress toward elimination of hepatitis B viurs transmission in the United States. *Vaccine* 1998;16(suppl): S48–S51.

29. Cohen MS. Sexually transmitted diseases enhance HIV transmission: No longer a hypothesis. *Lancet* 1998;351 (suppl III):5–7.

30. Fleming DT, Wasserheit. From epidemiological synergy to public health policy and practice: contribution of other sexually transmitted diseases to sexual transmission of HIV infection. *Sex Transm Infect* 1999;75:3–17.

31. Grosskurth H, Mosha F, Todd J, Mwijarubi E, Klokke A, Senkoro K, Mayaud P, Changalucha J, Nicoll A, ka-Gina G, Newell J, Mugeye K, Mabey D, Hayes R. Impact of improved treatment of sexually transmitted diseases on HIV infection in rural Tanzania: randomised controlled trial. *Lancet* 1995;346:530–536.

32. Cates W Jr. The epidemiology and control of sexually transmitted diseases in adolescents. *Adolescent Medicine: State of the Art Reviews.* 1990;1:410–427.

33. Centers for Disease Control. Trends in sexual risk behaviors among high school students—United States, 1991–1997. *MMWR* 1998;47:749–752.

34. Rosenberg MD, Gurvey JE, Adler N, Dunlop MBV, Ellen JM. Concurrent sex partners and risk for sexually transmitted diseases among adolescents. *Sex Transm Dis* 1999;26:208–212.

35. O'Reilly KR, Aral SO. Adolescence and sexual behavior: trends and implications for STD. *J Adolesc Health Care.* 1985;6:262–270.

36. Fortenberry JD. Health care seeking behaviors related to sexually transmitted diseases among adolescents. *Am J Public Health* 1997;87:417–420.

37. Brackbill RM, Sternberg MR, Fishbein M. Where do people go for treatment of sexually transmitted diseases? *Fam Planning Perspectives* 1999;31:10–15.

38. Rothenberg R, Bross DC, Vernon TM. Reporting of gonorrhea by private physicians: A behavioral study. *Am J Public Health* 1980;70:983–986.

39. Miller S, Exner TM, Williams SP, Ehrhardt AA. A gender-specific intervention for at-risk women in the USA. *AIDS Care* 2000;12:603–12.

40. Hooper RR. Cohort study of venereal disease: I. The risk of gonorrhea transmission from infected women to men. *Am J Epidemiol* 1978; 108:136–144.

41. Worm AM et al. Transmission of chlamydial infections to sexual partners. *Genitourin Med* 1987; 63:19–21.

42. Irwin DE, Thomas JC, Spitters CE, Leone PA, Stratton JD, Martin DH, Zenilman JM, Schwebke JR, Hook EW. Self-treatment patterns among clients attending sexually transmitted disease clinics and the effect of self-treatment on STD symptom duration. *Sex Transm Dis* 1997;24:372–377.

43. Hahn RA, Magder LS, Aral SO, Johnson RE, Larsen SA. Race and the prevalence of syphilis seroreactivity in the United States population: A national sero-epidemiologic study. *Am J Pub Health* 1989;79:467–470.

44. Mertz KJ, McQuillan GM, Levine WC, et al. A pilot study of the prevalence of chlamydial infection in a national household survey. *Sex Transm Dis* 1998;25:225–228.

45. Moran JS, Aral SO, Jenkins WC, Peterman TA, Alexander ER. The impact of sexually transmitted diseases on minority populations. *Pub Health Rep* 1989;104:560–565.

46. Toomey KE, Moran JS, Rafferty MP, Beckett GA. Epidemiological considerations of sexually transmitted diseases in underserved populations. *Infect Dis Clin North Am* 1993;7:739–752.

47. Aral SO, Soskolne V, Joesoef RM, O'Reilly KR. Sex partner recruitment as risk factor for STD: Clustering of risky modes. *Sex Transm Dis* 1991;18:10–17.

48. Wasser SC, Aral SO, Reed DS, Bowen GS. Assessing behavioral risk for HIV infection in family-planning and STD clinics: Similarities and differences. *Sex Transm Dis* 1989;16:178–183.

49. Aral SO, Wasserheit JN. Interactions among HIV, other sexually transmitted diseases, socioeconomic status, and poverty in women. In: O'Leary A and Jemmott LS (eds.). *Women at risk: Issues in the primary prevention of AIDS*. New York: Plenum Press, 1995;13–40.

50. Laumann EO, Youm Y. Racial/ethnic group differences in the prevalence of sexually transmitted diseases in the United States: A network explanation. *Sex Transm Dis* 1999:26:250–261.

51. Hillis SD, Nakashima A, Marchbanks PA, et al. Risk factors for recurrent Chlamydia trachomatis infections in women. *Am J Obstet Gynecol* 1994;170:801–806.

52. Hillis SD, Owens LM, Marchbanks PA, et al. Recurrent chlamydial infections increase the risks of hospitalization for ectopic pregnancy and pelvic inflammatory disease. *Am J Obstet Gynecol* 1997;176:103–107.

53. Aral SO. Sexual behavior in sexually transmitted disease research. An overview. *Sex Transm Dis* 1994;21:S59–S64.

54. Ghani AC, Swintin J, Garnett G. The role of sexual partnership networks in the epidemiology of gonorrhea. *Sex Transm Dis* 1997;24:45–56.

55. Edwards S, Carne C. Oral sex and the transmission of viral STIs. *Sex Transm Infect* 1998;74:6–10.

56. Edwards S, Carne C. Oral sex and transmission of non-viral STIs. *Sex Transm Infect* 1998;74:95–100.

57. Adimora AA, Schoenbach VJ, Martinson FEA, Donaldson KH, Fullilove RE, Aral SO. Social context of sexual relationships among rural African Americans. *Sex Transm Dis* 2001;28:69–76.

58. Louv WC et al. Oral contraceptive use and risk of chlamydial and gonococcal infections. *Am J Obstet Gynecol* 1989;160:396–400.

59. Burkman RT. Association between intrauterine device and pelvic inflammatory disease. *Obstet Gynecol* 1981;57:269–276.

60. Wolner-Hanssen P, Eschenbach DA, Paavonen J, Kiviat N, Stevens C, Critchlow C, et al. Association between vaginal douching and acute pelvic inflammatory disease. *JAMA* 1990;263:1936–1941.

61. Institute of Medicine. *The Hidden Epidemic: Confronting Sexually Transmitted Diseases.* Eng TR, Butler WT (eds). Washington DC, National Academy Press, 1997.

62. Gelberg L, Gallagher TC, Anderson RM, Koegel P. Competing priorities as a barrier to medical care among homeless adults in Los Angeles. *Am J Public Health* 1997;87:217–220.

63. Yorke JA, Hethcote HW, Nold A. Dynamics and control of the transmission of gonorrhea. *Sex Transm Dis* 1978;5:51–57.

64. Anderson RM, Garnett GP. Mathematical models of the transmission and control of sexually transmitted diseases. *Sex Transm Dis* 2000;27:636–643.

65. Martin DH, Mroczkowski TF, Dalu ZA, McCarty J, Jones RB, Hopkins SJ, Johnson RB, and the Azithromycin for Chlamydial Infections Study Group. A controlled trial of a single dose of azithromycin for the treatment of chlamydial urethritis and cervicitis. *N Engl J Med* 1992;327:921–925.

66. Wald A, Zeh J, Barnum G, Davis LG, Corey L. Suppression of subclinical shedding of herpes simplex virus type 2 with acyclovir. *Ann Intern Med* 1996;124:8–15.

67. American Academy of Pediatrics and American College of Obstetricians and Gynecologists. *Guidelines for Perinatal Care*, 4th ed. Washington, D.C., 1997.

68. U.S. Prevention Services Task Force. Screening for chlamydial infection. Recommendations and rationale. *Am J Prev Med* 2001;20(3S):90–94.

69. Scholes D, Stergachis A, Heidrich FE, Andrilla H, Holmes KK, Stamm WE. Prevention of pelvic inflammatory disease by screening for cervical chlamydial infection. *N Engl J Med* 1996;34:1362–1366.

70. Marrazzo JM, White CL, Krekeler B, Celum CL, Lafferty WE, Stamm WE, Handsfield HH. Community-based urine screening for *Chlamydia trachomatis* with a ligase chain reaction assay. *Ann Intern Med* 1997;127:796–803.

71. Wiesenfeld HC, Lowry DLB, Heine P, Krohn MA, Bittner H, Kellinger K, Schultz M, Sweet RL. Self-collection of vaginal swabs for the detection of chlamydia, gonorrhea, and trichomoniasis. *Sex Transm Dis* 2001;28:321–325.

72. Blank S, McDonnell DD, Rubin SR, Neal JJ, Brome MW, Masterson MB, Greenspan JR. New approach to syphilis control. *Sex Transm Dis* 1997;24:218–226.

73. Centers for Disease Control and Prevention. Syphilis screening among women arrestees at the Cook County jail — Chicago, 1996. *MMWR* 1998:47:432–433.

74. Manos MM, Kinney WK, Hurley LB, Sherman ME, Shieh-Ngai J, Kurman RJ, Ransley JE, Fetterman BJ, Hartinger JS, McIntosh KM, Pawlick GF, Hiatt RA. Identifying women with cervical neoplasia. Using human papillomavirus DNA testing for equivocal Papanicolaou results. *JAMA* 1999;281:1605–1610.

75. Oh MK, Boker JR, Genuardi FJ, Cloud GA, Reynolds J, Hodgens JB. Sexual contact tracing outcome in adolescent chlamydial and gonococcal cervicitis cases. *J Adolesc Health* 1996;18:4–9.

76. Rothenberg R, Kimbrough L, Lewis-Hardy R, Heath B, Williams OC, Tambe P, Johnson D, Schrader M. Social network methods for endemic foci of syphilis. *Sex Transm Dis* 2000;27:12–18.

77. Marrazzo JM, Celum CL, Hillis SD, Fine D, DeLisle S, Handsfield H. Performance and cost-effectiveness of selective screening criteria for *Chlamydia trachomatis* infection in women: implications for a national chlamydia control strategy. *Sex Transm Dis* 1997;24:131–141.

78. Jones CA, Knaup RC, Hayes M, Stoner BP. Urine screening for gonococcal and chlamydial infections at community-based organizations in a high-morbidity area. *Sex Transm Dis* 2000;27:146–151.

79. Heimberger TS, Chang H-G H, Birkhead GS, DiFerdinando GD, Greenberg AJ, Gunn R, Morse DL. High prevalence of syphilis detected through a jail screening program. *Arch Intern Med* 1993;153:1799–1804.

80. Todd CA, Haase C, Stoner BP. Emergency department screening for asymptomatic sexually transmitted infections. *Am J Public Health* 2001;91:461–464.

81. Gunn RA, Rolfs RT, Greenspan JR, Seidman RL, Wasserheit JN. The changing paradigm of sexually transmitted disease control in the era of managed health care. *JAMA* 1998;279:680–684.

82. Lytle CD, Routson LB, Seaborn GB, Dixon LG, Bushar HF, Cyr WH. An in vitro evaluation of condoms as barriers to a small virus. *Sex Transm Dis* 1997;24:161–164.

83. d'Oro LC, Parazzini F, Naldi L, La Vecchia C. Barrier methods of contraception, spermicides, and sexually transmitted diseases: a review. *Genitourin Med* 1994;70(6):410–417.

84. Wald A, Langerberg AGM, Link K, Izu AE, Ashley R, Warren T, Tyring S, Douglas Jr JM, Corey L. Effect of condoms on reducing the transmission of herpes simplex virus type 2 from men to women. *JAMA* 2001:285:3100–3106.

85. Roddy RE, Zekeng L, Ryan KA, Tamoufé U, Weir SS, Wong EL. A controlled trial of nonoxynol 9 film to reduce male-to-female transmission of sexually transmitted diseases. *N Engl J Med* 1998;339:504–510.

86. Rosenthal SL, Cohen SS, Stanberry LR. Topical microbicides. Current status and research considerations for adolescent girls. *Sex Transm Dis* 1998;25:368–377.

87. O'Donnell L, Doval SA, Vornfett R, O'Donnell CR. STD prevention and the challenge of gender and cultural diversity: knowledge, attitudes and risk behaviors among black and hispanic inner-city STD clinic patients. *Sex Transm Dis* 1994;24:137–148.

88. Kamb ML, Fishbein M, Douglas JM Jr, Rhodes F, Rogers J, Bolan G, Zenilman J, Hoxworth T, Malotte CK, Istesta M, Kent C, Lentz A, Graziano S, Byers RH, Peterman TA. Efficacy of risk-reduction counseling to prevent human immunodeficiency virus and sexually transmitted diseases: a randomized controlled trial. Project Respect Study Group. *JAMA* 1998 280:1161–1167.

89. Shain RN, Piper JM, Newton ER, Perdue ST, Ramos R, Champion JD, Guerra FA. A randomized, controlled trial of a behavioral intervention to prevent sexually transmitted disease among minority women. *N Engl J Med* 1999;340:93–100.

90. Kelly JA, St. Lawrence JS, Stevenson LY, Hauth AC, Kalichman SC, Diaz YE, et al. Community AIDS/HIV risk reduction: the effects of endorsements by popular people in three cities. *Am J Public Health* 1992;82:1483–1489.

91. Cohen DA, Farley TA, Bedimo-Etame JR, Scribner R, Waqrd W, Kendall, C, Rice J. Implementation of condom social marketing in Louisiana, 1993 to 1996. *Am J Public Health* 1999;89:204–208.

92. Kirby D, Short L, Collins J, Rugg D, Kolbe L, Howard M, Miller B, Sonenstein F, Zabin LS. School-based programs to reduce sexual risk behaviors: a review of effectiveness. *Public Health Rep* 1994;109:339–360.

93. Exner TM, et al. A review of HIV interventions for at-risk women. *AIDS Behav* 1997; 1:93–124.

94. Mast EE, Williams IT, Alter MJ, Margolis HS. Hepatitis B vaccination of adolescent and adult high-risk groups in the United States. *Vaccine* 1998;16:S27–S29.

95. Zimet GD, Mays RM, Fortenberry D. Vaccines against sexually transmitted diseases. Promise and problems of the magic bullets for prevention and control. *Sex Transm Dis* 2000;27:49–51.

96. Da Silva DM, Eiben GL, Fausch SC, Wakabayashi MT, Rudolf MP, Velders MP, Kast WM. Cervical cancer vaccines: Emerging concepts and developments. *J Cell Physiol* 2001:186:169–182.

97. Corey L, Langenberg AG, Ashley R, et al, for the Chiron HSV Vaccine Study Group. Recombinant glycoprotein vaccine for the prevention of genital HSV-2 infection: 2 randomized controlled trials. *JAMA* 1999;282:331–340.

ARTICLE 10

CHILD ABUSE AND NEGLECT

Patti R. Rosquist and Richard D. Krugman

INTRODUCTION

Whether one approaches family health from a medical, legal, mental health, or social perspective, child abuse and neglect are enormous and complicated problems. The incidence of child maltreatment is increasing despite recognition of the problem in medical literature for over a century. Recent federal legislation may exacerbate our ability to deal with the problem. As keys to prevention are slowly elucidated, much research remains to be done. Yet despite a large task at hand, the first step is the willingness to acknowledge that child abuse and neglect exist, and that its solution will require a public health approach.

INCIDENCE AND PREVALENCE

The precise incidence and prevalence of child abuse and neglect are difficult to determine. Nonetheless, recent studies are providing more reliable estimates. Despite a decrease in the incidence of non-inflicted trauma, there continues to be an increase in intentional injury.[1] Three million children are reported to child protective services in the United States each year. More than one million of these are confirmed as child abuse or neglect. According to 1993 case-level data on substantiated or indicated victims, 52% suffered from neglect, 20% were victims of physical abuse, 12% were victims of sexual abuse, 4% of emotional maltreatment, and 4% of medical neglect.

Almost 30% of victims of child maltreatment were less than 4 years of age, 25% were from 4 to 7 years old, 21% from 8 to 11, and 26% from 12 to 17 years old. The gender of maltreated children was roughly evenly split between males and females. Forty-three percent of victims of fatal child abuse were less than 1 year of age. Women were counted as perpetrators 1.6 times as often as men. Perpetrators are five times more likely to be relatives than non-relatives. More than half of the victims suffered from neglect.[2]

When following the incidence of child abuse and neglect over time, the National Incidence Study revealed that there have been significant increases in the incidence of child abuse. The number of abused and neglected children nearly doubled from 1986 to 1993. Girls were sexually abused three times more often than boys. Boys had a greater risk of serious injury. Children are consistently vulnerable to sexual abuse from at least as early as age 3. Family risk factors include single-parent families and poverty. Children in larger families were at greatest risk for neglect.[3]

The rate of victimization of children is about 15 per thousand. About 80% of perpetrators were parents of the victims. Depending on the source, between one and two thousand children die from severe child abuse each year.[3,4] Some researchers suggest that there is an 85% underestimation because of the way in which death certificates are recorded and because of incomplete investigations and inaccurate medical diagnoses.[4]

When a population was surveyed about a history of physical abuse or sexual abuse in childhood, it was found that childhood maltreatment was common: 30.2% of males and 21.1% of females reported a history of physical abuse; 12.8% of females and 4.3% of males reported a history of sexual abuse.[5]

EFFECTS OF CHILD ABUSE AND NEGLECT

These incidence and prevalence data tell only part of the story. In addition to the immediate suffering and cost, child maltreatment affects the mental and physical health and development of children for decades. For example, victims have increased rates of adolescent suicide, alcoholism, drug abuse, anxiety, depression, criminality, violence, and learning problems. Melton suggests that although the acute and chronic problem of child maltreatment is great, a broader and equally concerning perspective is that child abuse may reflect the decline of a society.[6] Although knowledge about the incidence, etiology, treatment, and prevention of abuse has increased in recent years, more information is needed.

HISTORIC PERSPECTIVE

In addition to incidence and prevalence data, a review of historic child abuse literature provides added perspective. In the United States, childrearing is personal and largely private except when there are social implications such as delinquency, divorce, and child abuse, or when it occurs in day care, scouting, or other settings. The founding fathers planned that resolution of most domestic conflicts rested with the states. Nonetheless, initial legislation to protect children began in 19th century England and 20th century United States with mandatory education.[7] The first report of skeletal injury from maltreatment was written by Tardieu. As a 19th century pathologist, and public health and forensic specialist, he described multiple fractures and other injuries in children that were inflicted by parents and others with authority over victims.[8] In 1874, Mary Ellen was removed from her abusive home after a writ of habeas corpus was invoked by an attorney from the American Society for the Prevention of Cruelty to Animals.[9]

In the early 20th century, the United States Supreme Court ruled against state interference in Meyer v. Nebraska (1923). Twenty-one years later, the court ruled that some limits could be placed on parental power in Prince v. Massachusetts (1944).

Throughout the 20th century more has been learned about normal behavior and development of children. Scientific and medical knowledge adds to insight handed down by family members.[7] In 1946, Caffey described infants with bone fractures and chronic subdural hematomas yet no history of trauma and suggested that injuries were possibly inflicted by care givers.[10] In 1953, Silverman determined that observed injuries were the result of repetitive trauma unrecognized through unawareness or denial by perpetrators.[11]

In 1962, Kempe published the first formal description and definition of the battered child syndrome.[12] With this foundation, scientific and medical knowledge has continued to expand, reporting laws have been passed, and intervention options explored. Yet, the causes of child abuse and neglect remain difficult to separate from broader social problems.

CAUSES OF CHILD ABUSE

With respect to one set of societal problems, it has been shown that alcohol and drug use is associated with an increased risk of homicide of other family members.[13] In another study, children born to women who used cocaine during pregnancy were at increased risk for maltreatment. The authors concluded that a mother's cocaine use is a marker of increased risk.[14] Yet, even discussions of discipline and parenting remain controversial. Corporal punishment of children remains actively debated by professionals dealing with children. As more information is gathered, the relationship between spanking and antisocial behavior may be established.[15] The effects of corporal punishment are difficult to separate from the family and social context.[16] Smith found that although harsh discipline was associated with lower IQ, harsh discipline plus low maternal warmth was associated with an even greater decline of IQ.[17] Bross notes that "most child maltreatment is not the product of insanity but rather an exaggeration of accepted practices."[7]

EFFECTS OF LEGISLATION

The spectrum of etiology, severity, and consequences of child maltreatment is very broad. Results extend from relatively subtle effects such as decreases in cognitive function to fatal child abuse where context is not relevant. With child maltreatment manifesting in so many ways, it is not surprising that opportunities for intervention, treatment, and prevention are many as well.

The effects of recent federal legislation may exacerbate some of the complex etiologies of child maltreatment. Specifically, welfare reform bill H.R. 3734, the

Personal Responsibility and Work Opportunity Reconciliation Act (PRWORA) of 1996, eliminates Emergency Assistance to Families with Children, and Aid to Families with Dependent Children (AFDC). This legislation allows for Temporary Assistance for Needy Families block grants of federal funds to the states. However, the act requires that states must have 25% of their welfare recipients engaged in work, that recipients must begin working within two years, and they are limited to five years of benefits for a lifetime. Some experts in child abuse and neglect have expressed concerns that these changes may increase the risk for child abuse and neglect. The incidence and severity of child abuse and neglect will need to be monitored as these legislative changes are implemented.

PREVENTION STRATEGIES

There is little agreement on what defines adequate care for our children—whether we speak as parents, citizens, or legislators. The standard of care may be set at various points from preventing additional harm after a crisis to affirmatively advocating for prevention of abuse. Some professionals are in a role to attempt to address preventing additional harm while others seek to prevent maltreatment from occurring.

Prevention strategies include both general and specific approaches. Examples of general approaches include community programs that address poverty and violence. Specific strategies include targeted interventions such as a violence prevention curriculum for children,[18] or prenatal and early childhood home visits. Such visits recently have been shown to reduce the number of subsequent pregnancies, use of welfare, child abuse and neglect, and criminal behavior. The effect is greater for women who are unmarried and from low socio-economic background.[19] Clearly, specific interventions have been shown to modify behavior.[1,18,19] Unfortunately, a systematic approach to the prevention of child abuse and neglect has not yet been studied.

Child Protection Research

Consequently, child abuse and neglect prevention research needs to be a funding priority. Regardless of one's role in child protection, decisions must frequently be made based on common sense, experience, and personal beliefs. Scientific studies may not have been done to provide a sound, literature-based decision-making process. These gaps in knowledge need to be filled by child protection research. There are many risk factors for abuse. Each of them represents an opportunity for a separate prevention strategy. Successful unintentional injury prevention strategies might be adapted to slow the increase in intentional injuries.[1] Specific needed areas of inquiry include evaluation of current prevention, intervention, and treatment programs; the perception of children of the current child protection system; and the relationship between domestic violence and child maltreatment.[6]

Education as Prevention

Perhaps a coordinated, systematic curriculum using existing resources could change attitudes and behavior in a cumulative way. In the meantime, the costs and benefits of many specific interventions remain to be tested. Perhaps children can learn skills that could enhance future parenting effectiveness and promote optimal child development of the next generation.

Beginning with primary and secondary education, some existing curricula teach conflict resolution skills and that violence is not an acceptable response to conflict. Secondary school students could be targeted for parenting education before they become parents. In early adulthood, susceptible individuals need access to drug, alcohol, and smoking-cessation treatment prior to becoming parents. In addition to targeted home visits, prenatal care addressing new-parent coping skills might prove helpful in decreasing the number of shaken babies.

The Role of Health Care Workers

Several general parenting issues can be addressed throughout childhood. At pediatric health supervision and immunization visits, health care providers can elicit concerns about behavior and offer age-appropriate anticipatory guidance. Parents need to know about community resources before abuse occurs.

When family dysfunction becomes apparent, early therapeutic intervention may be more effective than later intervention during adolescence. At times, hospitalization becomes necessary. A broader view of child protection to include identifying and building on family strengths may ameliorate the need for foster care in some instances. In the event of fatal child abuse, state fatality review teams can assist communities in identifying specific needs. In other words, many preventive and therapeutic interventions need to be explored in order to find the most cost-effective and humane strategy to approach the problem of child abuse and neglect. The results of such a strategy can only be evaluated by providing long-term follow-up for families.

COST OF CHILD PREVENTION

Cost is an important factor. How much does it cost to protect children? In 1992, more than 2 billion dollars were spent on foster care alone.[6] We also know that children identified as being at high risk for child abuse or neglect have significantly more hospitalizations.[20] But just as we must calculate the cost of protecting children we must also calculate the cost of not protecting them.

But what if child abuse and neglect were a genetic problem? Whether genetically determined or genetically influenced, the possibility that abusive or neglectful behavior was not merely a social problem could transform how society and health professionals deal with it. This intriguing possibility should keep anyone from being certain that he or she knows what needs to be done in an area so understudied.[21]

FUTURE POLICY

From this review of incidence, federal legislation, causes, and potential preventive strategies for child maltreatment, the need for a clear statement on child protection policy and focused child protection programs is clear. Such a policy must stem from informed public discussion, acknowledgment of the severity of the problem, and the need to support research. Each individual needs to know more about child abuse. For most of us, this means staying up to date on current literature. For society, it means investment in research, biomedical and biosocial, as well as a commitment to outcomes research on programs in place to help children. A comprehensive public policy should be based on known effective strategies, and it should support research to uncover additional approaches. These will likely include strengthening neighborhoods and improving parental competence. A system is needed that responds to parents' needs so they can get assistance prior to abuse. The task is large but necessary. After all, the prevention and treatment of child abuse are basic to the preservation of our communities.[22]

REFERENCES

1. Rivara FP, Grossman DC. Prevention of traumatic deaths to children in the United States: How far have we come and where do we need to go? *Pediatrics* 1997;97:791–797.

2. U.S. Department of Health and Human Services, National Center on Child Abuse and Neglect. *Child Abuse and Neglect Case-Level Data 1993: Working Paper 1.* Washington, D.C.: U.S. Government Printing Office; 1996.

3. U.S. Department of Health and Human Services, National Center on Child Abuse and Neglect. *Child Maltreatment 1995: Reports from the States to the National Child Abuse and Neglect Data System.* Washington, D.C.: U.S. Government Printing Office; 1997.

4. U.S. Advisory Board on Child Abuse and Neglect. *A Nation's Shame: Fatal Child Abuse and Neglect in the United States.* U.S. Government Printing Office, 1995.

5. MacMillan HL, Fleming JE, Trocme N, Boyle MH, Wong M, Racine YA, Beardslee WR, et al. Prevalence of child physical and sexual abuse in the community. *JAMA* 1997;278:131–135.

6. Melton GB, Flood MF. Research policy and child maltreatment: Developing the scientific foundation for effective protection of children. *Child Abuse and Neglect* 1994;18 (supplement): 1–28.

7. Bross D. Law and the abuse of children. *Currents in Modern Thought: Child Abuse and Society's Response* 1990; (6): 473–487.

8. Tardieu A. Etude medio-legale sur les services et mauvais traitments exerces surdes enfants. *Ann Hyg Publ Med Leg* 1860;13:361.

9. Lazoritz S, Shelman EA. Before Mary Ellen. *Child Abuse and Neglect* 1996;20:235–237.

10. Caffey J. Multiple fractures in the long bones of infants suffering from chronic subdural hematoma. *AJR* 1946;56:163

11. Silverman FN. The Roentgen manifestations of unrecognized skeletal trauma in infants. *AJR* 1953;69:413.

12. Kempe CH, Silverman FN, Steele BF, Droegmuler W, Silver HK. The battered child syndrome. *JAMA* 1962;181:17–24.

13. Rivara FP, Mueller BA, Somes G, Mendoza CT, Rushforth NB, Kellerman AL. Alcohol and illicit drug abuse and the risk of violent death in the home. *JAMA* 1997;278(7):569–575.

14. Leventhal JM, Forsyth BWC, Qi K, Johnson L, Schroeder D, Votto N. Maltreatment of children born to women who used cocaine during pregnancy: A population-based study. *Pediatrics* 1997;100(2):e7.

15. Straus MA, Sugarman DB, Giles-Sims J. Spanking by parents and subsequent antisocial behavior of children. *Arch Pediatr Adolesc Med* 1997;151:761–767.

16. Lindner Gunnoe M, Mariner CL. Toward a developmental-contextual model of the effects of parental spanking on children's aggression. *Ach Pediatr Adolesc Med* 1997;151:768–775.

17. Smith JR, Brooks-Gunn J. Correlates and consequences of harsh discipline for young children. *Arch Pediatr Adolesc Med* 1997;151:777–786.

18. Grossman DC, Neckerman HJ, Koepsell TD, Liu P, Asher KN, Beland K, et al. Effectiveness of a violence prevention curriculum among children in elementary school: A randomized controlled trial. *JAMA* 1997; 277:1605–1611.

19. Olds DL, Eckenrode J, Henderson CR, Kitzman H, Powers J, Cole R, et al. Long-term effects of home visitation on maternal life course and child abuse and neglect: Fifteen-year follow-up of a randomized trial. *JAMA* 1997; 278:637–643.

20. Krugman, RD. Editorial. Suppose It Were a Genetic Disorder? *Child Abuse and Neglect* 1997; 21:245–246.

21. Leventhal JM, Pew MC, Berg AT, Garber RB. Use of health services by children who were identified during the postpartum period as being at high risk of child abuse or neglect. *Pediatrics* 1996;97:331–335.

22. Krugman, RD. Future directions in preventing child abuse. *Child Abuse and Neglect* 1995;19:273–279.

BIBLIOGRAPHY

*Sedlak AJ, Broadhurst DD. *Executive Summary of the Third National Incidence Study of Child Abuse and Neglect.* U.S. Department of Health and Human Services, National Center on Child Abuse and Neglect, 1996.

*Sege RD, Perry C, Stigol L, Cohon L, Griffith J, Cohn M, et al. Short-term effectiveness of anticipatory guidance to reduce early childhood risks for subsequent violence. *Arch Pediatr Adolesc Med* 1997;151:392–397.

*U.S. Advisory Board on Child Abuse and Neglect. *Neighbors Helping Neighbors: A New National Strategy for the Protection of Children.* Washington, D.C.: U.S. Government Printing Office, 1993.

A R T I C L E   1 1

HOMELESS WOMEN AND THEIR CHILDREN IN THE 21ST CENTURY

Peter Sherman and Irwin Redlener

INTRODUCTION

In spite of an unprecedented growth in the economy and subsequent record low unemployment levels throughout most of the 1990s, the number of people who were homeless in the United States steadily increased. A slowdown in the economy that began in 2000 and continued through 2001 magnified the problem. Safety-net programs remain inadequate and a persistent unwillingness to address the lack of affordable housing means that the number of people who are homeless, particularly children, will increase over the next several years. Any long-term downturn in the nation's economy will greatly exacerbate this problem. In order to understand why this is so, it is important to have an understanding of the forces that create and maintain the condition of homelessness in families and how the condition of homelessness affects the well-being of children.

NUMBERS OF HOMELESS

Although it is well substantiated that homelessness is a major problem for many communities, it is not clear how many individuals are homeless in the United States. Estimates are in the range of 1.7–3 million per year, with the number varying according to the definition of homelessness and the methodology used to tabulate individuals.[1]

The most common method of counting the number of homeless individuals, point-in-time estimation, tends to underestimate the number of homeless persons. This is because this methodology focuses on the chronically homeless and misses many of those who are homeless for a short period of time. Many surveys do not count people who are homeless because they are doubled-up with other families or are living in hidden areas, such as cars, tunnels, or parks.

Retrospective studies provide a different picture. Link, in 1994, randomly surveyed a cross-section of people living in the United States, via telephone, to ask if they had ever experienced homelessness. Literal homelessness was defined as living in a park, abandoned building, street, train or bus station, shelter, or another temporary residence. Even though this methodology is likely to underestimate homelessness by missing those who do not have telephones and those who are currently homeless, the proportion reporting a history of homelessness was striking. Lifetime prevalence was 7.4% for literal homelessness and 14% if living doubled-up with others was included.[2] These were not just brief episodes of homelessness. Forty-six percent reported their length of homelessness to be between one month and a year and 13% were homeless for more than a year. This translates to over 13 million adult Americans reporting literal homelessness at some point in their lives. If one includes doubling-up the number increases to 26 million. This figure includes large numbers of single mothers and their children.

Several surveys show that the number of homeless families is reaching record levels. An Urban Institute report estimated that in 1996, 3.5 million people became homeless during the course of the year. This represented a 65% increase compared to 1987. Of these, 39% were children.[3] Therefore, nearly 2% of children in America are homeless each year. In 2000 the U.S. Conference of Mayors reported that the average demand for emergency shelter increased 15%, the largest one-year increase in the past decade. At the same time, requests for shelter by homeless families increased by 17%. In this survey families with children represented 36% of the homeless population.[4]

In July of 2001 the New York City Department of Homeless Services housed 6,252 families with 11,594 children in family homeless shelters. These numbers surpassed previous records set in the late 1980s and mid-1990s, when a maximum of 5,700 families were housed.[5]

CAUSES OF HOMELESSNESS

When single-parent families were queried about why they were homeless, 28% related it to housing problems, 20% to economic hardship, 31% to family and/or relationship problems, and 14% to drug use or violence.[6] However, to understand causes of homelessness it is necessary to step back and examine its roots in poverty, housing shortages, and the current labor market.

There are differing schools of thought concerning the causes of homelessness. One view is that it is caused by the combination of low wages and a shortage of affordable housing. Another view is that homeless families have certain psychosocial characteristics that make them vulnerable to housing loss. Both viewpoints are valid depending upon the type of population that is being studied. It is important to understand the difference between direct causes of homelessness, such as a deficiency of affordable housing, and characteristics that make people more vulnerable to homelessness, such as domestic violence.

In cities where the housing market is very tight and there is a paucity of low-income housing, one will find more families that are homeless due to economic factors. This is due to the fact that a relatively small loss of income can leave a person in the situation of not having access to affordable housing because such housing is exceedingly scarce. Cities that have a better supply of affordable housing will find more homelessness caused by psychosocial factors, as it is not the lack of affordable housing per se that causes homelessness, but rather the inability of the person to access housing because of individual circumstances. The interaction of these different factors may help explain the disparate findings reported in studies of homelessness. Cognizance of these factors is also important in designing programs that are responsive to an individual community's needs. Regardless of geographical variations, it is clear that there are forces pushing an unprecedented number of families into homelessness.

In 1996, 21% of children lived in poverty. This declined to 16% in 2000.[7] The largest decline was with children living in single parent families, with 45% in 1996 and 25% in 2000 fitting into this category.[7,8] Children of color are also disproportionately affected, though the news on this front has also been encouraging. In 1996, 66% of Hispanic and 62% of African American children, living in female-headed households, were living in poverty. This fell to 34% and 35%, respectively, in 2000.[7]

A clear and direct correlation exists between poverty and homelessness. The U.S. Department of Housing and Urban Development (HUD) places those families whose incomes are less than 50% of the median family income in their community and who are renters and do not receive federal housing assistance in the category of "worst-case housing needs." Between 1991 and 1997 there has been a 12% increase in this category. People of color are disproportionately affected. Worst-case housing needs among Hispanic working families with children rose 74% during this period and 31% among similar African Americans.[9] Among non-Hispanic white households there was only a 2% increase.[9] The fact that between 1991 and 1997 there was a 29% increase in the number of worst-case housing needs in families with children[9] sheds light on why there is an upsurge in the number of homeless families.[9]

Exuberance over decreases in the number of children living in poverty becomes somewhat muted when we examine the mechanism by which many are leaving poverty behind. For those who are working, poverty is fueled by a service economy that pays low wages and often provides only part-time work, with few or no benefits. Though unemployment (unemployed or those working part-time because they cannot find a full-time job) has decreased over the past decade from 6.8% in 1991 to 4% in 2000, underemployment affects a significant percentage of the workforce. In fact 6.2% of the labor force fit this category in 2000, compared to 9.6% in 1994.[10] The U.S. Conference of Mayors estimates that 26% of those who are homeless are employed.[4] That number was 22% in 1998.[11]

Though the minimum wage was raised to $5.15 as of September 1997, a single earner working full-time at minimum wage still has an income $4,000 below the poverty line.[12] As of 2000, 25% of the workforce was earning poverty-level hourly wages.[13] Though this is the lowest that this statistic has been in the past 20 years, homeless and near-homeless families are disproportionately represented in this group and are especially vulnerable. In 2000, the share of poor children living in a household headed by a full-time year-round worker was 37%, the highest level since this data was first collected in 1975.[14] As of 1997, one out of three children with worst-case housing needs lives in a family with someone working full-time at or above the minimum wage.[9]

Another important factor contributing to homelessness is that the number of families headed by single women, the population most vulnerable to becoming homeless, has soared. Sixty-eight percent of children lived with two parents in 1996, compared to 85% in 1976.[8] Twenty-five percent of children lived in single-parent families in 1997; however, in low-income families this number was 41%.[15] This trend has been fueled by rising divorce rates and a growing number of mothers who never marry.

The factor most central in this equation is a profound lack of affordable housing. Between 1973 and 1993, 2.2 million low-rent units were lost. At the same time, those requiring low-rent housing increased by 4.7 million. This has resulted in the largest shortage of low-rent housing on record.[16] The Section 8 housing program, a federal program that subsidizes rental costs for poor families, is unable to address this housing gap, due to insufficient funding. Over the past decade federal spending for housing assistance has decreased 78%.[17] Between 1977 and 1980 HUD was able to provide rental assistance to an average of 290,000 low-income households per year. Between 1981 and 1993 this number dropped to an average of 74,000 per year.[18] No new vouchers or certificates were issued in 1996 or 1997. Although in 1999 and 2000 there was a modest increase in Section 8 vouchers, the overall picture is bleak. The national average waiting time is 11 months for public housing and 28 months for Section 8 vouchers. There is an 8-year wait for public housing in New York City. In Washington, D.C. and Cleveland it is 5 years. The wait is 8 years for Section 8 housing in New York City and Washington, D.C., whereas in Los Angeles it is 10 years.[19]

The amount of housing that is affordable for extremely low-income families continues to drop. There was a 5% decline of affordable housing for families whose income was below 30% of area median income between 1991 and 1997. In other words, during 1997, for every 100 households in this category, there were only 36 affordable units. In 1991 this number was 41.[9] The national median housing wage, the amount a worker would have to earn per hour at full-time employment to afford a two-bedroom apartment at the Fair Market Rent is $13.75 an hour, more than twice the current minimum wage. The Fair Market Rent is the amount below which 40%—some areas use a 50% cut-off—of standard nonluxury units rent for and is calculated by the Department of Housing and Urban Development. This includes rent and utilities excluding phone. In New York City this figure is $17.57.[20] In this context, it is not surprising that in 2000 there was a 17% increase in demand for shelter across the country, and 76% of cities surveyed reported that they experienced this type of increase.[4]

One cannot examine the relationship between poverty and housing without attempting to understand how entitlements affect children and the profound changes that have been made in these programs over the past several years. Welfare (Aid to Families with Dependent Children) was replaced by Temporary Assistance to Needy Families (TANF) in 1997 and was designed to move adults from welfare into jobs and provide child care to assist with this transition. TANF and food stamp benefits place a family of three at approximately one-third of the poverty level and are only available for 5 years. Though there is controversy as to the degree with which families are able to successfully leave "welfare" and enter the job market, given that most wage earners are making $6.50 to $9.00 an hour, it is clear that these families are at risk for becoming homeless. On a positive note, though many families reported some hardship with housing, food, and health insurance, none reported a significant change in the use of emergency shelters.[21] One must monitor this in a cautionary fashion, given the cost and scarcity of affordable housing.

In summary, the combination of diminishing income, coupled with a decrease in affordable housing is working in concert to produce an epidemic of homeless families in the United States. It seems clear that this problem will continue to grow rather than abate unless there is an increase in housing stock along with wages that are compatible with costs of living.

Factors Putting Families at Risk for Homelessness

Numerous studies have examined homeless families, headed by single mothers, in an attempt to create a profile of the mother at risk for becoming homeless. By predicting which families are at risk for homelessness it would be possible to effectively target homelessness-prevention programs. Unfortunately, results are conflicting, principally because homeless families are not a homogeneous population. As previously indicated, there is a great deal of geographic variation in the root causes of homelessness, given that the housing and economic status of one locale may be very different from that of another. Another reason is that admission criteria for shelters vary considerably from one area to another. There is also a large variation in the allowable and actual length of stay among shelters. The profile of a family and the effects of homelessness may be very different in a family that stays in a shelter for a few days, compared to a family that is in residence for several months.

Another important reason for conflicting findings pertaining to the profile of homeless families is due to variation in study designs. Few studies actually compare homeless subjects with matched poor housed subjects. Without a comparison group it is not possible to separate out predisposing factors that are unique to homelessness. Even when control groups are used, they are often not well matched, making comparison difficult. Another methodological issue is that the number of families studied tends to be small, which decreases the ability of the study to statistically differentiate between the two populations.

In spite of these variations, research studies have uncovered much important information about risk factors. One study that examined a large number of homeless families, and used a case-control design to compare them with housed families who were receiving AFDC, found several interesting results. Predictors of homelessness were foster-care placement as a child and drug use by a respondent's primary female caretaker. Additional factors associated with homelessness were fewer social supports, frequent heroin or alcohol use, and mental health hospitalization within the past two years.[6] Other investigators have also found these factors identify homeless women.[17,22] Although they are powerful predictors, they still only identify a small subset of homeless women. Protective factors included being the lease holder of an apartment, receiving AFDC and/or a housing subsidy in the prior year, graduating from high school, and having a large nonprofessional support network.[23]

Numerous studies have found a correlation between homelessness and having a history of being abused as an adult or a child. Shinn found that 11.4% of homeless women had a history of being physically abused as a child compared to 6.5% of housed poor women. Twenty-seven percent of the homeless women had been abused or threatened as adults compared to 16.6% of housed women.[24] Several studies found higher rates of battering among homeless women when compared to housed women.[6,25,26]

Other investigators were unable to confirm these findings. Goodman found no difference in both childhood and adult episodes of both physical and sexual abuse in comparing the two groups.[27] Both groups had experienced strikingly high rates of abuse at some point during their lifetime, with approximately 90% of both populations reporting some form of physical or sexual abuse during their lifetimes. The investigator hypothesized that their study failed to find a difference between the populations because of the changing nature of the homeless population. Because housing had become scarcer since the previous studies were carried out, a greater number of higher functioning families were homeless. This tended to diminish the potential differences between housed and homeless poor families. The investigator also felt that the high prevalence rates of abuse found in their study was due to the use of a more sensitive instrument to measure abuse. The overall picture does suggest that a history of abuse is a common experience among homeless women.

Investigators have found significant differences between housed and homeless mothers regarding a history of living in foster care or a group home as a child, with homeless mothers reporting higher rates of both experiences.[22] Shinn found that 21.6% of homeless mothers reported running away as minors, compared to only 6.5% of housed mothers. In addition, a higher percentage of homeless mothers reported the experience, as children, of living on the street.[24]

These findings suggest that experiences interfering with a person's ability to form supportive relationships places a mother from an economically impoverished background at increased risk for homelessness, and in fact, other investigators have found the absence of a supportive network to be an important risk factor for homelessness. Shinn's study contacted families at their point of entry into the homeless shelter system to gather information about support networks. Thus, the study was able to capture the support system that existed for a person just prior to entering the homeless system. Homeless families were compared with families on welfare. The percentage of those with supportive family contacts was similar between the two groups. The study found that the homeless families had "used up" resources on which they could depend upon for housing in an emergency: 18.4% of the housed families had at least one contact where they could reside in an emergency, whereas only 4.4% of the homeless families had such a contact. For those under 30 years of age the difference was even more striking, being 27% and 4%, respectively.[24] Thus one can conjecture that it is not the direct lack of social support but rather the lack of a socially supportive network that can provide housing in an emergency that puts a family at risk for homelessness.

Bassuk found that homeless families moved much more frequently and had a much higher rate of living doubled-up just prior to being homeless. In addition, homeless mothers demonstrated a paucity of social supports. Twenty-two percent of homeless women were unable to name any individuals that they could turn to for support, compared to 2% of housed women. Only 26% of the homeless women could name three adult supports, compared to 74% of the housed women.[23] Wood also found similar differences with, for example, 37% of the homeless mothers naming a child less than 18 years old as a support, whereas only 13% of the housed mothers did so.[6]

Domestic Violence and Homelessness

One of the most common reasons for a women and her children becoming home-less is domestic violence. One survey that examined this issue in several cities found that 22% of families were homeless as a result of domestic violence. Among parents who lived with a spouse or partner, 57% reported domestic violence as the sole reason for their being homeless.[28] In another survey, 14 out of 25 cities identified domestic violence as a primary cause of homelessness.[4]

IMPACT OF HOMELESSNESS ON CHILDREN'S HEALTH AND DEVELOPMENT

Few studies compare the health of homeless children with poor housed children. Therefore, it is not clear whether there is a significant difference in the health of the two populations. When parents were asked to rate the health of their children, 13% of homeless children were reported to be in fair or poor health, compared to 3.2% of the general pediatric population and 6.5% of those living in poverty. However, 44% of the problems were clustered in 15% of the children.[29] Another investigator did not find any difference in the general health of homeless children compared to poor children.[30]

In addition, children who present to clinical services with complaints of an acute nature, such as an upper respiratory infection, are frequently found to have serious problems of a more chronic nature. For example, although the typical rate for a subspecialty referral in a pediatric setting is 1 out of 40 patient encounters,[31] the New York City Children's Health Project, which serves homeless children, reports that approximately 1 out of every 20 patient encounters results in a referral.[32]

The New York Children's Health Project has found several indicators of poor health in the homeless children. Twenty-nine percent were diagnosed with otitis media, 12.5% with obesity, 6.5% with nutritional failure to thrive, and 10% with iron deficiency anemia. It was also determined that only 49% of children 12–36 months of age were up to date with their immunizations.[33] Forty percent of children living in several homeless shelters in New York City had asthma. This is more than six times the national rate. Forty-three percent had symptoms consistent with moderate or severe asthma. Yet, very few of the children were receiving appropriate treatment.[34]

Alperstein found several areas of significant difference when comparing housed and homeless children; 3.8% of homeless children had a lead elevation above 30 mcg/dl, whereas this only occurred in 1.7% of housed poor children. Inpatient pediatric admission rates were 11.6/1,000 for homeless children and 7.5/1,000 for poor housed children. Twenty-seven percent of homeless children had delayed immunization, compared with 15% of housed children.[35] Eddins also found high rates of under-immunization with 27% of children less than five years old not immunized against DPT, 33% not immunized against polio, and 28% having never received an MMR.[36]

Of particular concern is the nutritional status of homeless children. When parents were asked if their children got enough food, 21% of the homeless families replied that there was insufficient food four days or more in the preceding month, because of lack of money, compared to 7% of housed poor families. Twenty-three percent of the homeless families reported hunger in their children, secondary to insufficient food resources compared with 4% of the housed poor. Fourteen percent of the homeless families stated that they ate in a fast food restaurant or convenience store at least four times per week, compared with 4% of housed families. Nine percent of the girls were at less than fifth percentile for weight for height, which is indicative of failure to thrive, and 12% of the children had weight for height greater than 95%, indicative of obesity.[35] Given the importance of adequate nutrition for development in the infant and young child and the risk factors associated with obesity in later life, these are disturbing findings.

Developmental, educational, and psychological outcomes in homeless children are equally worrisome. Homeless children have a higher rate of developmental delay when compared with housed poor children. Fifty-four percent of homeless children had at least one area of delay compared, in one study, with only 16% of housed children.[37] The greatest differences were found in the language and personal/social subscales. Rescorla found significant differences between homeless and housed children on receptive vocabulary and visual motor development among preschoolers. Yet, only 35% of the homeless children were enrolled in an early intervention program, compared with 85% of the housed children.[38] One report found 180,000 homeless preschool children do not attend school because of inadequate funding, lack of transportation to school, state noncompliance with federal law regarding barriers to school enrollment, and long waiting list for preschool spaces.[39]

The picture regarding school-age children is also of concern. Rubin found that homeless children scored significantly lower on the WRAT-R, a measure of academic achievement.[40] Another investigator found lower scores on the WISC-R, which reflects knowledge gained as the result of experience.[38] In another study 41% of homeless mothers reported that their children were failing or doing below average school work in comparison to 23% of housed mothers.[26] Because the differences found are related to a lack of knowledge rather than innate intelligence, these studies suggest that poor school performance may be due to a disruption in schooling, secondary to homelessness, rather than to innate differences in intelligence. The exact cause of this poor school performance, whether it is due to increased prevalence of illness, depression, or school absence, remains to be elucidated.

The Department of Education reported in 1989 that 30% of homeless children did not attend school.[41] The National Coalition for the Homeless in 1991 estimated this to be as high as 50%.[42] There has been much improvement in regard to this issue. A 1995 national study found that only 14% of homeless children were not attending school.[43] This improvement may be attributable to decreased barriers to school enrollment due to enforcement of the educational provisions of the McKinney Act. Congress enacted the McKinney Act in 1987 to provide funds for shelter, food, and health care of homeless people. Subtitle VII-B of the Act, as amended in 1990, requires that states receiving McKinney funding eliminate barriers to education for homeless children. Specifically, it is stated that homeless children have the same right to a free and appropriate education as housed children. States are required to revise any laws or regulations that might act as a barrier to education, and children are not to be separated from the mainstream school environment because they are homeless. Though many such barriers have been eliminated, a 1995 survey found four states with residency, five with prior school record, fifteen with immunization, fifteen with legal guardianship, and thirty with transportation requirements that hinder school enrollment for homeless children.

Evidence that homeless children may suffer from behavioral and psychological problems is persuasive. Using the Children's Depression Inventory, one study found the mean score of homeless children to be 10.3, while that of housed children was 8.3. A score of 9 indicates the need for psychiatric evaluation. Thirty-one percent of a group of homeless children, compared with 9% of housed children, scored at a level indicating the need for further evaluation when tested with the Children's Manifest Anxiety Scale.[26] Homeless preschoolers scored significantly higher on the Child Behavior Checklist compared to a group of housed children.[38] This test reflects anxiety, depression, and acting-out behavior.

It is clear, from the preceding studies, that *homelessness* creates an environment that is detrimental to both the physical and psychological well-being of a child. Removing a child from his or her community and all the elements that come with it, such as extended family, friends, school, and community supports, robs a child of the elements that are needed to develop and thrive.

LONG-TERM OUTCOME OF HOMELESSNESS UPON WOMEN AND CHILDREN

Current research demonstrates that homeless families are not a homogeneous population. Some families are homeless purely due to economic circumstances, such as losing a job, or the onset of an illness that overwhelms a person's financial resources. However, some homeless families fit more of a psychological profile, suggesting that factors such as mental illness, substance abuse, or lack of education are involved in the etiology of homelessness.

Less clear is whether the experience of homelessness, in itself, adversely affects a person's ability to function. Although differences in the psychological and developmental characteristics of homeless children compared to poor housed children have been identified, it is not clear whether this is the result of processes that occurred prior to homelessness or were precipitated by homelessness. Regardless of their etiology, these factors may continue to hamper the child's functioning even after the period of homelessness has ended.

It is also possible that homelessness adversely affects parents, therefore making future episodes of homelessness more likely. Do some adults become "institutionalized" once they enter the homeless system and lose skills needed to function autonomously? Clarification of these issues will be central to designing future homeless prevention programs.

ENDING HOMELESSNESS IN THE UNITED STATES

Further research is needed to better understand the effects that homelessness has on children, both acutely and long-term. In addition, more resources are needed in order to design and monitor interventions that will prevent the psychological and intellectual harm that results from placing children in this condition. However, such work is meaningless unless a concerted effort is made to provide affordable housing. Until this goal is placed on our political agenda and realized, we will continue to see increasing numbers of children who are scarred by growing up in an environment that is not conducive to normal health and development.

REFERENCES

1. Children's Defense Fund. *The State of America's Children Yearbook.* Washington, DC: Children's Defense Fund; 1994:37–44.

2. Link BG, Susser E, Stueve A, Phelan J, Moore RE, Stuening E. Lifetime and Five-Year Prevalence of Homelessness in the United States. *American Journal of Public Health* 1994;84:1907–12.

3. Urban Institute. *America's Homeless II: Population and Services.* February 2000.

4. U.S. Conference of Mayors. *A Status Report on Hunger and Homelessness in America's Cities 2000.* December 2000.

5. *New York Times.* Use of Shelters By Families Sets Record in City. August 1, 2001.

6. Wood D, Valdez RB, Hayshi T, Shen A. Homeless and Housed Families in Los Angeles: A Study Comparing Demographic, Economic, and Family Function Characteristics. *American Journal of Public Health* 1990;80:1049–52.

7. U.S Census Bureau. *Poverty in the United States 2000.* September 2001 (P60-214).

8. Federal Interagency Forum on Child and Family Statistics. *America's Children: Key National Indicators of Well-Being.* 1997.

9. U.S. Department of Housing and Urban Development. *Rental Housing Assistance—The Worsening Crisis.* 1999.

10. U.S. Department of Labor, Bureau of Labor Statistics. *Current Population Survey.* October 2001.

11. U.S. Conference of Mayors. *A Status Report on Hunger and Homelessness in America 1998.* December 1998.

12. Coalition on Human Needs. *The Minimum Wage.* June 2001.

13. Economic Policy Institute. Share of All Workers Earning Poverty-Level Hourly Wages. May 2001.

14. Children's Defense Fund. *Child Poverty in Working Families.* September 2001.

15. Urban Institute. *Children's Family Environment: Findings From the National Survey of America's Families.* October 2000.

16. Lazere, Edward. *In Short Supply: The Growing Affordable Housing Gap, 1995.* Center on Budget Policy and Priorities. Washington, D.C. 1995.

17. Nunez R. *Hopes, Dreams & Promises: The Future of Homeless Children in America.* Institute for Children and Poverty. 1994.

18. Department of Housing and Urban Development. *Waiting in Vain: An Update On America's Rental Housing Crisis.* 1999 (ACCN-HUD8693).

19. Department of Housing and Urban Development. *Section 8 Tenant-Based Housing Assistance: A Look Back After Thirty Years.* March 2000.

20. Twombly JG, Crowely S, Ferris N, Cushing ND. Out of Reach 2001: America's Growing Wage-Rent Disparity. *National Low Income Housing Coalition.* 2001.

21. Office of the Assistant Secretary for Planning and Evaluation, Department of Health and Human Services. *Status Report on Research on the Outcomes of Welfare Reform.* July 2001.

22. Bassuk EL, Weinreb LF, Buckner JC, Browne A, Salomon A, Bassuk SS. The Characteristics and Needs of Sheltered Homeless and Low-Income Housed Mothers. *JAMA.* 1996;276:64–66.

23. Bassuk EL, Buckner JC, Weinreb LF, Browne A, Bassuk SS, Dawson R, and Perloff JN. Homelessness in Female-Headed Families: Childhood and Adult Risk and Protective Factors. *American Journal of Public Health.* 1997;87:241–7.

24. Shinn MB, Knickman JR, Weitzman BC. Social Relationships and Vulnerability to Becoming Homeless Among Poor Families. *American Psychologist.* 1991;46:1180–7.

25. Weitzman BC, Knickman JR, Shinn M. Predictors of Shelter Use among Low-Income Families: Psychiatric History, Substance Abuse, and Victimization. *American Journal of Public Health.* 1992;82:1547–1550.

26. Bassuk EL, Rosenberg L. Why Does Family Homelessness Occur? A Case-Control Study. *American Journal of Public Health.* 1988;78:783–788.

27. Goodman LA. The Prevalence of Abuse Among Homeless and Housed Poor Mothers: A Comparison Study. *American Journal of Orthopsychiatry.* 1991;61:489–500.

28. Homes for the Homeless. *Ten Cities, A Snapshot of Family Homelessness Across America.* New York, 1998, The Institute for Children and Poverty.

29. Miller DS, Lin E. Children in Sheltered Homeless Families: Reported Health Status and Use of Health Services. *Pediatrics.* 1988;81:668–73.

30. Wood DL, Valdez RB, Hayshi T, Shen A. Health of Homeless Children and Housed, Poor Children. *Pediatrics.* 1990;86:858–866.

31. Forrest CB, Glade GB, Baker AE, et al. The Pediatric Primary-Specialty Care Interface: How Pediatricians Refer Children and Adolescents to Specialty Care. *Archives of Pediatrics and Adolescent Medicine.* 153;705–714:1999.

32. Grant R, Redlener K, Sherman P, Redlener I. *Urgent Needs for Specialist Care in a Homeless Pediatric Population.* Children's Health Fund. Manuscript in preparation.

33. Sherman P, Grant R, Redlener I. *The Health of Homeless Children Over the Past Decade.* Children's Health Fund. Manuscript in preparation.

34. McLean DM, Bowen S, Drezner K, Rowe A, et al. *Asthma Among Homeless Children: Undercounting and Undertreating the Underserved.* Submitted manuscript.

35. Alperstein G, Rappaport C, Flanigan JM. Health Problems of Homeless Children in New York City. *American Journal of Public Health* 1988;78:1232–1233.

36. Eddins E. Characteristics, Health Status and Service Needs of Sheltered Homeless Families. *The ABNF Journal* Spring 1993.

37. Bassuk EL, Rosenberg L. Psychosocial Characteristics of Homeless Children and Children With Homes. *Pediatrics* 1990;85:257–261.

38. Rescorla L, Parker R, Stolley P. Ability, Achievement, and Adjustment in Homeless Children. *American Journal of Orthopsychiatry.* 1991;61:210–20.

39. National Law Center on Homelessness and Poverty. *Blocks to Their Future: A Report on the Barriers to Preschool Education for Homeless Children.* Washington, DC. September 1997.

40. Rubin DH, Erickson CJ, San Augustin M, et al. Cognitive and Academic Functioning of Homeless Children Compared With Housed Children. *Pediatrics* 1996;97:289–94.

41. Bassuk EL. Homeless Families. *Scientific American* 1991.

42. National Coalition for the Homeless. *Education of Homeless Children and Youth.* February 1997.

43. Anderson LM, Janger MI, Panton KL. *An Evaluation of State and Local Efforts to Serve the Educational Needs of Homeless Children and Youth.* U.S. Department of Education.

ARTICLE 12

ENSURING SUBSTANCE ABUSE SERVICES FOR FAMILIES

Ellen Hutchins

INTRODUCTION

Substance abuse is a significant problem affecting many families in the United States. Alcohol and illicit drug use are associated with many of this country's most serious problems, including violence, injury, and HIV infection. Over the past decade, there has been an increase in the need for both prevention and treatment services, especially for women and adolescents. As new programs are being developed for these populations, there is a need to ensure that services provided are gender-specific and address issues relevant to the population. Managed care has given states new options as to how they will address substance abuse. This article examines the problem of substance abuse as it affects the maternal and child health population, provides some historical context for current trends, and recommendations for addressing the problem from a public health perspective.

The problem of substance abuse within families should concern all maternal and child health professionals, whether the issue involves a pregnant woman, an adolescent, or a male whose substance abuse affects other family members. Often it is unclear whose responsibility it is to address substance abuse and what role health providers and policymakers have to play. Frequently, health providers do not ask their patients about substance use and miss an opportunity to provide basic information and/or referrals to their patients who may be at risk for or using harmful substances.

Substance abuse is commonly viewed as an important social problem with health consequences for the individual; however, it also should be seen as a policy issue. Economic implications come into play when government resources are used to pay for drug prevention and treatment or building more prisons. Clearly, maternal and child health professionals should have a role in ensuring that substance abuse prevention and treatment services are available in their communities and that clients are not deterred from using these services because of punitive sanctions. This is even more important now as some managed-care plans will not pay for substance abuse assessments and/or treatment and as states decide how to address substance abuse treatment under their welfare reform programs.

ADOLESCENT SUBSTANCE USE

Among adolescents, alcohol is frequently the drug of choice. However, many adolescent alcohol abusers are also polydrug users.[1] Amphetamine use is prevalent among adolescents to promote weight loss, a common goal for teenage girls. Inhalants—found in adhesives, lighter fluid, spray paint, cleaning fluids, and cooking spray—may have been tried by as many as 22% of teenagers.[2,3] Some adolescents develop destructive behavior because of substance abuse. In the 1997 Monitoring the Future Study, a nationwide survey, more than 54% of respondents reported that they had consumed alcohol, and 23% reported that they had used marijuana, by the eighth grade.[4] The age at which one first drinks alcohol or tries other substances is predictive of later problems with these substances, with earlier use placing individuals at greater risk for later abuse.[5] The risk of pregnancy and sexually transmitted diseases increases when using substances. Studies have shown that the previous use of substances, including cigarettes, greatly increases the risk of early sexual involvement by adolescents. The higher the stage of drug use, the greater the likelihood of early sexual activity.[6]

PREVALENCE OF SUBSTANCE USE AMONG WOMEN, INCLUDING PREGNANT WOMEN

The problem of substance use during pregnancy significantly increased during the mid-to-late 1980s with the popularity of the inexpensive, smokable form of cocaine called "crack" among women of childbearing age. Prior to this time, substance abuse was seen as primarily affecting men. Both the highly addictive properties of cocaine and its popularity among women of childbearing age have contributed to large numbers of pregnant women giving birth to drug-exposed infants. Current nationally cited estimates report that 5.5% of all pregnant women use an illicit drug during pregnancy.[7] The development of drug-exposed infants may be compromised by either the biologic effects of prenatal exposure to cocaine or by social factors related to having a substance-using mother.[8]

SMOKING TRENDS AMONG ADOLESCENTS AND WOMEN

In 1998, 22% of women smoked cigarettes.[9] Smoking prevalence today is nearly three times higher among women who have only 9 to 11 years of education (32.9%) than among women with 16 or more years of education (11.2%). In 2000, 29.7% of high school senior girls reported having smoked within the past 30 days. Examining smoking trends by race/ethnicity indicates the following rates: 34.5% of American Indian or Alaskan Native women, 23.5% of Caucasians,

21.9% of African American women, 13.8% of Hispanics, and 11.2% of Asian/ Pacific Islanders.

Lung cancer is now the leading cause of cancer deaths among U.S. women; it surpassed breast cancer in 1987. Smoking during pregnancy remains a major public health problem despite increased knowledge of the adverse health effects of smoking during pregnancy. However, a higher percentage of women stop smoking during pregnancy than at other times in their lives. Using pregnancy-specific programs can increase smoking-cessation rates, which benefit both maternal and infant health.

RESEARCH FINDINGS

African American women have the highest rates of use for cocaine and other illicit substances, with the exception that white women younger than 25 have higher rates for marijuana use. Total rates of alcohol use are highest among whites. Substance users frequently use several drugs rather than only one substance such as cocaine. Although media attention has focused primarily on cocaine use among women, alcohol use during pregnancy also deserves the attention of health professionals, because fetal alcohol syndrome is completely preventable. In addition, the abuse of prescription drugs such as stimulants, sedatives, and analgesics has been frequently reported, although data are not reliable.

There is a need for more research to better understand the contribution of various factors to a pregnant woman's substance use during pregnancy. In one study examining psychosocial risk factors in the backgrounds of pregnant cocaine users, it was found that substance-using women were more likely to have a family history of alcohol or other drug problems, to have been introduced to drugs by a male partner, to be depressed, to have less social support, to have a current male partner who uses drugs or alcohol, and to have a less stable living situation.[10]

Additionally, there is a need for further evaluations to examine the most effective prevention and treatment strategies. Drug prevention strategies are usually school-based, thereby targeting only those adolescents who attend school. The most commonly cited prevention strategies include the Drug Abuse Resistance Education (DARE) program, conducted by police officers who talk to students about the dangers of drug use, and prevention approaches that teach adolescents about dealing with peer pressure and decision-making. Experimentation with alcohol, tobacco, and/or marijuana at early ages may lead to more serious illicit drug use. It is widely believed that pre-adolescents as well as adolescents need to be targeted in school-based prevention programs.

By the end of 1994, 95% of all cases of pediatric acquired immunodeficiency syndrome (AIDS) in New York State were being attributed to perinatal human immunodeficiency virus (HIV) from an infected mother.[11] The major contributing factors were the mother's intravenous drug use with contaminated needles or unprotected sex with an intravenous drug user.

MEDICAL EFFECTS ON THE NEWBORN

Findings in the early 1990s indicated that cocaine could have serious effects on the health of drug-exposed newborns. In the published peer-reviewed literature during this time period, sample sizes were small, and frequently there were no control groups for comparison. However, more recently in the past several years, studies have become much larger, allowing for multivariate analyses to be performed. These studies better isolated the unique contribution of cocaine while controlling for important variables such as maternal smoking, alcohol use, and home environment.

A systematic review of 36 studies assessing possible relationships between maternal cocaine use during pregnancy and several childhood outcomes found that crack/cocaine exposure *in utero* has not been demonstrated to affect physical growth; it does not appear to independently affect developmental scores in the first 6 years.[12] In summary, data are not convincing that *in utero* exposure to cocaine has major adverse developmental consequences in early childhood separate from those associated with other exposures and environmental risk, and the data suggest that the effects of tobacco and alcohol may be greater.

TREATMENT SERVICES

Frequently the debate has focused on whether addicted persons are worthy of services, because many view addiction as a moral weakness rather than a disease and believe that the government should not be spending funds on people who deliberately choose to ingest illicit substances. The public health point of view is that addiction is a chronic, relapsing condition that may require multiple admissions to a drug treatment program but is a worthy investment. Research has demonstrated that comprehensive care, including high-risk obstetrical care, psychosocial services, and addiction treatment can reduce complications associated with perinatal substance abuse.[13]

A 6-month follow-up of women who completed substance abuse treatment found that more were employed.[14] At the Families in Transition (FIT) program in Miami, Florida, all of the women were receiving welfare at the time of admission. Six to 12 months after discharge from treatment, 33% of the women moved off the welfare rolls, and an additional 19% reduced their welfare benefits through employment.[15] Many women substance abusers are the primary caretakers for their children, and research suggests that pregnant and postpartum women may not enter treatment if child care is not available.[16] Szuster and colleagues[17] report better retention rates for women who participated in treatment with their children compared with those in treatment without their children.

STATES' RESPONSES TO THE PROBLEM

There have been more than 160 cases in 23 states including the District of Columbia of prosecution of pregnant drug-using women, primarily involving cocaine use. However, many of these convicted cases have now been overturned. In 2001 the U.S. Supreme Court heard the case of Ferguson v. City of Charleston, which focused on whether the state of South Carolina has the right to test pregnant women for drugs without their knowledge.[18] The Supreme Court ruled 6–3 that the searches, which were conducted without warrants or probable cause, violated the Fourth Amendment in the absence of consent. It is too soon to know the impact that this decision will have on states' introducing legislation in the future around prenatal substance abuse. Over the past several years, many states have interpreted child protection laws to apply to prenatal substance abuse and have removed newborns from maternal custody on the basis of neonatal urine toxicology results.[19] Over the past decade, the trend has been to either incarcerate the drug-using woman or remove the child from her care, rather than expand drug-treatment capacity. Most states do not have sufficient drug-treatment capacity for addicted women seeking help. Only recently has there been more of an emphasis on expanding women's treatment programs to include their children.

Although incarcerating an addicted woman during her pregnancy may seem like the simplest and cheapest solution to the problem, treatment for one woman costs less than half the annual cost of incarceration.[20] Incarcerated women rarely receive drug treatment and may leave prison without having received any assistance for their drug problem. There is a need to increase the number of comprehensive, gender-specific treatment programs for substance abusing pregnant women and mothers and their children. Services that need to be addressed include psychosocial support, health care, child care, and aftercare support. Efforts to prosecute pregnant women who use alcohol and other drugs need to be eliminated, and more efforts need to be made to refer them into treatment. The experience of leading experts throughout the United States is that removal of infants in these cases is usually unnecessary and can be harmful to the child.[21]

By the early 1990s women constituted the fastest growing segment of the American population involved with the criminal justice system. More than 80% of the cases brought to prosecution involved women of color, specifically African American women. This may be due to the fact that these women rely on public hospitals and clinics more for their care, and more drug testing is done there. It is believed that punitive approaches by some states may have deterred some pregnant women from receiving prenatal care.

In a study by Chavkin,[22] it was found that the most common reasons for not seeking care were "having felt bad about using drugs" and having "felt guilty or embarassed about being a drug-using woman." Chavkin found that women were in need of aftercare, services for children, education, training, addiction services, on-site health care, housing, and food.

Successful programs based on the family unification model should be expanded. One example is Operation PAR (Parental Awareness and Responsibility) in St. Petersburg, Florida. Through its long-term residential program, children from infancy to 10 years can live with their mother while she is receiving treatment.

SCREENING ISSUES

Staff training is important to address staff attitudes toward serving substance-using adolescents and women. Staff should include representation from the culture served, as well as provide bilingual services when needed. Consumer input is also desirable to ensure that services and approaches are reaching the population targeted. Compared to awareness of risks from drug abuse and cigarette smoking during pregnancy, clinical screening for alcohol use during routine prenatal care has received less attention.[23] In a survey of obstetrician-gynecologists on their patients' alcohol use during pregnancy, 97% reported that they ask their prenatal patients about alcohol use.[24] However, only 30% felt very prepared to assess pregnant women's alcohol use, and 83% say they need information on thresholds at which prenatal drinking poses specific threats to the pregnancy or the fetus. Heavy drinking during pregnancy is more frequent among women who are over 35 years, unmarried, of low income, and lack prenatal care.

Prenatal and family planning clinics need to screen all women for alcohol and illicit substances using simple self-report questionnaires. Staff need to be trained in how to administer these questionnaires in a nonjudgmental way. The purpose of screening should be to identify women in need of counseling or referral, not to use this information to report them to authorities. To be useful, the screening process must be brief, easily conducted and interpreted, highly sensitive and specific, and inexpensive to administer. A screening tool is not designed to diagnose alcohol problems, but can determine if a patient is at risk for alcohol problems and would benefit from a more comprehensive evaluation by a specialist. Screening can easily be incorporated into prenatal care using brief questionnaires designed to be administered face-to-face, patient-to-provider.

A recent study of 2,066 Medicaid-eligible pregnant women revealed that women who smoked in the month before pregnancy were about 11 times more likely to currently use drugs than women who had never smoked.[25] Another study found similar findings, that women who smoked at least half a pack a day during pregnancy were 10 times more likely to also be using illicit substances.[26]

Similarly, it was found that past alcohol use was associated with a greater risk of substance use during pregnancy, with women who drank being 41 times more likely to currently use either drugs or alcohol or both than women who had never drunk alcohol.

Innovative outreach services are important to identify those who may not access services on their own and should include homeless and battered women's shelters. Alcohol and drug treatment are successful strategies that need to be addressed to end welfare dependency and increase employment-related outcomes. Outreach programs are especially important now with states developing Medicaid managed-care contracts, which frequently do not cover outreach to those clients who do not seek medical services on their own.

SUMMARY

Many of the policies enacted to deter substance abuse by imposing punitive sanctions have in fact deterred women from coming into the health system. More policies need to be developed that encourage women to seek preventive and treatment services. Policy responses should not be developed without a detailed assessment of a state's resources in areas such as drug treatment, family support services, child protective services, and foster care. It is important that managed-care plans include assessment and treatment of addiction problems. Substance abuse affects an entire family, and if untreated, has extensive consequences. Maternal and child health professionals have a role in ensuring that policies and services encourage the identification and early treatment of this problem.

REFERENCES

1. Martin, C.S., Arria, A.M., Mezzich, A.C., and Bukstein, O.G. Patterns of polydrug use in adolescent alcohol abusers. *American Journal of Drug and Alcohol Abuse* 1993;19(4):511–521.

2. Dinwiddie, S.H. Abuse of inhalants: A review. *Addiction.* 1994; 89(8):925–939.

3. National Institute on Drug Abuse. *Drug use among 8th, 10th, and 12th graders.* NIDA Notes 11(1). (NIH Publication No. 96-3478). Washington, D.C: U.S. Government Printing Office, 1996.

4. Johnston, L., O'Malley, P., and Bachman, J. *National survey results on drug use from the Monitoring the Future Study, 1975-1997, Volume I: Secondary School Students.* Rockville, MD: National Institute on Drug Abuse, 1998.

5. Gruber, E., DiClemente, R., Anderson, M., and Lodico, M. Early drinking onset and its association with alcohol use and problem behavior in late adolescence. *Preventive Medicine,* 1996; 25:293–300.

6. Gilmore, M.R., Butler, S., Lohr, M.J., and Gilchrist, L. Substance use and other factors associated with risky sexual behavior, among pregnant adolescents. *Family Planning Perspectives.* 1992;24:255–261.

7. U.S. Department of Health and Human Services. D*rug use among women delivering live births: 1992.* (NIH Publication No. 96-3819). National Institute on Drug Abuse, National Pregnancy and Health Survey, Rockville, MD:1996.

8. Hutchins, E. Drug use during pregnancy. *Journal of Drug Issues* 1997; 27:463–485.

9. *Women and Smoking: A Report of the Surgeon General—2001.* U.S. Department of Health and Human Services, Centers for Disease Control and Prevention, Atlanta: 2001.

10. Hutchins, E., and DiPietro, J. Psychosocial risk factors associated with cocaine use during pregnancy: A case-control study. *Obstetrics and Gynecology* 1997; 90(1):142–147.

11. *Program advisory: Use of zidovudine to reduce perinatal HIV transmission in HRSA-funded programs.* U.S. Department of Health and Human Services, Rockville, MD: 1995.

12. Frank, D., Augustyn, M., Knight, W., Pell, T., and Zuckerman, B. *Growth: Development and behavior in early childhood following prenatal cocaine exposure: A systematic review.* JAMA. 2001, 285(12):1613–1625.

13. Kaltenbach, K., and Finnegan, L. Prevention and treatment issues for pregnant cocaine-dependent women and their infants. *Annals of the New York Academy of Sciences.* June 21, 1998.

14. Stevens, S., and Arbiter, N. A therapeutic community for substance-abusing pregnant women and women with children: Process and outcome. *Journal of Psychoactive Drugs* 1995:27(1):49–56.

15. Young, N.K. *Alcohol and other drug treatment: Policy choices in welfare reform.* Washington, D.C.: National Association of State Alcohol and Drug Abuse Directors, 1996.

16. Smith, I., Dent, D., Coles, C., and Falek, A. A comparison study of treated and untreated pregnant and postpartum cocaine-abusing women. *Journal of Substance Abuse Treatment* 1992; 9(4):343–348.

17. Szuster, R.R., Rich, L.L., Chung, A., and Bisconer, S.W. Treatment retention in women's residential chemical dependency treatment: The effect of admission with children. *Substance Use and Misuse.* 1996; 31:1001–1013.

18. Center for Reproductive Law and Policy Press Release. *U.S. Supreme Court affirms right to confidential medical care.* New York. March 21, 2001.

19. Layton, C., Breitbart, V., Rawding, N., Chavkin, W., Fisher, W., & Wise, P. *Integrating the needs of women and children: Addressing perinatal drug exposure and perinatal HIV infection.* Washington, DC: National Association of County Health Officials, 1994.

20. Young, N.K., and Gardner, S.L. *Implementing welfare reform: Solutions to the substance abuse problem.* Washington, DC: Children and Family Futures and Drug Strategies, 1996.

21. National Council of Juvenile and Family Court Judges. *Protocol for making reasonable efforts to preserve families in drug-related dependence cases.* Reno, NV: National Council of Juvenile and Family Court Judges, 1992.

22. Chavkin, W., Paone, D., Friedman, Pl, and Wilets, I. Reframing the debate: Toward effective treatment for inner city drug-abusing mothers. *Bulletin of the New York Academy of Medicine.* 1993; 70:50–68.

23. Morse, B., and Hutchins, E. Reducing complications from alcohol use during pregnancy through screening. *JAMWA.* 2000; 55(4):225–228.

24. Diekman, S., Floyd, L., Decoufle, P., Schulkin, J. et al. A survey of Obstetrician-gynecologists on their patients' alcohol use during pregnancy. *Obstetrics and Gynecology* 2000; 95(5): 756–763.

25. Chasnoff, I., Neuman, K., Thornton, C., and Callaghan, A. Screening for substance use in pregnancy: A practical approach for the primary care physician. *American Journal of Obstetrics and Gynecology;* 18(4), 752–756.

26. Hutchins, E., and DiPietro, J. Psychosocial risk factors associated with cocaine use during pregnancy: A case-control study. *Obstetrics and Gynecology* 1997; 90(1):142–147.

ARTICLE 13

INFANT MORTALITY IN THE UNITED STATES: LEVELS, TRENDS, AND INTERVENTIONS

Marian F. MacDorman, Solomon Iyasu, and T. J. Mathews

INTRODUCTION

Infant mortality is an important indicator of the health of a nation, as it is associated with a variety of factors such as maternal health, quality and access to medical care, socio-economic conditions, and public health practices.[1-3] Although the infant mortality rate in the United States has declined about 14-fold since the beginning of this century,[1-3] it is still considerably higher than that of a number of other industrialized nations.[4-5] Within the United States, large and persistent differences in infant mortality rates by race and ethnicity demonstrate that not all groups have uniformly benefited from the social and medical advances driving the infant mortality decline.[6] This article presents an overview of patterns and trends in infant mortality, identifies areas in which substantial progress has been made and areas in which improvement is needed, and finally discusses selected local and national programs to improve pregnancy outcomes and reduce infant mortality.

Data discussed in this chapter are based primarily on the linked birth/infant death data sets produced by the Centers for Disease Control and Prevention's National Center for Health Statistics.[6] In these data sets the information from the birth certificate is linked to the information from the death certificate for each infant who dies in the United States. The purpose of the linkage is to utilize the many additional variables available from the birth certificate to conduct more detailed analyses of infant mortality patterns.

TRENDS AND INTERNATIONAL COMPARISONS

The U.S. infant mortality rate has declined approximately 14-fold during the 20th century. Although precise data are not available from 1900, it is estimated that at least 100 out of 1,000 babies born in that year died before their first birthday.[7]

This compares to an infant mortality rate of 7.2 infant deaths per 1,000 live births in 1998.[6] Despite this large decline, the problem of infant mortality remains substantial. In 1998, there were 28,371 deaths to children under 1 year of age in the United States.[8] Each of these deaths represents a personal tragedy for parents, siblings, and other family members.

Although the overall decline during the 20th century has been impressive, recent declines in infant mortality in the United States have not kept pace with declines in other countries. As a result, the United States' international ranking in infant mortality has fallen from 11th lowest in 1960 to 27th lowest in 1997 (Table 1).[4] In 1997, Sweden had the lowest infant mortality rate (3.6), followed by Japan (3.7) and Singapore (3.8). The Swedish rate was half the U.S. rate of 7.2. The low infant mortality rates achieved by other countries suggest that despite large declines in U.S. infant mortality, there is still a great deal of room for improvement.

Variations by Race and Ethnicity

Another indication that further improvements in U.S. infant mortality are possible is the large variation in infant mortality rates by mother's race and ethnicity. Infant mortality rates for the U.S. race/ethnic groups with the lowest rates (Japanese, 3.5; Cuban, 3.6; Chinese, 4.0) are comparable to those for the countries with the lowest rates, while the highest rate—13.9 for infants of non-Hispanic black mothers—was nearly four times that for U.S. Japanese mothers (Figure 1). Rates were intermediate for infants of Central and South American

FIGURE 1

Infant mortality rates by race and ethnicity, 1998

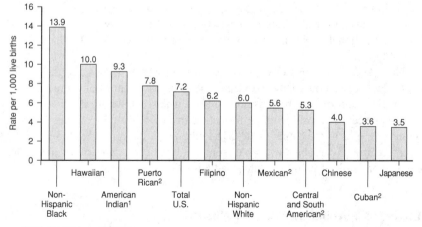

¹ Includes Aleuts and Eskimos.
² Persons of Hispanic origin may be of any race.

Source: Centers for Disease Control and Prevention, *National Center for Health Statistics,* National Vital Statistics System.

TABLE 1 INFANT MORTALITY RATES AND INTERNATIONAL RANKINGS: SELECTED COUNTRIES, 1960 AND 1997

	Infant mortality rates[1]		International rankings[2]	
Country[3]	1960	1997[4]	1960	1997
Australia	20.2	5.3	4	12
Austria	37.5	4.7	23	8
Belgium	31.2	6.1	19	22
Bulgaria	45.1	17.5	29	37
Canada	27.3	5.3	14	12
Chile	125.1	10.5	35	32
Costa Rica	74.3	14.2	32	35
Cuba	37.3	7.2	22	27
Czech Republic	—	5.9	—	19
Czechoslovakia	23.5	—	10	—
Denmark	21.5	5.3	7	12
England and Wales	21.8	5.9	8	19
Finland	21.0	3.9	5	4
France	27.4	4.8	15	9
Germany[5]	35.0	4.9	21	10
Greece	40.1	6.4	24	24
Hong Kong	41.5	3.9	25	4
Hungary	47.6	9.9	30	29
Ireland	29.3	6.2	16	23
Israel	31.0	6.0	18	21
Italy	43.9	5.5	28	16
Japan	30.4	3.7	17	2
Kuwait	—	11.5	—	34
Netherlands	17.9	5.0	2	11
New Zealand	22.6	6.5	9	26
Northern Ireland	27.2	5.6	13	18
Norway	18.9	4.1	3	6
Poland	56.1	10.2	31	31
Portugal	77.5	6.4	34	24
Puerto Rico	43.3	11.3	26	33
Romania	75.7	22.0	33	38
Russia[6]	—	17.3	—	36
Scotland	26.4	5.3	12	12
Singapore	34.8	3.8	20	3
Slovakia	—	9.9	—	29
Spain	43.7	5.5	27	16
Sweden	16.6	3.6	1	1
Switzerland	21.1	4.5	6	7
United States	26.0	7.2	11	27

— Data not available.
[1] Infant deaths per 1,000 live births.
[2] Rankings are from lowest to highest infant mortality rates. Some of the variation in infant mortality rates is due to differences among countries in distinguishing between fetal and infant deaths.
[3] Refers to countries, territories, cities, or geographic areas with at least 1 million population and with "complete" counts of live births and infant deaths as indicated in the United Nations Demographic Yearbook.
[4] Rates for Kuwait, Slovakia, and Spain are for 1996.
[5] Rates presented for the years prior to the reunification of Germany were calculated by combining information from the Federal Republic of Germany and the German Democratic Republic.
[6] Excludes infants born alive after less than 28 weeks' gestation, of less than 1,000 grams in weight and 35 centimeters in length, who die within 7 days of birth.
Source: Adapted from *Health, United States, 2001,* table 26.

(5.3), Mexican (5.6), non-Hispanic white (6.0), and Filipino (6.2) mothers, but higher for Puerto Rican (7.8), American Indian (9.3), and Hawaiian (10.0) mothers.

Differences in infant mortality by race and ethnicity reflect in part differences in maternal socio-demographic and behavioral risk factors. For example, infant mortality rates are higher than the U.S. average for teenage and for unmarried mothers, those with lower educational levels, those who smoke during pregnancy, or who do not obtain adequate prenatal care.[6] The race/ethnic groups with the lowest infant mortality rates tend to have a smaller percentage of births to women with some or all of these characteristics, while the race/ethnic groups with the highest infant mortality rates tend to have a higher percentage of births to women with some or all of these characteristics (Table 2). For example, Japanese, Chinese, and Cuban mothers were more likely than the U.S. average to begin prenatal care in the first trimester, less likely to smoke during pregnancy, had fewer teen and nonmarital births, were less likely to have a fourth or higher-order birth, and were more likely to have completed high school. Conversely, a higher percentage of the births to non-Hispanic black, Puerto Rican, and American Indian

TABLE 2 PERCENT OF LIVE BIRTHS WITH SELECTED CHARACTERISTICS BY MATERNAL RACE AND ETHNICITY, UNITED STATES, 1998 LINKED FILE

	First Trimester Prenatal Care	Teen Births	Fourth and Higher-Order Births	Births to Unmarried Mothers	Mothers with 12+ Years of Education	Maternal Smoking during Pregnancy[1]	Low Birthweight
All races/ethnicities[2]	82.8%	12.5%	10.5%	32.8%	78.1%	12.9%	7.6%
Non-Hispanic white	87.9	9.4	8.5	21.9	87.2	16.2	6.6
Non-Hispanic black	73.3	21.6	15.0	69.3	73.3	9.6	13.2
American Indian	68.8	20.9	19.5	59.3	67.3	20.2	6.9
Chinese	88.5	0.9	2.4	6.4	88.6	0.8	5.4
Japanese	90.2	2.4	4.3	9.7	97.6	4.8	7.5
Hawaiian	78.8	18.8	14.7	51.1	81.5	16.8	7.2
Filipino	84.2	6.2	7.2	19.7	93.1	3.3	8.2
Mexican	72.8	17.5	14.7	39.6	44.8	2.8	6.0
Puerto Rican	76.9	21.9	12.3	59.5	64.1	10.7	9.7
Cuban	91.8	6.9	5.7	24.8	87.0	3.7	6.5
Central and South American	78.0	10.3	11.1	42.0	61.5	1.5	6.5

[1] Excludes data for California, Indiana, New York State (but includes New York City), and South Dakota, which did not report maternal smoking on the birth certificate.
[2] Includes races/ethnicities not listed separately.

mothers occurred to mothers who did not receive adequate prenatal care, were unmarried or teenagers, were having fourth or higher-order births, and had not completed high school. The percentage of mothers who smoked was substantially higher for American Indians, compared to the overall population, suggesting that maternal smoking may play a role in their elevated infant mortality rates. However, smoking was less common among non-Hispanic black and Puerto Rican mothers than for the overall population, suggesting that smoking played a relatively smaller role in their elevated infant mortality rates.

In contrast, the percentage of infants born at low birthweight was substantially higher than the U.S. average for non-Hispanic black (13.2) and Puerto Rican (9.7) mothers, suggesting the contribution of low birthweight to the elevated infant mortality rates for these groups. This is consistent with previous research that has demonstrated that three-quarters of the black–white gap in infant mortality was due to deaths among low-birthweight infants.[9] The percentage of low-birthweight infants was 6.9 for American Indian mothers, slightly lower than the U.S. average (7.6). However, the risk factors discussed above do not fully explain race and ethnic differences. For example, Schoendorf et al. found higher low-birthweight and infant mortality rates among college-educated black than white mothers, even after controlling for parity, maternal age, marital status, and prenatal care.[10]

Differences in income and access to health care between race and ethnic groups may also contribute to differences in infant mortality. In 1999, 37% of black families with children under 6 years of age had incomes below the poverty level, compared to 31% for Hispanic, and 10% for white families.[11] Black and Hispanic families were also less likely than non-Hispanic white families to have health insurance that covers the cost of prenatal and infant health care.[12]

Although the factors considered above play a role in infant mortality, other social and cultural factors are also important. This is illustrated by the Mexican population, which has an infant mortality rate and percentage of low-birthweight births lower than the U.S. average, despite lower income and health insurance levels and a higher prevalence of most risk factors except maternal smoking (Table 2). Previous studies have related the generally favorable birth outcomes for Mexican women to their lower levels of smoking and alcohol use and more favorable weight gain profiles,[13] as well as to a greater degree of familial integration, which may provide increased social support for pregnant women and new mothers.[14] The findings of lower infant mortality rates for mothers born outside the 50 states and D.C. than for those born in the 50 states and D.C. tend to support this hypothesis, as well as suggesting a gradual dilution of this traditional cultural framework with more time spent in the United States.[15-16]

Variations by Birthweight and Period of Gestation

Birthweight and period of gestation are the two most important predictors of an infant's subsequent health and survival. Obviously, the two variables are closely interrelated. For example, in 1998, two-thirds of all low-birthweight births (less than 2,500 grams or 5 lbs 8 oz) occurred among infants born preterm (at less than 37 completed weeks of gestation). Although period of gestation is actually the conceptually antecedent measure and thus the one most amenable to intervention, birthweight is often easier to measure, and thus is often discussed in summary analyses.

Infants born too soon or too small have a much greater risk of death and disability than those born at full term (37–41 weeks of gestation) or with birthweights of 2,500 grams or more. In 1998, 65% of all infant deaths occurred to the 7.6% of infants born at low birthweight; 51% of all infant deaths occurred among the 1.5% of infants born at very low birthweight (less than 1,500 grams or 3 lbs 4 oz). Similarly, 65% of all infant deaths occurred among the 11.6% of infants born preterm; 52% of all infant deaths occurred among the 2.0% of infants born very preterm (< 32 completed weeks of gestation).

Table 3 shows the mortality rates for infants born at various birthweights. The infant mortality rate for very-low-birthweight infants was 250.0, over 90 times the rate of 2.6 for infants with birthweights of 2,500 grams or more. The rate for moderately low-birthweight infants (those with birthweights of 1,500–2,499 grams) was 16.5, more than six times the rate for infants with birthweights of 2,500 grams or more. Patterns by period of gestation were similar.[6]

The infant mortality rate for a given population can be partitioned into two key components: the birthweight distribution and birthweight-specific mortality rates (the mortality rate for infants at a given weight). The percentage of low-birthweight births relates mostly to prenatal factors such as the proportion of multiple births, preexisting maternal risk factors such as very young or elevated maternal age, behavioral risk factors such as smoking, and medical risk factors such as hypertension. Variations in birthweight-specific infant mortality rates for low-birthweight infants reflect in large part the quality and availability of neonatal intensive care, while those for normal birthweight infants reflect the influences of these and other factors (for example, postneonatal mortality attributable to sudden infant death syndrome or injuries). The infant mortality rate can decrease when either the percentage of low-birthweight births decreases or birthweight-specific mortality rates decrease. Since the percentage of low-birthweight births has increased since the mid-1980s (from 6.8% in 1985 to 7.6% in 1998), all of the decline in the infant mortality rate since 1985 is attributable to declines in birthweight-specific infant mortality rates.

Over the past three decades, the United States has been very successful in improving neonatal care for low-birthweight infants, including the regionalization of neonatal intensive care units and medical advances in the treatment of preterm infants with immature lung development.[17–19] Mortality rates for low-birthweight and very-low-birthweight infants have declined by more than one-third since 1985.[6,20] However, we have been unsuccessful in reducing the percent-

Table 3 INFANT MORTALITY RATES BY BIRTHWEIGHT, UNITED STATES, 1998 LINKED FILE

Birthweight	Infant Mortality Rate[1]
Less than 2,500 grams	61.5
Less than 1,500 grams	250.0
Less than 500 grams	868.2
500–749 grams	485.6
750–999 grams	157.4
1,000–1,249 grams	71.5
1,250–1,499 grams	50.0
1,500–1,999 grams	28.7
2,000–2,499 grams	12.5
2,500 grams or more	2.6
2,500–2,999 grams	4.8
3,000–3,499 grams	2.5
3,500–3,999 grams	1.8
4,000–4,499 grams	1.6
4,500–4,999 grams	1.9
5,000 grams or more	4.4

[1]Infant deaths per 1,000 live births.

age of preterm and low-birthweight births even though prevention efforts have the potential to save many more infant lives than do further improvements in neonatal care.

Much research over the past two decades has been devoted to preventing preterm delivery,[21] yet the percentage of infants born preterm or at low birthweight has been increasing. Preterm birth is a complex problem with multiple etiologies, but factors that may contribute to preterm birth include maternal reproductive tract infection, stress, socio-economic deprivation, insufficient access to health care, and maternal smoking, among others.[22] An increase in the proportion of multiple births, in large part due to increasing use of assisted reproductive therapies, has also played a role.[23] Another factor that has received relatively little attention is the effect of medical interventions, such as induction of labor, on the preterm birth rate. Medical interventions have been demonstrated to affect the percentage of preterm and low-birthweight births in Canada and other countries.[24-25] Although some argue that an induction of labor at 35 or 36 weeks of gestation has relatively little adverse effect on the infant's chance for survival, Kramer et al. have demonstrated that even infants born just a couple of weeks early have higher mortality rates and are responsible for an important fraction of infant deaths.[26]

Maternal Smoking during Pregnancy

Among the many maternal risk factors discussed above, one deserves special mention in that it is entirely preventable and it has a large adverse effect on infant mortality. In 1998, the infant mortality rate for babies born to smokers was 10.9, 60% higher than for nonsmokers (6.8) for a reporting area comprising 46 states, New York City, and the District of Columbia (D.C.).[6] Overall, 12.9% of mothers smoked in 1998 (Table 2). Tobacco use during pregnancy causes the passage of substances such as nicotine, hydrogen cyanide, and carbon monoxide from the placenta into the fetal blood supply. These substances restrict the growing infant's access to oxygen and can lead to adverse pregnancy outcomes such as low birthweight, preterm delivery, intrauterine growth retardation, and infant mortality.[27-28]

Leading Causes of Death

Table 4 presents infant mortality rates for the five leading causes of infant death by maternal race and ethnicity. Overall, the three leading causes of infant death—congenital anomalies, disorders relating to short gestation and unspecified low birthweight, and sudden infant death syndrome (SIDS)—taken together accounted for nearly half (46%) of all infant deaths in the United States in 1998. The fourth and fifth leading causes—newborn affected by maternal complications of pregnancy (maternal complications) and respiratory distress syndrome (RDS)—each accounted for about 5% of all infant deaths in 1998. Since 1990, mortality declined for four of the five leading causes of infant death. Infant mortality declined most rapidly for SIDS (45%) and RDS (52%).[8,29] The rapid decline in SIDS coincides with the implementation of the Back to Sleep campaign to reduce SIDS by placing infants on their back to sleep (discussed in more detail below).[30] The rapid decline in RDS coincides with the widespread adoption around 1990 of new medicines such as exogenous surfactant and antenatal corticosteroids developed to treat this condition, particularly among very-low-birthweight infants.[17-19] Infant mortality declined more slowly for congenital anomalies (20%) and maternal complications (14%) from 1990–98. In contrast, the infant mortality rate from low birthweight actually increased by 8% during the time period, reflecting the increase in the percentage of preterm and low-birthweight births.[8,29]

Important differences also exist in cause-specific infant mortality rates by race and ethnicity and these differences help to explain the overall differences in infant mortality by race and ethnicity. For four of the five leading causes of death, infant

TABLE 4 INFANT MORTALITY RATES* FOR THE FIVE LEADING CAUSES OF INFANT DEATH, BY RACE AND HISPANIC ORIGIN OF MOTHER: UNITED STATES, 1998 LINKED FILE

Causes of Death (ICD-9)	All Races/Ethnicities[1]		Non-Hispanic White		Non-Hispanic Black		American Indian[2]		Asian and Pacific Islander		Hispanic	
	Rank	Rate	Rank	Rate	Rank	Rate	Rank	Rate	Rank	Rate	Rank	Rate
All causes	—	718.6	—	597.9	—	1,388.1	—	933.7	—	553.7	—	575.5
Congenital anomalies (740–759)	1	158.3	1	154.6	2	182.6	1	171.3	1	152.3	1	149.9
Disorders related to short gestation and unspecified low birthweight (765)	2	103.8	2	69.2	1	279.9	3	91.9	2	81.1	2	74.2
Sudden infant death syndrome (798)	3	71.7	3	66.4	3	140.0	2	151.5	3	39.4	3	37.4
Newborn affected by maternal complications of pregnancy (761)	4	34.2	4	27.9	4	74.7		**	4	29.0	5	19.6
Respiratory distress syndrome (769)	5	33.1	5	26.0	5	71.0		**	5	20.9	4	28.6

* Rates per 1,000 live births in specified group.
** Figure does not meet standard of reliability of precision; based on fewer than 20 deaths in the numerator.
— Category not applicable.
1 Includes other races/ethnicities not listed separately.
2 Includes Aleuts and Eskimos.

Source: Centers for Disease Control and Prevention, *National Center for Health Statistics*, National Vital Statistics System.

mortality rates were highest for non-Hispanic black mothers, while SIDS rates were highest for American Indian mothers. For infants of non-Hispanic black mothers, the mortality rate for low birthweight was four times that for infants of non-Hispanic white mothers. For SIDS, RDS, and maternal complications, rates were 2.1–2.7 times higher for non-Hispanic black than for non-Hispanic white mothers.

For infants of American Indian mothers, the SIDS rate was 151.5, 2.3 times that for infants of non-Hispanic white mothers, and the highest among all race and ethnic groups. American Indian women were more likely than any other race/ethnic group to smoke during pregnancy (Table 2) and smoking probably contributes to their high SIDS rates. Overall, infants of mothers who smoke during pregnancy have SIDS rates nearly four times those for nonsmokers.[31] As most SIDS occurs during the postneonatal period (from 28 days through 11 months of age), the high SIDS rate for infants of American Indian mothers accounts for much of their elevated risk of postneonatal mortality. For infants of Asian or Pacific Islander and Hispanic mothers, SIDS rates were 40% to 44% lower than those for non-Hispanic white mothers.

An examination of cause-specific differences in infant mortality rates among race and ethnic groups can help researchers understand overall differences in infant mortality rates between these groups. For example, 27% of the elevated infant mortality rate for infants of non-Hispanic black mothers, when compared with non-Hispanic white mothers, can be accounted for by their higher infant mortality from the cause-of-death category low birthweight, and a further 9% can be accounted for by differences in SIDS. In other words, if non-Hispanic black infant mortality rates for low birthweight and SIDS could be reduced to non-Hispanic white levels, the difference in the infant mortality rate between non-Hispanic black and white mothers would be reduced by 36%. For infants of American Indian mothers, 25% of their elevated infant mortality rate, when compared with non-Hispanic white mothers, can be accounted for by their higher SIDS rates. If American Indian SIDS mortality could be reduced to non-Hispanic white levels, the difference in the infant mortality rate between American Indian and non-Hispanic white mothers would be reduced by one-fourth. Comparisons such as these can be helpful in targeting prevention efforts, and in assessing the potential effects of intervention efforts, particularly as a number of the recent interventions discussed below have been targeted towards reducing infant mortality from particular causes of death.

Geographic Variations

Table 5 presents infant mortality rates for the years 1996 to 1998 combined by race and Hispanic origin for the 50 States and D.C. State-specific rates were calculated for infants of Hispanic, non-Hispanic white, and non-Hispanic black mothers for all states with at least 20 infant deaths in the specified group. Overall infant mortality rates ranged from a low of 4.5 infant deaths per 1,000 live births in New Hampshire to a high of 10.5 per 1,000 live births in Mississippi (in D.C.

TABLE 5 INFANT MORTALITY RATES,* BY RACE AND HISPANIC ORIGIN OF MOTHER: UNITED STATES AND EACH STATE, 1996–98 LINKED FILES

	All races[1]	Non-Hispanic White	Non-Hispanic Black	Hispanic[2]
United States	7.2	6.0	13.9	5.9
Alabama	10.0	7.7	14.7	8.4
Alaska	6.9	5.4	**	**
Arizona	7.4	6.9	14.0	7.4
Arkansas	9.0	7.8	13.6	8.4
California	5.9	5.3	12.2	5.4
Colorado	6.8	6.2	13.9	7.3
Connecticut	6.8	4.9	15.0	9.0
Delaware	8.4	6.7	15.2	**
District of Columbia	13.8	**	17.2	**
Florida	7.3	6.1	12.4	4.9
Georgia	8.7	6.3	13.7	5.6
Hawaii	6.5	5.5	**	6.9
Idaho	7.0	6.6	**	7.3
Illinois	8.5	6.3	17.1	6.9
Indiana	8.1	7.2	15.2	7.5
Iowa	6.5	6.2	16.3	5.2
Kansas	7.6	7.1	14.5	6.3
Kentucky	7.3	6.8	12.4	**
Louisiana	9.2	6.6	13.1	**
Maine	5.3	5.2	**	**
Maryland	8.6	5.7	14.4	5.8
Massachusetts	5.1	4.4	10.7	6.4
Michigan	8.2	6.2	15.8	6.8
Minnesota	5.9	5.4	12.3	6.2
Mississippi	10.5	7.0	14.6	**
Missouri	7.6	6.2	15.5	5.7
Montana	7.1	6.5	**	**
Nebraska	7.8	7.2	17.0	8.6
Nevada	6.6	6.7	12.9	5.1
New Hampshire	4.5	4.2	**	*
New Jersey	6.5	4.3	14.1	6.7
New Mexico	6.6	6.4	**	6.6
New York	6.6	4.5	12.6	6.0
North Carolina	9.2	7.0	15.8	6.0
North Dakota	6.8	6.4	**	*
Ohio	7.8	6.6	14.5	7.8
Oklahoma	8.1	7.6	14.2	5.8
Oregon	5.5	5.3	10.3	6.1
Pennsylvania	7.5	6.0	15.8	8.7
Rhode Island	6.5	4.8	9.9	9.5
South Carolina	9.2	6.0	14.8	8.3
South Dakota	7.4	6.1	**	**
Tennessee	8.4	6.6	15.2	6.8
Texas	6.3	6.0	10.7	5.6
Utah	5.9	5.6	**	6.5
Vermont	6.7	6.4	**	**
Virginia	7.7	5.9	13.5	5.9
Washington	5.7	5.3	11.4	5.0
West Virginia	8.3	8.0	15.1	**
Wisconsin	7.0	5.7	16.6	10.3
Wyoming	6.6	6.0	**	**

* Infant deaths per 1,000 live births.
** Figure does not meet standards of reliability or precision; based on fewer than 20 deaths in the numerator.
[1] Includes births not shown separately.
[2] Persons of Hispanic origin may be of any race.
Source: Centers for Disease Control and Prevention, *National Center for Health Statistics,* National Vital Statistics System.

the rate was 13.8). For infants of non-Hispanic white mothers, rates ranged from 4.2 in New Hampshire to 8.0 in West Virginia. Rates for infants of non-Hispanic black mothers ranged from 9.9 in Rhode Island to 17.1 in Illinois (in D.C. the rate was 17.2). Thirteen states and D.C. had infant mortality rates at or above 15.0 for non-Hispanic black mothers. Infant mortality rates for Hispanic mothers ranged from 4.9 in Florida to a rate more than twice that in Wisconsin (10.3).

Variations in infant mortality rates by state are influenced by the population composition of the state. For example, states with larger populations of non-Hispanic black mothers (who have higher infant mortality rates than other populations) generally had higher infant mortality rates. Large variations by state in the percentage of the population with limited educational attainment, living in poverty, and with access to health insurance can also help to explain these differences.[11–12,32]

EXAMPLES OF INNOVATIVE HEALTH INTERVENTIONS TO REDUCE INFANT MORTALITY

In the past decade, there have been a number of initiatives designed to reduce infant mortality in the United States at the local, state, or national levels, some of which are discussed in other chapters of this book. The purpose here is not to provide a comprehensive list of such projects, but to give several examples of innovative programs which have had a positive impact on reducing infant mortality.

Black Infant Health Project, California

In 1990, California initiated the Black Infant Health (BIH) Project, a statewide demonstration and implementation program to improve birth outcomes among African Americans in California.[33] The pilot phase of the program was conducted between 1990 and 1993 in four counties, following which six best practices and intervention models were identified. The six-model interventions were (1) prenatal care outreach (using community workers to locate and link women to services), (2) case management (using public health nurses to coordinate referrals, services, and follow-up), (3) social support and empowerment (group and individual support using the Mandala of Health Model), (4) health behavior modification (individual and group curriculum), (5) recognition of the role of men (skills training programs that address positive health and well-being, parenting, jobs/vocational issues), and (6) prevention (curriculum for adolescents to reduce risk-taking behaviors, increase social skills, and enhance self-esteem and family life). At the completion of the pilot phase, a comprehensive statewide program implementing these best practice interventions was implemented in the 17 local jurisdictions where 95% of births to African American women occur. Concomitant with program implementation, screening tools, training in management information systems, and a strong evaluation plan were developed.

An evaluation of the project from 1994–98 identified important successes and lessons. BIH succeeded in reaching high-risk and hard-to-reach groups. Overall, BIH was associated with a reduction in very-low-birthweight (< 1,500 GMS) and very premature (< 32 weeks) births in the target population. A possible mechanism for this positive impact may be through the empowerment of women to recognize and respond to symptoms and signs of premature labor as soon as they become apparent. The evaluation found that coordination with health care providers was a crucial element in all the intervention models. Although each selected model was associated with a positive outcome, the lessons from the BIH underscored the need to choose intervention models based on the identified needs of local communities. No single practice or intervention model was found to be effective in all jurisdictions.

The National Back to Sleep Campaign

One of the most successful interventions to reduce infant mortality in the past decade has been the relatively simple and low-cost intervention of placing babies to sleep on their back to reduce the risk of SIDS. The cause of SIDS is still unknown but the since the beginning of the 1990s, ample epidemiological evidence had accumulated that suggested an increased risk of SIDS associated with placing infants to sleep prone (on their stomach). Additional evidence indicated that SIDS mortality declined markedly in countries where public educational campaigns to encourage parents to place infants on their back to sleep were mounted.

In 1992, the American Academy of Pediatrics (AAP) issued a statement recommending that healthy infants be placed to sleep on their backs. In 1994, a national public educational campaign, the Back to Sleep (BTS) campaign was launched to encourage parents, care-givers, and health professionals to place infants on their backs to sleep. The BTS campaign was sponsored by the U.S. Public Health Service in partnership with the American Academy of Pediatrics, the National SIDS Alliance, and other federal and nonfederal groups but has since included partnerships with industry. This public and private partnership has proven to be effective in discouraging prone positioning in the United States, and has been accompanied by substantial declines in SIDS mortality.

At the beginning of the campaign, about 70% of infants were usually placed to sleep in the prone position. By 1998, the proportion of prone sleepers was reduced to fewer than 20%.[30,34] Concomitant with the change in sleep positioning, the SIDS mortality rate declined by over 40%. This represented a decline from approximately 5,000–6,000 annual SIDS deaths to about 3,000 deaths by 1998.

The BTS campaign is composed of general media public educational campaigns and targeted outreach activities. The media campaign included radio and television public service announcements and print advertisements, which since the mid-1990s have included a minority outreach component (targeting African American and Hispanic families). Brochures for parents and health professionals were prepared and distributed widely, including to newborn nurseries, nursing organizations, and to members of the American Academy of Pediatrics and the American College of Obstetrics and Gynecology. Partnerships with industry resulted in the BTS logo and the Back to Sleep recommendation being displayed on baby consumer products.

Folic Acid Supplementation and Fortification

In 1992, the U.S. Public Health Service recommended that all women of child-bearing age consume 400 micrograms of folic acid each day to decrease the risk of neural tube defects, such as spina bifida and anencephaly.[35] Numerous scientific studies have shown that folic acid dramatically reduces these serious birth defects of the brain and spinal cord. In 1996, the Food and Drug Administration (FDA) authorized the addition of folic acid to enriched grain products, an authorization that became mandatory in 1998.[36] Fortification is estimated to provide an additional 100 micrograms of folic acid to the diet of reproductive-aged women and helps more women attain the necessary 400 micrograms of folic acid daily. Women can also get the necessary 400 micrograms by taking a vitamin containing folic acid daily. This level of folic acid can prevent 50% to 70% of these serious birth defects, but only if women consume folic acid before and during early pregnancy. CDC researchers recently reported a 19% decline in the birth prevalence of NTDs in the United States among births conceived after mandatory folic acid fortification.[37]

Perinatal Periods of Risk Approach

The reduction of infant mortality is an important public health goal. Although there has been much success in reducing the U.S. infant mortality rate, significant geographic and race/ethnic differences persist. Nowhere are these differences more apparent than in the large metropolitan cities of the United States. Understanding the reasons for the excess infant mortality in American cities, and the development of appropriate prevention strategies to reduce these deaths has been hampered by several problems. Among these problems is the lack of a suitable public health tool that is simple, validated, widely accepted, and action-oriented that communities can use at the local level to address infant mortality. To fill this gap, new approaches to combat the problem of infant mortality must be developed and tested.

In 1997, CityMatCH (association of urban health departments focused on the health of women, children, and families) began testing a new approach that adapts the World Health Organization's Perinatal Periods of Risk (PPOR) approach.[38] The PPOR approach has been used in developed and developing countries for over a decade. CityMatCH in partnership with the Centers for Disease Control and Prevention and the National March of Dimes began a multicity program to test, validate, and adapt the PPOR approach for use in U.S. urban settings. After testing the feasibility of the PPOR approach in three cities—Boston, Seattle, and Honolulu—CityMatCH has expanded this innovative and promising approach to

14 new cities to develop and test new tools and practices, and to better define the best practices of using this approach.

The PPOR approach has five logical steps that must be followed in sequence:

1. *Engaging community partners.* The goal is to mobilize community support and participation in the assessment of the problem and development of solutions.

2. *Mapping feto-infant mortality.* The goal is to assess the problem of feto-infant mortality in the target community using a simple analytic framework that employs two routinely collected data elements: age at death and birthweight. In the CityMatCH program, a two-dimensional matrix of age at death subdivided fetal, neonatal, or postneonatal deaths by two major birthweight categories: very low birthweight (500–1,499 grams) and higher birth weight (> 1,500 grams). This matrix provides a prevention map for feto-infant mortality. Fetal deaths less than 24 weeks of gestation and infant deaths with birthweights of less than 500 grams are excluded because of potential reporting inaccuracies. The PPOR approach categorizes the six cells into four primary prevention groups that link risk with potential prevention strategies (Figure 2). The results of this assessment suggest four areas of community investments in prevention activities: improving maternal health/preventing prematurity, maternal care, newborn care, and infant health.

FIGURE 2

Relationship between feto-infant mortality and potential prevention strategies in the Perinatal Periods of Risk approach

Birthweight	Age at Death		
	Fetal	Neonatal	Postneonatal
500–1,499 g	Maternal Health/Prematurity		
1,500+ g	Maternal Care	Newborn Care	Infant Health

3. *Focusing on reduction of the overall feto-infant mortality rate.* The goal is to ensure that the overall focus is on reducing the total feto-infant mortality rate after careful examination of the individual components that make up the rate.

4. *Identifying potential "opportunity gaps."* The goal is to estimate the prevention potential by calculating excess mortality in each of the primary prevention groups by using a suitable internal or external reference for comparison. A common internal comparison group used in this approach is deaths to low-risk women (non-Hispanic white women who are 20 or more years of age and have 13 or more years of education).

5. *Targeting prevention and further studies.* The final step of the PPOR approach is to direct and target assessment and program efforts related to the group or groups that contribute the most to the excess deaths. In other words, target efforts in which the opportunity gap is the greatest, given that each community has limited health care dollars for prevention. These program activities may include further studies, fetal and infant mortality reviews (FIMR), or prevention activities targeted at those groups that experience the most excess deaths. This step also includes developing plans for monitoring and evaluation of the program impact.

CHALLENGES FOR THE 21ST CENTURY

Despite the dramatic decline in infant mortality during the 20th century, important challenges remain. Two of the biggest challenges for the future are to reduce the proportion of preterm and low-birthweight births, and to reduce the large and persistent differences in infant mortality by race and ethnicity. Obviously, these two goals are closely interrelated, as excess mortality from low-birthweight births accounts for much of the black–white infant mortality gap.[9]

Although further research is needed into the causes of these problems, there are actions that can be taken now to reduce infant mortality in the United States, based on what is already known about risk factors for infant mortality (Figure 3). All of the interventions listed in Figure 3 are available to varying degrees within the United States—the challenge is to make all services available to every woman who needs them. Beyond this, it may be helpful to examine the larger context of social, economic, psychological, and environmental factors affecting infant mortality. For example, the California Black Infant Health Project has identified social support and empowerment of women as a major pathway to infant mortality reduction in their project. Also, although data on poverty are not available from vital statistics, research has shown a relationship between poverty and infant mortality;[39] therefore, poverty reduction efforts may also help to reduce infant mortality.

FIGURE 3

Opportunities to reduce maternal and infant mortality

Prevention measures to reduce maternal and infant mortality and to promote the health of all childbearing-aged women and their newborns should start before conception and continue through the postpartum period. Some of these prevention measures include the following:

Before conception

- Screen women for health risks and pre-existing chronic conditions such as diabetes, hypertension, and sexually transmitted diseases.
- Counsel women about contraception and provide access to effective family planning services (to prevent unintended pregnancies and unnecessary abortions).
- Counsel women about the benefits of good nutrition; encourage women especially to consume adequate amounts of folic acid supplements (to prevent neural tube defects) and iron.
- Advise women to avoid alcohol, tobacco, and illicit drugs.
- Advise women about the value of regular physical exercise.

During pregnancy

- Provide women with early access to high-quality care throughout pregnancy, labor, and delivery. Such care includes risk-appropriate care, treatment for complications, and the use of antenatal corticosteroids when appropriate.
- Monitor and, when appropriate, treat pre-existing chronic conditions.
- Screen for and, when appropriate, treat reproductive tract infections including bacterial vaginosis, group B streptococcus infections, and human immunodeficiency virus.
- Vaccinate women against influenza, if appropriate.
- Continue counseling against use of tobacco, alcohol, and illicit drugs.
- Continue counseling about nutrition and physical exercise.
- Educate women about the early signs of pregnancy-related problems.

During postpartum period

- Vaccinate newborns at age-appropriate times.
- Provide information about well-baby care and benefits of breastfeeding.
- Warn parents about exposing infants to secondhand smoke.
- Counsel parents about placing infants to sleep on their backs.
- Educate parents about how to protect their infants from exposure to infectious diseases and harmful substances.

Source: Centers for Disease Control and Prevention. Opportunities to reduce maternal and infant mortality. In: Achievements in public health, 1900–1999: Healthier mothers and babies. *MMWR* 48(38): 856. 1999.

REFERENCES

1. Wegman, ME. Infant mortality in the 20th century: Dramatic but uneven progress. *J Nutr* 131: 401s–408s. 2001.

2. Centers for Disease Control and Prevention, Division of Reproductive Health. Achievements in public health, 1900–1999: Healthier mothers and babies. *MMWR* 48(38): 849–858. 1999.

3. Guyer B, Freedman MA, Strobino DM, Sondik EJ. Annual summary of vital statistics: Trends in the health of Americans during the 20th century. *Pediatrics* 106: 1307–1317. 2000.

4. National Center for Health Statistics. *Health, United States, 2001.* Hyattsville, MD. 2001.

5. Guyer B, MacDorman MF, Martin JA, Peters KD, Strobino DM. Annual summary of vital statistics—1997. *Pediatrics* 102: 1333–1349. 1998.

6. Mathews TJ, Curtin SC, MacDorman MF. *Infant mortality statistics from the 1998 period linked birth/infant death data set.* National vital statistics reports; vol. 48 no. 12, Hyattsville, MD: National Center for Health Statistics. 2000.

7. Meckel RA. *Save the babies: American public health reform and the prevention of infant mortality, 1850–1929.* Baltimore, MD: The Johns Hopkins University Press, 1990.

8. Murphy SL. *Deaths: Final data for 1998.* National vital statistics reports; vol. 48 no. 11. Hyattsville, MD: National Center for Health Statistics. 2000.

9. Iyasu S, Becerra JE, Rowley DL, Hogue CJ. The impact of very low birthweight on the black–white infant mortality gap. *Am J Prev Med* 1992;8:271–7.

10. Schoendorf KC, Hogue CJ, Kleinman JC, Rowley D. Mortality among infants of black as compared with white college-educated parents. *N Engl J Med* 1992;326:1522–6.

11. Dalaker J, Proctor BD, U.S. Census Bureau. *Current population reports, series P60-210, Poverty in the United States, 1999.* U.S. Government Printing Office, Washington, D.C. 2000.

12. Mills R, U.S. Census Bureau. *Current population reports, series P60-211, Health insurance coverage, 1999.* U.S. Government Printing Office, Washington, D.C. 2000.

13. Mendoza FS, Ventura SJ, Valdez RB, et al. Selected measures of health status for Mexican-American, mainland Puerto Rican, and Cuban-American children. *JAMA* 265(2): 227–232. 1991.

14. Scribner R, Dwyer JH. Acculturation and low birthweight among Latinos in the Hispanic HANES. *Am J Public Health* 79:1263–76. 1989.

15. English PB, Kharrazi M, Guendelman S. Pregnancy outcomes and risk factors in Mexican Americans: The effect of language use and mother's birthplace. *Ethnicity Dis* 7:229–240. 1997.

16. Singh GK, Yu SM. Adverse pregnancy outcomes: Differences between U.S.- and foreign-born women in major U.S. racial and ethnic groups. *Am J Public Health* 86:837–43. 1996.

17. Schoendorf KC, Kiely JL. Birthweight and age-specific analysis of the 1990 US infant mortality drop—Was it surfactant? *Arch Pediatr Adolesc Med* 1997:129–134.

18. Schwartz RM, Luby Am, Scanlon JW, Kellogg RJ. Effect of surfactant on morbidity, mortality, and resource use in newborn infants weighing 500–1500 g. *N Engl J Med* 1994;330:1476–80.

19. National Institutes of Health. *Antenatal corticosteroids revisited: Repeat courses.* NIH Consensus Statement Online, 2000 August 17-18, 17(2): 1–10.

20. MacDorman MF, Atkinson JO. *Infant mortality statistics from the linked birth/infant death data set—1995 period data.* Monthly vital statistics report; vol. 46 no. 6 supp. 2. Hyattsville, MD: National Center for Health Statistics. 1998.

21. Alexander GR, Ed. Proceedings of an international conference on preterm birth: etiology, mechanisms and prevention. *Prenatal and Neonatal Medicine* 1998;3:1–190.

22. Alexander GR. Preterm birth: Etiology, mechanisms and prevention. *Prenatal and Neonatal Medicine* 1998:3:3–9.

23. Ventura SJ, Martin JA, Curtin SC, Menacker F, Hamilton BE. *Births: Final data for 1999.* National vital statistics reports, vol. 49 no. 1. Hyattsville, MD: National Center for Health Statistics. 2001.

24. Joseph KS, Kramer MS, Marcoux S, Ohlsson A, Wen SW, Allen A, Platt R. Determinants of preterm birth rates in Canada from 1981 through 1983 and from 1992 through 1994. *N Engl J Med* 1998;339:1434–1439.

25. Daltveit AK, Vollset SE, Skjaerven R, Irgens LM. Impact of multiple births and elective deliveries on the trends in low birth weight in Norway, 1967–1995. *American Journal of Epidemiology* 1999;129:1128–1133.

26. Kramer MS, Demissie K, Yang H, Platt RW, Sauve R, Liston R. The contribution of mild and moderate preterm birth to infant mortality. *JAMA* 2000;284: 843–849.

27. Wilcox AJ. Birthweight and perinatal mortality: The effect of maternal smoking. *Am J Epidemiol* 1993;137:1098–1104.

28. U.S. Department of Health and Human Services. W*omen and Smoking. A Report of the Surgeon General.* Rockville (MD): U.S. Department of Health and Human Services, Public Health Service, Office of the Surgeon General, 2001.

29. National Center for Health Statistics. *Vital Statistics of the United States, 1990, vol. II, mortality, part A.* Washington, D.C.: Public Health Service. 1994.

30. Willinger M, Hoffman HJ, Wu KT, et al. Factors associated with the transition to nonprone sleep positions of infants in the United States: the National Infant Sleep Position Study. *JAMA* 1998;280:329–335.

31. National Center for Health Statistics. *1998 Perinatal mortality data file.* CD-ROM Series 20 no. 18. National Center for Health Statistics, December 2000.

32. Bird ST. Separate black and white infant mortality models: Differences in the importance of structural variables. *Soc Sci Med* 1995. 41(11):1507–1512.

33. California Black Infant Health Program Evaluation Report, *Program Planning and Implementation 1994.* July, 1999 (prepared by San Diego State University, Graduate School of Public Health).

34. Willinger M, Ko CW, Hoffman HJ, Kessler RC. Corwin MJ. Factors associated with caregivers' choice of infant sleep position, 1994–1998: The National Infant Sleep Position Study. *JAMA* 283(16):2135–42, 2000 Apr 26.

35. CDC. Recommendations for the use of folic acid to reduce the number of cases of spina bifida and other neural tube defects. *Morb Mortal Wkly Rep* 1992:41(RR-14):1–7.

36. FDA. Food Standards. *Federal Register* 1996;61:8781–8797.

37. Honein MA, Paulozzi LJ, Mathews TJ, Erickson JD, Wong LC. Impact of Folic Acid Fortification of the U.S. Food Supply on the Occurrence of Neural Tube Defects. *JAMA* 285(23):2981–2986. 2001.

38. Perinatal Periods of Risk Approach (PPOR), http://www.citymatch.org.

39. CDC. Poverty and Infant Mortality—United States, 1988. *Morb Mortal Wkly Rep* 1995:44;922–927.

U NIT 5

POLICY IMPLICATIONS

INTRODUCTION

In previous chapters, the background for MCH policies has been reviewed and brought up-to-date. This unit provides an overview of those policies and their implications. It is clear that objectives for the early 21st century will be influenced by a growing knowledge of genetics, an increased reliance on evidence-based strategies, and a commitment to reducing disparities. Market and social forces, funding for research, and support for community-based preventive services are all critical issues influencing policy. These issues must be addressed in order to provide for physical health, mental health, and social well-being—the World Health Organization definition of health.

Social policy changes, including the switch from AFDC to TANF, the addition of SCHIP, and the inroads of managed-care organizations, have coincided with a growing number of children and families unable to receive needed care. Title V agencies have proven to be flexible and adaptive, taking on a widening role as well as greater formal responsibility for the core functions of public health. Devolution of responsibility for decision making from the federal government to states and localities has fostered new opportunities, especially for urban maternal and child health (MCH) programs. Challenges remain; these include welfare-to-work job shortfalls, Medicaid managed-care struggles, and local resource-use disagreements, all of which will require innovative solutions. We will need system change, collaboration, seamless connections, political will, and new levels of government and public accountability.

With increased support, MCH early programmatic priorities will include expanded services to all family members, increased quality of child care, expanded programs for adolescents, outreach and services for immigrant children, and full attention to marginal-income children with special health care needs (CSHCN) and children served by university-affiliated programs. The implications of gene research will extend far into the 21st century and will affect health overall and maternal and child health in particular.

ARTICLE 1

PREVENTION FOR HEALTH

Solomon Iyasu and Hani K. Atrash

INTRODUCTION

"An ounce of prevention is worth a pound of cure." "A stitch in time saves nine." Prevention enjoys a wonderful reputation among the general public, and deservedly so. What could be more straightforward, less subject to doubt, than the idea that health professionals and the public alike should try to prevent disease wherever and whenever possible? Yet, when clinicians, public health practitioners, and policy makers grapple with the idea of prevention, we find they often disagree about what the word means, what kinds of preventive services should be offered, and how we should pay for preventive care. To resolve some of these differences and strengthen our preventive services overall, we suggest that a well-considered conceptual framework is needed to properly define the relationship between preventive services and our goals for the public's health and quality of life.

Given the variety of views of those who work in the health sector, whether they are dealing with individual patients or populations, a good starting point for a conceptual framework would be a comprehensive, yet easily understood, definition of health that is acceptable to all. With that definition in place, one could decide what prevention should cover. Currently, the most widely accepted definition is that developed by the World Health Organization (WHO): "The state of complete physical, mental, and social well-being and not merely the absence of disease." If we make this the goal of prevention, we see that one-on-one clinical interventions such as immunization and the early detection of specific illnesses make up only part of the picture. We must include a variety of other services that cover those who already are burdened with disease, for example, and we must consider what preventive services can be offered to increase the social and mental well-being of persons at every age. We can conclude that many in the society have conceptualized prevention too narrowly, and, correspondingly, we may assume that prevention research has neglected many areas where it should properly be engaged.

In this article we discuss some of the past, current, and future conceptual frameworks for prevention, the role of research, and the challenges facing us in the new millennium as we seek to make prevention an even stronger force in our society.

FRAMEWORKS FOR PREVENTION

Primary, Secondary, Tertiary Prevention

Traditionally, three levels of prevention have been defined: primary, secondary, and tertiary. Primary prevention is directed at people without the disease(s) of interest; secondary, at early detection and treatment for those who have the disorder; and tertiary, at prevention of complications.

- In *primary prevention*, the causes or risk factors for the disease or condition are usually well known. Interventions here include immunizations, supplementation with folic acid, use of automobile seatbelts, and educating school students to prevent tobacco use. Epidemiologically, primary prevention lowers the incidence of the diseases (new cases) and is what the public usually thinks of as prevention.
- *Secondary prevention* may permit a greater likelihood of cure or at least longer survival than would otherwise have been possible. This type of prevention is directed at asymptomatic persons or those whose symptoms are nonspecific for the disease or condition but who have developed early biologic evidence that they are affected. It generally does not reduce incidence, but if treatment is curative it can reduce prevalence. Very often, secondary prevention takes the form of screening asymptomatic persons, such as testing for iron deficiency, screening for lead poisoning in children or breast and cervical cancer in women, measuring prenatally an expectant woman's blood pressure or hematocrit, or screening for metabolic disease such as phenylketonuria.
- *Tertiary prevention*, if successful, may improve the quality of life and sometimes lengthen survival of the person with the condition. It does not change incidence but would raise prevalence if the initiative succeeds in lengthening the patient's life. Examples of tertiary prevention include aggressive treatment of early rheumatoid arthritis to prevent joint destruction, administering antibiotics to women with premature rupture of membranes to prevent chorioamnionitis, giving corticosteroids to women in or at risk of preterm labor to prevent respiratory distress syndrome and intraventricular hemorrhage in the newborn, and closely managing blood glucose concentrations in persons with type I diabetes to delay onset of renal disease.

Because the aim of primary prevention is to prevent a disease before it occurs, many see it as the only true form of prevention. Such a belief is shortsighted, however, and fits poorly with the WHO definition of health. That definition compels us to look at the entire population, not just those who are apparently untouched by disease. Thus, even the older person with poorly managed diabetes whose health and quality of life have been severely compromised by retinopathy and neuropathy, for example, is still a candidate for prevention.

Universal, Selective, Indicated Prevention

A less well-known but still commonly used framework for prevention is Gordon's characterization of preventive interventions as universal, selective, or indicated. *Universal preventive* interventions target the general public or a whole population group that has not been identified as universally at risk. For example, women of childbearing age (risk of giving birth to a baby with neural tube defect resulting from inadequate intake of folic acid). *Selective prevention* targets persons or population subgroups whose risk of a disorder is significantly above average (risk may be imminent or over the lifetime). Such subgroups could include pregnant women with a prior history of gestational diabetes (elevated risk of gestational diabetes in subsequent pregnancies) or sedentary persons with a high body mass index (elevated risk for cardiovascular disease and type II diabetes mellitus). *Indicated prevention* targets high-risk persons identified as having either minimal but detectable signs or symptoms that foreshadow a disease or who, although not meeting diagnostic criteria, have biologic markers indicating predisposition for a disease (e.g., a woman with an abnormal Pap smear indicating a pre-cancerous cervix, a woman with a family history of breast cancer who has a mutation of the *BRCA1* or *BRCA2* gene). This definition excludes all individuals with full-blown disorders and is even less accommodating than the traditional designations of primary, secondary, and tertiary prevention.

Paradigm Shift in Prevention

With the significant reduction in recent decades in single-factor health conditions (e.g., infectious diseases), and with a more intensified focus on quality of life, prevention has undergone a shift in emphasis from targeting specific health conditions to taking comprehensive approaches that simultaneously deal with multiple risk factors at numerous levels to prevent a variety of conditions. For example, the current standards of prenatal care call for multiple preventive measures to help improve pregnancy outcomes through (1) early detection, (2) management of several medical conditions, and (3) educational efforts to modify risky behaviors. These preventive measures include early detection and treatment of such conditions as anemia; pre-eclampsia; fetal distress; gestational diabetes; and counseling pregnant women about diet, exercise, family planning, and the dangers of smoking, drinking, and using illicit substances. Many of these interventions are being implemented at multiple levels such as the individual, family, community health care system, and policy levels. Moreover, many of the health threats are being addressed using strategies that go beyond clinical interventions. These strategies recognize the role of individual behaviors, social and environmental factors, public health policy, and legislation.

MODERN PREVENTION SCIENCE AND RESEARCH

With so many prevention measures being recommended for routine implementation, questions have arisen about their effectiveness, cost, safety, benefit, equity, ethics, and associated moral issues. Those concerns have been accompanied in turn, by a demand for accountability from an increasingly aware public. As a consequence, we have seen a dramatic increase in research activities to provide a scientific basis to support or abandon recommended interventions. Such activities are commonly referred to as *prevention research*, which has three components.

- *Pre-intervention research* or *risk-factor research* involves basic social, behavioral, preclinical, clinical, and epidemiological/public health studies that form the building blocks for preventive intervention research. This first component includes research on risk and protective factors as well as processes to (1) identify basic mechanisms of biological, behavioral, and psychosocial change; (2) elucidate factors that increase or decrease the likelihood of developing target outcomes; and (3) develop and test models of processes that mediate and moderate the translation of risk into disease, its course, and its consequences. In addition, pre-intervention research includes translating results from the preceding three areas into intervention development research. This research is aimed at (a) promoting research methods innovation and development, and (b) designing, pilot testing, refining, and analyzing new preventive intervention strategies before testing them in efficacy trials. The focus of study in pre-intervention research may range from individual-level to population-level outcomes, as in epidemiological and other public health research.

- *Preventive intervention research* is the core of prevention research because of its great potential for directly improving public health. It consists of trials of the *efficacy* and *effectiveness* of preventive interventions. These interventions might study participants who currently have (1) no symptoms of disease; (2) subclinical symptoms; (3) a diagnosed disease with previous symptoms. (For this group the emphasis is on prevention of relapse or recurrence.) (4) Participants might also have a diagnosed condition with full-blown clinical disease. This is a group for whom the emphasis is on preventing comorbidity or disability. The choice of prevention targets will depend on scientific opportunity, pre-intervention knowledge base, and the public health burden of the condition to be prevented. The prevention targets might include individuals and broader levels of the social environment such as families, work or school settings, communities, and their social norms and policies.

  Efficacy trials test the extent to which a specific intervention produces positive results under near-ideal conditions (the experimental condition). Effectiveness trials, in contrast, test how well an intervention works under natural settings, with the objective of evaluating the generalizability of intervention effects for a defined population or service setting. Effectiveness trials may also include economic analysis, such as cost-benefit studies. Both efficacy and effectiveness studies can involve randomized controlled trials and both can focus on individual-level or population-level outcomes in community-based trials.

- *Preventive service-systems research* is concerned with the study of effective preventive interventions within service systems. Here the focus is on the interactive effects of preventive interventions with organizational aspects of the service environment, such as the characteristics and skills of those providing care and of the populations being served, organizational culture and climate, and methods of financing services.

  Preventive service systems research can include studies of (1) policies and procedures that facilitate or hinder the adoption and implementation of effective interventions, as well as research on the technology of effective dissemination; (2) the effects of age, gender, and ethnicity, as well as those socio-cultural factors that affect access to or use of available preventive interventions; and (3) the costs associated with the delivery of preventive interventions as well as methods of financing. The focus of preventive service-systems research is on contextual and system-level outcomes.

PREVENTION IN THE 21ST CENTURY

In the 21st century, prevention is likely to be significantly shaped by several forces including even more rapid advances in molecular genetics, a greater interest in and demand for evidence-based clinical and community-based preventive strategies, and a national commitment to eliminate geographic and racial/ethnic disparities in health.

Genetics: Opportunities for Prevention

The last decade of the 20th century saw the completion of the mapping and sequencing of the human genome, a feat that has raised the tantalizing prospect of preventing and curing many devastating diseases that are genetically determined or influenced. Genes can play a role in disease causation in multiple ways, from directly causing a disease through a single-gene disorder to increasing the odds of disease through gene–gene or gene–environment interaction.

In the coming decades, we are likely to see a large array of genetic tests to predict single-gene disorders and to identify susceptibility to genetically influenced diseases. More than ever, individualized and targeted primary prevention among infants and children who are genetically at risk will be a routine part of clinical practice. Currently, primary prevention applications (carrier detection, premarital counseling, prenatal diagnosis, and termination) are limited to single-gene disorders such as Tay-Sachs disease or chromosomal disorders such as Down syndrome.

The greatest potential for prevention lies in the far more common gene-influenced disorders than these rare single-gene disorders. Reducing the risk of neural tube defect through folic acid fortification of food is a prime illustration of the role of primary prevention in genetically influenced disorders. An important goal will be the understanding of gene–gene interactions and the environmental triggers that increase the likelihood of adverse health outcomes in genetically susceptible individuals. Future preventive interventions may thus involve the identification and removal of environmental triggers (exogenous factors) to pre-empt expression of the disease-producing genotype. Direct genetic manipulation or alteration to prevent polygenically determined diseases is far in the future, but such intervention technologies are likely to come fairly sooner for single-gene conditions.

From a public health policy perspective, the emergence of the genomic era has raised fundamental ethical, legal, and pychosocial issues. A major ethical question is whether or not individuals should be tested for conditions for which no known prevention or control technologies are available. Legal issues have to deal with potential misuse of genetic test results such as denying employment or health insurance or failing to keep genetic test results confidential. At this time we do not know a great deal about possible adverse psychological impacts on the persons examined and other family members from the release of test results. Finally, adequate procedures and regulations to guide population-based genetic prevention programs have not been developed. Before these issues are resolved, offering population-based genetic prevention programs remains unrealistic.

Evidence-Based Clinical and Community Preventive Interventions

The organization, financing, and delivery of health care are changing rapidly in response to market and social forces. Some of the pressures shaping the health care system are cost containment, a need to do more with fewer health care dollars, an increasing focus on health promotion and disease prevention, and the adoption of new technologies that are shifting services to nontraditional settings. In addition, the public is increasingly well informed and demands greater accountability and equity of access for preventive health care services. One of the ways health care providers are adapting and responding to these new demands is by offering new population-based preventive services while maintaining their traditional role of treating disease.

In the United States, efforts are under way to develop a Guide to Community Preventive Services, with the hope of recommending a set of effective evidence-based population-based interventions. The Guide to Clinical Preventive Services was published in 1988 and this new effort should result in a companion set of recommendations to apply in community settings.

WHERE WE STAND

The potential to develop preventive services that embrace people of all ages, both the sick and the well, is greater than it has ever been. If we can agree that prevention should have as its goal the World Health Organization's conception of health, we should be better prepared to deliver the level and scope of preventive services that Americans need and deserve. When we consider as well the scientific advances already made and those that are in the offing, we can be sure that the first few decades of the new millennium will see a revolution in prevention. But significant barriers remain, including inadequate financing for prevention research, lack of payment for preventive services, and insufficient organizational and system support to implement delivery of community-based preventive services.

REFERENCES

Gordon R S. An operational classification of disease prevention. *Public Health Rep.* 1983;98:107–109.

Gordon R S. An operational classification of disease prevention. In Sternbert JA, Silverman MM, eds. *Preventing Mental Disorders: A Research Perspective* 1987:20–26 DHHS publication no. ADM 87-1492. Washington, DC: U.S. Government Printing Office.

Khoury M J. From genes to public health: the applications of genetic technology in disease prevention. Genetics Working Group. *Am J Public Health.* 1996;86:1717–1722.

McGinnis J M, Foege W. Guide to community preventive services: harnessing the science. *Am J Prev Med.* 2000;18(1 suppl):1–2.

U.S. Preventive Services Task Force. *Guide to Clinical Preventive Services*, 2nd ed. Baltimore, MD: Williams and Wilkins, 1996.

Wertz D C, Fanos J H, Reilly P R. Genetic testing for children and adolescents. Who decides. *JAMA.* 1994;272:875–881.

ARTICLE 2

MATERNAL AND CHILD HEALTH: BACK TO THE FUTURE

Karen VanLandeghem and Catherine A. Hess

INTRODUCTION

In the mid-1990s, major changes in health and welfare systems had dramatic impact on women, children, youth, and families. Welfare reform brought about significant changes in the social service delivery system that had for many years supported low-income women, children, and their families. Prior to welfare reform, low-income families could indefinitely receive cash assistance support; afterwards, states were required to impose strict work requirements and implement a five-year lifetime limit on receipt of benefits funded with federal dollars.[1] In addition, the historic link between welfare and Medicaid eligibility ended. Although efforts to create a universal health insurance program were never realized, the endeavor laid the groundwork for passage of the State Children's Health Insurance Program (SCHIP) as part of the Balanced Budget Act (BBA) of 1997. The BBA not only included provisions allowing states to expand health insurance coverage for children, but also made some of the most significant changes to Medicaid since its inception.[2]

The vast changes brought by these new laws were further compounded in states and communities by shifts toward managed care delivery systems, state agency restructuring, and an emphasis on greater autonomy in implementing federal laws and reforms. In addition, public health advocates achieved a monumental victory and states a windfall of additional funding as a result of the 1998 tobacco settlement.[3] These developments were followed by an extremely strong economy between 1997 and 1999, with broad-based reductions in poverty rates, greater work among single parents, and a small decline in the percentage of children living in single parent households.[4]

Reforms in health and welfare systems were converging at state and local levels, requiring policy makers and other key stakeholders to make rapid assessments and decisions. These reforms brought new challenges and opportunities for improving the health of women, children, and youth, including children with special health care needs due to chronic or disabling conditions. Prior to these reforms, many states had served as laboratories and proving grounds for change efforts to cut health care costs, increase access to and availability of health care, and streamline service delivery systems. In the aftermath of these reforms, some states pioneered further system and program changes while others struggled with new program start-ups and with revamping infrastructures responsive to a changing environment.

State and local health and welfare agencies, managed-care organizations, community-based organizations, legislators, advocates, consumers, and others have critical roles in the design and implementation of service delivery systems for women, children, and their families. Specifically, state Title V Maternal and Child Health (MCH) Services Block-Grant programs[5] are at the core of public health agency efforts for women, children, and youth. Amidst all of these rapid systemic changes, public health and maternal and child health in particular, were closely examining what their roles would be in this new environment. Maternal and child health programs were at a critical crossroads.

A HISTORICAL CONTEXT FOR THE CHANGING ROLE OF
TITLE V MATERNAL AND CHILD HEALTH SERVICES BLOCK-GRANT PROGRAMS

In 1988, a landmark Institute of Medicine (IOM) study declared public health to be "in disarray."[6] The dramatic changes in health and social welfare policies and services of the 1990s added to the decade-long challenge to reinvigorate and reinvent public health. Long viewed by much of the public and many policy makers as health care of last resort for the poor, public health agencies, including MCH programs and professionals, struggled to redefine their images and roles in the mold laid out by the IOM. The IOM formulated three core functions for public health—assessment, policy development, and assurance. This last function of ensuring the availability of services needed to improve health could be accomplished through a variety of means other than directly providing services.

In 1989, the most significant changes occurred in Title V of the Social Security Act since it was amended in 1981 to create the Maternal and Child Health Services Block-Grant legislation. Some of the 1989 changes, such as linking the purpose of the program to achievement of national health objectives and requiring comprehensive needs assessments, were consistent with the future directions outlined by the IOM. Others, particularly addition of language explicitly stating the program's purpose as one of providing and not just ensuring care, seemed to push the program's thrust more in line with the common perception of public health programs' role as providers of care for the poor.

This tension in roles continued throughout the 1990s. National and state momentum in the first half of the decade toward comprehensive health care reform, including universal coverage, propelled federal, state, and local public health agencies to realign their roles and build their capacities to carry out core public health functions. Anticipating a diminished need, if any, to be providers of last resort, public health agencies focused on how to better articulate and enlist public and political support for core functions. In the aftermath of the failure of comprehensive reforms, public health achieved minimal success in gaining such support.

As the focus for reform shifted to the private sector and cost-containment-driven managed-care arrangements, public health agencies increasingly were confronted by the possibility of losing Medicaid-insured clients, largely women and children. To many, there appeared to be a choice: to focus on strengthening capacities to carry out core public health functions, or to pursue aggressively and competitively a continued role in providing health care services to Medicaid-insured clients.

The changing health care marketplace took the place of comprehensive public reforms in stimulating redefinition of public health roles, but it did not solve one of the fundamental problems in the system—the growing numbers of uninsured. The percentage of uninsured Americans had been steadily increasing since at least 1987. Despite a recent modest decline in the number of uninsured Americans—the first such decline after 12 years of steady increases—there are now nearly 43 million uninsured Americans.[7] Welfare reform, by severing the link between cash and medical aid, might push those numbers even higher. In fact, reports examining the effects of these many reforms indicate that the gains in coverage due to the State Children's Health Insurance Program were offset by losses of coverage to welfare reform. To many, neither the promises nor the obstacles brought by the reforms of the mid-1990s have been fully realized or seen.[8]

In spite of public health recognizing the need to reinvent itself in light of the health and welfare reforms of the 1990s, public health continues to face some of the same challenges it faced prior to these reforms. One factor that contributes to maintaining and improving health status is access to health care. If public health is to ensure that all populations have access to health care, it must address the access needs of uninsured, underinsured, and underserved groups. To address effectively the primary contributors to preventable morbidity and mortality, public health must also focus on improving capacities and support for less publicly visible functions such as research, surveillance, and investigation and control measures on a population basis. On an individual level, public health must include services such as outreach, health education and counseling, and home visiting, which are often not reimbursable.

The years since the inception of these reforms show that many public health agencies, including maternal and child health programs, have evolved to meet the needs of a changing health care delivery environment while simultaneously strengthening and refining core programs and mission. Certainly, state Title V programs have participated in health and welfare system reforms in varying degrees. As health insurance coverage for children has expanded under SCHIP, public health has had to be less engaged in the development of these programs and can focus on more traditional public health programs such as home visiting. Where necessary, however, state Title V programs still provide and pay for health care services.

Nonetheless, reforms have prompted Title V programs to further strengthen core public health functions and in turn, retool some of the fundamental roots of maternal and child health.

The maternal and child health field is seeing programs expand to address new causes of morbidity and mortality such as mental illness and domestic violence, areas not always considered public health arenas. Moreover, many MCH programs are evolving to embrace a family and community health perspective. These programs are choosing this broader framework because it affords increased fiscal opportunity and flexibility, improved health status and service delivery, increased opportunities for broader education and prevention efforts, and improved avenues for collaboration. The reforms of the 1990s have given way to more effective and consistent ways of state MCH program data collection and reporting, and tools for helping states re-examine their roles in light of public health core functions. Parallel efforts are also occurring in public health overall.

MATERNAL AND CHILD HEALTH PROGRAMS SINCE 1990

The remainder of this article highlights examples of MCH program activities and directions since the reforms and influences of the 1990s. These few examples illustrate how states have risen to the challenges to invigorate public health services and roles to promote the health and well-being of women, children, and youth including those with special health care needs. The examples here reflect recent practices and structures of some state Title V Maternal and Child Health Service Block-Grant programs; however, it is important to note that many of the systems and programs here continue to evolve.[9]

The Rhode Island Family Health Approach

Until the 1980s, Rhode Island's Division of Family Health was a traditional Title V program, comprised of a maternal and child health section, and a children with special health care needs program. In 1988, the division's mission was expanded with the addition of the Special Supplemental Nutrition Program for Women, Infants and Children (WIC), followed by Early Intervention, Immunization, and school health services in the 1990s. Title V funding makes up only 5% of the Division's budget, yet the principles and focus of the federal Title V legislation are found not only in the organizational structure, but in the Division's approach and philosophy.

In 1997, the Adolescence and Young Adult Health Unit was created to address the needs of school-age youth and young adults. The Unit administers many categorical programs designed to assist this population. One of the Unit's new programs, the Men 2 B Role Model Support Capacity Program, is used to demonstrate how the Division of Family Health, and more specifically, the Rhode Island Title V program, has used a family health approach in its efforts to meet the broad and diverse needs of the young adult male population. The program trains and supports a cadre of men who live and/or work with boys in five Rhode Island cities where risk factors for teen pregnancy are the highest. The program's goals are to reduce the teen pregnancy rate, the proportion of school-aged youth who have engaged in sexual intercourse, the incidence of 15–19-year-olds who have contracted sexually transmitted diseases, and other related indicators. The Rhode Island Division of Family Health, in its comprehensive approach to family health, has also focused on family involvement in program development, policy making, outreach, and evaluation.

The Louisiana Infant Mental Health Program

During the last five years, Louisiana's Title V program has shifted from direct service delivery to broader core public health functions. The catalyst has been the program's focus on systems building efforts in the area of mental health. In 1995, simultaneous needs assessments by the state's Title V agency and the Department of Social Services revealed that parenting education and family support systems were a major need. This finding led to the initiation of the Infant Mental Health Initiative to train local parish nurses in infant social and emotional development and attachment theories and practice. The training also addresses child rearing and disorders influenced by family violence. With support from the Title V MCH Services Block Grant and the Louisiana State University Department of Psychiatry, the program's goal is to train nurses statewide in parenting education and in how to conduct mental health assessments as part of a well-child, WIC, or EPSDT clinic visit.

One result of this effort has been major improvements in data collection. As a result of the Infant Mental Health Program, the Child Health Record—the medical record that local public health nurses complete during a clinic visit—has been expanded to include information about the infant's mental health, abuse, domestic violence, and maternal functioning and emotional status. Also, what began as a training initiative to address infant mental health issues has grown to address the health and psychosocial needs of Louisiana's high-risk families. Comprehensive home-visiting programs have been established in four of the nine regions of the state, relying on the clinic nurses trained by the Infant Mental Health Initiative.

Together, the Infant Mental Health Initiative and the home-visiting program revealed an even bigger need in the state for a mental health infrastructure and referral systems where young children and their families with more complex mental health issues can receive more in-depth intervention and services. This resulted in partnerships between Title V and the Louisiana Office of Mental Health, which previously had focused on older children. The biggest lesson learned by the state was the tremendous mental health needs of high-risk families and the important role public health can play in system building and accessing resources for these families. Given the success of the Infant Mental Health Initiative, the subsequent development of the Home Visiting Program, and a resulting partnership with the Office of Mental Health, great potential exists for even more successful system-building in the future.

Healthy Families Lead to Healthy Children

Massachusetts' Title V program is based on the philosophy that healthy families lead to healthy children. In fact, a family health unit linked to maternal and child health and children with special health care needs has been in existence in Massachusetts since the mid-1970s. In 1991, the Bureau of Family and Community Health was created, bringing Title V, the Preventive Health Services Block-Grant, the Primary Care program, and other key women's, children's, and family-related programs under one organizational umbrella.

The philosophy is best illustrated by the evolution of three state programs: the Massachusetts Women's Health program, the FOR families home-visitation program, and the shift of the Bureau's Division of Special Needs to address not only children with special health needs and disabilities but also adults with disabilities. In each instance, unique approaches to address the broader needs of families have been the focus.

The Women's Health program has broadened its reach far beyond reproductive health, offering services to decrease women's morbidity and mortality, such as cardiovascular prevention programs targeting young women, and services to promote knowledge and well-being among women, in such areas as occupational health and wellness programs. The FOR home-visiting program represents an important partnership between the state welfare agency and the Bureau of Community and Family Health to assist families transitioning from welfare to work. The project is supported by federal Temporary Assistance to Needy Families (TANF) funds, but relies on the expertise of the Bureau to offer comprehensive home visiting services to the most vulnerable families with multiple needs. The Division of Special Needs is especially noteworthy for having assumed responsibilities beyond those of the Children with Special Health Care Needs (CSHCN) program. This has been done in areas including the Initiative for Youth with Disabilities Program, which assists adolescents with disabilities in transitioning to adulthood, and through many other efforts that focus on the broader needs of families of CSHCN and the needs of adults with disabilities.

SUMMARY

Public health agencies including MCH programs continue to struggle in a dynamic environment with the most appropriate and effective mix of roles and functions to achieve their missions of protecting and promoting health and well-being. One thing is clear—MCH programs have continued to evolve and have remained flexible and adaptive over nearly a century. MCH programs have revisited roots that pre-date Title V of the Social Security Act in collecting and effectively utilizing data and public policy to effect conditions related to the health and well-being of women, children, youth, and families. In turn, they are embracing ever-widening concerns, such as mental health and violence prevention, that increasingly are facing today's families and communities.

REFERENCES

1. AFDC (Aid to Families with Dependent Children), the former cash-assistance welfare program, was a federal entitlement. Those eligible for AFDC were automatically eligible for Medicaid. Under welfare reform, AFDC was replaced by TANF (Temporary Assistance for Needy Families), and the historic link between welfare and Medicaid eligibility ended. TANF replaced AFDC, Job Opportunity and Basic Skills (JOBS) program, and Emergency Assistance with a block grant to the states. TANF-funded assistance is not an individual entitlement under federal law. States are required to apply strict work requirements, and there is a five-year lifetime limit on receipt of benefits funded with federal TANF dollars.

2. The Balanced Budget Act of 1997 (P.S. 105-33), 111 Stat. 251 (1997), Title IV, Subtitle J. State Children's Health Insurance Program, Sections 4901-4923, includes provisions for establishing separate state children's health insurance programs, expanding Medicaid coverage, implementing presumptive Medicaid eligibility for children, continuing Medicaid eligibility for children losing Supplemental Security Income (SSI) benefits, and creating special diabetes programs for children.

3. In 1998, the state Attorneys General reached a historic settlement proposal, which among other mandates would contribute $1.5 billion over five years for public education, pay $250 million for a foundation dedicated to reducing teen smoking, and pay states $12 billion in "up-front" money over five years.

4. Wigton, A. and Weil, A., *Snapshots of America's Families II: A View of the Nation and 13 States from the National Survey of America's Families,* Washington, DC: Urban Institute, 1999.

5. Authorized under Title V of the Social Security Act, the Maternal and Child Health (MCH) Services Block Grant focuses broadly on the health of women, infants, children, and youth. In 1981, Title V's categorical programs were consolidated under block-grant legislation, and states were given increased discretion in the use of funds. Amendments in 1989 included important changes that improved accountability while maintaining flexibility.

6. Institute of Health. Summary and recommendations. In *The Future of Public Health,* Washington, DC: National Academy Press, 1988, p. 8.

7. Mills, R.J., *Health Insurance Coverage: 1999,* Washington, DC: U.S. Census Bureau, September 2000.

8. Wigton, A., and Weil, A., *Snapshots of America's Families II: A View of the Nation and 13 States from the National Survey of America's Families,* Washington, DC: Urban Institute, 1999.

9. State examples were excerpted from Whitehand L, VanLandeghem K, and Kagan, J: *Family Health: The Next Generation of MCH?* Washington, DC: Association of Maternal and Child Health Programs, September, 2001.

ARTICLE 3

SOCIAL POLICY REFORM AND AMERICA'S CITIES: RISK AND OPPORTUNITY FOR MATERNAL AND CHILD HEALTH

Magda G. Peck and Debora Barnes-Josiah

INTRODUCTION

This article was prepared before the terrorist attacks of September 11, 2001, on the World Trade Center and the Pentagon. The social reforms described in the chapter now share the stage with a national mobilization against further attacks, with threats of bioterrorism, and a significantly weakened national economy. The resulting financial and social challenges to America's largest cities have added a massive new uncertainty to the lives of the women, children, and families of these cities. Yet, their daily lives go on. Recent events do not supersede the original message of this chapter, but rather reveal additional stresses to the complex fabric of the national safety net. It is in urban areas that these changes are most likely to manifest. In these changes are both risk and opportunity.

OVERVIEW OF RECENT CHANGES

The last years of the 20th century saw winds of change sweeping through American social welfare policy, transforming health and human services approaches that had been in place for over a half-century. Although these reforms affect every community, America's cities are the principal stage upon which the drama of changing social policy is playing out. Sharing the spotlight in this drama are managed care, welfare reform, and the State Child Health Insurance Program (SCHIP).

During the last decade, managed care became a permanent part of nearly every major urban community and a cornerstone to state Medicaid policy. City and county health departments, long-standing safety-net providers to the most vulnerable, continue to shift their role from direct delivery of services to low-

527

income families and children to population-based assurance and assessment. Welfare reform mandates able-bodied citizens to work first, eliminating entitlement to public sector support for those most in need. The State Child Health Insurance Program offers states the opportunity to extend insurance coverage to large numbers of children who remain uninsured. New social reforms continue to strive for further cost restraints, balancing savings against the need to assure a safety net for those most vulnerable.

This article describes the social, economic, and demographic factors that converge in urban communities; it is there that changes in national health and social policy are being played out. It first examines the impact of three recent reforms—managed care, welfare reform, and child health insurance legislation—on health and human services for families and children in America's cities. It next identifies underlying issues that intensify the vulnerability of urban women, children, and families under these reforms—"devolution" of decision-making authority to states and localities for major social programs, public demand for greater public sector accountability, and public perception of the role of government to protect the vulnerable. Last, it outlines broad recommendations to assure the health of women, children, and families in America's cities, in anticipation of continued social policy reform.

THE URBAN CONVERGENCE OF MATERNAL AND CHILD HEALTH RISKS

Urban communities host populations that bear a disproportionate burden of adverse maternal and child health risks and outcomes. In 2000, America's metropolitan areas were home to 80.6% of all children under 18 years and 57 million families, or 79.3% of all families in the United States.[1] Ongoing demographic and economic trends in American cities amplify the already considerable risks associated with U.S. urban residence. In 1999, 16.4% of residents of central cities were living in poverty, compared to 8.3% outside the central city and 14.3% outside of metropolitan areas.[2] The 50 largest cities were home to one-half of all American children who live in distressed neighborhoods (defined by community concentration of poverty, female-headed families, unemployment, and welfare dependency), and the child poverty rate in these cities increased from 18% to 27% between 1969 and 1989. Minority Americans are also more likely to live in cities. According to newly released Census 2000 data, 39% of all Blacks and 36% of all Hispanics lived in the 100 largest cities, compared to 14% of Whites. Residential segregation and concentrations of poverty are the hallmarks of urban minority poverty. Detailed income and poverty data from the 2000 census are not yet available. However, figures are likely to resemble those from the 1990 census, where the concentration of poverty was found most intense for African Americans: 42% of those living in the 100 largest cities lived in census tracts where 40% or more of residents were poor. Urban minority populations are all too often concentrated within poor communities that cannot support a strong enough economic base to nurture a comprehensive neighborhood fabric of commerce and services.[3]

There is no national system for compiling important indicators of wellness or morbidity at the city level.[4] However, compiled secondary data suggest that the largest cities are host to the highest rates of key social ills such as infant mortality, low birth weight, asthma, AIDS, and firearm homicides.[4-9] According to a 2001 Child Trends/KidsCount Special Report on children, seven of the eight leading measures of child well-being in the 50 largest U.S. cities are worse than the measures for the nation as a whole.[10]

Not surprisingly, the greatest proportion of those benefiting from welfare and other social policy reforms are in the nation's largest cities. Residents of the 23 central cities with over 500,000 residents account for only 12% of the nation's population, yet 17% of the nation's poor live in these cities. The counties that contain the 10 largest cities in the United States accounted for 22% of the entire national AFDC caseload in 1993, but only 14% of the population. This pattern of urban concentration has likely continued, and is most pronounced in states with a single large city (e.g., New York City and Chicago).[11]

RECENT HEALTH AND WELFARE REFORMS: AN URBAN PERSPECTIVE

The challenges of transitioning people from welfare to work are daunting for rural as well as urban areas. However, the largest caseloads of welfare recipients have been in cities, as well as the largest proportion of long-term recipients who were likely to be more difficult to move from welfare to work.

Welfare Reform's Uncharted Urban Course

Congressional enactment of the Personal Responsibility and Work Opportunities Reconciliation Act of 1996 (PRWORA) ended a national policy of entitlement to welfare crafted over a half-century ago to cushion the nation's most vulnerable families and children from the adverse effects of poverty. Reform in the nation's welfare system signaled a shift in the role of federal public assistance to the poor from a guaranteed safety net of benefits to one of transitional assistance to bridge the gap between welfare and work. The law replaced the long-standing Aid to Families with Dependent Children (AFDC) program with a single cash welfare block grant to states—Temporary Assistance for Needy Families (TANF)—while imposing strict guidelines on eligibility, duration of benefits, and work participation. In short, welfare reform changed the rules on whom the government will help, what help will be offered, for how long, and how the help will be administered.

At welfare's peak and prior to reform, nearly half (48%) of welfare recipients lived in the 89 largest American urban areas.[12] By 1999, these areas accounted for 58% of welfare cases. This concentration of recipients into urban areas resulted from a combination of local, state, and federal policies as well as demographic and market factors; it occurred at the same time as the overall numbers of cases declined both nationally and in cities.[13,14] Personal characteristics including education, skill level, and previous amount of time on welfare combine with state-specific policies to determine whether recipients become welfare "stayers" or "leavers." Some of the "leavers" do so voluntarily, some not. Remaining recipients are more likely now to be "hard-to-serve," with multiple barriers to self-sufficiency, yet they are still facing strict time limits and work requirements. Cities, the common point of entry for new immigrants, are also home to the largest numbers of immigrant populations—both legal and undocumented—whose eligibility for benefits changed significantly under welfare reform but whose barriers to employment did not.

However, the act of leaving the welfare rolls does not automatically mean economic independence. In addition to the declines in urban economies, "leavers" find other barriers to employment, including racial bias in hiring and a frequent "spatial mismatch" between residences and jobs. That is, economic expansion has increasingly occurred outside of the inner city, and so work opportunities for urban welfare recipients are often a considerable distance from their residence. This spatial mismatch increases commuting times and challenges existing public transportation routes. Quality, affordable child care, an essential ingredient for working mothers of young children, is in short supply in many urban communities. Further, early studies projected a deficit of low-skill jobs in cities for former recipients, although these fears have eased somewhat.[15] Nonetheless, early indications are that the goal of moving urban women off of welfare may be easier than the goal of ending dependence and promoting economic self-sufficiency.

Recent surveys by the U.S. Conference of Mayors (USCM) suggest that in the short run, the burden of welfare reform has been acutely felt in urban communities. The USCM 1997 Task Force on Welfare-to-Work reported (1) job shortfalls in 34 major cities, (2) early problems with transportation and child care, and (3) that an estimated average of only 27% of low-skill jobs in their cities provided health insurance.[16] The Mayors' Task Force on Hunger and Homelessness subsequently reported that the number of cities projecting increased requests in the next year for emergency food assistance by families with children dropped from over 95% in 1997 to 65% in 2000, a trend that, while encouraging, still reflects an unacceptable level of urban hunger.[17] Paradoxically, some city officials reported that the then strong economy had little or no effect on hunger or homelessness, that jobs that were available were low paying and lacked necessary benefits, and even that a strong economy actually increased hunger through effects on affordable housing.

State Child Health Insurance Program—Title XXI and Cities

The 1996 PRWORA was followed by the Balanced Budget Act of 1997 (P.L.105-33), codifying a new State Child Health Insurance Program (SCHIP) as Title XXI of the Social Security Act.[18] SCHIP was designed to improve children's access to both public and private health insurance through active case finding of eligible children and the provision of financial assistance to states to provide subsidized child health assistance. Each state had to decide by the year 2000 whether to expand its existing Medicaid program to further extend coverage to uninsured children, to design its own insurance product for children, or to use some combination of the two. Further details of these options can be found elsewhere in this volume.

As of mid-2001, 15 states and six districts and territories had chosen to expand their Medicaid programs using SCHIP funds; the rest created a partial or fully non-Medicaid SCHIP program.[19] During the first years of the programs, states have been working to improve coverage and reduce barriers to enrollment. Policies such as elimination of assets tests for children, using joint applications for Medicaid and the state CHIP program, innovative outreach programs, and presumptive eligibility have led to substantive increases in the number of U.S. children that are insured.[20,21] Yet, some 10 million children remained uninsured at the end of 1999.

SCHIP has tremendous implications for urban communities, where the largest numbers of uninsured and immigrant children reside. Safeguards for urban mothers and children may be better assured in cities where existing Medicaid programs have created successful networks to reach eligible, low-income children. However, the large numbers of eligible children that remain uninsured are a clear indication that all needs are not being met. Concerns continue about systematic obstacles—some bureaucratic, some arbitrary—that effectively prevent access. The focus to date on examining the creation and impact of the SCHIP programs at the state level may also mask inequalities occurring at the local level: Who are the children being left out and where do they live? Are barriers to covering eligible children greater in cities?

Managed Care and Medicaid: How Have Cities Fared?

America's inner cities continue to be the bellwether of consequences and opportunities under Medicaid managed care. The experience of large employers in controlling health care costs by adopting the managed-care model of health care delivery proved attractive to states as well. The Balanced Budget Act of 1997 that created the children's health insurance programs also contained provisions steering Medicaid into managed care. Over the past decade, state Medicaid agencies have embraced managed care as a mechanism to control costs, assure access, and improve performance and quality. Nowhere is this more apparent than in America's central cities, whose high concentrations of low-income women and children are prime targets for the growth of Medicaid managed care.[22] In a 1994 national survey of major urban health departments, 61% of city and county health departments serving cities with at least 100,000 population reported that Medicaid managed care was in place or would be implemented within one year, a figure that had increased to 84% by 1997.[23,24]

Central to concerns about Medicaid managed care is how the changes will affect the nation's safety net of health care to urban women, children, and adolescents, as well as uninsured and other vulnerable patients.[25,26] Issues include assuring access to care, assuring appropriate emphasis on primary and preventive care, maintaining quality care despite pressures to control costs, securing the participation of quality providers, helping consumers achieve satisfaction, and managing enrollment and disenrollment as clients move across systems and in and out of eligibility.[27] Urban health departments in jurisdictions where

Medicaid managed care was being implemented reported problems in each of these dimensions in the early stages of implementation.[23] The logistics of the managed-care transition for local health departments and other essential community providers—including public hospitals, publicly funded family planning providers, community and migrant health centers, and physicians serving minority patients—are considerable challenges to the urban safety net.[26] Urban health departments typically have less revenue but are responsible for populations with diverse challenges: less healthy inner-city residents needing more costly care; groups with special needs including physical, literacy, and language barriers; and mobile populations that strain continuous enrollment criteria. Essential community providers face a clash between their responsibilities for providing uncompensated care and the principles of managed care.[22]

FACTORS INTENSIFYING THE URBAN IMPACT OF SOCIAL REFORMS

The social, demographic, and economic conditions described above are intensified by three factors underlying health and welfare reform in America's cities: *public perception* of government's role and capacity to meet the needs of vulnerable populations; demand for increased public sector *accountability* for outcomes; and *devolution of decision-making authority* for social programs to the states. These factors converge to heighten the challenges facing urban communities.

Public Perceptions of Government's Role

Americans differ from those in other industrialized countries in their attitudes about the role of government in caring for the poor. A 1991 poll of Western nations showed that in the other countries studied, at least 50% of adults completely agreed with the statement: "It is the responsibility of the government to take care of very poor people who can't take care of themselves"; only 23% of American adults surveyed completely agreed.[28] This uniquely American view underscores the public's ambivalence about the role of government in caring for those who may not be able to care for themselves. In their description of underlying beliefs that shape public preferences in social policy, Blendon and colleagues identified the preference that both government and people share responsibility for self-sufficiency.[29] Surveys and polls have reported that a majority (57%) of Americans feel that responsibility for making sure that nonworking low-income people have a minimum standard of living should be shared between the government and the people themselves, friends, and volunteer agencies. How well this sharing of responsibilities works depends in part on the size of the government's share and the capacity of others to make up the difference, a balance more fragile in America's cities. In an era of increased pressure to reduce the size of government and cap state and local taxes, public perception influences the amount of state revenue allocated to health insurance for low-income women and children. Similarly, state welfare policy is shaped in part by public opinion about those dependent upon the public sector, and it is fueled by beliefs about whether welfare encourages teenage childbearing, undermines families, or inhibits the work ethic. State welfare policy is also shaped by social values about key social issues such as mothers of small children working outside the home, quality child care, and benefits to resident immigrants.

Accountability: Increased Public Demand for Measurable Results

The public is increasingly asking all levels of government to ensure that their tax dollars are being well spent in a way that is similar to the accountability demanded in the nonprofit sector. This demand for accountability, to know exactly what public and private dollars are buying and what specific effects these expenditures are having, is one of the driving forces of health and welfare reform. It suggests public doubt about government's capacity to efficiently provide effective services to the poor and needy that will make a measurable difference. Federal moves towards private-sector participation in social reform, including the push for faith-based initiatives, are expected but are as yet untested.

Two challenges exist in the measurement of maternal and child health outcomes in this era of accountability: (1) Do we have the ability to measure community-wide results? (2) Can we agree upon the definition of what makes for successful outcomes? For example, managed-care organizations under contract with Medicaid have the capacity to measure service utilization of two-year-olds continuously enrolled in their plan. From an urban public health perspective, such measures are necessary but insufficient to describe the health and well-being of the overall population of Medicaid-eligible and/or enrolled toddlers. The ability of state and local health departments to fulfill their core function of monitoring the health of the broader populations is thus a key to accountability.[30] Another key is acceptance of appropriate measures of success. Even though the sharply reduced number of able-bodied adults on the welfare roles is hailed as success for welfare reform,[31] the full story remains untold in terms of intended and unintended consequences on families' and children's health and well-being.

The New Federalism: Devolution of Authority to States

The term "new federalism" describes the changing relationship between national and state governments, based on the theory that state and local governments can do a better job of providing services for their residents. Devolution entails passing policy responsibilities from the federal to state and local governments, thus enhancing the responsiveness and efficiency of government.[32] This wave of devolution is shifting the most difficult decisions about how to meet the health and social needs of vulnerable populations from the federal to state level. The stakes of the many decisions states have in the new social programs are highest for urban areas, in part because of their disproportionate share of targeted children and immigrants.

Political forces affect whether and how well each state addresses its changing role in urban health and social needs. Decades of increasing suburbanization and urban flight, and of periodic redistricting of state legislatures after the decennial censuses, have fueled new regional politics, with greater Republican strength and an increase in suburban power in many state houses at the expense of urban districts. Cities' efforts to shift their disproportionate burden for general assistance to the states have become less successful amid divisive regional politics. Where state policy makers respond inadequately to the urban agenda and governors push tax cuts and reduce social spending to attract new business, cities and urban counties will be left to bear the costs of social transformation. Alternatively, some states opt to pass and devolve part or all of the burden of welfare reform directly to the cities, many of whom would not be prepared or willing to absorb the full burden of program design, implementation, and evaluation. As Annie E. Casey Foundation President Douglas Nelson noted, "[I]t may be fair to predict that the willingness of states to rise to the challenge of making troubled city neighborhoods a priority for innovation and investment will largely determine whether devolution itself succeeds or fails."[33]

This brief examination of the new federalism would be incomplete without mention of one of the newest players on the stage—the proposed role of faith-based institutions in providing social services in communities across the country. The 1996 welfare reform law contained provisions on "charitable choice," which allows religious organizations to receive federal funds for faith-based delivery of social services. One of President George W. Bush's first acts in office was the creation of a White House office focused on helping religious or faith-based groups obtain federal funds. The new White House Office of Faith-Based and Community Initiatives is so far off to a slow start, amidst controversy over the legality of such funding, concerns about possible discrimination based on clients' religious and other personal preferences, which religions would be allowed to participate, where the locus of accountability would lie, and indeed whether distinguishing an organization's "religious activities" from its "social service programs" would undercut its effectiveness and its own identity. However, in the absence of government funding, religious organizations have been a traditional and important purveyor of services in America's cities. Whether officially recognizing and promoting this relationship improves or detracts from urban health remains to be seen.

FINDING OPPORTUNITY:
RECOMMENDED STRATEGIES FOR SAFEGUARDING CITIES' HEALTH

The triple play of managed care, welfare reform, and child health insurance offer fresh challenges to urban communities to rethink the organization, financing, and delivery of health and human services for their most vulnerable populations. The potential ill consequences of this triple feature challenge state and federal governments to reach out in partnership to the cities to shape and support effective solutions. What must be done to safeguard the health and well-being of urban women, infants, children, and adolescents, given the changing policies and the recent shift at the national level to a more conservative administration? We propose several themes for change.

- *Leverage social reform's opportunities to foster community-wide systems change for healthier children and families.* Urban communities that actively embrace the meaning of reform—social or political improvement; to make better by removing faults or defects—are those best positioned to safeguard the health and well-being of women, children, and families.

  Experience with managed care has helped some cities better mobilize for welfare reform's sweeping changes and be poised to shape Title XXI. The Ramsey County Community Partnership for Welfare Reform developed early consensus on outcomes for families and children in the St. Paul, Minnesota area: *people who cannot work or who are working in jobs that do not support their families will be supported by the community; people receiving cash assistance who can work will be working in jobs that support their families before time limits.*[34] Milwaukee's effective working relationship between city and state government, forged in part through managed-care trials, positioned the city to be a major player in the development of BadgerCare, Wisconsin's Child Health Insurance Program.[35] Coalitions and collaboratives formed in recent years to build healthier cities and communities may have stronger, more timely community-wide responses to welfare reform and Title XXI. The San Francisco Starting Points Initiative, one of over a dozen Carnegie Corporation of New York–funded initiatives to mobilize communities on behalf of young children, provided the city with key information and analysis for local decision making on welfare reform.[36] Proactively, public health and human services agencies in states and some localities, notably Wake County (Raleigh), North Carolina, have reorganized for greater efficiency and accountability.[37,38] Reform gives communities the chance to shape lasting, systems-level solutions that build on their actual assets and resources.

  Achieving optimal outreach and enrollment in health insurance programs needs the continuing engagement of the full array of urban safety-net providers (disproportionate-share hospitals, local health department clinics, federally funded health centers, and other local agencies) to effectively identify eligible children, particularly those hardest to reach. Of equal importance is the capacity of providers to provide all children enrolled through Title XXI with comprehensive, quality primary and preventive health care, and to provide children with special health care needs with the full array of health care services they require. Although an insurance card is necessary to get in the provider door, it is insufficient to assure receipt and utilization of needed care. The acute challenge for urban communities continues to be assuring a seamless connection of outreach, eligibility, enrollment, and utilization of comprehensive systems of care, that can lead to improved health outcomes for more children.

- *Rekindle political will at the local, state, and national level to safeguard and promote the health and well-being of all children and families in America's cities.* As long as social reforms are perceived as being about people who are different, there will be insufficient political will to assure the health and well-being of those most likely to be affected. As former Housing and Urban Development Secretary Henry Cisneros has asserted, "What this country lacks is not the capacity to end the isolation of the minority poor; it lacks the will."[39] Poor families have long been judged by the majority as weak in their lack of self-sufficiency, undeserving in their dependency on government. The transformation of AFDC into a work-based program may foster new political will for the working poor. Child Health Insurance under Title XXI gives an opportunity for bridging our efforts between the poorest and the working middle class.

  One proposed strategy for breaking the isolation of the urban poor is to link the fates of the cities and suburbs for maternal and child health. It has been argued that given their interdependence, cities and suburbs do best when they interact and make use of respective and complementary strengths.[40] Suburbs that surround healthy cities tend to be healthier than those that surround sick cities. Only when those in the outer city acknowledge and understand that central city political boundaries do not seal off problems associated with air pollution or childhood poverty or epidemic interpersonal violence among youth can metropolitan alliances be forged to address interconnected concerns.

  Another strategy is to have cities advocate for further devolution from the state to the local level of health and human services. Some health policymakers advocate for greater flexibility in the use of funding in exchange for greater accountability for specified outcomes accountability, as the heart of a new deal between states and localities.[41] Urban governments and equivalent emerging local governance entities will need to prepare for and assure their readiness to assume the responsibility for local social policy decision making and accountability. This readiness includes the setting of clear, measurable outcomes and the capacity to develop and use results-based budgets, in the context of community-wide consensus of a vision for children and families.[42]

- *Strengthen the capacity of the urban public health sector to do its essential governmental roles effectively.* Assessment, monitoring, and assurance—the core functions of public health—should prove invaluable during the continued social changes of this new century. With greater capacity building in outcomes accountability and the effective use of data, more urban health departments can become the valued and empowered lead agency. That agency could facilitate community-wide consensus on measures and methods for assessing local impacts of managed care, welfare reform and child health insurance, and related social reforms. Indeed, several urban health departments, like San Diego County, have forged partnerships with managed-care organizations to better utilize their capacities in assessment.[43] Critical to this strategy is strong collaboration between state and federal government to assure compatible methods in monitoring the health and well-being of its women, children, and families in an era of reform. Recent consensus on the core functions of public health specific to maternal and child health, forged among leading public health institutions, gives an excellent framework for moving ahead.[30]

CONCLUSION

The complete history of late 20th century health and welfare reform has yet to be written. Yet, the tumultuous beginning of the 21st century may make that history merely a footnote to a completely new, evolving social order. As was true a century ago, all that is right and wrong in new health and welfare policy will manifest on the stage of urban America. Public health must continue to play an essential advocacy role for systems change to safeguard the health of women, children, and families along the way, for, as Ehlinger has noted wisely, "The fate of our cities eventually will become the fate of us all."[44]

REFERENCES

1. U.S. Census Bureau, Census 2000.

2. U.S. Census Bureau, March 1999 and 2000 Current Population Surveys.

3. Fossett, J.W., and Perloff, J.D. *The "New" health reform and access to care: The problem of the inner city.* Report to the Kaiser Commission on the Future of Medicaid, Washington, DC, December, 1995.

4. Benbow, N., Wang, Y., and Whitman, S. *Big cities health inventory, 1997: The health of urban U.S.A.* Chicago: Chicago Department of Health, 1997.

5. Andrulis, D. *Urban Social Health Indicators.* Washington, DC: National Public Health and Hospitals Institute, 1995.

6. Andrulis, D. *The Urban Health Penalty: New Dimensions and Directions in Inner City Health Care.* Washington, DC: National Public Health and Hospitals Institute, 1996.

7. CityLights 6(3/4). *Special Report on Low Birthweight in U.S. Cities, 1993–1995.* Omaha, NE: CityMatCH at the University of Nebraska Medical Center, 1998.

8. Heagarty, M.C. Urban maternal and child health services. In: H.M. Wallace, R.P. Nelson, and P.J. Sweeney (eds.). *Maternal and Child Health Practices.* 4th edition. Oakland CA: Third Party Publishing Company, 1994.

9. U.S. Department of Health and Human Services, Health Resources and Services Administration. *Child health USA.* Rockville, MD: DHHS, 1997.

10. The Annie E. Casey Foundation. *Child Trends KIDS COUNT Special Report. City trends—Conditions of babies and their families in America's largest cities (1990–1998).* Baltimore, MD: Annie E. Casey Foundation, 2001.

11. Weir, M. Is Anybody Listening? The uncertain future of welfare reform in the cities. *The Brookings Review.* Winter, 1997;15(1):30–33.

12. Allen, K., and Kirby, M. *Unfinished Business: Why Cities Matter to Welfare Reform. Center on Urban & Metropolitan Policy.* Washington, DC: The Brookings Institution, July 2000.

13. Brookings Institution. *The State of Welfare Caseloads in America's Cities: 1999. Center on Urban & Metropolitan Policy.* Washington, DC: The Brookings Institution, February, 1999.

14. Katz, B., and Allen, K. Cities Matter—Shifting the Focus of Welfare Reform. *Brookings Review.* Summer, 2001;19(3):30–33.

15. Lerman, R.I., and Ratcliffe, C. *Did metropolitan areas absorb welfare recipients without displacing other workers?* Assessing the New Federalism, Series A, No. A-45. Washington, DC: The Urban Institute, November 2000.

16. U.S. Conference of Mayors. *Implementing welfare reform in America's cities.* Washington, DC: U.S. Conference of Mayors, 1997.

17. U.S. Conference of Mayors. *A status report on hunger and homelessness in America's cities.* Washington, DC: U.S. Conference of Mayors, 2000.

18. Rosenbaum, S., Johnson, K., Sonosky, C., Markus, A., and DeGraw, C. *Issue brief—An overview of the state children's health insurance program.* Washington, DC: The George Washington University Medical Center, Center for Health Policy Research, September, 1997.

19. Health Care Financing Administration. State Child Health Insurance Program Plan Activity Map. http://www.hcfa.gov/init/chip-map.htm. Accessed 9/4/2001.

20. Alberga, J., DeFrancesco, L., Molinari, S., and Wheatley, B. *State of the States Report.* Washington, DC: Academy for Health Services Research and Health Policy, January, 2001.

21. American Academy of Pediatrics. Implementation Principles and Strategies for the State Children's Health Insurance Program (RE100035). *Pediatrics.* May, 2001;107(5):1214–1220.

22. Darnell, J., Rosenbaum, S., Scarpulla-Nolan, L., Zuvekas, A., and Budetti, P. *Access to Care among Low-Income, Inner-City, Minority Populations: The Impact of Managed Care on the Urban Minority Poor and Essential Community Providers.* Report to the Commonwealth Fund by the Center for Health Policy Research. Washington, DC: The George Washington University, December, 1995.

23. Peck, M.G., and Hubbert, E.H. *Changing the Rules: Medicaid Managed Care and MCH in U.S. Cities.* Omaha, NE: CityMatCH at the University of Nebraska Medical Center, 1994.

24. Simpson, P., Garrett-Brown, N., and Peck, M.G. *A Second Look at Medicaid Managed Care, MCH, and Urban Health Departments: Changing the Rules II.* Omaha, NE: CityMatCH at the University of Nebraska Medical Center, 1998.

25. Andrulis, D.P. Community, service, and policy strategies to improve health care access in the changing urban environment. *American Journal of Public Health.* June, 2000;90(6):858–862.

26. Lewin, M.E., and Altman, S. *America's Health Care Safety Net: Intact but Endangered.* Washington, DC: National Academy Press, 2000.

27. Fox, H.B., and McManus, M.A.: *Medicaid managed care arrangements and their impact on children and adolescents: A briefing report.* Washington, DC: The Child and Adolescent Health Policy Center, 1992.

28. Times Mirror Center for the People and the Press Poll. Storrs, CT: Roper Center for Public Opinion Research, May 1991. (Cited in Blendon et al. p. 1066.)

29. Blendon, R.J., Altman, D.E., Benson, J., Brodie, M., James, M., and Chervinsky, G. The public and the welfare reform debate. *Archives of Pediatric and Adolescent Medicine.* 1995;149:1065–1069.

30. Grason, H.A., and Guyer, B. *Public MCH programs functions framework: Essential public health services to promote maternal and child health in America.* Baltimore, MD: Johns Hopkins University, 1995.

31. Broder, J.M. Big social changes revive the false God of numbers. *The New York Times.* August 17, 1997, Section 4(1).

32. Watson, K., and Gold, S.D. *The other side of devolution: Shifting relationships between state and local governments.* Washington, DC: The Urban Institute, Assessing the New Federalism, 1997.

33. Annie E. Casey Foundation. *City kids count: Data on the well-being of children in large cities.* Baltimore, MD: Annie E. Casey Foundation, 1997.

34. Fulton, R. *From windows to worries: The Ramsey County experience.* Presented at the 1997 Urban MCH Leadership Conference. Atlanta, GA, September 1997.

35. Nannis, P. Commissioner of Health, Milwaukee Health Department. *Personal communication.* November 1997.

36. Mihaly, L.K. *Impact of federal welfare reform on children in San Francisco.* San Francisco, CA: Starting Points Initiative, Mayor's Office of Children, Youth and Their Families, May, 1997.

37. Maralit, M., Orloff, T.M., and Desonia, R. *Transforming state health agencies to meet current and future challenges.* Washington, DC: National Governors' Association, 1997.

38. CityLights 6(3/4). *Reorganization, re-engineering, restructuring, right-sizing: Public health leadership in the reorganization of government.* Omaha, NE: CityMatCH at the University of Nebraska Medical Center, January, 1998.

39. Cisneros, H.G. Regionalism: The new geography of opportunity. *National Civic Review.* 1996;85(2):35–48.

40. Savitch, H.V., Collins, D., Sanders, D., and Markham, J.P. Ties that bind: Central cities, suburbs, and the new metropolitan region. *Economic Development Quarterly.* November, 1993;7(4):341–347.

41. Center for the Study of Social Policy. *Trading outcome accountability for fund flexibility.* Washington, DC: 1995.

42. Friedman, M. *A Strategy map for results-based budgeting: Moving from theory to practice.* Washington, DC: The Finance Project, 1996.

43. Center for Studying Health System Change. *Issue brief: Tracking changes in the public health system.* Number 2. Washington, DC: September, 1996.

A R T I C L E   4

STEPS FOR THE FUTURE

Naomi M. Morris

INTRODUCTION

This is a challenging time for those of us who feel obligated to help create and sustain "a society where children are wanted and born with optimal health, receive quality care, and are nurtured lovingly and sensitively as they mature into healthy, productive adults."[1] Current statistics show millions of children and their mothers still without health insurance; great disparities among survival and morbidity data by race/ethnicity; incomplete immunization patterns; serious behavior problems in school children that suggest unmet needs for mental health and social services; risky behaviors, including the use of cigarettes, alcohol, and drugs in young adolescents, to say nothing of high-risk sexual behavior inviting unwanted pregnancies and STDs including HIV; and violence (data in Unit 1, Article 1; Unit 3, Article 6; Unit 4, Articles 3, 8, 9, 10). The relationship between the well-being of children and the need for healthy, productive adults in society is the basic political reason for financial support to the field of maternal and child health (MCH); such support is seen in various forms in all developed countries.

Most nations realize that the children are their future, although agreement with this idea never eliminates the need for visible advocacy. This realization, however, justifies funding of a variety of health and social support programs throughout the family life cycle, including preconception services and maternity and infant care that extends through childhood to young adulthood. Healthy children, in a supportive, stimulating environment within a safe community to which they and their parents are connected have a good chance of growing up to become good citizens of that community and of their country, and this is part of the vision to which American MCH professionals are committed. Unfortunately, there are recent changes in the American family (data in Unit 1, Articles 4 and 5; Unit 2, Articles 1, 2, and 3) that greatly increase social support and health care needs, magnified by changes in the economy and world unrest since 9/11/01.

In the last chapter of the first edition of this book, Vince Hutchins cited Wilbur Cohen's prediction that major social legislation can be expected to occur about

540

every thirty years, going back to the Progressive Movement just after the turn of the century.[2] Cohen was the main architect of the Social Security Act (SSA) of 1935 and contributed to the inclusion of Medicare and Medicaid in the SSA in 1965. Hutchins concluded that Welfare Reform enacted in 1996 and Title XXI of the Social Security Act (The State Children's Health Insurance Program, SCHIP or CHIP, 1997) were "the most important family policy initiatives in the past 30 years." He suggested, given the tendency for legislators, after interest peaks and significant legislation is passed, to ignore an area until new problems build up and action is again sparked by people who urgently want to do something about them, that the next great advance would not be until 2025.

Cohen had predicted that by 1995 "every single person in the United States will be insured for comprehensive health benefits." However, in 1999 42 million people remained uninsured.[3] Although Welfare Reform in 1996 decoupled Medicaid eligibility from cash assistance, many parents who no longer received welfare payments believed that their children were no longer eligible for Medicaid. On the other hand, the enactment of SCHIP the next year expanded the eligibility for health services far beyond former Medicaid guidelines for child coverage in many states. After increasing efforts at outreach there are many more children now participating in Medicaid and, as of October, 2000, 3.3 million children were enrolled in SCHIP.[4] However, the more than 10 million uninsured children under 19 are of continuing concern, as are uninsured parents, especially mothers (working fathers may have insurance that is limited to themselves). Over 9 million parents are uninsured nationwide; nearly three-quarters of uninsured children eligible for Medicaid or SCHIP have at least one uninsured parent.[5]

HEALTH INSURANCE

The cost of services has long been a barrier to accessing care for many families. The role of the Social Security Act and its Title V in helping families is described in Unit 2, Article 4. Some safety-net Title V–funded health services are shrinking as local health agencies make the switch to population-based services simultaneous with the growth of Medicaid managed care and the expansion of coverage through SCHIP. Unit 3, Article 3 gives a progress report on SCHIP. Unfortunately, many children whose parents do not realize they are still eligible for Medicaid assistance or for SCHIP have been left out, and outreach programs have not succeeded in finding them all. A survey in Colorado found the major reasons for parents not enrolling their children included the ownership of other insurance, the parents' belief that their income was too high for eligibility, and the large amount of paperwork associated with the enrollment process.[6]

MediKids

To remedy this situation important legislation was proposed—the MediKids Health Insurance Act of 2001. Endorsed by the American Academy of Pediatrics and various advocacy organizations, the ideas embodied in it would guarantee health care coverage for all children, much as Medicare does for seniors. *Enrollment would be automatic at birth* for every child born after December 31, 2002, regardless of family income. Parents could substitute other insurance, including private, Medicaid, or SCHIP if one of these were preferred. Benefits would be comprehensive, similar to Medicare, and based on Medicaid EPSDT (Early Periodic Screening, Diagnosis and Treatment). Children would be covered through age 22 years. Premiums would be graduated, related to income, and collected at income tax filing.[7] If successful according to the phase-in plan, by 2007 all individuals 22 and under would be eligible.

FamilyCare

MediKids is a logical step beyond SCHIP. A related step in the direction of universal coverage for health insurance has already occurred in a few states: the opening of SCHIP programs to parents of the eligible children. About one-third of mothers with a family income less than 200% of poverty lack health insurance. Legislation, "FamilyCare," has been proposed that would allow the federal government to increase SCHIP funding specifically to expand coverage for parents of children in Medicaid and SCHIP. This would enable more states to assist needy parents.[8] Unspent SCHIP dollars now have to be returned to the federal government, but the FamilyCare project could be supported using those dollars as the state contribution. The Commonwealth Fund Report noted that when low-income parents are insured, their children are nearly twice as likely to have health insurance as children with uninsured parents.[5] Therefore, it is assumed that helping the parents helps enroll more children.

MediKids, a More Inclusive Version

The mechanism to recruit children at birth through MediKids offers great promise. Along with FamilyCare, the passage of this legislation would be an important step in the direction of a process to guarantee health insurance for all families. The growing interest in providing complete coverage for all children is clear. A more inclusive version of MediKids has already appeared, and more may come. On May 23, 2001, Senator Dodd of Connecticut and Representative Miller of California introduced the Act to Leave No Child Behind (S. 940 and H.R. 1990). Health-related provisions include the creation of a Medicare-like guarantee of coverage of all children through age 21, with the same name, MediKids. This Act expands SCHIP to 300% of poverty, with eligibility through age 21, and improves services for children enrolled in Medicaid, making sure all have the benefits of EPSDT. There are other specific provisions related to asthma, lead poisoning, and environmental health risks to children.[9] If, like SCHIP, MediKids becomes part of the Social Security Act or takes the place of SCHIP, its relationship to other programs for children and families would be clearly established, and it would not have to be reconsidered every few years for continuation of appropriations. The role for MCH professionals is to educate all stakeholders including other professionals and the public about the needs and the possibilities, to help develop and support the legislation, and to continue to foster collaboration among communities and all members of the care-providing infrastructure, so that we will not have to wait for the year 2025 for all children to be covered.

FAMILY HEALTH: WOMEN

Welfare reform has reduced the access of low-income women to health care (discussed in Unit 2, Article 3). In a recent re-organization, the Maternal and Child Health Bureau (MCHB) has given more serious recognition to the family surrounding a child. The family is the infant's first environment, a small, intimate, and protective one, and it remains extremely important as the child grows up. Therefore, the health of the entire family, not just that of the mother, is important. It has become seen as clearly appropriate for the field of MCH to expand its attention beyond the perinatal period and the childbearing years, to take more responsibility for women's health throughout adulthood. Women are potential childbearers for a long time, and even if they do not eventually have children or any additional children, their continuing health is relevant to their families and society as well as to themselves. The MCHB through its Office of Women's Health now has a Division of Perinatal Systems and Women's Health (DPSWH); the point is made that more than biomedical and simplistic social factors influence a woman's ability to reproduce, care for her family, and reach her personal capacity for a successful, socially beneficial, and rewarding life. The draft for the five-year Women's Health Plan (2001–2006) suggests that pregnancy and prenatal care "provide important windows of opportunity" to reach women, but says that care-providing systems for females also must reach women who are not or won't become pregnant. Elsewhere in the DPSWH five-year draft, the Vision Statement suggests "all women and their families" should receive "comprehensive, coordinated, supportive, culturally and linguistically appropriate, quality health care provided in a family-oriented and community-centered setting that enables them to lead healthy and productive lives."[10]

From Maternal Health to Women's Health

The DPSWH five-year health plan FY 2001–2006 mainly addresses service needs of women of reproductive age, but several objectives and activities deal with "collaboration with federal, state, and local entities that address the needs of very young women and women beyond their reproductive years," in line with the intent to meet the needs of individuals throughout their lives. For example, information about preventive health behaviors is relevant to older women as well as to those who are younger. The expansion of services for women is a very significant step, greatly increasing the domain of MCHB to "W"CHB. Actually accepting responsibility for the health of all women would be a huge undertaking when life expectancy and gerontological issues are considered, even limiting the services to prevention and health promotion. Perhaps it will be appropriate to draw the line at age 65, when Medicare provides support for needed health services. Or perhaps not, since Medicare is only health insurance! It will be interesting to see what services and policies evolve in the next decade, and how this new focus on women within MCHB is integrated into the delivery of other MCH services.

FAMILY HEALTH: THE MALE IN MCH

Except for selected services for adolescent males, only one member of the family was not specifically named in MCH plans intended to ultimately improve children's well-being. The question was raised: "Where is the male in MCH?" In the first edition of this book, before the latest reorganization of the MCHB and the publication of the Women's Health Plan, Vince Hutchins said, "[T]he involvement of families has been strengthened and institutionalized ..." by working with public and private agencies and family associations, and "the reality and perception of male involvement in these programs [related to children] have changed positively over recent years." Although suggested by some, the name of the Bureau was not changed to *family* health partly because of the emotional appeal of mothers and children critical for political and public support, Dr. Hutchins noted. He said that the objective of greater family involvement including that of males "was accomplished through policy emphasis rather than a name change." However, since that time, fathers have actually been named in the definition of the MCH population, as stated by Vince Hutchins himself in a more recent publication: "The MCH population includes all of America's pregnant women, infants, children, adolescents and their families, including women of reproductive age, fathers, and children with special health care needs."[11]

Integrating Services for Men

The question is how to integrate services for the male into MCH, and what services would be appropriate. Services for the father aside from his role in relation to the child, domestic violence, or possibly to his partner and family planning are not mentioned except within the general goals and objectives of MCHB to provide leadership "to improve access to comprehensive, culturally sensitive, quality health care" for the MCH population, defined above. Objectives for the year 2003 include eliminating barriers and health disparities, assuring quality of care, and improving the health infrastructure and system.[11] These objectives, if accomplished, will certainly reach beyond traditional services for mothers and children.

Data Gathering

Although recommendations or perhaps referrals for services could be made in clinical settings at his partner's request, in this situation the male would not benefit from any organizational responsibility for his receipt of services or well-being. Perhaps regularly recording a reasonable amount of specific data about the health of fathers (or male partners) in MCH data sets would better define males' needs and impart to the male member of the household a feeling that he too is important. Collecting more data would cost something, but not as much as adding services beyond referrals for males. It would make sense in the context of supporting family health in a comprehensive way to record data about the adult male partner in the household, and in so doing, gain a better understanding of the entire family. The goal would be to support family functioning for the benefit of the children primarily and to support the function of each adult as well.

Gaps in Coverage

Further thought about providing some services for fathers or women's partners leads to the realization that nonfathers or those not partnering women would be entirely left out of the system. In all fairness, this does not seem right. Further, insurance coverage for health services for males per se is not elaborated upon in the recent documents. The gap between Medicaid or SCHIP and Medicare exists for all males since none receives special health services during "the childbearing years." What is needed is incorporation of the already defined pattern of recommended preventive services for males to be covered along with illness by the new FamilyCare insurance extension of SCHIP and its later successors. Collaboration with the American College of Preventive Medicine could help MCHB sponsor the appropriate pattern. Perhaps Title XXII of the Social Security Act will be the final piece of legislation that fills in all the gaps, *maybe in 2025.*

PROGRAMMATIC PRIORITIES, IN ORDER OF IMPORTANCE:
I. CHILD CARE

Unit 2, Article 5, describes the problem very well and makes valuable recommendations. Because of its high priority, this topic merits more discussion at this point. Child care, particularly from infancy up to school age, is an essential MCH service. Recent research has demonstrated the tremendous capacity of the newborn's brain to remember and learn, making "0–3" programs especially important. With two-thirds of infants' mothers in the workforce, a large number of children are dependent on day care, since only about half are cared for by other family members or relatives.[2] Some are left in small group homes and some in facilities with special programs. But high-quality infant care is scarce. Early Head Start (0–3) has appeared in some areas and its benefits have been clearly shown, but there are not enough programs operating to begin to reach all babies who could benefit. Head Start, in existence for several decades with similarly demonstrated long-range positive effects, usually serving children 3 or 4 years old, is now variable in quality.

An Issue of Quality

According to the *Chicago Tribune*[12] it costs $5 billion annually to enroll 857,000 children in Head Start across the United States, and in Chicago alone there are 500 sites with 18,000 children enrolled. Half of these sites, although not identified as Early Head Start, take children under 3 and are located in private homes, where the care probably does not differ from that in traditional day care. Traditional day care lacks the programmatic changes incorporated into the better experimental programs, and often is little better than baby sitting. Head Start funding makes possible the incorporation of "hot meals, health care, and social activities"; this comprehensive model is what has made Head Start unique and not just another day care program. Criticism of Head Start programs in Chicago is focused on the inadequacy of the educational component, which should help children arrive at school ready to read. Apparently, in Chicago more than one agency has jurisdiction over Head Start projects. The City's Department of Human Services has developed some, and the Chicago Public Schools has started others. The latter employs only state certified teachers with bachelor's degrees, not true of the former. These problems are not unique to Chicago, although the names of agencies and programs may differ. States require licensing of day care homes and centers, but not all day care locations are licensed, and licensing requirements vary by state. Theoretically, licensing allows the state to monitor what is happening in day care locations and give advice to the operators. However, there is often not the number of state personnel necessary to carry this out frequently enough to be meaningful, and the requirements for licensing are usually focused on safety and nutrition, not on education.

Early Day Care as Part of Public Education?

The important point is that there are insufficient high-quality day care positions that parents can afford. In addition to the fact that there are few Early Head Start programs, and that Head Start for 3- and 4-year-olds serves only about 40% of eligible poor children, there is a financial contradiction in ordinary day care that makes it necessary for the present situation to be seriously assessed and changed. Ordinary day care workers tend to be women with limited education, lacking training for the work, whereas in experimental programs the providers have studied early child development in order to foster it through educational processes. Ordinary day care workers' earnings are low, in the poverty range, partly because parents cannot afford to pay very much for day care services. The parents whose children would benefit the most from well-designed educational programs are least able to afford this level of care. Women with higher incomes can sometimes find good quality day care for their children, but they pay a lot for it. The more common cycle of low provider income, low fees, and low quality must be interrupted.

Logically, early day care/preschool should be part of the public education system, with appropriately educated caretakers/teachers. Funding for public schools would have to be increased to subsidize early childhood education for the number of children potentially to be served. Some European school systems begin with 3-year-olds. This might be a good starting point for a new system of public education in the United States. Early Head Start, or 0–3 programs, might remain more limited for select populations in need, but would definitely benefit from being incorporated into the educational system with trained caretakers and adequate public funding. In addition, there must be increased resources to support well-educated and well-trained day care providers for all children 0–3 in need of day care.

The Role of MCH Professionals

The importance to society of early stimulation and competent care of very young children cannot be overstated. Since women in the work force cannot afford, and sometimes do not wish, to remain at home, MCH professionals need to explain and publicize at every opportunity the differences that have been shown between the development and behavior of children who have had appropriate stimulation and care, and those who have not. Fewer risky and destructive actions, better health, higher levels of completed education, and more positive contributions to society and community life represent tremendous cost benefits to be gained from excellent early childhood education and experiences.[13] If other developed countries can do this, the United States can do this as well; without such an investment our other investments in education beyond the preschool years will not be as fruitful.

PROGRAMMATIC PRIORITIES: II. ADOLESCENTS

Unit 3, Article 6, reports that 31% of youth have a chronic illness or handicap. Barriers to adequate health care include lack of insurance, lack of confidentiality, and failure of the care provider (as in Medicaid managed care) to cover all treatable aspects called for in EPSDT. Although all the conditions are important, of major concern is the prevention of problems related to sexuality; these problems should be totally preventable.

Effectiveness of Current Programs

Recent articles report fewer births to adolescents, more use of condoms for protection, and more use of other birth control methods. Yet the United States still has higher rates of teen births and adolescent abortions than many other developed countries.[14] The National Campaign to Prevent Teen Pregnancy has reported that an intensive program combining sex education, comprehensive health care, and activities such as tutoring does impact sexual behavior, contraceptive use, pregnancy, and births among girls for as long as three years. The effectiveness of abstinence-only programs is not clear.[15] But providing information and making condoms or other contraceptives available in schools "[do] not hasten or increase sexual activity." Policies in other developed countries have long included education and accessible birth control; we must replicate the newer U.S. intensive programs until they are in every middle and high school for the benefit of our teens and nation. Teen pregnancy starts the cycle that leads to unfortunate infant and child development and then to too-early nonmarital pregnancy in the next generation. This cycle must be stopped.

The Roles of Professionals and Parents

Again, the role for MCH professionals is education and collaboration in programs to the extent that we can help. Parents also need help to do their part, with reference materials and education. Their role is very important as early sex educators, but many lack vocabulary and understanding necessary to act. While the children are young, health care providers including MCH personnel can assist in the anticipatory training of parents. Research has shown that later, with older children, if knowledgeable parents just take an interest in adolescents' daily activities, risky behaviors of all types are less apt to occur.[16] When the incorporation of all the programs and parental education is universal and routine, we should expect to see great improvement in our statistics.

PROGRAMMATIC PRIORITIES: III. SCHOOL-AGED CHILDREN

Once children are regularly attending school, a setting away from home, where they are observed by teachers during various activities, special needs and health problems may be noted.

School-Based Health Services

In the last decade a large number of schools have established clinics or comprehensive health services on site. By 1998 there were 1,154 schools around the country with broad arrays of services, one of every two receiving some state funding.[11] Some of these school-based health services have been incorporated into managed-care organizations, including those that accept Medicaid, or are served by integrated service networks of providers who work for universities, health departments, or community clinics. These school-based health services and their linkages have facilitated comprehensive exams, anticipatory guidance, immunizations, care for inter-current illness or minor emergencies, care for chronic problems such as diabetes and asthma, and record-keeping at a convenient location. School nurse practitioners have played a large role in the operation of these health centers, with physicians responsible for consultation and overall supervision.

Need for Mental Health Care

One service that usually has not been available for grade school children is mental health care. Undiagnosed behavior problems often result in extra visits to the health care system without resolution of underlying causes. Rates of psychosocial disorders may be as high as 27% among 4- to 16-year-olds, and 13% among preschool children, according to a recent review of the literature.[17] Teachers have a prolonged opportunity to observe children's behavior. Children who cause disruption in the school or do not seem interested in schoolwork or their classmates may have emotional problems. Sometimes they have been diagnosed as having ADHD and have been put on medication; recently, there is concern that this diagnosis and treatment are overused. (Unit 4, Article 7, discusses ADHD.) Comprehensive mental health services provided early in the course of behavior problems could help families and may reduce the likelihood of risky behavior, such as use of alcohol, drugs, weapons, and violence later on. A specific group of children who could benefit from mental health services are those in foster care (see Unit 2, Article 6).

Services provided at school could also include oral health care (see Unit 4, Article 4), and education for injury prevention (see Unit 4, Article 6). School-aged children at times need Emergency Medical Services, which often are not prepared for children's special needs (see Unit 4, Article 5).

PROGRAMMATIC PRIORITIES:
IV. IMMIGRANT CHILDREN IN SCHOOL

The children of illegal immigrants are another group who need services, but since they are not eligible for public insurance in most states and their parents are not apt to have private insurance, they may have no source of health care outside of school. Documented Hispanic immigrants are more apt to have no health insurance than other minority groups, so their children need services as well. Taking care of these children may be problematic in terms of payment for their services, but from the public health and school perspective their care is essential. New solutions need to be found for the provision of health care to immigrant families, even if they are illegally present in the United States. Some, but not all, states do provide some health care to undocumented immigrants. More local jurisdictions should organize comprehensive services to meet the health needs of all immigrants. Their health care actually protects the citizen population from infectious diseases brought in from other countries, such as tuberculosis and childhood diseases no longer common here because of immunization, and it keeps adults in the workforce. Federal matching support should eventually be obtained for the purpose of protecting the public's health, as well as on behalf of the children and their families.

PROGRAMMATIC PRIORITIES:
V. INCARCERATED TEENS

Hopefully, in the first decade of the new millennium the need for incarcerating teens will be reduced as preventive efforts in earlier school years begin to succeed. However, at the present time there are many children who have "earned" jail and prison time for violence and other illegal behavior. Studies of health services in jails reveal much to be desired; the priorities of the institutions do not noticeably include the health of the prisoners, although nominally, some services are available. Teens who still have the potential for turning their lives around deserve medical and psychiatric health care to the extent that these might make a difference for the future. Public health agencies need to include surveillance of prisoners' health—especially that of youth—and rehabilitation as important parts of their responsibilities, so that these young lives are not just thrown away. Coordination between the juvenile justice system and local public health authorities should be fostered.

PROGRAMMATIC PRIORITIES:
VI. CHILDREN WITH SPECIAL HEALTH CARE NEEDS

As medical science advances and it becomes possible to correct more and more congenital anomalies and illnesses that might once have led to crippling, Title V funds flowing through the appropriate state agencies contribute significantly to the expensive surgery and other care needed by children with special health care needs (CSHCN). These funds also contribute to the research that leads to the definitions of best care. Over the years the number of conditions covered has steadily increased, although the types of problems vary from state to state. The contributions of CSHCN agencies have included the definitions of comprehensive, coordinated care; a medical home; and family-centered, community-based, culturally appropriate services.

A Definition

Defined as "those who have or are at increased risk for a chronic physical, developmental, behavioral, or emotional condition and who also require health and related services of a type or amount beyond that required by children generally," children with special health care needs constituted about 17% of low-income children in 1994, with one-third of those having a disability limiting their school or play activities.[2] That means that about one-sixth of children eligible for SCHIP are CSHCN. Attention must be paid to ensuring that these children are both enrolled in SCHIP and provided all the services that would benefit them. These services should be those they would have received if evaluated and served under the auspices of a CSHCN agency. Those served by Medicaid managed care might not receive all the care that they need, according to information in Unit 3, Article 5.

University-Affiliated Programs or Facilities

The broad definition for CSHCN appears to include children who might be seen within university-affiliated programs (UAPs) or facilities (UAFs), which traditionally have provided diagnostic and other services for children judged at developmental risk. UAPs (but not all of them) have been funded with Title V funds and state funds (usually in the mental health category), and because of a strong research tradition, funded with large research grants and sometimes foundation support. Their services sometimes expand into the provision of special equipment for assisting mobility and communication. In the future UAPs (or UAFs) should be part of a collaborative network serving CHSCN and children at developmental risk, for children whose needs might meet both definitions in some states and who would benefit from referral.

PROGRAMMATIC PRIORITIES:
VII. GENETICS

One of the most dramatic scientific advances at the beginning of the new millennium has been the complete definition of the human genome. Experimentation on animals has shown that genetic makeup of the next generation can be altered by the removal or insertion of genes. In fact, it has been shown that an animal may be cloned; that is, an offspring may be produced by inserting nuclear material from the desired animal's body cell into the nucleus of a female's egg cell from which the original nuclear contents have been removed, and then planting this cell into the female's womb to develop.

Now and in the Future

State-level genetics units keep track of genetics-related diseases in newborns and try to epidemiologically pin down causes of sudden appearances of higher than usual rates of specific congenital problems such as cleft lip or cystic fibrosis. They have responsibilities for ordering diagnostic tests or providing assistance for families trying to find out what is wrong with a child. However, state-level genetics units as yet really have had limited responsibilities. These genetics units in the future may find themselves a focal point for discussions of what it is ethical to do in the modification of genes. Discussions among researchers currently begin with how to avoid a genetic problem that runs in the family, but end with the notion that there is no limitation to what could be programmed into the next generation. At this point in time, the lab procedures are filled with uncertainty; success rates in animals are not 100%. We are not close to being able to carry out the imaginative ideas related to genes sometimes mentioned in the media. But the discussions must begin.

Closer Connections

The state-level genetics units should become more closely connected to the service networks of care providers, professional organizations, related governmental agencies, collaborating community groups, and parent groups. They have special understanding that must be shared; hopefully, their deliberations can balance the giddy enthusiasm that has celebrated the final mapping of the human genome.

SUMMARY

Problems in the present economy, the impact of direction changes from the White House, and funding shortages at the Health Resources and Services Administration (HRSA) may have unfortunate effects on health indicators for the well-being of children and families. Together with reductions in health care utilization (related to some misunderstanding of the Welfare to Work policy) and our improving abilities to collect and use data (a process which must be supported and advanced in every program we attempt), we may be politically able to increase resources to help mothers, children, and families, including children with special health care needs, sooner than we thought a Republican administration might have allowed. Any sign of serious economic downturn and increase in poor health indicators might precipitate extension of the MediKids and Family Care ideas and even fulfill Wilbur Cohen's prophecy of health care for all before 2025. However, it is likely that progress will continue to occur in small steps, with children and parents first being guaranteed coverage somewhat like Medicare covering the elderly; the last to have total guaranteed coverage by health insurance will likely be those who are neither children nor parents, nor living in absolute poverty. It is hard not to believe that coverage for all will eventually come, since other developed countries have long had systems that provide health care for all their citizens.

Adding goals related to women who are not childbearing has increased the tasks to be accomplished by the MCH Bureau. Outreach and education regarding health promotion promise to be the first efforts, along with increasing public knowledge of the health needs of all women. At the same time, the word "fathers" has been added to the definition of the MCH population. Services directed to the male will enhance maternal and child or family well-being, but exactly what services fathers will receive is not clear. Regardless, the child will remain the central beneficiary of services to the parents.

Considering the status of women in our nation today, and our knowledge of brain development in the youngest infants, improvement of day care services and early education is of highest priority. Making these services consistently part of the educational system, and paying day care operators a decent wage, seem a logical solution to the weaknesses in the current nonsystem. Then there will be an incentive for day care operators to have appropriate education for their extremely important responsibility, and they will be deserving of higher remuneration.

By our current measures, teen parenthood is not wise or beneficial to the mom or the baby. And risky behaviors of types other than premature parenthood are not desirable. Teens start out with potential, but without adequate preparation beginning much earlier, at home and in school, they can destroy their own futures, and fill the future of our country with a need for more jails, more police, more tranquilizers, and less respect from the rest of the world than we have today. Research has shown programs of promise. Some of them need to start in grade school or before; high school is too late for most, since troubled students drop out. The programs will be expensive but, in the long run, not as expensive as failing to change the direction in which destructive teens seem headed.

Immigrant children enter the school system with multiple handicaps. Even if their parents are in the United States illegally, helping the children will largely help the larger population, as well as them. Change will occur in state-by-state decisions in the immediate future, but hopefully attention from the federal level will be eventually focused on immigrant children; health care for these children will enhance their chances to play a productive role in society.

Children with special health care needs require special attention if they are in the SCHIP category, since a CSHCN designation may require a change in their care providers. State agencies should ensure that these children receive all the services that would benefit them, regardless of primary care provider. Since UAPs sometimes serve children who fit CSHCN categories, bringing them into the care-providing networks within states and communities would benefit the clients of the several agencies and care providers involved.

Perhaps the most difficult, thoughtful decisions will come in the next several decades as the implications for gene transfer and potential modification of an individual's human genome are discussed. For no field does this have more relevance than for maternal and child health. All MCH professionals should attempt to educate themselves on this topic to the extent possible and participate in discussions at every level dealing with the ramifications for human reproduction and the future.

ACKNOWLEDGMENT

Sincere thanks go to Bernard Turnock, MD, MPH, and Arden Handler, Dr PH, for reading and commenting on an earlier version of this chapter.

REFERENCES

1. Van Dyck PC: Forward. Vision, Strategic Plan, MCHB 1999, in Hutchins V: *Maternal and Child Health at the Millennium.* Department of Health and Human Services (DHHS), Health Resources and Services Administration (HRSA), Maternal and Child Health Bureau (MCHB). Released in April, 2001.

2. Hutchins V: Summing Up, in *Health and Welfare for Families in the 21st Century.* Senior Ed. Helen M. Wallace; Eds. Gordon Green, Kenneth J. Jaros, Lisa L. Paine, Mary Story. Jones and Bartlett Publishers, Inc. 1999.

3. Kaiser Commission on Medicaid and the Uninsured (2000). *Health Insurance Coverage in America:1999 Update.* [on line] http://www.kff.org/content/2001/2222.

4. Nelson RP et al.: Implementation Principles and Strategies for the State Children's Health Insurance Program. *Pediatrics* 107(5):1214–1220, May, 2001.

5. Commonwealth Fund Report: http://www.cmwf.org/media/releases/lambrew_release05302001.asp.

6. Kempe A et al.: Barriers to Enrollment in the State Children's Health Insurance Program. *Ambulatory Pediatrics,* 1(3):169–177, May–June 2001.

7. Tharp M: Washington Report: Health Care. *AAP News,* 18(5) May, 2001.

8. Guyer A et al.: *Millions of Mothers Lack Health Insurance* http://www.cbpp.org/5-10-01health--pr.htm.

9. Children's Defense Fund, *Child Health Information Project,* June 4, 2001.

10. Division of Perinatal Systems and Women's Health (DPSWH): *Draft DPSWH 5-Year Women's Health Plan, FY 2001–2006,* Executive Summary, October, 2000. HRSA, MCHB, DPSWH.

11. Hutchins V: *Maternal and Child Health at the Millennium.* DHHS, HRSA, MCHB. Released April, 2001.

12. Quintanilla R: *Head Start reformers say program has lost its way. Chicago Tribune* Metro Section 4, May 20, 2001.

13. Kotulak R: Teaching Them Early. Madigan CM: An expert urges greater investment in young students. In Perspective, *Chicago Tribune,* June 3, 2001.

14. MacKay AP, Fingerhut LA, Duran CR: *Adolescent Health Chartbook.* Health, U.S., 2000. Hyattsville, MD. NCHS 2000.

15. Kirby D: *The National Campaign to Prevent Teen Pregnancy.* Press release May 30, 2001.

16. DiClemente RJ et al.: Parental Monitoring: Association with Adolescents' Risk Behaviors. *Pediatrics* 107(6):1363–1368, June 2001.

17. Hawkins-Walsh E: Turning primary care providers' attention to child behavior: A review of the literature. *Journal of Pediatric Health Care* 15(3):115–122, 2001.

GLOSSARY

abstinence: refers to abstaining from sexual intercourse.

Access Initiative: a type of innovative programming which improves the availability of, and access of individuals to necessary health care services.

activities of daily living (ADL): activities related to basic self care and functions necessary for independent living, i.e., feeding, dressing, walking, bathing, toileting.

acute care: a pattern of health care in which an individual is treated for an immediate or severe physical or mental condition.

Americans With Disabilities Act of 1990 (ADA): federal statute designed to prevent discrimination and promote equal opportunities in the areas of employment, access to public services, and access to transportation and telecommunications services for persons with physical, sensory, or mental disabilities.

anecdotal evidence: information reported from individuals based on their personal experience, but not obtained from methodologically rigorous research.

assessment: one of public health's three core functions, calls for regularly and systematically collecting, analyzing, and making available information on the health of a community, including statistics on health status, community health needs, and epidemiological and other studies of health problems.

attention deficit hyperactivity disorder (ADHD): a disorder in children characterized by impulsive behavior, lack of attention, extreme physical activity, and lack of attention.

battered child syndrome: having a pattern of abusing children, as applied to an individual or a family.

battering: physically abusive behavior.

block grant: method by which government agencies fund states or localities to provide health and welfare services. Although block grants are for specific types of services they carry minimal regulations and offer considerable flexibility in how the monies are allocated, as compared to categorical or program specific funding.

cap: a specific limitation on funding or services.

capitation: payment to providers of a fixed amount for each person served, regardless of the actual amount and type of services provided, as compared to a fee for service reimbursement.

case control design: retrospective study design for the purpose of estimating the cause-effect relationship between suspected risk factor and a disease or condition.

case management: a system used by insurance companies and managed care organizations to ensure that individuals receive appropriate, timely and reasonable services; involves a procedure to plan, obtain, coordinate and monitor services on behalf of a client or patient.

categorical program: health or social services programs supported through funding that must be allocated to very narrowly specified service needs; usually targeted to specific groups at particular risk.

Centers for Medicare & Medicaid Services (CMS): the component (formerly named Health Care Financing Administration (HCFA)) within the U.S. Department of Health and Human Services which oversees Medicare, Medicaid, and the Child Health Insurance program (CHIP); and which assesses the nations health care programs and finances.

child abuse/maltreatment: the physical, sexual, or emotional maltreatment of a child. Abuse may be overt or covert and often results in permanent physical or psychiatric injury, mental impairment, and sometimes can result in death.

Child Health Insurance Program (CHIP): federal legislation passed in 1997 which provides funding to states to set up programs to provide health insurance for uninsured children.

child neglect: the failure by parents or other caregivers to provide the basic needs of a child by physical or emotional deprivation that interferes with normal growth and development, or that places a child in jeopardy.

Children's Defense Fund (CDF): a national advocacy and educational organization focusing on the health and welfare of children.

children with special health care needs: children with physical or developmental disabilities.

chronic disease: long standing persistent disease or condition.

Congressional Budget Office (CBO): the component of the federal legislative branch that provides to Congress fiscal information, and economic analysis data and reports.

Continuing Disability Review (CDR): a periodic examination conducted by the Social Security Administration to determine whether the health of a person receiving disability benefits has improved to the point where they are no longer considered disabled.

co-payment: a pre-determined fee that an individual or family pays for services or goods in addition to what is covered by insurance.

cost-based reimbursement: payment for health care services which reflects the actual cost of providing the service.

cost-benefit analysis: an approach to evaluation that converts outcomes into monetary terms (dollars) so that both costs and outcomes are expressed in economic terms.

cost shifting: balancing revenue loss or underpayment from certain groups of patients with overpayment or profit resulting from other groups.

cultural competence: the ability to provide services or care that is sensitive and responsive to cultural differences, assumes an awareness of one's own culture, and possession of skills that assist in the provision of services that are culturally appropriate in responding to unique cultural differences, such as race and ethnicity, national origin, religion, age, sexual orientation and physical or mental disability.

culture of poverty: the set of values, norms, motivations, social and environmental factors that inhibit the ability of poor individuals and families to pursue alternatives which may lead to improved economic independence.

dependent enrollment period: time period during which a health insurance policy holder is allowed to enroll a dependent child for health care coverage.

developmental screening: limited examination or testing of a child by a health care professional for the purpose of determining possible developmental delay, and facilitating an appropriate referral.

Disability Determination Services (DDS) agency: agency (usually at state level) which adjudicates the disability claims of applicants for Social Security benefits.

disproportionate share hospitals: hospitals that serve a disproportionate number of low income patients with special needs. These hospitals may receive supplemental reimbursement as part of the Medicaid program.

early discharge: discharge from inpatient hospital care at the earliest possible time, taking into account key medical factors.

Early Intervention Services: applies to children of school age or younger who have, or are at risk of developing a handicapping condition or other special need that may affect development. Early intervention consists of a range of remedial or preventive services to both the child and family.

Employee Retirement Income Security Act (ERISA): 1974 federal legislation which regulated private pension plans; also called Pension Reform Act.

employer based coverage: health insurance available as part of job related benefits package.

entitlement: financial support, goods, or services to which individuals of groups are entitled by virtue of their specific status. Examples of federally mandated entitlement programs are Social Security and Medicare.

EPSDT Program: Early Periodic Screening, Diagnosis, and Treatment program; federal program which supports screening of children for developmental disabilities, and subsequent referral for treatment.

ethnographic: using approaches and methods based in ethnography, i.e. participant observation, case studies; qualitative research.

etiology: underlying causes of a problem or condition.

exclusions: medical services that are either not covered or are limited in an individuals' insurance coverage.

federally qualified health centers: community health centers, migrant health centers and health care for the homeless clinics which receive federal grants under the Public Health Services Act, Section 330.

fee for service: a reimbursement mechanism based on payment for a unit of specific services rendered.

fetal alcohol syndrome: refers to the various deleterious effects of excessive maternal alcohol consumption on the unborn infant.

frail elderly: older individuals suffering from physical, cognitive or emotional impairments which may limit their ability to provide entirely for their own needs.

gatekeepers: a health care provider or case manager who screens and approves specialty care and hospital services

general assistance (GA): term referring to state or local programs providing public assistance benefits to low income persons.

Government Accounting Office (GAO): the investigative arm of the Congress charged with examining matters relating to the receipt and disbursement of public funds; performs audits and evaluations of government programs and activities.

grandfathered: exempted from a regulation, requirement, or rule change based on the fact that an individual or group of individuals was already engaged in the relevant activity.

hallucinogen: the group of drugs which may cause hallucinations when ingested.

Health Care Financing Administration (HCFA): renamed in 2001 as the Centers for Medicare & Medicaid Services (CMS), the component within the U.S. Department of Health and Human Services which oversees Medicare and Medicaid, and which assesses the nations health care programs and finances.

Health Maintenance Organization (HMO): a common form of a managed care organization; a pre-paid or capitated health care plan in which services are provided by physicians and other health care providers employed by, or under contract to the HMO.

Healthy People 2000/2010: the national disease prevention and health promotion agenda that includes some 300 national health objectives to be achieved by the year 2000, addressing improved health status, risk reduction, and utilization of preventive health services. HP 2010 addresses the 2010 objectives.

home visiting: a health or social service provided in the client's place of residence for the purpose of promoting, maintaining, or restoring health and well being; or for minimizing the effects of illness and disability.

horizontally integrated system: a system of linked organizations at the same stage of the production process; examples include hospital–hospital or hospital–nursing home combinations; mergers occur to achieve economies of scale, improve utilization of resources, enhance access to capital and extend the scope of the market.

hospital based home health: home health care services operated directly by a hospital, as opposed to services provided by free standing (for-profit or non-profit) organizations.

human capital investment: investment in programs and activities directly related to individual productivity and well being; i.e., education, job development, health promotion and medical care.

I&R databases and services: information and referral programs designed to link (through hotline, clearinghouses, etc.) individuals with necessary information and services.

incentive program: programs that employ cash or in-kind incentives to encourage participation or to reward positive behaviors.

incidence: the number of new cases of a disease or condition in a population over a specific period of time.

indemnity based insurance: with indemnity plans, the individual pays a pre-determined percentage of the cost of health care and the insuring company pays the additional percentage; fees for services are defined by providers and vary; individuals retain the freedom to choose any hospital or physician.

indicator: a measure of health status or a health outcome.

individual functional assessment (IFA): an assessment of the effects of an individual's disability on their functioning.

Individuals With Disabilities Education Act (IDEA): federal legislation passed in 1975 and re-authorized in 1990 requiring that children have access to free and appropriate public education regardless of disability.

inhalants: vapors that are inhaled or sniffed (i.e. glue, solvents, gasoline) for the purpose of intoxication.

in-kind assistance: goods or services that act in lieu of cash; i.e., vouchers, food stamps; matching contributions.

intentional injury: an injury arising from purposeful action, such as interpersonal or self-directed violence.

long term care: the provision of health and social services over an extended period to individuals who are functionally impaired; typically involves provision of some level of assistance with various activities of daily living.

low birth weight (LBW): weight at birth of less than 2500 grams, regardless of gestational age.

maladaptive behavior: behavior that is inconsistent with reasonable functioning in the environment and with accomplishing personal goals.

managed care: a general term used to refer to the organization of health care providers into systems that accept set fees for services or capitated fees for each patient enrolled.

mandatory eligibility: requiring the eligibility of certain individuals of groups of individuals for benefits or services.

matching funds: money that must be provided by states or localities to match all or some portion of a federal (or state) allocation; these funds must be provided in order to receive the full allocation.

means test: an assessment of the income and assets of an individual or family to determine eligibility for certain health and welfare benefits and services.

Medicaid: the U.S. federal program, established in 1965, that provides medical care benefits for individuals and families of very low income; funding is provided by states and the federal government and programs are typically administered by state welfare departments.

Medicaid agency: the specific agency at the state or local level which has responsibility for administration of the Medicaid program.

Medicaid denials: denial of reimbursement to providers for services delivered to Medicaid clients; denials typically result from fiscal and administrative review of records and determination that services were not necessary.

medical savings accounts: a tax-exempt account established by individuals for the purpose of paying for future medical expenses.

medically determinable impairment: a disability that is identifiable and diagnosable through regular medical procedures.

Medicare: the U. S. national health care insurance program established in 1965 for the elderly.

mental disorder: impaired cognitive or psychosocial functioning resulting from any of a range of causes; major categories of mental disorder are: personality disorders, psychosis, mood disorders, and organic mental disorders.

monitoring: ongoing assessment and evaluation of an intervention that provides continuous feedback on performance.

National Center for Health Statistics (NCHS): the federal government's principal vital and health statistics agency; part of the Centers for Disease Control and Prevention.

negative income tax: the concept that if the income of poor families fell below a certain level, they could be reimbursed up to that amount from the federal government as part of the federal income tax system.

non-marital childbearing: giving birth to a child while not being officially married.

Omnibus Budget Reconciliation Act (OBRA): 1989 federal legislation that increased eligibility levels for Medicaid, and made significant changes in the design and implementation of the MCH Services Block Grant.

outreach: activities of social welfare and health care workers designed to inform the community of services, and to engage eligible target groups to take advantage of services and benefits.

PL 104-193: the federal Personal Responsibility and Work Opportunity Reconciliation Act of 1996.

Point of Service Plan (POS): a version of a managed care plan which offers the individual a choice of providers outside of the plan at a higher co-payment rate.

population based public health services: interventions aimed at disease prevention and health promotion that affect an entire population and extend beyond medical treatment by targeting underlying risks such as tobacco, drug and alcohol use; diet and sedentary life styles; and environmental factors.

population based screening: the process of discovering characteristics known to be associated with health problems; its purpose is to identify individuals who are at high risk for health problems or who have unrecognized conditions.

portability: refers to the degree to which health insurance coverage can remain with the individual in an uninterrupted form as their employment and economic status change.

poverty by choice theories: a set of theories that postulate that those in poverty are comfortable with their situation and will make little or no attempt to change their status.

poverty level: a measure (taking into account the cost of living index) of the amount of money required by an individual or a family to live at a minimum subsistence level.

pre-existing conditions: medical conditions (either chronic or acute) which exist prior to the enrollment into a health insurance plan.

Preferred Provider Organization (PPO): a group of health care providers who have agreed by contract to furnish services to members of a health plan (MCO) at discounted rates.

presumptive eligibility: a mechanism for speeding up or eliminating the eligibility determination process for health or welfare services; this process assumes that individuals with certain characteristics are eligible and therefore foregoing any form of means test.

prevalence: measure of the number of individuals or the rate having a disease or condition at a given point in time.

preventive care: services designed to prevent diseases or conditions, or to identify risks for diseases or conditions.

primary care: basic or general health care focused on the point at which a patient ideally first seeks assistance from the medical care system; usually deals with care of the simpler and more common illnesses; the primary care provider should also assume on-going responsibility for the patient in maintaining health and treating disease; such care is generally provided by physicians but is increasingly provided by other personnel such as nurse practitioners or physicians assistants.

primary prevention: prevention strategies that seek to prevent the onset of disease or injury, generally through reducing exposure or risk factor levels; these strategies can reduce or eliminate causative risk factors (risk reduction).

protective factors: characteristics of an individual or their environment that make them less likely to experience certain conditions, illnesses or experiences.

reduced fertility: reduction in the birth rate.

reproductive health care: gynecological and obstetric services.

Respiratory Distress Syndrome: a lung disorder caused by a lack of pulmonary surfactant, that primarily affects premature infants and causes increasing difficulty in breathing.

risk factors: characteristics of the individual or their environment which put them at greater likelihood of experiencing certain conditions, illnesses or experiences.

safety net: basic social welfare and health programs that serve individuals without access to other sources of support or care.

sanction: a provision which penalizes an individual (or a system) for not conforming.

secondary prevention: prevention strategies that seek to identify and control disease processes in their early stages before signs and symptoms develop (screening and treatment).

Section 1902(r)(2): a part of the Medicaid legislation under which states may modify the Medicaid plan to incrementally increase eligibility.

self-efficacy: an individual's belief that they have the ability to accomplish certain tasks and reach certain objectives.

skilled nursing home care: long term residential and treatment facilities characterized by intensive health care services provide by highly trained and experienced nursing providers.

smokeless tobacco: chewing tobacco and snuff.

social capital: social value; the general value or worth to society, in non monetary terms, of a resource, commodity or a service.

social insurance: government operated insurance programs that set aside money in trust (contributions from individuals and employers) to insure individuals in the event of disability, death, unemployment and retirement.

social networks: links between individuals and other individuals and institutions within their social environment.

SSA: U.S. Social Security Administration.

stagflation: national economic situation characterized by inflation without economic growth (stagnation).

standard deviation: a statistical measure indicating characteristics of the distribution of a data set.

statutory rape: consensual sexual relationship with someone under the age of consent.

STD: sexually transmitted disease (i.e. syphilis, gonorrhea, chlamydia).

sub-acute care: a level of medical care following acute care service, requiring less intensive services, and often functions as a transition phase to rehabilitation services or to placement in residential care, or return home.

Sudden Infant Death Syndrome (SIDS): diagnosis given for the sudden death of an infant under one year of age, that after a complete investigation, remains unexplained.

Sullivan vs. Zebley: A 1984 case heard before the Supreme Court which resulted in the development by the U.S. Department of Health and Human Services and the Social Security Administration of a new process of determining disability among children.

supplemental medical insurance: health or long term care insurance purchased to supplement or expand coverage available through existing health care plan; "Medigap" plans are available to help cover costs not covered by Medicare.

Supplemental Security Income (SSI): the federally supported program which provides cash assistance to individuals with a variety of disabilities; although it is administered primarily by the Social Security Administration, eligibility is not related to previous work record.

surfactin: a lipoprotein which when given via direct tracheal instillation to newborns suffering from respiratory distress syndrome, favorably alters the lung mechanics and improves oxygenation.

surveillance: systematic monitoring of the health status of a population.

technology dependent: reliant on certain medical equipment (i.e., ventilator, communicator) to perform certain activities of daily living and to maintain quality of life.

Temporary Assistance for Needy Families (TANF): welfare to work programs established at the state level which comply with 1996 federal legislation.

tertiary prevention: prevention strategies that prevent disability by restoring individuals to their optimal level of functioning after a disease or injury is established and damage is done.

third party payor: an insurance company or government agency that provides payment to providers for services delivered to clients or patients.

three drug cocktails: combination of drugs used in regimen to treat individuals with AIDS.

Title XXI: Title XXI of the Balanced Budget Act of 1997; creates the States' Children's Health Insurance Program (SCHIP).

Title V agency: the organization at the state or local level which is responsible for the administration of the Title V Block Grant funds for the designated jurisdiction.

trimester: a period of three months (either 1st, 2nd, or 3rd) during pregnancy.

unintentional injury: injury arising from unintentional events.

U.S. Conference of Mayors: founded in 1932; the official nonpartisan organization of cities with populations of 30,000 or more.

vaginal delivery: child birth not requiring Caesarian section.

vertically integrated system: systems involving the linking of organizations at related stages of the production process (i.e. hospital- insurance company); vertical integration enables organizations to move toward providing multiple levels, and more coordinated and comprehensive services.

very low birth weight (VLBW): weight at birth of less than 1000 grams, regardless of gestational age.

vulnerable populations: groups of individuals that are at risk for certain negative conditions or circumstances.

waiver (1115/1915b): permissions granted to state Medicaid agencies to attempt innovative pilot programming to encourage Medicaid eligibility and to make systems more efficient.

War on Poverty: a series of major health and welfare programs enacted nationally in the 1960s during the administration of Lyndon B. Johnson.

weight for height: the ratio of weight to height; an indicator of infant development.

welfare state: a country or jurisdiction where the government guarantees as a right essential goods, services, and opportunities (including income) to its residents.

welfare to work programs: the type of welfare/public assistance programs which require recipients to participate in some type of employment in order to maintain their eligibility for benefits.

WIC Program: U.S. Special Supplemental Food Program for Women, Infants, and Children that provides food assistance to women and children at risk for nutritional problems.

workfare: an approach to public assistance programming which requires recipients either to work or to receive job training in order to be eligible for benefits.

Year 2000/2010 targets: specific quantitative health objectives for the nation as stated in the document Healthy People 2000 and Healthy People 2010.

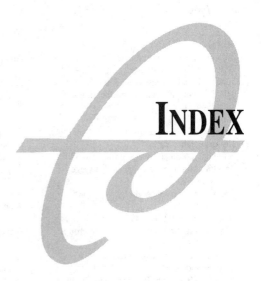

INDEX